Articular Cartilage of the Knee

Harpal K. Gahunia
Allan E. Gross
Kenneth P. H. Pritzker
Paul S. Babyn
Lucas Murnaghan
Editors

Articular Cartilage of the Knee

Health, Disease and Therapy

Springer

Editors
Harpal K. Gahunia, MSc, PhD
President and CEO
Orthopaedic Science Consulting Services
Oakville, ON, Canada

Kenneth P. H. Pritzker, MD, FRCPC
Professor Emeritus
Department of Laboratory Medicine and Pathobiology, Department of Surgery, and Institute of Biomaterials and Biomedical Engineering
University of Toronto
Toronto, ON, Canada

Department of Pathology and Laboratory Medicine
Mount Sinai Hospital
Toronto, ON, Canada

Lucas Murnaghan, MD, MEd, FRCSC
Assistant Professor
Division of Orthopaedic Surgery
University of Toronto
Toronto, ON, Canada

Division of Orthopaedic Surgery
The Hospital for Sick Children and Women's College Hospital
Toronto, ON, Canada

Allan E. Gross, MD, FRCSC, O ONT
Professor
Division of Orthopaedic Surgery
University of Toronto
Toronto, ON, Canada

Gluskin Granovsky Division of Orthopaedics
Joseph and Wolf Lebovic Health Complex, Mount Sinai Hospital
Toronto, ON, Canada

Paul S. Babyn, MDCM, FRCPC
Physician Executive
Saskatchewan Health Authority
Department Head of Medical Imaging
University of Saskatchewan and Saskatoon Health Region
Saskatoon, SK, Canada

ISBN 978-1-4939-7585-3 ISBN 978-1-4939-7587-7 (eBook)
https://doi.org/10.1007/978-1-4939-7587-7

This Springer imprint is published by the registered company Springer Science+Business Media, LLC part of Springer Nature.
The registered company address is: 233 Spring Street, New York, NY 10013, U.S.A.

To all the staff at Mount Sinai Hospital, Toronto, ON, Canada, who over many years have participated in the cartilage transplant program.

To the very many physicians and scientists who have developed knowledge about knee articular cartilage in health, disease, and therapy.

To current and future trainees who will extend our understanding of articular cartilage for the benefit of patients afflicted with knee articular cartilage injury and disease.

To my daughter, Vinique Dhian Wolski, and husband, Dr. Vince Wolski, for their unwavering support, understanding, and encouragement.

Foreword

It is a privilege for me to write the foreword for this book entitled "*Articular Cartilage of the Knee: Health, Injury and Therapy*", edited by Dr. Allan Gross and his colleagues from Toronto, along with world-renowned contributors in the field of articular cartilage. The scope of this excellent book is extensive, and is a timely and much needed state-of-the-art survey that covers every aspect of knee articular cartilage, from its genesis through the various stages of growth, aging, trauma and therapy. The basic science and diagnostic imaging techniques are discussed along with treatment interventions, beginning with conservative options, followed by well-established treatments as well as cutting-edge, innovative surgical approaches, including cellular repair, allografts and implant matrices. This multi-disciplinary text is aimed at a wide audience and will be an exceptional reference volume for an in-depth knowledge of articular cartilage of knee. Also, with its extensive bibliography, it will serve as an ideal cross-reference for healthcare professionals, scientists, bioengineers as well as clinical and basic research trainees. Further, the book's comprehensive focus on multiple aspects of the life cycle of articular cartilage sets it apart from other publications on this topic.

Appropriate management of patients with injuries and diseases affecting the knee articular cartilage relies heavily on an armamentarium of sophisticated imaging and surgical techniques, and clinical trials. Repair of articular cartilage of the knee remains challenging despite recent advances in knowledge and technology. Whilst investigations of the biochemical factors that modulate chondrocyte behaviour was of prime focus in the past, the paradigm has now shifted towards a more holistic approach directed at maintaining articular cartilage health and treating knee articular cartilage injury/disease through better characterization of the effects of biomechanical forces on chondrocytes, adjacent tissues and the knee joint as well as the altered articular cartilage physiology due to aging and disease. This book addresses various challenges in articular cartilage therapy, describing in detail the current trends and techniques, the pros and cons of each technique followed by future directions in the field. It is my hope and expectation that the articular cartilage community will eventually succeed in developing innovative techniques to diagnose, prevent and treat disorders of the articular cartilage of the knee, and so control the modern scourge of osteoarthritis. This book will augment that progress, and I recommend it most strongly to all those interested in articular cartilage of the knee.

George C. Bentley,
DSC, FRCSE, MB, ChM, F Med SCi

Professor Emeritus and Director,
Institute of Orthopaedics
and Musculo-Skeletal Science,
University College, London, UK

Consultant Orthopaedic Surgeon,
Royal National Orthopaedic Hospital,
Stanmore, UK

Preface

With the rapid growth of knowledge of the pathophysiology underlying knee diseases and the recognized pivotal role of articular cartilage as the target tissue for bearing of forces, the need and opportunity to compile this comprehensive book on knee articular cartilage from the health and disease perspective is timely.

This book strives to provide an understanding of the various stages and the life cycle of knee articular cartilage from its genesis through its growth and development, aging (in health and disease), injury, degeneration from disease, and responses to therapy (nonsurgical and surgical repair, including the use of cell- or non-cell-based biocompatible matrix implants). Overall, we aimed to create a compendium of current knowledge of articular cartilage of the knee in health, disease, and therapy. The comprehensive focus of this book on diverse aspects of articular cartilage of the knee sets it apart from other books available on articular cartilage.

This book is the first to encompass a broad spectrum of knee articular cartilage-associated disciplines, such as orthopedic surgery, sports medicine, rheumatology, musculoskeletal imaging, pathology, knee rehabilitation, basic science, and cartilage engineering. Under the broad umbrella of "Articular Cartilage of the Knee", this multidisciplinary book is recommended for those engaged or interested in the field of knee articular cartilage biology, diagnostic imaging, engineering, and clinical strategies for treatment of injured or diseased articular cartilage. Clinicians, clinical researchers, basic scientists, cartilage engineers, postdoctoral fellows, and graduate students will benefit from its insights as it is a one-book reference for all articular cartilage specialities.

This book is organized into 8 parts with a total of 19 chapters, which collectively encompass a broad number of disciplines and several review topics related to knee articular cartilage. Each chapter is self-contained, can be read independently, and is supplied with a comprehensive reference list.

Part I (Normal Articular Cartilage) includes the overview of normal knee articular cartilage three-dimensional structure and intrinsic properties as well as growth and development. The *first chapter* by Gahunia and Pritzker describes in-depth the macromolecular composition and structure of knee articular cartilage and its unique biomechanical properties. The authors emphasize the unique structural and biomechanical symbiotic relationship between the chondrocytes and their pericellular environment along with the extracellular matrix of the various zones. A current understanding of the key molecular and genetic participants during the various stages of growth and development of articular and epiphyseal cartilage is elucidated in Chap. 2 by Las Heras and Gahunia.

Part II (Aging and Degeneration of Articular Cartilage) includes chapters that elucidate the knee articular cartilage normal homeostasis and its alterations during aging, degeneration, and disease. In Chap. 3, Pritzker and Gahunia discuss chondrocytes as the key cellular mediators for cartilage homeostasis and aging of mature chondrocytes and their surrounding extracellular matrix that is reflective of metabolic changes related solely with the passage of time. Clinically, these changes can manifest as decreased capacity to withstand mechanical forces leading to degenerative arthritis. In Chap. 4, Gahunia and Pritzker provide a thorough understanding of the specific roles of the various articular cartilage matrix component biomarkers. The role of mechanical stress on articular cartilage resulting in a cascade of mechanosensitive events within the extracellular matrix which then stimulates the mechanoreceptors at the chondrocyte surface is highlighted.

Part III (Knee Articular Cartilage Injury: Evaluation and Assessment) includes chapters that discuss traumatic articular cartilage injuries and their diagnosis, evaluation, and assessment using magnetic resonance imaging and arthroscopy. In Chap. 5, Ellis presents the natural history and incidence of traumatic and sports-related articular cartilage injuries with associated risk factors. From an orthopedic surgeon's perspective, the importance of identifying the size, depth, and anatomic location of the lesion, patient's age, activity level, clinical presentation, the use of appropriate classification system, and association with other knee tissue injuries prior to assigning the treatment strategies for knee cartilage repair is discussed. In Chap. 6, Thawait, Andreisek, and Chhabra highlight the technical considerations when using magnetic resonance imaging and appearances of the wide spectrum of injury-related pathologies. The assessment and classification systems of chondral lesions using arthroscopy that guide treatment algorithms are reviewed by Dwyer and Theodoropoulos in Chap. 7. The authors discuss articular cartilage injury patterns seen with common knee pathology and trauma.

Part IV (Repair of Knee Articular Cartilage Injury: Nonsurgical Approaches) is devoted to the current knowledge of conservative treatment of knee articular cartilage lesions. Pharmacologic management for articular cartilage injury and osteoarthritis should always be considered as supplemental to conservative approaches related to physical and/or rehabilitative exercises. In Chap. 8, Houpt, Gahunia, and Pritzker discuss the efficacy of lifestyle modifications, weight loss, and active physical therapy in reducing symptoms following knee injury and facilitating knee articular cartilage repair. In Chap. 9, Houpt, Pritzker, and Gahunia review the current oral, topical, and intra-articular pharmacologic agents, and their use for the management of knee articular cartilage injury and for the treatment of osteoarthritic symptoms.

In *Part V (Repair of Knee Articular Cartilage: Surgical Approaches)*, the most up-to-date strategies for the treatment, repair, and reconstruction of knee articular cartilage defects are discussed in a series of highly informative chapters. Building on already established techniques, Gross and his colleagues explore state-of-the-art surgical techniques that have come to the forefront within the last decade including cell and cartilage transplantation. Also, early and midterm results from clinical trials are reviewed. In Chap. 10, Popkin describes the natural history and discusses the current surgical treatment options for osteochondritis dissecans. In Chap. 11, Chahal, Benedict, and Gross provide a comprehensive approach to evaluating patients with articular cartilage defects and describe the treatment options and algorithms. Patient- and defect-specific factors pertinent to surgical decision making are discussed along with an evidence-based and technical overview of common surgical approaches. In Chap. 12, Rogers, Chahal, and Gross emphasize on the patient-focused diagnosis and treatment options and provide a comprehensive synopsis of the biopsychosocial approach toward primary and secondary clinical outcome measurement following articular cartilage repair surgery.

The focus of *Part VI (Qualitative and Quantitative Assessment of Articular Cartilage Repair)* is to highlight the magnetic resonance imaging and histopathological imaging techniques, and assessment tools to visualize and assess knee articular cartilage repair and disease at post- and during treatment stage. In Chap. 13, Chhabra, Thawait, and Andreisek review the role of MRI for the preoperative diagnosis of knee cartilage injury and postoperative follow-up as it relates to the visualization, characterization, and assessment of cartilage repair tissue. Also, the authors provide an understanding of the currently used cartilage repair scoring system. In Chap. 14, Trattnig, Welsch, Röhrich, Schreiner, and Zalaudek highlight how both morphological and biochemical MRI can provide quantitative data and to what degree this data is associated with clinical outcome in articular cartilage repair and disease. Also, the authors provided an understanding of how to employ the latest MR techniques, such as permeability imaging and susceptibility imaging. In Chap. 15, Pritzker and Gahunia discuss the standardized histopathological methods for the assessment, evaluation, and classification of knee articular cartilage lesions and repair.

The chapters included in *Part VII (Research in Articular Cartilage Repair and Cartilage Bioengineering)* showcase the recent cartilage engineering strategies in transplantation for cell-based and non-cell-seeded scaffolds for cartilage repair. The current and future approaches pertaining to the rationale and clinical studies underlying the use of human-derived cells for chondral and osteochondral repair are eloquently reviewed by Mollon, Kandel, and Theodoropoulos in Chap. 16. This chapter provides an in-depth understanding of the biology of cell-seeded tissue-engineered matrices that will help with the development of new products and clinical applications. The relevance of non-cell-seeded tissue-engineered scaffolds with and without the use of exogenous agents is discussed in-depth by Starecki, Gott, Schwartz, Sgaglione, and Grande in Chap. 17. The authors highlight the characteristic features of a successful cartilage scaffold. Further assessment and investigation of the commercially available bioengineered cartilage grafts including cell-based therapies, the use of particulate articular cartilage, as well as examples of scaffold and synthetic materials that can be used in isolation is overviewed by Rogers, Chahal, and Gross in Chap. 18.

Finally, in *Part VIII (Future Prospects for Knee Articular Cartilage Therapy)* and concluding Chap. 19 of this book, Gahunia, Gross, and Pritzker succinctly summarize the book contents and suggest future directions for knee articular cartilage research and practice.

In addition to the wealth of information covered in the various chapters, four appendixes (A to D) are included to provide readers with an easy access to the commonly used scoring systems for knee cartilage assessment. *Appendix A* includes the arthroscopic classification systems for chondral injuries (Outerbridge, Modified Outerbridge, Noyes, and International Cartilage Repair Society) and chondral repair (International Cartilage Repair Society and Oswestry). *Appendix B* provides access to six of the current most commonly used outcome assessment tools developed for patients to assess their view about their knee health either post-injury, to evaluate the efficacy of pharmacological intervention, preoperative and post-surgery follow-up assessments (cartilage repair or knee arthroplasty), or during the course of disease such as osteoarthritis. A total of nine commonly used measures of knee function are included. These scoring tools are used to assess one or more of the following criteria: pain, symptoms, activities of daily living, sports, quality of life, and physical health value. Magnetic resonance imaging evaluation systems for chondral injuries and repair are outlined in *Appendix C*. There are three main MRI evaluation systems currently used, namely, International Cartilage Repair Society as well as two- and three-dimensional magnetic resonance observation of cartilage repair tissue scores. Finally, *Appendix D* includes the histopathological classification systems to assess cartilage lesions and repair. This unique approach of grouping all the currently used scoring systems will enable the readers to develop a better understanding of the various aspects of cartilage biology and injury from the perspective of different disciplines.

My co-editors and I envisage that this book will help stimulate scientific research among physicians, scientists, and researchers with an active interest in the field of knee articular cartilage biology as well as diagnosis and treatment of joint diseases. This continuing translation of clinical and basic sciences to healthcare and clinical practice, in turn, will serve to lead to the development of more effective treatment strategies for those afflicted by knee joint injuries and disorders.

Toronto, ON, Canada Allan E. Gross, MD, FRCSC, O ONT

Acknowledgments

Attempting to highlight the complexities of knee articular cartilage in health and disease is a daunting task. We are much indebted to our world-renowned experts and contributors of each chapter for their thoughtful and scholarly input. It is wonderful to have contributions from worldwide leaders in the fields of orthopedic surgery, radiology, rheumatology, pathology, epidemiology, rehabilitation science, basic science, and cartilage engineering who came together to offer their expertise and invaluable insights toward this large and complex topic of knee articular cartilage in health, disease, diagnosis, therapy, and healing. Through their dedication and highly collaborative efforts, they have made this comprehensive and authoritative book possible.

We extend our appreciation to Kristopher Spring (Senior Editor, Springer Nature) for his great enthusiasm, patience, and support for this book from concept until completion. Also, we extend our deepest gratitude to Atma Biswal (Project Manager, Content Solutions, Spi Global), Mario Gabriele (Sr. Project Manager, Content Solutions, Spi Global), and Krishnan Sathyamurthy (Production Editor, Springer Nature), and their editorial and production staff for all their hard work, dedication, and patience in ensuring the success and timely publication of this book. We thank Maureen Alexander (Springer Developmental Editor) who worked with much passion and has been instrumental in ensuring that the book structure and content is at its best. The state-of-the-art illustrations would not have been possible without the contributions of Danny Aguilar (Medical Graphic Artist-illustrator, JD Graphics Solutions, Toronto, Canada) who worked with deep dedication to ensure the accuracy and high-quality production of the schematics.

Contents

Part V Repair of Knee Articular Cartilage: Surgical Approaches

Contributors

Gustav Andreisek, MD, MBA Professor, Head MSK and MR Imaging, Department of Radiology, University Hospital Zurich, University of Zurich, Zurich, Switzerland

Swiss Center for Musculoskeletal Imaging, Balgrist Campus AG, Zurich, Switzerland

Department of Radiology, St Claraspital, Basel, Switzerland

Department of Radiology, Spital Thurgau AG, Cantonal Hospital, Munsterlingen, Switzerland

Jaskarndip Chahal, MD, FRCSC, MSc, MBA Assistant Professor, Division of Orthopaedic Surgery, University of Toronto, Toronto, ON, Canada

University of Toronto Orthopaedic Sports Medicine and University Health Network Arthritis Program, Toronto, ON, Canada

Division of Orthopaedic Surgery, Toronto Western Hospital and Women's College Hospital, Toronto, ON, Canada

Avneesh B. Chhabra, MBBS, MD Associate Professor, Department of Radiology and Orthopaedic Surgery, University of Texas Southwestern Medical Center, Dallas, TX, USA

Department of Musculoskeletal Radiology, Parkland Health and Hospital System, Dallas, TX, USA

Tim Dwyer, MBBS, FRACS, FRCSC, PhD Assistant Professor, Division of Orthopaedics, University of Toronto, Toronto, ON, Canada

University of Toronto Orthopaedic Sports Medicine, Women's College Hospital, Toronto, ON, Canada

Division of Orthopaedic Surgery, Women's College Hospital and Mount Sinai Hospital, Toronto, ON, Canada

Henry B. Ellis Jr, MD Assistant Professor, Department of Orthopaedic Surgery, University of Texas Southwestern Medical Center, Dallas, TX, USA

Department of Orthopaedic Surgery, Children's Health Dallas and Texas Scottish Rite Hospital for Children, Dallas, TX, USA

Harpal K. Gahunia, MSc, PhD President and CEO, Orthopaedic Science Consulting Services, Oakville, ON, Canada

Michael A. Gott, MD Westchester Health Orthopaedics and Sports Medicine, Westchester Sport and Spine, White Plains Hospital, White Plains, NY, USA

Daniel A. Grande, PhD Director, Orthopaedic Research Laboratory, Feinstein Institute for Medical Research, North Shore-LIJ Health System, Manhasset, NY, USA

Associate Professor, Center for Bioelectronic Medicine, Feinstein Institute for Medical Research, North Shore-LIJ Health System, Manhasset, NY, USA

Associate Professor, Department of Molecular Medicine and Orthopaedic Surgery, Donald and Barbara Zucker School of Medicine at Hofstra-Northwell, Hempstead, NY, USA

Department of Orthopaedic Surgery, Long Island Jewish Medical Center, Northwell Health, New Hyde Park, NY, USA

Allan E. Gross, MD, FRCSC, O ONT Professor, Division of Orthopaedic Surgery, University of Toronto, Toronto, ON, Canada

Gluskin Granovsky Division of Orthopaedics, Joseph and Wolf Lebovic Health Complex, Mount Sinai Hospital, Toronto, ON, Canada

Joseph B. Houpt, MD, FRCPC Faculty of Medicine, University of Toronto, Toronto, ON, Canada

Rita Kandel, MD Professor, Department of Laboratory Medicine and Pathology, Department of Surgery, and Institute of Biomaterials and Biomedical Engineering, University of Toronto, Toronto, ON, Canada

Pathologist-in-Chief, Department of Pathology and Laboratory Medicine, Mount Sinai Hospital, Toronto, ON, Canada

Associate Member, Lunenfeld-Tanenbaum Research Institute, Mount Sinai Hospital, Toronto, ON, Canada

Facundo Las Heras, MD, PhD Departamento de Anatomia Patologica, Clinica Las Condes, Santiago, Chile

Pathology Department, University of Chile, Santiago, Chile

Brent Mollon, MD, FRCSC, MSc Department of Orthopaedics, Orillia Soldiers' Memorial Hospital, Orillia, ON, Canada

Simcoe-Muskoka Orthopaedics, Orillia, ON, Canada

Charles A. Popkin, MD Assistant Professor, Orthopedic Surgery and Sports Medicine, Columbia University Medical Center, New York, NY, USA

Department of Orthopedic Surgery, Sports Medicine Center for the Developing Athlete, Presbyterian Morgan Stanley Children's Hospital, New York, NY, USA

Kenneth P. H. Pritzker, MD, FRCPC Professor Emeritus, Department of Laboratory Medicine and Pathobiology, Department of Surgery, and Institute of Biomaterials and Biomedical Engineering, University of Toronto, Toronto, ON, Canada

Department of Pathology and Laboratory Medicine, Mount Sinai Hospital, Toronto, ON, Canada

Benedict A. Rogers, MA, MSc, MRCGP, DipLMC, DipSEM, FRCS (Orth), PhD Honorary Reader, Brighton and Sussex Medical School, Brighton, UK

Trauma and Orthopaedics Department, Brighton and Sussex University Hospitals NHS Trust, Brighton, UK

Sebastian Röhrich, MD High Field MR Centre, Department of Biomedical Imaging and Image-Guided Therapy, Computational Imaging Research Laboratory, Medical University of Vienna, Vienna, Austria

Markus M. Schreiner, MD Department of Orthopaedics and Trauma Surgery, Medical University of Vienna, Vienna, Austria

High Field MR Centre, Department of Biomedical Imaging and Image-Guided Therapy, Computational Imaging Research Laboratory, Medical University of Vienna, Vienna, Austria

John A. Schwartz, MD Orthopaedic Research Center, Colorado State University, Fort Collins, CO, USA

Orthopaedic Research Laboratory, Feinstein Institute for Medical Research, North Shore-LIJ Health System, Manhasset, NY, USA

Nicholas A. Sgaglione, MD Department of Orthopaedic Surgery, Long Island Jewish Medical Center, Northwell Health, New Hyde Park, NY, USA

Department of Molecular Medicine and Orthopaedic Surgery, Donald and Barbara Zucker School of Medicine at Hofstra-Northwell, Hempstead, NY, USA

Mikael Starecki, MD Resurgens Orthopaedics, West Cobb, Marietta, GA, USA

Department of Orthopaedic Surgery, East-West Surgery Center, Wellstar Cobb Hospital and Wellstar Douglas Hospital, Austell, GA, USA

Gaurav K. Thawait, MBBS, MD Associate Professor, Russell H. Morgan Department of Radiology and Radiological Science, Johns Hopkins University, Baltimore, MD, USA

Department of Biomedical Engineering, Johns Hopkins University, Baltimore, MD, USA

John S. Theodoropoulos, MD, FRCSC, MSc Assistant Professor, Division of Orthopaedic Surgery, University of Toronto, Toronto, ON, Canada

University of Toronto Orthopaedic Sports Medicine Program, Women's College Hospital, Toronto, ON, Canada

Division of Orthopaedic Surgery, Women's College Hospital and Mount Sinai Hospital, Toronto, ON, Canada

Siegfried Trattnig, MD Professor, High Field MR Center, Department of Biomedical Imaging and Image-Guided Therapy, Medical University of Vienna, Vienna, Austria

Austrian Cluster for Tissue Regeneration, Vienna, Austria

Christian Doppler Laboratory for Clinical Molecular MR Imaging, Vienna, Austria

Götz H. Welsch, MD Professor, Department of Athletics and Sports Medicine, University Medical Center Hamburg-Eppendorf, Hamburg, Germany

Head of Medical Management, UKE Athleticum, Division of Orthopaedic Sports Medicine, University Hospital of Hamburg-Eppendorf, Hamburg, Germany

Martin Zalaudek, MD Department of Orthopaedics and Trauma Surgery, Medical University of Vienna, Vienna, Austria

High Field MR Center, Department of Biomedical, Imaging and Image-Guided Therapy, Medical University of Vienna, Vienna, Austria

Abbreviations

2D	Two-dimensional
3D	Three-dimensional
4D	Four-dimensional
AAOS	American Academy of Orthopaedic Surgeons
AC	Articular cartilage
ACI	Autologous chondrocyte implantation
ACIG	Articular Cartilage Imaging Group
ACL	Anterior cruciate ligament
ACLR	Anterior cruciate ligament reconstruction
ADAMTS	Disintegrin and metalloproteinases with thrombospondin motifs
ADL	Activities of daily living
AECC	Articular-epiphyseal cartilage complex
AGEs	Advanced glycation end products
ALK5	Activin receptor like kinase 5
ALP	Alkaline phosphatase
AMIC	Autologous matrix-induced chondrogenesis
AMZ	Anteromedialization
AO	Association for Osteosynthesis
AOSSM	American Orthopaedic Society for Sports Medicine
AP	Anteroposterior
ApoA-1	Apolipoprotein A-1
ARGS	Alanine-arginine-glycine-serine
AS	Arthroscopic surgery
ASC	Adipose-derived stromal cells
ASIF	Association for the Study of Internal Fixation
BLOKS	Boston-Leeds Osteoarthritis Knee Scoring System
BMAC	Bone marrow aspirate concentrate
BME	Bone marrow edema
BMI	Body mass index
bmMSCs	Bone marrow-derived mesenchymal stromal cells
BMP	Bone morphogenetic protein
BMPR	Bone morphogenetic protein receptor
BMS	Bone marrow stimulation

BW	Body weight
C2C	Collagen type II C-terminal cleavage product
C4S	Chondroitin-4-sulfate
C6S	Chondroitin-6-sulfate
Ca^{++}	Calcium ion
CAIS	Cartilage autograft implantation system
cAMP	Cyclic adenosine monophosphate
CCI	Characterized chondrocyte implantation
CCL	Chemokine (C-C motif) ligand
CCL3	Chemokine (C-C motif) ligand 3
C-Col10	C-terminus of collagen type X
CEST	Chemical exchange-dependent saturation transfer
CIIM or C2M	Metalloproteinase-derived collagen type II neoepitope
CILP	Cartilage intermediate layer protein
CILP-2	Cartilage intermediate layer protein 2
CM	Chondromalacia
CMGP	Cartilage matrix glycoprotein (also termed chondronectin)
CMP	Cartilage matrix protein (also termed Matrilin-1)
CNR	Contrast to noise ratio
COMP	Cartilage oligomeric matrix protein
CPM	Continuous passive motion
CPMG	Carr-Purcell-Meiboom-Gill (MR sequence)
CPPD	Calcium pyrophosphate dihydrate
CRD	Cartilage Repair Device
CROAKS	Cartilage repair osteoarthritis knee score
CRP	C-reactive protein
CS	Chondroitin sulfate
CSΔdi-4S	Chondroitin-4-sulfate delta disaccharides
CSΔdi-6S	Chondroitin-6-sulfate delta disaccharides
CT	Computed tomography
CTX-II	C-terminal telopeptide collagen type II
CX3CL-1	Fractalkine
CXCL	Chemokine interferon gamma inducible protein
CXCL-10	Chemokine interferon gamma inducible protein 10
DeNovo NT	DeNovo Natural tissue
DESS	Dual excitation steady-state (also termed double echo steady-state)
DFVO	Distal femoral varus osteotomy
dGEMRIC	Delayed gadolinium-enhanced magnetic resonance imaging of cartilage
DM1	Type 1 diabetes mellitus
DNA	Deoxyribonucleic acid
Dpyd	Deoxypyridinoline
DS	Dermatan sulfate
DS-PGI	Biglycan
DS-PGII or PG40	Decorin
DTI	Diffusion tensor imaging
DVL	Dishevelled type proteins

DWI	Diffusion-weighted imaging
DZ	Deep zone (also termed radial zone or Zone 3)
EB	Embryoid body
ECM	Extracellular matrix
EGF	Epidermal growth factor
EO	Endochondral ossification
EPOS	European Paediatric Orthopaedic Society
EQ-5D	European Quality of Life-5 Dimensions
ESCs	Embryonic stem cells
ESSKA	European Society of Sports Traumatology, Knee Surgery and Arthroscopy
EUA	Examination under anaesthesia
FACIT	Fibril-associated collagen with interrupted triple helix
FCD	Fixed charge density
FDA	Food and Drug Administration
FEMR	Fluctuating equilibrium magnetic resonance
FFE	Fast field echo
FGF	Fibroblast growth factor
FGFr-2	Fibroblast growth factor-2
FGFr-2, -3, -8	Fibroblast growth factor receptor-2, -3, -8
FGFr-3	Fibroblast growth factor-3
Fib 3	Fibulin 3 peptide
Fib 3-1	Fibulin 3 peptide-1
Fib 3-2	Fibulin 3 peptide-2
FIESTA	Fast imaging using steady-state acquisition
FISP	Fast imaging with steady-state precession
FLASH	Fast low angle shot
FN	Fibronectin
FOV	Field of view
fs	Fat suppressed
FSE	Fast spin echo
FSTL1	Follistatin-like glycoprotein 1
FVDIPEN	Neoepitope generated by MMP cleavage of aggrecan (Amino acids – Phe-Val-Asp-Ile-Pro-Glu-Asn)
GAG	Glycosaminoglycan
gagCEST	Glycosaminoglycan chemical exchange-dependent saturation transfer
Gd-DTPA^{2-}	Gadolinium diethylenetriamine pentaacetate anion
GE	Gradient echo
GH	Growth hormone
GI	Gastrointestinal
GP	Growth plate
GRASS	Gradient-recalled echo acquired in steady state
GRE	Gradient recalled echo
HA	Hyaluronic acid (also termed hyaluronan)
HABR	Hyaluronic acid binding region
HABR-FMDIPEN	Aggrecan fragments from HABR

HC-gp39	Human cartilage glycoprotein-39 (also termed YKL-40)
HELIX II	Helical peptide of collagen type II
hESCs	Human embryonic stem cells
HETE-15	15-Hydroxyeicosatetraenoic acid
HGF	Hepatocyte growth factor
HH	Hedgehog
HIF-1α	Hypoxia-inducible factor-1-alpha
HLA	Human leukocyte antigens
HS	Heparan sulfate
HSS	Hospital for Special Surgery
IA	Inflammatory arthritis
ICC	Intra-class correlation coefficient
ICF	International Classification of Functioning, Disability and Health
ICIDH	International Classification of Impairments, Disabilities and Handicaps
ICRS	International Cartilage Repair Society (Since 2018, renamed as "International Cartilage Regeneration and Joint Preservation Society")
IDEAL	Iterative decomposition of water and fat with echo asymmetry and least-squares estimation
IGF	Insulin-like growth factor
IH	Indian hedgehog
IHH	Indian hedgehog homologue
IKDC	International Knee Documentation Committee
Il	Interleukin
Il-1β	Interleukin-1 beta
iPSCs	Induced pluripotent stem cells
IR	Inversion recovery
IT	Iliotibial
ITM	Interterritorial matrix
JAAOS	Journal of the American Academy of Orthopedic Surgeons
KL	Kellgren-Lawrence Score
KOOS	Knee Injury and Osteoarthritis Outcome Score
KOSS	Knee Osteoarthritis Scoring System
KS	Keratan sulfate
KSS	Knee Society Score
LEF-1	Lymphoid enhancer-binding factor-1
LFC	Lateral femoral condyle
LI	Lequesne Index
LMT	Lateral meniscal tear
LTP	Lateral tibial plateau
MACI	Matrix-induced autologous chondrocyte implantation
MACT	Matrix-associated autologous chondrocyte transplantation
MAT	Meniscal allograft transplantation
MCID	Minimal clinically important difference

MCP-1	Monocyte chemotactic protein 1
MDSCs	Muscle-derived stem cells
MEDIC	Multiple echo data image combination
MFC	Medial femoral condyle
MFX	Microfracture
MGP	Matrix Gla-protein
MMP	Matrix metalloproteinase (also termed matrixin)
MMP-1	Matrix metalloproteinase-1 (also termed collagenase)
MMP-3	Matrix metalloproteinase-3 (also termed stromelysin)
MMT	Medial meniscal tear
MOAKS	Magnetic Resonance Imaging Osteoarthritis Knee Score
MOCART	Magnetic Resonance Observation of Cartilage Repair Tissue
MOON	Multicenter Orthopaedic Outcomes Network
MOW HTO	Medial opening wedge high tibial osteotomy
MPR	Multiplanar reconstruction
MR	Magnetic resonance
MRI	Magnetic resonance imaging
mRNA	Messenger ribonucleic acid
MSCs	Mesenchymal stem cells
MT	Magnetization transfer
MT1-MMP	Membrane type 1 metalloproteinase
MTC	Magnetization transfer contrast
MTP	Medial tibial plateau
MTR	Magnetization transfer ratio
MTRasym	Asymmetric magnetization transfer ratio
MW	Molecular weight
MZ	Middle zone (also termed transitional zone or Zone 2)
N-CAM	Neural cell adhesion molecule
NIH	National Institutes of Health
NMR	Nuclear magnetic resonance
NOG	Noggin-type TGF-β inactivating polypeptide
NOTCH	A family of type-1 transmembrane highly conserved cell signaling proteins
NSAID	Nonsteroidal anti-inflammatory drug
NTX-1	N-terminal telopeptide of collagen type 1
OA	Osteoarthritis
OARSI	OsteoArthritis Research Society International
OAT	Osteochondral autograft transplantation
OATS	Osteochondral autograft transfer system
OC	Osteochondral
OCA	Osteochondral allograft
OCD	Osteochondritis dissecans
OKS	Oxford Knee Score
ON	Osteonecrosis
OSN	Osteonectin
OP	Osteogenic protein

OR	Operating room
ORIF	Open reduction internal fixation
p	Plasma
PA	Posteroanterior
PACS	Picture archiving and communication system
PASE	Physical Activity Scale for the Elderly
PASS	Patient acceptable symptomatic state
PCL	Posterior cruciate ligament
PCM	Pericellular matrix
PDGF	Platelet-derived growth factor
PDO	Polydiaxanone
PDW	Proton density-weighted
PECL	Poly-epsilon-caprolactone
PEMF	Pulsed electromagnetic field
PF	Patellofemoral
PFJ	Patellofemoral joint
PG	Proteoglycan
PGA	Polyglycolic acid
PGE2	Prostaglandin E2
PG-M	Versican (also termed Vcan or chondroitin sulfate proteoglycan core protein 2 or chondroitin sulfate proteoglycan 2 ie CSPG2)
PGs	Proteoglycans
PIICP	Procollagen type II C-terminal propeptide
PIINP	Procollagen type II N-terminal propeptide
PIPP	Perceived Impact of Problem Profile
PLA	Polylactic acid
PLA2	Phospholipase A2
PLGA	Polylactic co-glycolic acid
PLLA	Poly-L-lactic acid
PRG4	Proteoglycan 4
PRO	Patient-reported outcome
PROMs	Patient-reported outcome measures
PRP	Platelet-rich plasma
PsA	Psoriatic arthritis
PTA	Post-traumatic arthritis
PTH	Parathyroid hormone
PTHrP	Parathyroid hormone–related peptide
PTOA	Post-traumatic osteoarthritis
Pyd	Pyridinoline
QALYs	Quality-adjusted life years
QoL	Quality of life
RA	Rheumatoid arthritis
RAGE	Receptor for advanced glycation end products
RANK	Receptor activator of nuclear factor kB
RCTs	Randomized controlled trials
RGD	Arginine, Glycine and Aspartate
ROA	Radiographic osteoarthritis

ROCK	Research in Osteochondritis Dissecans of the Knee
ROI	Region of interest
ROM	Range of motion
ROS	Reactive oxygen species
RTP	Return to play
RUNx2	Runt-related transcription factor
s	Serum
SA-Gel	Sodium alginate and gelatin
SAPLs	Surface-active phospholipids
SAR	Specific absorption rate
SDF-1	Stromal cell-derived factor-1
SE	Spin echo
SEM	Scanning electron microscopy
SF or sf	Synovial fluid
SF-36	36-Item Short-Form Health Survey
SFA	French Society of Arthroscopy (Société Francaise d' Arthroscopie)
sFRP1	Secreted frizzled-related protein 1
SHG	Second harmonic generation
SHH	Sonic hedgehog
SMAD	A family of protein homologs – the term is a portmanteau to the gene products of the *Caenorhabditis elegans* gene SMA for small body size and the Drosophila gene "Mothers Against Decapentaplegic" (MAD)
SMSCs	Synovium-derived mesenchymal stem cells
SNR	Signal to noise ratio
SPACE	Sampling perfection with application optimized contrasts using different flip angle evolutions
SPARC	Secreted protein acidic and rich in cysteine
SPGR	Spoiled gradient-recalled
SSEA	Stage-specific embryonic antigen
SSFP	Steady-state free precession
STIR	Short-tau (TI) inversion recovery
SZ	Superficial zone (also termed lamina splendens or Zone 1)
SZP	Superficial zone protein
T	Tesla
T1	Longitudinal relaxation time (also termed spin-lattice relaxation time)
T2	Transverse relaxation time (also termed spin-spin relaxation time)
T2W	T2-weighted
TA	Acquisition time
TAS	Tegner Activity Scale
TE	Echo time (MR sequence)
TE	Tissue engineering
TESS	Triple-echo steady-state
TGF	Transforming growth factor

TGF-β	Transforming growth factor-beta
TI	Inversion time
TIMP	Tissue inhibitor of metalloproteinase
TIMP-1	Tissue inhibitor of metalloproteinases type I
TKA	Total knee arthroplasty
TM	Territorial matrix
TNAP	Tissue nonspecific alkaline phosphatase
TN-C	Tenascin-C
TNF	Tumor necrosis factor
TNF-Rs	Tumor necrosis factor-receptors
TNF-α	Tumor necrosis factor-alpha
TR	Repetition time
True-FISP	True fast imaging with steady-state precession
TSE	Turbo-spin-echo
TTTG	Tibial tuberosity-trochlear groove
u	Urine
ucMGP	Uncarboxylated matrix Gla-protein
ucMSC	Umbilical cord matrix-derived stromal cells
UTE	Ultrashort echo time
VAS	Visual Analog Scale
VEGF	Vascular endothelial growth factor
VHAS	Visual Histologic Assessment Scale
VIBE	Volumetric interpolated breath-hold examination
VIPR	Vastly undersampled isotropic projection (radiology)
VISTA	Volumetric isotropic T2-weighted acquisition
WASSR	Water saturation shift referencing
Wnt	Wingless-related integration site signaling protein
WOMAC	Western Ontario and McMaster Universities osteoarthritis Index
WOMET	Western Ontario Meniscal Evaluation Tool
WORMS	Whole-organ Magnetic Resonance Imaging Score
YKL-40	Human cartilage glycoprotein-39
ZCC	Zone of calcified cartilage (also termed Zone 4)
Δdi-DS	Dermatan sulfate delta disaccharides
Δdi-HA	Hyaluronic acid delta disaccharides

Part I

Normal Articular Cartilage

Structure and Function of Articular Cartilage

1

Harpal K. Gahunia and Kenneth P. H. Pritzker

1.1 Introduction

In synovial joints, articular cartilage is a smooth, wear-resistant lubricated surface that caps the bones, allowing them to glide over one another with minimal friction and to absorb impact forces. The articular cartilage faces the joint cavity on one side and is linked to the subchondral bone plate via a narrow layer of calcified cartilage tissue on the other side. Articular cartilage, also referred to as *hyaline cartilage* because of its amorphous glassy macroscopic appearance, is a uniquely ordered, highly specialized connective tissue with biophysical properties consistent with its ability to withstand high compressive forces. The synovial fluid (SF) plays an important role in cartilage nourishment, joint lubrication and wear resistance [1]. Articular cartilage is maintained through long-range diffusion of nutrients from the adjacent connective tissue blood vessels and SF [2]. In addition, diffusion of substances from blood vessels in the subchondral bone can also contribute to cartilage nourishment in immature tissues prior to complete calcification of the growth plate. In neonates and early childhood, cartilage canals connect the cartilage and subchondral bone, and contribute to cartilage nourishment. During growth and development, the cartilage canals extend as branches of blood vessels to the immature articular cartilage [3–5]. Although these canals are abundant in young cartilage, with increasing age, their number decreases and they are absent in mature cartilage [3]. Adult cartilage is typically avascular, alymphatic and aneural, and it is nourished primarily by the diffusion of nutrients from SF through the articular surface [6].

This chapter is organized into two main sections. The first section comprehensively presents the structure, composition and architecture of articular cartilage. The three-dimensional (3D) complexity of articular cartilage due to its horizontal zone heterogeneity from the articular surface to the subchondral bone and its extracellular matrix (ECM) compartmentalization from the vicinity of chondrocytes outwards are presented in depth. The second section of this chapter is focused on the varied function of articular cartilage, with emphasis on the critical role played by the articular surface as well as the chondrocytes and their microenvironment. During mobility and cartilage compression, the important role played

H. K. Gahunia, MSc, PhD (✉)
Orthopaedic Science Consulting Services,
Oakville, ON, Canada
e-mail: harpal.gahunia@utotonto.ca

K. P. H. Pritzker, MD, FRCPC
Department of Laboratory Medicine and Pathobiology,
Department of Surgery, and Institute of
Biomaterials and Biomedical Engineering,
University of Toronto, Toronto, ON, Canada

Department of Pathology and Laboratory Medicine,
Mount Sinai Hospital, Toronto, ON, Canada

H. K. Gahunia et al. (eds.), *Articular Cartilage of the Knee*,
https://doi.org/10.1007/978-1-4939-7587-7_1

by the SF and surface lubricating molecules is thoroughly discussed. Also presented are the various lubrication mechanisms as these relate to the human knee.

1.2 Articular Cartilage Structure and Composition

Articular cartilage is a dynamic, highly hydrated tissue comprised of cells, the chondrocytes (2–5% cartilage wet weight), which are embedded in the ECM (95–98% cartilage wet weight) secreted and maintained by the chondrocytes. The ECM of cartilage is a resilient gel comprised of tissue fluid with small molecular weight (MW) ions and macromolecular composition, mainly of collagen type II and proteoglycans (PGs). The unique biological and biomechanical properties of articular cartilage depend on the architecture of collagen fibres, the composition of PGs as large MW solutes, and interactions between the ECM and the chondrocytes that maintain the cartilage function and homeostasis [7, 8].

1.2.1 Chondrocytes and Chondrons

Chondrocytes are the only cell type found in articular cartilage. The chondrocyte morphology varies from flat, discoid-shaped cells at the articular surface to round or polygonal with increasing cartilage depth. Using confocal microscopy, the morphometric analysis of cadaver (age 23–49 years) medial femoral condyle articular cartilage (mean depth 2.4 mm) determined the chondrocyte volume density as 1.7% and the mean chondrocyte diameter was 13 μm [9]. The chondrocyte has intracellular morphologic features characteristic of a metabolically active cell, consistent with its role in the synthesis and turnover of ECM components (Fig. 1.1). Chondrocytes are responsible for generating and maintaining the cartilaginous extracellular environment. Deviation from the normal articular cartilage homeostasis, due to injury, aging or disease, is reflected in the chondrocyte ultrastructure [10–12].

Chondrons are the microanatomical, micromechanical and metabolically active

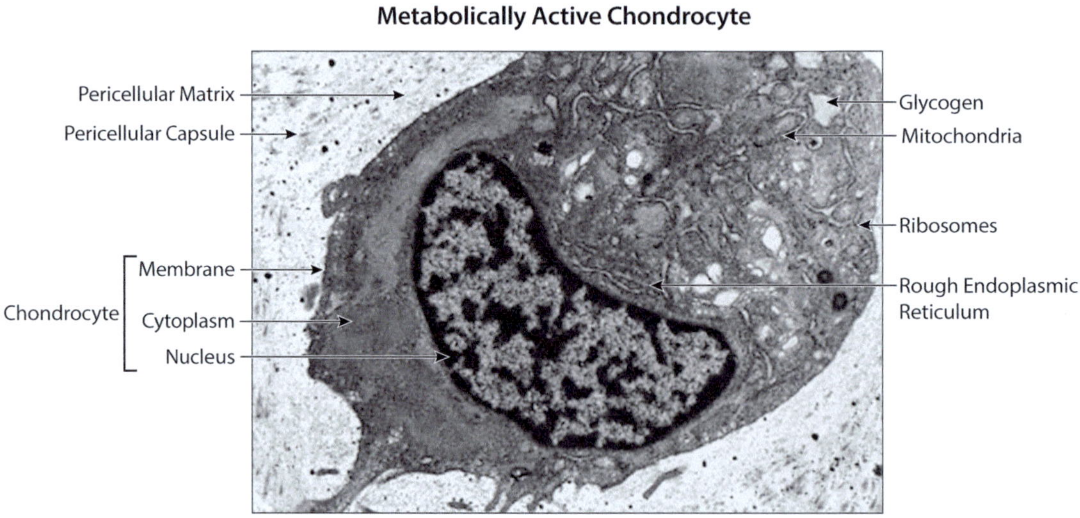

Fig. 1.1 Electron microscopy of a metabolically active chondrocyte showing the intracellular structures (abundant rough endoplasmic reticulum, free ribosomes, mitochondria and glycogen) and its pericellular environment (matrix and capsule). Magnification ×5000

functional units of articular cartilage. Due to the nature of mature cartilage, the immediate pericellular microenvironment of the chondrocytes plays a critical role in maintaining the homeostasis of the articular cartilage [13–15]. Anatomically, the chondron comprises a chondrocyte and its pericellular microenvironment (Fig. 1.2) [15]. Morphologically, the chondrocyte surface membrane is surrounded by a transparent glycocalyx at the outer periphery of which is a thin pericellular matrix (PCM) that becomes more distinct as cartilage matures. The PCM is composed of a mixture of collagen types VI and IX along with small PGs and glycoproteins [16–18]. The PCM in turn is surrounded and enclosed by a fibrillar pericellular capsule [19, 20]. Usually, chondrocytes of mature cartilage fill the chondron with little PCM seen between the chondrocyte and the chondron capsule. During histological processing the chondrocytes slightly shrink, hence an empty space referred to as "lacuna" is seen between the chondrocyte membrane and chondron capsule.

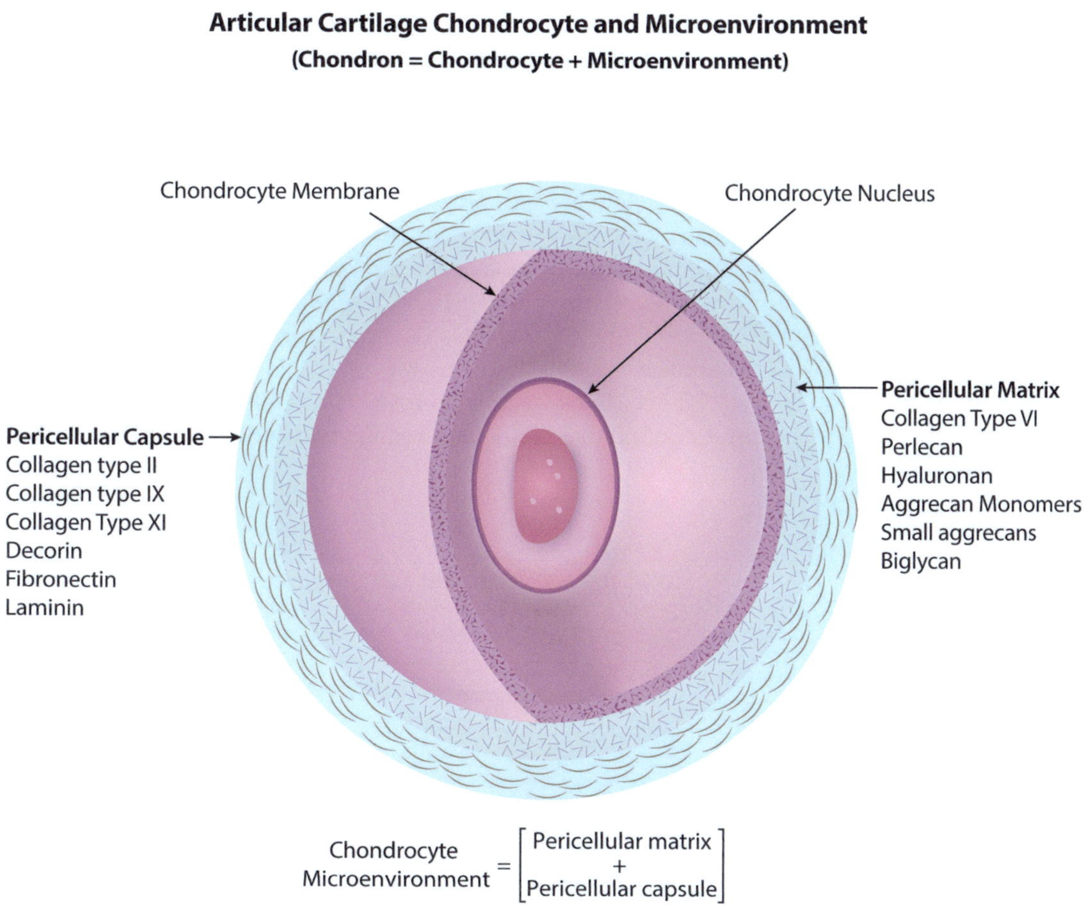

Fig. 1.2 Schematic diagram depicting a chondron composed of articular cartilage chondrocyte and its microenvironment. The chondrocyte membrane is surrounded by a thin pericellular matrix comprised of collagen type VI and other small proteoglycans and glycoproteins. The pericellular matrix is surrounded and enclosed by a fibrillar pericellular capsule of collagens and non-collagenous proteins. (Schematic created by Dr. Harpal K. Gahunia, and graphic illustration by Danny Aguilar, JD Graphics Solutions, East York, Ontario, Canada)

1.2.2 Extracellular Matrix

The physicochemical properties of articular cartilage depend on the structure, organization and concentration of the ECM macromolecules (20% to 25% of the cartilage wet weight) and their interactions with the tissue fluid (70% to 80% of the cartilage wet weight) that contains small MW ions (Fig. 1.3). The tissue fluid plays an important role in joint lubrication, wear resistance, and enables nutrients and oxygen to diffuse through the cartilage matrix from the cartilage surface to its cells located at varying depth [1].

The mature ECM is composed of predominantly collagen type II bundles together with non-collagenous proteins, ions (primarily Na^+ and Cl^- ions) and soluble, negatively charged PG molecules. Depending on the age and anatomic location of articular cartilage, the PGs could approximately constitute 50% of the dry weight, whereas the total collagen may constitute 24% of the dry weight (Fig. 1.4). In humans, collagen type II is the principal fibrillar macromolecule, representing 90–95% of the total collagen in articular cartilage, whereas other cartilage-specific and cartilage-non-specific collagens constitute 5–10% of the total collagen (about 1% of the dry weight) [21–23]. The turnover of normal adult cartilage collagen type II is extremely low with a half-life of > 100 years, whereas PGs and aggrecans continue to be synthesized and secreted into the ECM with the normal turnover for a large monomer corresponding to a half-life of 3.4 years [24–26]. Depending on age, the non-collagenous proteins including glycoproteins could form about 25% of the ECM dry weight. These non-collagenous proteins include fibronectin, laminin, tenascin, chondronectin, cartilage oligomeric matrix protein (COMP) and cartilage matrix glycoprotein (CMGP) [7, 27–33].

1.2.2.1 Proteoglycans

Proteoglycans, a diverse family of molecules, are strongly hydrophilic, and this property facilitates the lubrication of the joint bearing surfaces. Articular cartilage PGs vary in size, glycosaminoglycan (GAG) content and functional properties [34, 35]. These PG molecules are present as soluble PG monomers or as PG aggregates, which together with tissue fluid molecules are associated with the collagen fibres (Fig. 1.5, Table 1.1). The large aggregating PGs (such as aggrecan and versican) form 50% to 58% of the total PGs, whereas non-aggregating PGs form 40% of the total PGs [37, 60]. The non-aggregating cartilage PGs include

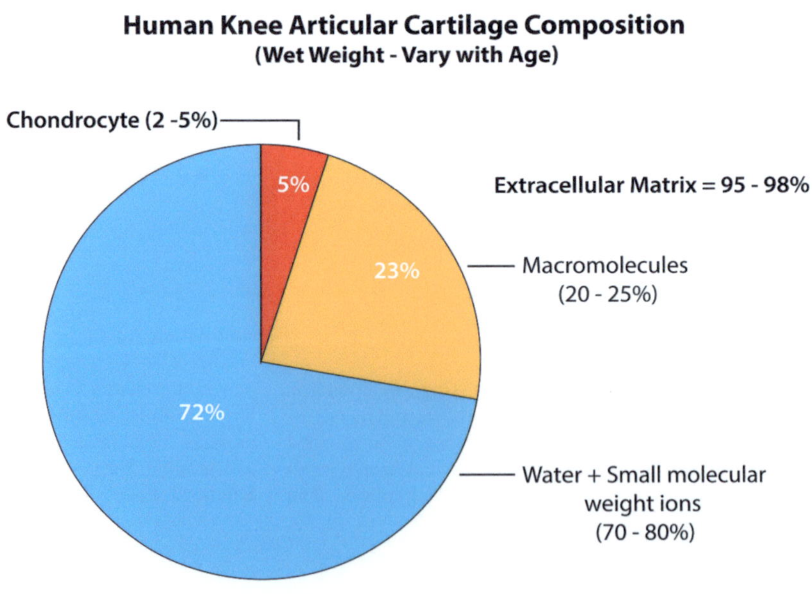

Fig. 1.3 Articular cartilage wet weight composition in the human adult knee. The chondrocytes consist of only 2–5% of wet weight, whereas the extracellular matrix consists of 95–98%, of which tissue fluid and small molecular weight ions occupy the majority of extracellular matrix. Note that wet weight of knee articular cartilage macromolecules varies with age and anatomic location

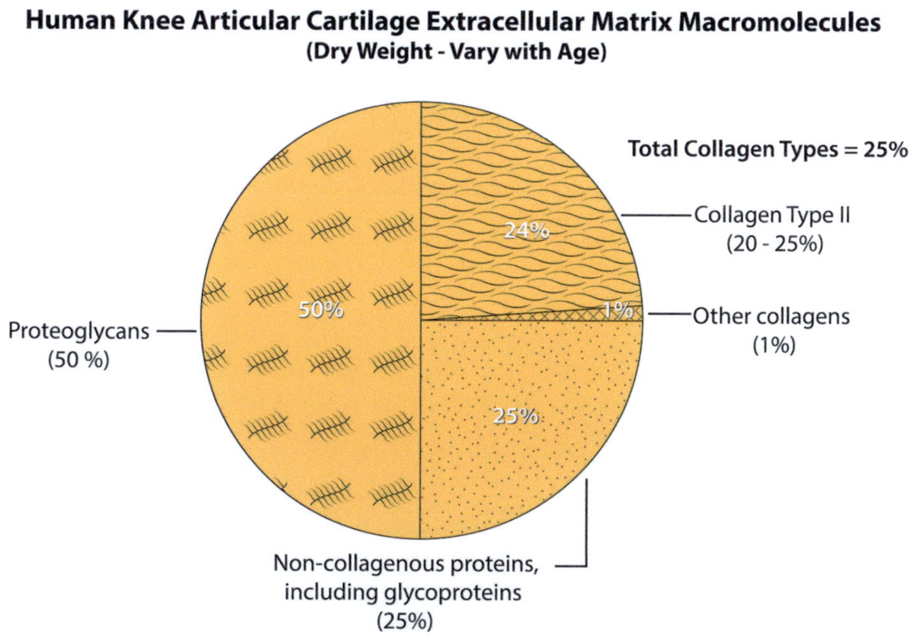

Fig. 1.4 Schematic representation of the articular cartilage extracellular matrix macromolecules dry weight composition in the human adult knee. Note that dry weight of articular cartilage molecules varies with age and anatomic location

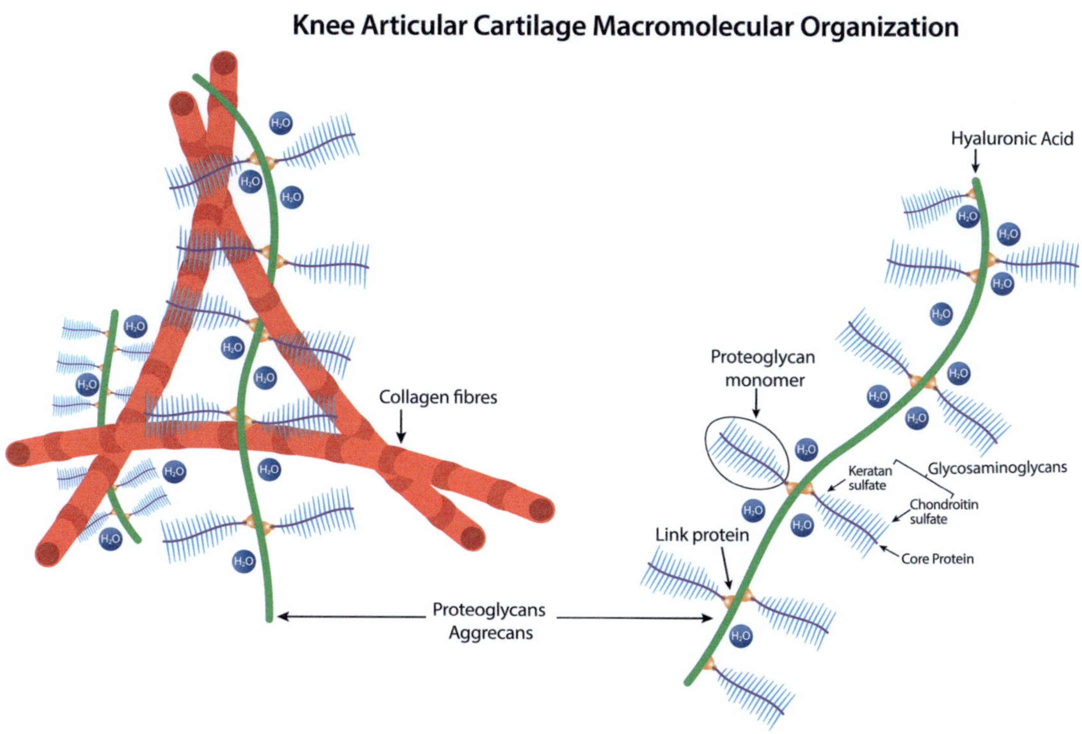

Fig. 1.5 Schematic diagram showing the articular cartilage collagen and aggrecan interaction and organization. The proteoglycan monomer consists of a protein core with covalently bonded glycosaminoglycan side chains, namely, chondroitin sulfate and keratan sulfate. These monomers are non-covalently attached to the hyaluronic acid backbone via HA-binding region which is further stabilized by the link protein. (Schematic created by Dr. Harpal K. Gahunia, and graphic illustration by Danny Aguilar, JD Graphics Solutions, East York, Ontario, Canada)

Table 1.1 Knee articular cartilage glycosaminoglycans and proteoglycans: basic structure, location and functions

Glycan Type	Alternating Copolymer Disaccharide Repeating Units (Basic Structure)	Molecular Weight (Kilodaltons)	Extracellular Matrix Localization	Function
		Hyaluronan – Binding Proteoglycans		
Chondroitin Sulfate (CS)			ITM	Structural constituents; Highly sulfated GAGs providing negative charge for enhanced hydration and biomechanical properties; Provides viscoelastic properties
1. Chondroitin-4-sulfate (C4S)	β -1,4-linked d-glucuronic acid and β -1,3-linked N-acetyl-β -galactosamine-4-O-sulfate	5–50		
2. Chondroitin-6-sulfate (C6S)	β -1,4-linked d-glucuronic acid and β -1,3-linked N-acetyl-β -galactosamine-6-O-sulfate	5–50		
Keratan Sulfate (KS)	β-N-acetyl-D-glucosamine and β -1,3-linked poly-N-acetyllactosamine	5–15	ITM	Highly sulfated GAGs providing negative charge for enhanced hydration and biomechanical properties; Binds to many ECM constituents, particularly fibrillar collagens to stabilise collagen network
Dermatan Sulfate (DS)	β -1,3- or β -1,4-linked N-acetyl galactosamine-4-O-sulfate and either L-iduronic acid or D-glucuronic acid	87×10^3 to 285×10^3 with ~ 45×10^3 Protein core	ITM	Interacts with fibrillar collagens; Important in matrix organisation
Hyaluronic Acid (HA, also known as hyaluronan)	β-D-(1-4)-N-Acetyl-D-glucosamine β-D-(1-3)-Glucuronic acid	4–8000	PCM; ITM	Structural constituents; Stabilises large aggrecan formation; Facilitates cell-ECM interactions; Provides viscoelastic properties; Retains water and maintains osmotic pressure
Proteoglycan Monomer (PG)	Protein core with CS and KS GAG chains	1×10^3 to 3×10^3 with ~ 200 to 250 Protein core	AC ECM; Predominant PG in SZ	Structural constituents; Facilitates joint lubrication; Load-bearing properties
Proteoglycan Link Protein	Consists of three domains: A, B1 and B2 with structural analogy to G1 region of aggrecan; Has one or two N-linked oligosaccharide chains that may have variable sialic acid contents	54	ECM	Stabilizes the binding of PG monomer to HA; Concentration of link protein significantly influence aggrecan aggregation, aggregate stability, and uniformity of aggrecan spacing; Domain A interacts with the G1 region of aggrecan and both B domains interact with HA; Complex formed by aggrecan, link protein and HA stabilizes soluble aggrecans in collagen network; Helps protect PG aggregates from degradation

(continued)

Table 1.1 (continued)

Glycan Type	Alternating Copolymer Disaccharide Repeating Units (Basic Structure)	Molecular Weight (Kilodaltons)	Extracellular Matrix Localization	Function
Proteoglycan Aggregates	HA with attached PGs	> 2 × 10^5	PCM, small size; TM, medium size; ITM, large size	Principal load-bearing PGs; Facilitates joint lubrication; Important in mediating chondrocyte-chondrocyte and chondrocyte-matrix interactions
1. Aggrecan	Supramolecule with as much as 50 PG monomers bound to HA	3 × 10^3 to 3 × 10^6	ITM	Provides viscoelastic properties; Provides osmotic resistance to compressive loads
2. Versican (also known as PG-M)	Large ECM molecule with CS PGs	> 1 × 10^3 with > 200 protein cores	ITM	Participates in matrix organization during chondrogenesis; Mediates cell adhesion and migration; Promotes cell growth
		Pericellular Proteoglycans		
Perlecan	Protein core with CS / HS side chains	~ 500 Protein core	PCM	Promotes chondrocyte attachment; Modulates activity of several growth factors; Promotes chondrogenesis; Maintains chondrogenic differentiation
Heparan Sulfate (HS)	D-Glucuronic acid or L-iduronic acid D-Glucosamine or N-acetyl-D-glucosamine	75 × 10^3	Cell surface; PCM	Major modifiers of growth factors; Interacts with other HS PGs and with PCM laminins and collagen type IV; Important role in chondrogenesis
		Small Leucine-Rich Repeat Proteoglycans		
Biglycan (also known as DS-PGI has > 65% homology to decorin)	Carries two CS or DS side chain	100 with 38 protein core	PCM	Interacts with collagen type VI; Binds to and modulates TGF-β bioactivity; Affects the Wnt signalling pathway
Decorin (also known as PG40 and DS-PGII)	Carries one CS or DS side chain	72 with 36 protein core	ITM of SZ	Associates with collagen fibrils and regulates collagen fibrillogenesis and structure; Controls cell growth; Interacts with other proteins; Mediates interaction between collagen and PG; Binds to and modulates TGF-β bioactivity
Fibromodulin (homologous to biglycan and decorin)	Carries up to four N-linked KS side chains. Some molecules contain KS chains exclusively capped with α(2-3)-linked sialic acid	59	ITM of AC: Most abundant in SZ	Forms strong association with collagen fibrils; Regulates collagen fibril diameter and fibrillogenesis; Involved in collagen cross-linking; Binds and sequesters growth factors during cartilage remodelling

(continued)

Table 1.1 (continued)

Glycan Type	Alternating Copolymer Disaccharide Repeating Units (Basic Structure)	Molecular Weight (Kilodaltons)	Extracellular Matrix Localization	Function
Lumican	Contains ten tandem leucine-rich repeats; Carries four N-linked sites within the leucine-rich domain of the horse-shoe-shaped protein core that can be substituted with KS	40	ECM	Helps stabilise collagen fibrils and orient fibrillogenesis; Binds to ECM collagen molecules within a collagen fibril, thus helping keep adjacent fibrils apart
Chondroadherin	Contains eleven leucine-rich repeats flanked by cysteine-rich regions	38	PCM; ECM	Provides a link between chondrocytes and ECM via specific interactions with α2β1 integrins and heparin sulfate chains; Promotes attachment of chondrocytes to ECM; Regulates chondrocyte growth and proliferation; Binds to collagen types II and VI, influencing fibrillogenesis
		Other Proteoglycans		
Lubricin	Attachment site for a CS chain	227	Surface of SZ	Forms protective layer on SZ to maintain surface integrity; Allows extensive hydration; Responsible for lubrication; Reduces friction and wear

References: [31, 34, 36–59]
AC, *Articular cartilage*; ECM, *Extracellular matrix*; GAGs, *Glycosaminoglycans*; PCM, *Pericellular matrix*; TM, *Territorial matrix*; ITM, *Interterritorial matrix*; TGF-β, *Transforming growth factor*; SZ, *Superficial zone*

biglycan, decorin, fibromodulin, lumican and perlecan [44, 49, 61].

In articular cartilage, the heterogeneity of PG structure and function is a reflection not only of the variation in protein core but also variation in the type and size of the GAG chains. The variation in the position of sulfation can also increase diversity in the chemical and physical properties of the GAG chains. PG monomers are composed of a protein core onto which one or more highly sulfated GAG side chains are covalently bonded. The GAG molecules are unbranched chains of repeating disaccharides, which confer negative charge to the cartilage matrix. The concentration of the negative charge is known as *fixed charge density* (FCD). The cartilage FCD with tissue fluid is primarily responsible for maintaining the compressive properties of articular cartilage. The GAG groups present in the articular cartilage PGs are mainly chondroitin sulfate (CS, 87%), which exists both as chondroitin-4-sulfate (C4S) and chondroitin-6-sulfate (C6S). Other GAGs present in AC are keratan sulfate (KS, 6%) and hyaluronic acid (HA), also called hyaluronan. Each PG molecule can consist of over 100 CS chains, 20-40 KS and 40 O- and N-linked oligosaccharides [62]. The CS chains are covalently attached to the protein core via a xylose residue linkage to specific serine residues, whereas KS chains are attached to protein via N- and O-linked glycosidic linkages to asparagine or serine/threonine, respectively. As one moves away from the chondrocytes towards the interterritorial matrix (ITM), CS PGs and dermatan sulfate (DS) PGs predominate [37]. HA is a large polyanionic molecule that can have a MW up to 6 million Daltons. HA is the only GAG that is not bound to a core protein and is non-sulfated. The HA receptor on the surface of chondrocyte serves as the critical link for the retention of the HA-PG aggregates to the chondrocyte cell surface and plays an important role in PCM assembly and retention [63–65].

The majority of PG molecules in articular cartilage are aggrecans with varying composition and size, hence the propensity to aggregate into large supramolecular complexes [66]. These macromolecular composites are heavily sulfated with the negatively charged GAG side chains that attract water molecules with associated cations. Aggrecans generate a densely packed hydrated gel, intertwined in the collagen fibril network along with other PGs and glycoproteins [62]. An aggrecan molecule is a composite macromolecule comprising of a central HA to which several PG monomers are non-covalently attached (Fig. 1.6). The core protein of aggrecan has a MW of approximately 230 kDa and consists of three globular domains, G1, G2 and G3, with three interglobular regions [44, 67]. Each PG molecule of an aggrecan binds with HA backbone via the HA-binding region (G1 domain) of their core protein at the N-terminal domain (Table 1.2). This interaction between aggrecan and HA is further stabilized by the link protein which consists of about 100 amino acids in length

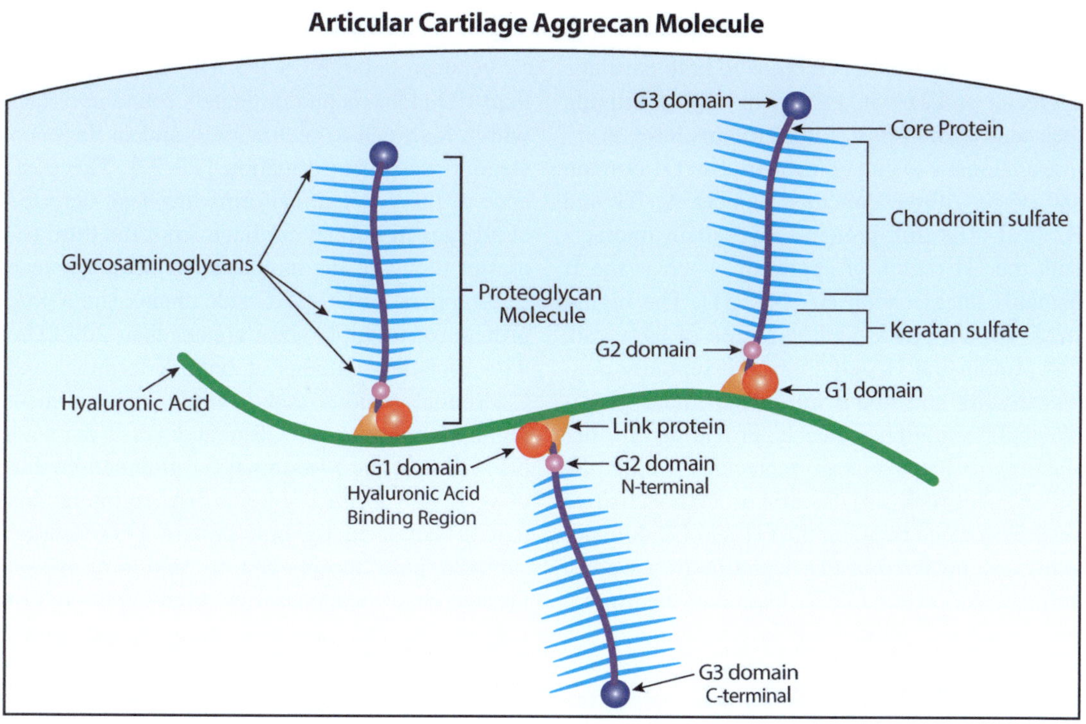

Fig. 1.6 Schematic diagram of articular cartilage aggrecan molecule showing the backbone hyaluronic acid (HA). Each aggrecan molecule consists of three domains, namely HA-binding, N-terminal and C-terminal domains, also referred to as G1, G2 and G3 domains, respectively. Each aggrecan molecule attaches to the HA backbone via G1 domain and is stabilized by link protein. (Courtesy of Dr. Harpal K. Gahunia and graphic illustration by Danny Aguilar, JD Graphics Solutions, East York, Ontario, Canada)

Table 1.2 Aggrecan globular structure domains play an important role in anchoring the proteoglycans to other extracellular molecules

G1 domain	G2 domain	G3 domain
	Domain Location	
• Amino terminus of core protein	• Amino terminus of core protein	• Carboxyl terminus of core protein
	Domain Functions	
• Binds HA; • Forms ternary complex with HA and link protein to stabilise aggrecan molecule; • Mediates interactions between chondrocyte and ECM	• Unique to aggrecan; • Involved in regulating aggrecan production; • Inhibits product secretion	• Links aggrecan complexes to ECM components; • Enhances GAG modification such as GAG chain attachment and product secretion; • Binding domain for galactose present on collagen type II, cell surface or other ECM constituents; • Interacts with tenascin and sulfated glycolipids; • Enhances product secretion (alone or in combination with KS or CS domain); • Promotes GAG chain attachment

References: [37, 62, 67–72]
CS, *Chondroitin sulfate*; ECM, *Extracellular matrix*; GAG, *Glycosaminoglycan*; HA, *Hyaluronic acid*; KS, *Keratan sulfate*

with a characteristic sequence comprising four disulfide-bonded Cys residues [42]. Link protein is a 45 kDa molecule that binds to both cartilage aggrecan and HA in ECM, thereby stabilizing their aggregation [50]. Link proteins have structure analogous to that of the aggrecan G1 domain and possess three domains, namely A, B1 and B2 [73]. The link protein's A domain interacts with the G1 region of aggrecan, whereas the B domains interact with HA [42, 51]. The highly stable tripartite HA-binding region of aggrecan, link protein and HA complex is essentially non-dissociating and non-displaceable under physiological conditions, hence providing further stability to the aggrecan molecules within the collagen network [44]. Several protease-sensitive sites are located between the G1 and G2 domain, which are involved in PG depletion observed in arthritis. Following the G2 domain of the protein core is a small region rich in KS chains and a largest region with > 100 covalently linked CS chains [37]. Following the CS-rich region, the G3 domain is located towards the C-terminal of the protein core. The G3 domain serves as the binding domain for the galactose present on chondrocytes or cartilage ECM molecules, which has the ability to interact with tenascins, fibulins and sulfated glycolipids [74].

Versican, a large CS PG with a MW of more than 1000 kDa, is predominately found in tissues with a high cell-to-matrix ratio and in the early stage of cartilage formation [75–77]. The presence of the versican isoforms has been detected at all ages in normal cartilage from the third trimester foetus to the mature adult [43]. Versican is comprised of CS GAG side chains and a core protein (of multiple sizes greater than 200 kDa) with globular domains at both N-terminal and C-terminal regions and central CS-attachment regions consisting of CS-α and CS-β domains [75, 77, 78]. The N-terminal G1 globular domain of versican specifically binds HA, an interaction that is stabilised by link protein [79]. During synovial joint morphogenesis and precartilage mesenchymal condensations, high expression of versican and HA have been shown to facilitate a highly hydrated environment that promotes cell proliferation and migration as well as the formation/organisation of the articular surface [76]. The versican-HA complexes surrounding cells serve an important role in controlling cell shape and cell division [80, 81].

Perlecan is a modular heparan sulfate (HS) and/or CS-substituted PG with a protein core size between 400 kDa and 500 kDa [49, 82]. Perlecan is a predominant component of articular cartilage and epiphyseal plate during long bone growth and development. Perlecan shows a PCM distribution through all age groups. It was also found in the ITM of newborn to 19-month-old stifle articular cartilage of merino sheep. A significant age-dependent decline in perlecan levels in the articular cartilage and epiphyseal plate cartilage has been documented [61]. In human knee articular cartilage, perlecan is densely distributed in the fetal (12–14 weeks) PCM with diffuse localization in the ITM, whereas postnatal (2–7 months) and mature (55–64 years) femoral cartilage showed strong pericellular localizations [83]. HS PGs are attached to different core proteins and are associated with the chondrocyte surface and its pericellular environment molecules [84]. The vast structural diversity of HS GAG chains enables it to bind and interact with a wide variety of chondrocyte surface and ECM proteins such as growth factors, chemokines and morphogens [84].

Biglycan, decorin, fibromodulin and lumican are members of a family of structurally related small leucine-rich PGs called the small CS/DS PGs, which differ in GAG composition and function [34, 37]. These molecules play significant roles in matrix assembly and stabilization, and metabolic regulation of articular cartilage, such as collagen fibrillogenesis and binding of matrix molecules, e.g. fibronectin and growth factors [85, 86]. Biglycan (also known as DS-PGI), a 100 kDa molecule with a core protein of 38 kDa, is the predominant small PG of cartilage and contains two chains of CS/DS. Biglycan is localized to the PCM, where it may interact with collagen type VI [34, 53]. Decorin, also known as PG40 and DS-PGII, is a 74 kDa PG with a core protein of 36 kDa, which possesses one DS chain. Decorin is present throughout the ITM, with increased amounts in the superficial zone (SZ) of articular cartilage, and is thought to mediate interactions between aggregating PGs [46, 54, 86]. Fibromodulin, a 59 kDa PG bearing several KS chains, represents 0.1–0.3% of the cartilage wet weight. It has a characteristic amino acid composition, with 14% of its residues being made up of leucine [87]. Fibromodulin is present in ECM and interacts with the collagen type II fibrils to assist in fibrillogenesis and interfibril interactions [34]. The presence of non-collagenous proteins on the cartilage surface in normal bovine and human samples revealed abundant fibromodulin and a small amount of fibronectin, decorin and biglycan [88]. Lumican, a 40 kDa PG with four major intramolecular domains, is present in the ECM of articular cartilage [39, 89, 90]. Lumican is expressed at low levels in the juvenile, immature cartilage and in the form of a PG molecule. However, in adult articular cartilage, lumican is expressed at high levels and exists predominantly in a glycoprotein form lacking KS [90, 91]. Lumican binds within collagen fibrils to help stabilize and organize the collagen fibrils, orient fibrillogenesis and maintain the collagen fibril circumferential growth [47]. Chondroadherin is a 38 kDa, cell-binding, leucine-rich repeat protein found in the territorial matrix (TM) of articular cartilage [92–94]. Chondroadherin regulates the chondrocyte growth and proliferation, and promotes the attachment of chondrocytes to ECM. This chondroadherin-chondrocyte interaction is thought to maintain the adult chondrocyte phenotype and cartilage homeostasis [95]. It mediates adhesion of chondrocytes by providing a link between chondrocytes and ECM via specific $\alpha2\beta1$ integrins (on chondrocyte surface) and HS chains (within ECM) [96]. In the ECM, chondroadherin interacts with collagen types II and VI, influencing collagen fibrillogenesis [93]. Other PGs, such as lubricin, proteoglycan 4 (PGR4) and superficial zone protein (SZP), will be discussed in depth in the section pertaining to lubrication molecule.

1.2.2.2 Collagens

Collagens are the major proteinaceous constituents of articular cartilage. Collagens are secreted by the chondrocytes as a procollagen molecule, which are then processed in the ECM by enzymatic cleavage of the C- and N-propeptides [97]. Although propeptide removal is required for fibrils to grow normally, partially processed N-procollagen can also assemble into thin collagen fibrils [98, 99]. In the ECM, the collagen molecules copolymerize to form a fibrillar framework and are stabilized by covalent cross-links formed between adjacent collagen chains (intramolecular cross-link) and adjacent collagen molecules (intermolecular cross-link) [100, 101].

Several collagen types are known to exist in articular cartilage, which can be classified as fibrillar, microfibrillar or non-fibrillar based on distinct sets of polypeptide chains that can form homo- or heterotrimeric assemblies (Table 1.3). Cartilage collagens capable of forming fibrillar networks include collagen types II, XI and XXVII, whereas collagen type VI is the only microfibrillar cartilage collagen [104, 131, 142]. The non-fibrillar collagens include two subcategories: collagens that are capable of forming hexagonal networks (such as types IV and X) and collagens that associate with the surface of various fibrils also referred to as fibril-associated collagen with interrupted triple helix (FACIT, such as types IX, XII, XIV, XVI and XXII).

Of all cartilage collagens, types II, IX and XI are articular cartilage-specific and form a cross-linked copolymer core network in developing cartilage [22, 103, 152]. Collagen type II is the principal molecule that provides high tensile strength to the cartilaginous matrix and maintains cartilage integrity by providing resiliency [102, 153, 154]. Collagen type II is important for the establishment of temporal and spatial organization with other matrix components such as the aggrecan. Although both collagen types II and XI are structurally closely related, they differ primarily in their N-propeptides [131]. Collagen type XI contributes to about 1–2% of the total collagen and is incorporated in the collagen type II fibre in a ratio of about 1:30 in mature tissues [21]. Collagen type XI is thought to mediate physical interactions between collagen fibrils and PGs in cartilage as well as to regulate the size of the collagen type II fibres [104, 106, 107]. Collagen type XXVII is located at the site of transition from cartilage to bone and growth plate matrix surrounding the proliferative chondrocytes [104, 109–112]. During endochondral ossification, collagen type XXVII plays an important structural role in the PCM of the growth plate, is required for the organization of the proliferative zone and facilitates cartilage to bone transition [109, 110]. Collagen type VI, a large disulfide-bonded microfibrillar molecule concentrated in the PCM, represents 1–2% of the total collagen [104, 113, 114, 119, 155]. Collagen type VI mediates the attachment of chondrocytes to the macromolecular framework of the cartilage PCM, maintains chondrocyte morphology, regulates chondrocyte swelling, protects chondrocyte from apoptosis and facilitates chondrocyte-ECM and intermolecular interactions [115, 116, 118].

The two articular cartilage non-fibrillar and hexagonal network-forming collagens are type IV and type X. Collagen type IV is predominantly found in the PCM where it co-localizes with laminin and binds with perlecan, and is also located as a discrete layer on the surface of articular cartilage [30, 82, 120, 121]. Being abundant in the pericellular area, collagen type IV maintains the chondrocyte phenotype and viability, as well as the matrix integrity where it also binds to fibronectin [30]. Collagen type X is a short homotrimeric collagen constituting 1% of all cartilage collagens. Collagen Type X is present in the zone of calcified cartilage (ZCC) of the articular-epiphyseal cartilage complex (AECC) and the growth plate surrounding the hypertrophic chondrocytes, as well as the transitional zone (also called the calcified zone that exists between the articular cartilage and the subchondral bone) at the site of collagen fibril arcades [22, 133–135]. Collagen type X is synthesized and deposited largely by chondrocytes of hypertrophic cartilage, and the onset of collagen type X expression occurs before calcification becomes apparent [136]. Collagen type X interacts with anchorin CII [137]. Collagen type X plays an important role in the development of the growth plate, endochondral ossification and mature cartilage remodelling and calcification [132, 138].

Collagen type IX represents 1% of the collagens in adult articular cartilage and at least 10% in fetal cartilage [22]. Collagen type IX is located on the outside of the collagen type II fibril to which it is covalently cross-linked and is shown to co-localize with fibronectin [105, 122, 127, 128]. It is also distributed in ECM without association with collagen type II and is covalently cross-linked to other molecules of collagen type IX [125, 129–131]. Because of the presence of CS or DS GAG chains on its α2(IX) chain, collagen type IX is also considered as a PG. These

Table 1.3 Articular cartilage collagen types, characteristic features and functions

Collagen Type	Molecular Structure	Molecular Weight (Kilodaltons)	Articular Cartilage Location	Characteristics and Functions	References
Fibrillar Collagens					
Collagen Type II	$\alpha1(II)_3$	290	Predominant ECM collagen	Articular cartilage-specific collagen; Provides main framework of articular cartilage with soluble PGs; Provides cartilage with tensile strength	[21, 22, 102, 103]
Collagen Type XI	α1(XI) α2(XI) α3(XI)	300	Predominantly pericellular capsule; ECM	Articular cartilage-specific collagen; Regulates cartilage formation; Mediates physical interaction between collagen type II fibrils and PGs; Binds to heparin, HS and DS	[21, 22, 103–108]
Collagen Type XXVII	$\alpha1(XXVII)_3$	185	Site of transition from cartilage to bone; Present in growth plate matrix surrounding proliferative chondrocytes	Facilitates transition of cartilage to bone during endochondral ossification; Key structural role in PCM of growth plate; Essential for growth plate proliferative zone organisation	[104, 109–112]
Microfibrillar Collagens					
Collagen Type VI	α1(VI) α2(VI) α3(VI)	500–550	Predominantly PCM	Forms a network bridge anchoring chondrocytes to PCM; Maintains chondrocyte morphology and protects chondrocytes from apoptosis; Facilitates cell-ECM and intermolecular interactions; Binds to collagen types II, IV and XIV, biglycan, decorin, perlecan, fibronectin, tenascin	[104, 113–119]
Non-Fibrillar Collagens					
Collagen Type IV	$\alpha1(IV)_2$ α2(IV)	161	Predominantly PCM; Discrete layer on the articular cartilage surface (hexagonal network forming collagen)	Maintains chondrocyte phenotype and viability; Binds to perlecan, fibronectin and TGF-β	[30, 82, 104, 120, 121]
Collagen Type IX	α1(IX) α2(IX) α3(IX)	250	Predominantly pericellular capsule (FACIT collagen)	Articular cartilage-specific collagen; Formation of stable collagen network; Maintains cartilage matrix organisation and integrity; Interacts with matrilin-3; Binds to collagen types II and XII, fibronectin and fibromodulin	[21, 22, 103, 105, 108, 122–131]

(continued)

Table 1.3 (continued)

Collagen Type	Molecular Structure	Molecular Weight (Kilodaltons)	Articular Cartilage Location	Characteristics and Functions	References
Collagen Type X	$\alpha 1(X)_3$	170	Predominantly ZCC; Hypertrophic chondrocytes of growth plate; Transitional zone at the site of collagen fibril arcades (hexagonal network-forming collagen)	Regulates chondrocyte metabolism and interacts with hypertrophic chondrocytes; Modifies ECM for calcification; Facilitates and regulates endochondral ossification; Maintains cartilage stiffness and participate in remodeling of articular cartilage; Facilitates collagen type II fibrils and chondrocyte removal from the matrix during vascular invasion; Binds to anchorin CII	[22, 103, 132–138]
Collagen Type XII	$\alpha 1(XII)_3$	340–350	Predominantly articular surface and around cartilage canals; Physically bound to collagen fibril surfaces (FACIT collagen)	Mediates interactions between fibrils and other matrix macromolecules/cells; Promotes collagen alignment or stabilise organised fibril orientation; Binds with decorin, fibromodulin, tenascin and COMP	[103, 139–143]
Collagen Type XIV	$\alpha 1(XIV)_3$	220	Uniform throughout ECM; Associated with and physically bound to collagen fibril surfaces (FACIT collagen)	Facilitate collagen fibrillogenesis; Maintains cartilage integrity and mechanical properties; Interacts with collagen types II and VI, and COMP; Binds to DS chain of decorin and to HS chain of perlecan	[103, 104, 141, 144, 145]
Collagen Type XVI	$\alpha 1(XVI)_3$	160	Predominantly TM (FACIT collagen collagen)	Organises the ECM by stabilising collagen type II fibrils, anchoring microfibrils; Mediates intracellular signalling affecting cell adhesion and proliferation; Binds to collagen type II, collagen type XI and fibronectin	[104, 146–150]
Collagen Type XXII	$\alpha 1(XXII)_3$	200	SZ surface at the articular cartilage- synovial fluid junction (FACIT collagen)	Associated with extrafibrillar matrix of cartilage; Interacts with microfibrils, collagen type VI; Binds to integrins	[151]

COMP, *Cartilage oligomeric matrix protein*; DS, *Dermatan sulfate*; ECM, *Extracellular matrix*; FACIT, *Fibril-associated collagens with interrupted triple helices*; HS, *Heparan sulfate*; PCM, *Pericellular matrix*; PGs, *Proteoglycans*; SZ, *Superficial zone*; TGF-β, *Transforming growth factor-beta*; TM, *Territorial matrix*; ZCC, *Zone of calcified cartilage*

GAG chains in collagen type IX are thought to stabilize collagen type II fibril structure [22, 103, 124]. Collagen type IX interacts with matrilin-3, fibromodulin and collagen type XII [123]. Collagen type XII is a homotrimer with two collagenous domains flanked by three non-collagenous regions [143]. It is localized (non-covalently) on the surface of collagen type II and is distributed in areas of articular cartilage ECM with more organized fibril orientation [103, 140]. During cartilage growth and development, collagen type XII is relatively more abundantly distributed in the SZ and upper middle zone (MZ) compared to the deeper zones [140]. Its presence has also been detected around the cartilage canals [141]. Collagen type XII binds with decorin, fibromodulin, tenascin and COMP [139]. Collagen type XII is thought to connect collagen fibrils to other ECM molecules and regulate ECM organization and mechanical properties of collagen fibril bundles in articular cartilage [139, 142].

Collagen type XIV is a homotrimeric molecule with a triple helical disulfide-bonded domain, which shares structural homologies with some domains of collagen types IX and XII [104, 141, 144, 156]. Collagen type XIV is distributed uniformly in articular cartilage ECM, especially in regions of high mechanical stress, where it interacts with collagen types II and VI, and COMP [103, 104, 141]. Also, collagen type XIV is known to bind to the DS chain of decorin and to the HS chain of perlecan [144]. Collagen type XVI structurally belongs to the FACIT family and shares a limited sequence homology to the non-cartilage collagen type XIX [104, 146]. Collagen type XVI is mainly distributed in the TM of chondrocytes, where it acts as an adaptor protein and can be incorporated into distinct suprastructural aggregates [147–149]. It interacts with cartilage ECM large fibrillar components, organizes macromolecular networking, and hence plays a role in modulating and maintaining the cartilage ECM integrity and stability [148]. Collagen type XXII structurally belongs to the FACIT protein family and is located at the articular cartilage-SF junction [151]. Although rare, collagen type XXII is associated with the cartilage extrafibrillar matrix [104].

1.2.2.3 Non-Collagenous Proteins and Glycoproteins

Small non-collagenous proteins and glycoproteins are present in the cartilage ECM, which are thought to be crucial for modulating several fibril properties (Table 1.4). Non-collagenous proteins in cartilage ECM, such as cartilage matrix glycoprotein, matrix Gla protein, anchorin CII and chondronectin, are known to mediate the attachment of chondrocytes to collagen type II or aggrecan, thus stabilizing the cartilage matrix [29, 32, 33, 161, 168, 174, 175, 191, 196–198].

Matrix Gla protein (MGP) is a vitamin K-dependent 10–14 kDa protein, which was initially isolated from bone but now is known to be present in cartilage [31, 161, 162, 199]. MGP contains the unusual amino acid gamma-carboxyglutamic acid [162]. In newborn and immature articular cartilage, MGP is located diffusely throughout the cartilage ECM and in late hypertrophic and calcifying-zone chondrocytes of the growth plate, whereas in adult cartilage MGP is primarily located in the chondrocytes and the PCM [160]. MGP binds to chondrocyte surface through integrin [200]. MGP has affinity for hydroxyapatite and plays an important role as a regulator (inhibitor) of cartilage calcification.

Cartilage matrix protein (CMP, also termed matrilin-1) is a 148 kDa cartilage-specific protein composed of three identical disulfide-bonded subunits [166, 201]. CMP is distributed in the articular cartilage ECM where it binds to and bridges collagen type II fibrils and interacts with aggrecan [164, 197, 202, 203]. The amount of CMP covalently attached to aggrecan increases with age [203]. CMP acts as an adhesion molecule for chondrocytes, serving a structural role [164]. Although suppressed under physiologic conditions, chondrocytes can synthesize CMP and its expression is upregulated in response to arthritic stimuli [204]. Matrilin-2 is a 106 kDa protein localized on the articular cartilage surface and hypertrophic chondrocytes of the growth plate [167]. Matrilin-2 is involved in the development and homeostasis of ECM network and acts as an adapter molecule connecting proteins and PGs in ECM. Furthermore, it shows age-dependent expression [167]. Matrilin-2 is also

Table 1.4 Articular cartilage non-collagenous proteins and glycoproteins

Molecules	Molecular Weight (Kilodalton)	Articular Cartilage Location (Adult)	Characteristics and Functions	References
			Non-collagenous Proteins	
Matrix Gla Protein (MGP)	10–14	PCM	Primarily present in PCM in carboxylated form; Acts as ECM mineralization inhibitor when present in carboxylated form; Synthesis is vitamin K2-dependent; Chondrocytes show significant attachment to MGP	[157–162]
Matrilin-1 (also termed cartilage matrix glycoprotein, CMGP)	148	Cartilage ITM; Limited levels in PCM or absent	Articular cartilage-specific; Involved in formation of ECM filamentous network; Acts as an adhesion molecule for chondrocytes, hence plays a structural role; Binds to $\alpha 1\beta 1$ integrin, aggrecans, collagen type II and itself	[163, 164–166]
Matrilin-2	106	Articular cartilage surface; Hypertrophic chondrocytes of growth plate	Involved in the formation of ECM filamentous network; Involved in ECM homeostasis	[163, 167–169]
Matrilin-3	240	PCM and ITM of growth plate; Chondrocytes and ECM of SZ and upper MZ in mature articular cartilage	Articular cartilage-specific; Involved in formation of ECM filamentous network; Integration into cartilage fibrils occur both directly with collagen tye IX and indirectly with COMP; Filaments anchored via interactions with chondrocytes or PCM components; Helps preserve the PCM	[163, 167, 170, 171]
Anchorin CII (also termed Annexin V)	31	Chondrocyte membrane; Mainly localized in upper third of articular cartilage and almost none in DZ	Binds with N-telopeptide of collagen type II to facilitate adhesion of chondrocytes to ECM collagen via anchorin CII receptors on chondrocyte surface	[172–175]
Chondrocalcin	69	Longitudinal septa of lower hypertrophic zone in growth plate and AECC; Fetal articular cartilage; Adult ZCC	Calcium-binding protein released from type II procollagen $\alpha 1$ after secretion by chondrocytes; Participates in collagen fibre formation; Exhibits electrostatic interactions with PG sulfate groups, hence affecting articular cartilage organisation and osmotic properties	[31, 176, 177]
Cartilage Intermediate Layer Protein (CLIP)	92	Interterritorial matrix of AC lower half of middle zone	More abundant in adult AC than in immature AC; Increased concentration with age; Induces expression of $TGF\beta$ in aging cartilage	[178, 179]

			Glycoproteins	
Cartilage Oligomeric Matrix Protein (COMP)	524	Fetal articular cartilage, PCM; Immature cartilage, proliferating and hypertrophic chondrocytes; Adult cartilage, uniform distribution, TM and ITM	Helps anchor chondrocytes to the matrix and facilitates ECM formation; Promotes strong anchoring of lubricin/ PRG4 in a favourable confirmation to facilitate joint lubrication; Prevents vascularization of cartilage; Facilitates repair process; Differentially regulated by TGF-β in the various cartilage zones	[7, 31, 33, 180, 181]
Human Cartilage Glycoprotein (HC gp-39), also known as YKL-40	38–40	ECM (low level)	Major secretary glycoprotein product of human chondrocytes; Not present in normal ECM but detected at high level of articular cartilage remodelling and disease (RA and OA); Plays an important structural role in enabling the chondrocytes to adapt and respond to changes in their environment; Induction occurs rapidly upon changes in the normal cartilage environment	[182–184]
Fibronectin (FN)	440	Thin layer on articular cartilage surface; Low levels in normal cartilage PCM and TM	Binds directly to collagen before mediating interaction of chondrocytes with ECM; Influences interactions between chondrocytes and ECM; Helps regulate local IGF levels; Mediates enhanced wear protection of lubricin during shear	[7, 28, 31, 185–187]
Tenascin	220 & 320 (two size variants)	Predominantly PCM of developing cartilage; Present in TM and ITM of DZ	Articular cartilage calcification inhibitor; Assists in HA cross-linking to create high-order structure in ECM; Influences between chondrocytes and ECM, and assists in assembly of cartilage ECM from component molecules	[7, 31, 186, 188–190]
Chondronectin	180	Predominantly associated with chondrocyte or PCM	Interacts with articular cartilage PG monomer to efficiently and specifically mediate attachment of chondrocytes to collagen type II; Helps maintain chondrocyte phenotype through its specific interactions between chondrocytes, collagen type II and PCM	[28, 31, 191–193]
Vitronectin	160	ECM	Promotes chondrocyte adhesion; Binds to GAGs and chondrocyte surface via integrin αVβ3	[159, 194, 195]

AECC, *Articular-epiphyseal cartilage complex*; DZ, *Deep zone*; ECM, *Extracellular matrix*; HA, *Hyaluronic acid*; IGF, *Insulin-like growth factor*; ITM, *Interterritorial matrix*; MZ, *Middle zone*; OA, *Osteoarthritis*; PCM, *Pericellular matrix*; PGs, *Proteoglycans*; PRG4, *Proteoglycan 4*; RA, *Rheumatoid arthritis*; SZ, *Superficial zone*; TM, *Territorial matrix*; TGF-β, *Transforming Growth Factor - Beta*; ZCC, *Zone of calcified cartilage* overexpressed on the articular surface as well as the proliferating and hypertrophic zones of diseased articular cartilage. Its expression is increased in the early stage of OA [167]. Matrilin-3, a 240 kDa protein, contains von Willebrand factor A-like domains and is able to form hetero-oligomers with matrilin-1 [170]. Matrilin-3 is found in the PCM and ITM of the growth plate as well as in low concentration in mature articular cartilage chondrocytes and ECM of SZ and upper MZ [170, 205, 206]. It mediates the interactions between cartilage fibrils and ECM. The integration of matrilin-3 into cartilage fibrils occurs directly via interaction with collagen IX and indirectly with COMP serving as an adapter [123]. Matrilin-3 expression is increased in OA articular cartilage [170, 207].

Anchorin CII, also referred to as cartilage annexin V, is a 31 kDa non-collagenous protein found on the chondrocyte surface and ECM of the proliferating and resting zones of fetal growth plate [174]. Anchorin II mediates association of chondrocytes with collagen type II of the PCM and binds at the N-telopeptide region of collagen type II [137, 172, 174]. It also co-localizes and binds to collagen type X and chondrocalcin in the ECM of calcifying cartilage [137]. The enhanced expression and tissue distribution of anchorin II is an indicator of chondrocyte metabolic activity alterations and phenotypic changes associated with articular cartilage destruction, pathological mineralization and joint diseases [175, 208–210]. Chondrocalcin, a 70 kDa calcium-binding protein with two subunits, is located in developing fetal cartilage ECM, the longitudinal septa of lower hypertrophic zone ECM of both the growth plate and articular-epiphyseal cartilage complex (AECC), and calcified articular cartilage, where high demand for calcification is required [211–213]. Its strong affinity for hydroxyapatite suggests that chondrocalcin plays a fundamental role in the calcification of cartilage matrix in endochondral ossification. It is also present in small amounts in non-calcifying articular cartilage and is associated with areas where high concentrations of PG and link proteins are detected [176, 213]. Release of chondrocalcin as the carboxypropeptide of collagen type II occurs after its parent molecule, procollagen type II, is secreted by chondrocytes, indicating its association with new collagen synthesis and fibre formation [31]. However, ex vivo human cartilage explants demonstrated internalization of chondrocalcin by chondrocytes, which in turn triggered cartilage destruction via an interleukin-1β (Il-1β) dependent pathway in vitro; hence, its association with cartilage destruction [45, 214, 215]. Cartilage intermediate layer protein (CILP), a 92 kDa protein specifically synthesized and secreted by articular cartilage chondrocytes, contains a single polypeptide chain substituted with N-linked oligosaccharides [179]. CILP is located in the articular cartilage ITM of the lower 2/3rd MZ but is absent from the SZ and DZ [179]. Its concentration varies with age, being lower in articular cartilage of young individuals [178]. Increased CILP expression in hypertrophic chondrocytes and in chondrocytes derived from aged cartilage compared to young cartilage suggests that CILP promotes the formation of calcium pyrophosphate dehydrate (CPPD) crystals in aged cartilage and is responsible for the immune response involved in joint disease pathogenesis [178, 216–219].

Although glycoproteins form a small fraction (2–5%) of the cartilage ECM, they play an important role in matrix assembly and/or regulation of matrix metabolism. The matrix glycoproteins contain distinct and functionally active peptide domains that allow interactions with chondrocyte surface receptors as well as other ECM molecules. Cartilage oligomeric matrix protein, a disulfide-bonded homopentameric 524 kDa multidomain ECM glycoprotein, is markedly anionic due to its high content of aspartic and glutamic amino acid residues, and due to its substitution with negatively charged sugars [33, 220]. COMP helps anchor chondrocytes to the matrix and facilitates ECM formation during chondrogenesis, and it persists in mature cartilage. It strongly adheres to the cartilage surface lubricating protein, lubricin, providing molecular synergy in knee lubrication [180, 221, 222]. In fetal articular cartilage, COMP is localized to chondrocyte PCM [223]. During articular cartilage growth, COMP is abundantly expressed in the proliferating and hypertrophic chondrocytes of the growth plate and AECC [224]. In mature cartilage, COMP synthesis is differentially regulated by TGF-β1 in the various cartilage zones, is preferentially localized in the TM and ITM surrounding the chondrocytes, and it prevents the vascularization of the articular cartilage [31, 33, 181, 223, 225]. Further, COMP is a cartilage matrix biomarker that is detected in the SF, blood and serum samples and has been shown to be useful in assessing mechanical loading-induced cartilage changes in sports, cartilage injury and disease [221, 226–234]. Human cartilage glycoprotein (HC-gp39), also termed YKL-40, is a 38–40 kDa glycoprotein [183, 184, 235–239]. It is a major secretory glycoprotein of human chondrocytes and synovial fibroblasts, which was originally identified in the whey secretions of nonlactating cows [236, 239, 240]. In normal human cartilage, HC-gp39 levels are low, but its secretion is enhanced in both inflammatory and degenerative disease [236, 241]. HC-gp39 induces the synthesis of both SOX9 and collagen type II, and has been suggested to promote the maintenance or expression of a chondrocytic phenotype as well as play a role in articular cartilage remodelling [237, 242]. Fibronectin (FN) is an ECM glycoprotein which is composed of two similar disulfide-linked polypeptide chains of approximately 220 kDa each. FN is thought to effect cell adhesion, morphology, migration and differentiation as well as matrix assembly [243–245]. FN plays a significant role in the adhesion of chondrocytes to ECM and is implicated in tissue repair [187]. FN mediates enhanced wear protection of lubricin during shear [246]. Tenascins are oligomeric glycoproteins that function in processes such as wound repair and formation of bone and cartilage [190, 247]. Tenascins are expressed in 220 and 320 kDa forms in articular cartilage and are located predominantly in the TM and ITM of DZ [185, 186, 190]. Tenascins are involved in the assembly of the cartilage matrix, and they are thought to influence interactions between the chondrocytes and the matrix [7, 188]. Tenascins facilitate the HA cross-linking to create a higher order level of structured HA that may regulate cartilage inflammation and also function as cartilage calcification inhibitors [31, 188]. Chondronectin is a 180 kDa cartilage glycoprotein that requires interaction with cartilage PG for it to specifically mediate the attachment of chondrocytes to collagen type II [31, 191, 192, 248]. This specific interaction is essential for the maintenance of the chondrocyte phenotype [193]. Chondronectin is predominantly associated with the chondrocyte and PCM [28]. Vitronectin is a 160 kDa glycoprotein found in the articular cartilage ECM. Vitronectin binds to GAGs, and through its tripeptide sequence consisting of arginine, glycine and aspartate (RGD) it binds to the integrin receptor αVβ3 on the chondrocyte surface [159, 194, 195]. It mediates the inflammatory and repair reactions at the site of cartilage injury. Vitronectin plays a role in cartilage healing and remodelling.

1.2.3 Articular Cartilage Fluorescent Molecules

Intrinsic fluorescent molecules are found within the articular cartilage matrix. Interaction of the lysines and modified lysines can generate complex heterocyclic compounds, some of which have fluorescent properties. Cartilage collagens provide tensile strength and resiliency to the cartilage matrix [153, 154]. Collagen fibrils are stabilized by covalent cross-links formed between adjacent collagen chains (intramolecular cross-link) and adjacent collagen molecules (intermolecular cross-link). Cross-linking of collagen fibrils is initiated extracellularly via lysyl oxidase, a 30 kDa copper-requiring enzyme [249]. This enzyme catalyses the oxidative deamination of certain -NH_2 groups in collagen and acts on specific lysine or hydroxylysine residues in the telopeptide region at each end of the collagen molecule, eventually resulting in the formation of mature cross-links [250, 251]. Intramolecular cross-links in collagen are derived from lysine side chains at the nonhelical region near the N-terminal.

Two types of pyridinium collagen cross-links have been identified in mature articular cartilage, namely, the pyridinoline (Pyd) and deoxypyridinoline (Dpyd). These are naturally fluorescent compounds formed by condensation of two hydroxylysine residues and one lysine residue, i.e. between residues near the N-terminal of one collagen molecule and the C-terminal of another. Four residues in each collagen molecule can participate in these cross-links: a lysine near the N-terminal, a lysine near the C-terminal and hydroxylysines in helical regions near the ends of the molecule (residues 87 and 930). Pyd was first isolated from rat tail tendon and characterized in the mid-1970s [252, 253]. Pyd is present in collagen-containing tissues such as the cartilage, synovial membrane, meniscus, bone and ligament [254, 255]. Animal studies showed that the Pyd content per collagen in fetus and newborns is low but increased markedly with the growth of the animal [256]. In humans, the amount of Pyd is five to ten times more abundant in cartilage than in bone, and its concentration remains relatively constant in adult cartilage with age [257–259]. On the other hand, Dpyd content is more abundant in bone compared to articular cartilage.

Yet another cross-linking molecule, pentosidine, was isolated from senescent human articular cartilage. Fluorophores are formed by the non-enzymatic glycosylation and fructosylation of certain proteins such as native collagen [260, 261]. Glycation (non-enzymatic glycosylation), cross-linking and fluorophore formation of collagen occur both in vivo and in vitro [260, 262]. Pentosidine, a condensation product of arginine, lysine and ribose, is an end product of advanced glycation [263]. Characterization of pentosidine isolated from human dura mater revealed its formation by sequential glycosylation and oxidation reactions [264]. As shown in various collagen-rich tissues such as dura mater, skin, ocular lens and cartilage, the amount of pentosidine per collagen molecule in human articular cartilage also increases linearly with age [258, 262, 265–267]. Lipofuscin is a heterogeneous group of glycopeptides, likely oxidation products, which accumulate in articular cartilage with age. These fluorescent molecules are responsible for the yellow coloration of aging cartilage [268].

1.3 Articular Cartilage Heterogeneity and Compartmentalization

During the process of endochondral ossification, articular cartilage maturation stages can be identified by macroscopic and microscopic changes. As a function of the articular cartilage depth from the articulating surface, the horizontal and parallel histologic lamination, referred to as zones, differs in immature children and adolescent cartilage versus mature adult cartilage (Fig. 1.7 and Table 1.5). Biochemical and biomechanical stimulation of the chondrocytes from the various zones leads to the synthesis of a distinct set of matrix components, and these cells are also responsible for the organization and maintenance of ECM. The differences between the various histologic zones of skeletally immature and mature articular cartilage are based on chondrocyte morphology, orientation and distribution as well as collagen and PG concentration, and collagen architecture and fibre diameter. Although not visualized histologically, there is also variation in the tissue fluid content.

In addition to zonal heterogeneity, the complexity of articular cartilage ECM is conferred by the compartmentalisation and circumferential differentiation of matrix components into pericellular, territorial and interterritorial matrices around each chondrocyte.

In normal adult articular cartilage, chondrocytes account for less than 5% of the tissue wet weight, and cellularity decreases progressively with aging. The relative concentration of GAGs varies markedly with age with a preponderance of C4S and little KS in immature cartilage and an appreciable increase in KS content and a corresponding fall in C4S with advancing age [269]. These variations in the depth-dependent structure and biochemical composition of cartilage could explain the varied cartilage function in such processes as aging, repair and degeneration.

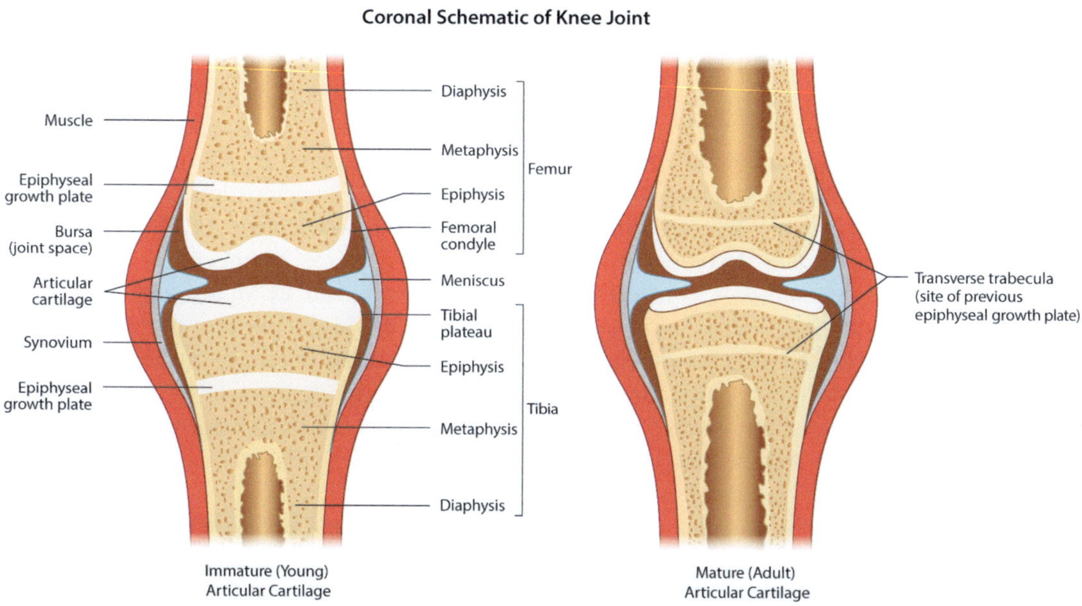

Fig. 1.7 Coronal illustrations of the human knee showing the articular cartilage, other tissues and synovial bursa in the skeletally immature (left) and mature (right) joint. Note the thick immature articular-epiphyseal cartilage complex and epiphyseal growth plate in young children and adolescents in comparison to the thin articular cartilage and absence of epiphyseal growth plate in adults. At skeletal maturity, the transverse trabecula (right) replaces the previous epiphyseal growth plate (left) of the immature joint. (Courtesy of Dr. Harpal K. Gahunia, and graphic illustration by Danny Aguilar, JD Graphics Solutions, East York, Ontario, Canada)

Table 1.5 Characteristic features of immature and mature articular cartilage

	Structure/ Macromolecules	Articular Cartilage Matrix Characteristics: Immature *Children and Skeletally Immature Adolescents*	Articular Cartilage Matrix Characteristics: Mature *Young and Old Adults*
Articular Cartilage	Extracellular Matrix Homeostasis	Synthesis outweighs degradation	Synthesis is finely balanced by controlled matrix degradation
	Thickness	Relative to knee size, thick articular epiphyseal cartilage complex which decreases with skeletal maturation	Relative to knee size, thin articular cartilage which further decreases with age
	Morphology	***Two distinct zones*** *forming complex* Articular cartilage zone Epihyseal cartilage zone	***Four distinct zones*** Superficial zone (uncalcified) Middle zone (uncalcified) Deep zone (uncalcified) Zone of calcified cartilage
	Tidemark	Absent initially but develops with cartilage maturation	Well demarcated tidemark
	Calcified zone	Hypertrophic / apoptopic chondrocytes in calcified matrix characteristic of endochondral ossification	Rounded chondrocytes nesting in uncalcified lacunae are embedded in calcified matrix
	Vascularity	Present but decreases with cartilage maturation	Absent (avascular)
Growth Plate	Zones	***Five distinct zones*** Resting zone Proliferation zone Maturation zone Calcification zone Ossification zone	***Absent*** Remnant is primary tensile bone trabecula called "transverse trabecula"

1.3.1 Immature Articular-Epiphyseal Cartilage Complex

At birth, the immature articular cartilage is very thick, homogenous, hypercellular and highly vascularized, occupying the majority of the epiphysis. With growth and development, the immature cartilage cellularity is considerably reduced, especially in the DZ, and AECC eventually forms a cap over the articulating ends of the epiphyses of femoral condyle and tibial plateau. Diffusion of nutrients into the AECC proceeds from the articular surface and also from blood vessels penetrating the epiphyseal cartilage component from the subchondral one. AECC shares some morphological and biochemical features of the epiphyseal plate, also known as the growth plate, which is described in depth in Chap. 2.

In children and skeletally immature individuals, the AECC is comprised of articular cartilage component adjacent to the joint space and epiphyseal cartilage component subjacent to the subchondral bone (Fig. 1.8). The articular cartilage component is thick, homogenous and unstratified, with chondrocytes distributed in the ECM in a random, isotropic pattern, whereas the epiphyseal component is stratified into distinctive zones with characteristic features typical of the epiphyseal growth plate. As AECC matures, a much higher degree of anisotropy is achieved where the cells and ECM macromolecules are architecturally, biochemically and biomechanically characterized in clearly defined zones. The articular cartilage component of AECC persists into adult life, whereas its epiphyseal component is resorbed by bone remodelling.

1.3.1.1 Articular Cartilage Component

The articular cartilage component of the AECC extends from the articular surface to the epiphyseal component. This zone is homogenous with a random distribution of numerous small, rounded chondrocytes. Depending on the stage of maturity, the parallel collagen fibres at the surface may extend up to 40% of the depth of articular component.

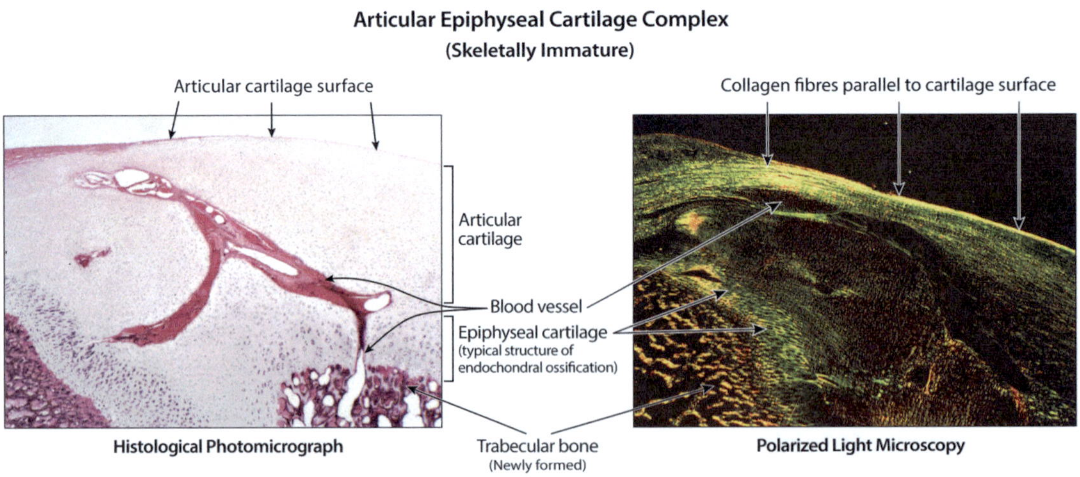

Fig. 1.8 Articular-epiphyseal cartilage complex (AECC) from a skeletally immature knee stained with Haematoxylin and Eosin (left) and picrosirius red with polarized light (right). The histological photomicrograph (left) shows the presence of thick articular cartilage component extending from the articular surface up to two-thirds of the total AECC thickness. The epiphyseal component at the lower one-third of AECC exhibits features typical of an epiphyseal growth plate with newly formed trabecular bone towards the epiphysis. The corresponding articular cartilage section when visualized using polarized light microscopy (right) reveals the parallel alignment of thin collagen fibres at the cartilage surface

1.3.1.2 Epiphyseal Cartilage Component

The epiphyseal cartilage component of the AECC extends from the articular cartilage component to the junction of subchondral bone with characteristic features typical of the epiphyseal growth plate. The epiphyseal component consists of five morphologically distinct zones. The *zone of resting chondrocytes* consists of cells that are capable of replicating at a slow rate. These cells are small and flat or round, atypical of the chondrocyte morphology. The *zone of proliferation* consists of cells that are actively undergoing mitosis, hence providing a continuing supply of new chondrocytes. The *zone of maturation* consists of enlarged chondrocytes. The *zone of hypertrophy* consists of chondrocytes that accumulate glycogen and lipid, and secrete alkaline phosphatase to the surrounding ECM. The *zone of calcification* lies adjacent to the newly formed trabecula of the subchondral bone and is characterized by apoptotic chondrocytes and an ECM rich in insoluble salts with traces of bone trabeculae and vascular infiltration. Unlike mature articular cartilage, the epiphyseal cartilage component lacks the interface to the tidemark and calcified cartilage.

1.3.2 Skeletally Mature Articular Cartilage Zones

The heterogeneous uncalcified adult cartilage can be distinguished microscopically into three zones, which are parallel to, and extend from the articular surface to the tidemark (Fig. 1.9). Uncalcified articular cartilage exhibits heterogeneity in the ECM macromolecular composition, collagen organization, and chondrocyte size, shape, aggregation and metabolic activity [270–274]. This uncalcified articular cartilage is attached to the subchondral bone plate via tidemark and a narrow zone of calcified cartilage, which is considered as zone 4 of the articular cartilage (Fig. 1.10).

1.3.2.1 Zone 1: Superficial Zone

The superficial zone, also referred to as lamina splendens or Zone 1, is adjacent to the joint space. Depending on age, SZ is about 200 μm thick, and constitute 10–20% of the total uncalcified adult articular cartilage. SZ is characterized by small, flat or ellipsoid chondrocytes with their long axis parallel to the cartilage surface (Fig. 1.11). Thin collagen type II fibrils with fibril diameter 30–35 nm are densely packed and oriented parallel to the articular surface. The PG content of articular cartilage is lowest in SZ.

Normally, the SZ consists of two sub-laminae. The upper chondrocyte-devoid lamina forming the articular cartilage surface is comprised of a thin collagen fibre sheet with minimal amount of small GAGs and lubricating molecules. The lower lamina is characterized by flat chondrocytes and fibrillar collagen network mostly formed by aggregation of small fibres of collagen types II (80%), IX (10%) and XI (10%), which are densely packed and aligned parallel to the cartilage surface (Fig. 1.12) [131, 275, 276].

1.3.2.2 Zone 2: Middle Zone

The middle or transitional zone constitutes 40–60% of the total uncalcified cartilage thickness. The MZ consists of randomly distributed chondrocytes that are round or oblong with the long axis perpendicular to the cartilage surface (Fig. 1.13). The bundles of collagen type II fibrils form an oblique transitional network in the MZ and appear as arcades when visualized using polarized light microscopy. At the upper one-third of zone 2, the thin collagen fibrils are oriented oblique to tangential to the articular surface, whereas at the lower two-thirds, the thick collagen fibrils are mostly perpendicular to the cartilage surface (Fig. 1.12).

1.3.2.3 Zone 3: Deep Zone

The deep or radial zone constitutes about 20–30% of the total uncalcified cartilage thickness. The chondrocytes are round, largest and oriented in characteristic longitudinal columns perpendicular to the tidemark. The DZ chondrocytes synthesize alkaline phosphatase that is likely involved in the calcification of the subjacent ZCC [277]. The collagen type II bundles are also thickest in the uncalcified cartilage with fibril diameter of 40–80 nm. These collagen

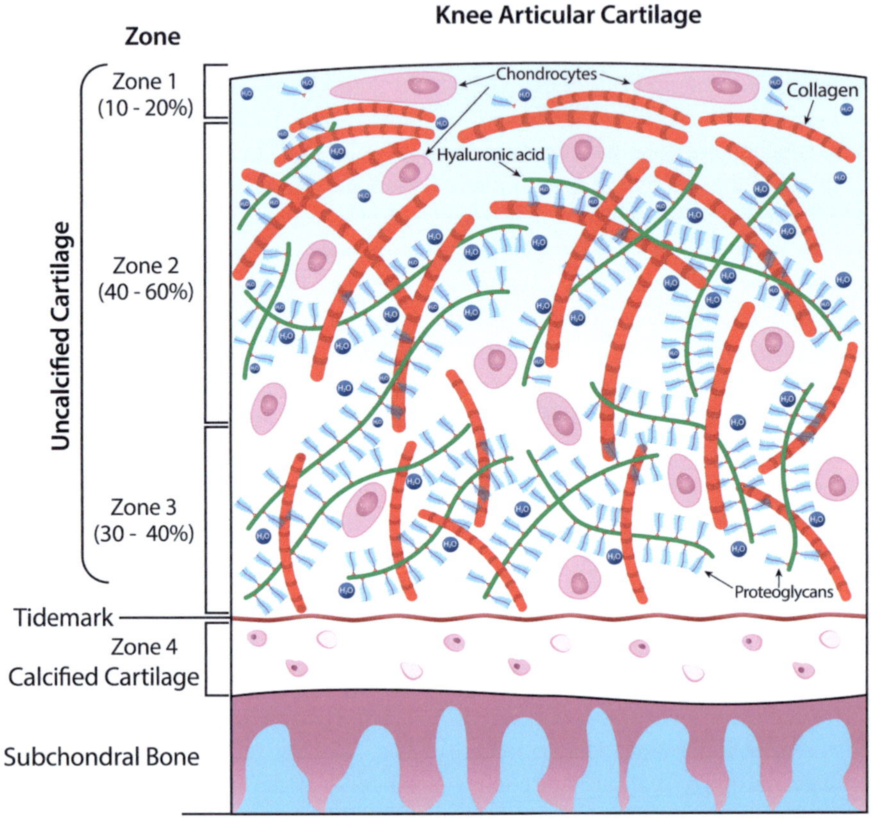

Fig. 1.9 Schematic representation of adult knee articular cartilage depicts a complex architecture of its constituent macromolecules with morphologically distinct layered heterogeneity from the cartilage surface to the subchondral bone. The uncalcified cartilage is comprised of three zones (zone 1 to zone 3) which is attached to the subchondral bone via a narrow layer of calcified cartilage (zone 4). The interface between uncalcified and calcified cartilage is demarcated by a thin calcified line termed tidemark. (Schematic created by Dr. Harpal K. Gahunia, and graphic illustration by Danny Aguilar, JD Graphics Solutions, East York, Ontario, Canada)

bundles form the base of the gothic arch and are oriented perpendicular to the articular surface as well as the tidemark.

1.3.2.4 Tidemark

The interface between the uncalcified cartilage and the calcified cartilage is demarcated by a 2–5 μm thick, densely basophilic calcified line referred to as the "tidemark" (Fig. 1.9) [278–280]. The tidemark is typically absent in immature cartilage and develops with skeletal maturation. In adults, tidemark originates, by chondrocyte activity, in areas exposed to either loading or pulling [279]. Tidemark is a dynamic structure formed within the collagen type II positive, uncalcified cartilage matrix [280].

1.3.2.5 Zone 4: Zone of Calcified Cartilage

The zone of calcified cartilage, also referred to as zone 4, is about 100–250 μm thick. The ZCC is located between the tidemark and subchondral bone, thus forming a tight bonding and integrating structure of the uncalcified cartilage to bone [280] (Figs. 1.11 and 1.12). The thickness of ZCC varies with the local distribution of loading in the knee [281]. The ZCC is characterized by chondrocytes that are round, smallest in size and embedded in a heavily calcified matrix. These chondrocytes are positive for alkaline phosphatase and are surrounded by a nest of collagen fibres [279]. Within ZCC, collagen type II fibres become structurally cemented to collagen type I osteoid tissue deposited by osteoblasts [280].

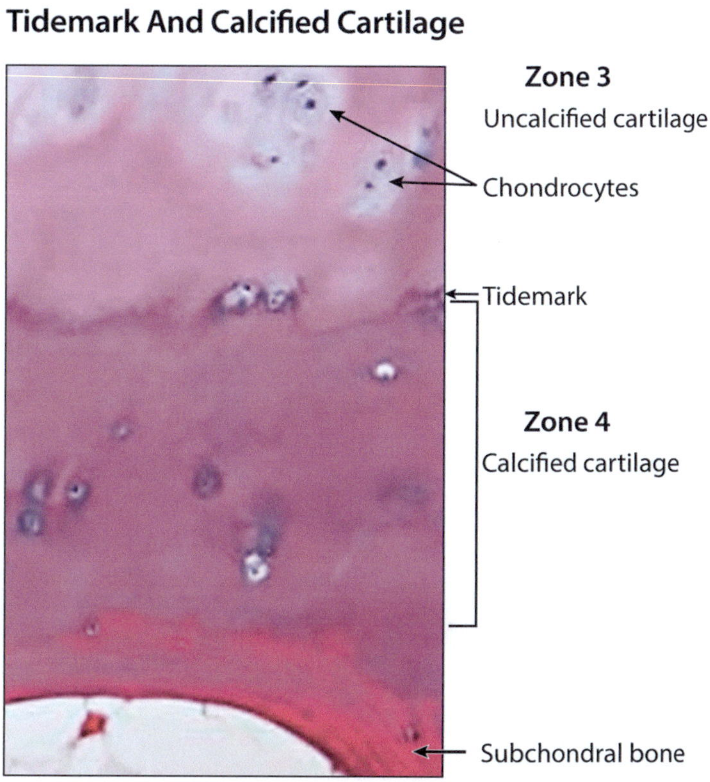

Fig. 1.10 Histological section of adult human tibial plateau articular cartilage showing the basophilic thin line of calcified tidemark, which demarcates the interface between uncalcified and calcified cartilage. Note the large round chondrocytes of uncalcified cartilage in zone 3 in comparison to the smaller, round chondrocytes embedded in the calcified cartilage. Some of the chondrocytes in the calcified cartilage are necrotic (H&E, 5 μm, original magnification: x20)

Three-dimensional reconstructions of normal knee cartilage above and below the tidemark demonstrated prolongations of DZ uncalcified cartilage that may extend through the ZCC up to the subchondral bone, observed in cross-section as islands of uncalcified cartilage [282]. Although demarcating the uncalcified from calcified cartilage, the tidemark in this region usually appears as an irregularly undulating line.

1.3.3 Macromolecular Variation of Uncalcified Articular Cartilage Zones

Polarized light, transmission electron and scanning electron microscopic studies of adult human articular cartilage revealed the spatial orientation and fibril diameter of collagen in the various zones [13, 276, 283, 284]. The arcade architectural concept of cartilage collagen is based on the 3D orientation and organization of collagen fibrils within the various observable zones (Fig. 1.14). The collagen fibril diameter is thin in the SZ where the small fibrils are densely packed and lie approximately parallel to the plane of the cartilage surface [285]. The fibril diameter increases from the SZ towards the DZ. Collagen fibres in the MZ form arcade-like architecture, whereas the DZ collagen is more loosely packed and is oriented perpendicular to the tidemark [286]. The collagen cross-links between collagen fibres increase with depth through the cartilage thickness [287].

Biochemical variations in tissue fluid, PG and collagen content between the cartilage zones have been reported [288–291]. In adult human cartilage, the fluid content decreases from 80% to 74% in the SZ to 65–67% in the DZ [7, 292]. The PG content is lowest in the SZ and most abundant in the MZ [293, 294] (Fig. 1.15). HA is more abundant in the superficial and middle zones than the DZ [291]. The concentrations of HA and DS are high in the MZ, whereas those of CS and KS

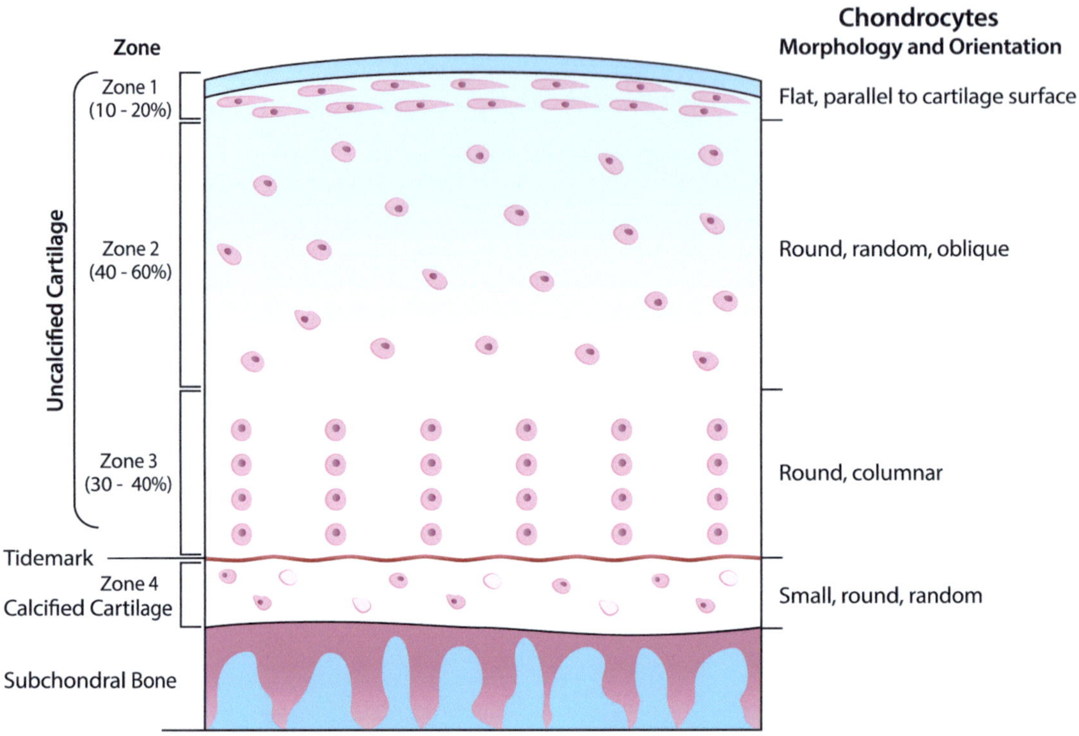

Fig. 1.11 Schematic representation of articular cartilage chondrocyte morphology and orientation within the zones. Zone 1 is characterized by small, flat, discoid or ellipsoid chondrocytes with their long axis parallel to the cartilage surface. Zone 2 consists of an obliquely oriented, random distribution of round or oblong chondrocytes with the long axis perpendicular to the cartilage surface. Zone 3 chondrocytes are round and largest in size with columnar distribution, whereas those within the zone of calcified cartilage (zone 4) are smallest in size, round and randomly distributed. Some of the chondrocytes show empty lacunae indicative of cell death. (Schematic created by Dr. Harpal K. Gahunia, and graphic illustration by Danny Aguilar, JD Graphics Solutions, East York, Ontario, Canada)

are high in the DZ [291]. The collagen type II content is highest in the SZ and lowest in the MZ [283]. Both decorin and biglycan decrease with articular cartilage depth from the SZ to DZ [295].

1.3.4 Articular Cartilage Extracellular Matrix and Chondrocyte Microenvironment

Articular cartilage ECM and chondrocyte microenvironment studies have revealed a clear subdivision of the middle and deep zones into pericellular, territorial and interterritorial matrices [16, 19, 20, 296, 297] (Fig. 1.16a, b, Table 1.6).

1.3.4.1 Pericellular Matrix

The chondrocyte and its pericellular microenvironment (i.e. pericellular matrix and pericellular capsule) are collectively referred to as a "chondron" [13, 20, 296]. Each chondrocyte cell membrane is immediately surrounded by a narrow PCM, which is characterized by the abundance of PGs and absence of fibrillar collagens. The PCM is predominantly composed of microfibrillar collagen type VI, and other molecules include perlecan, hyaluronan, aggrecan monomers and small aggregates, chondronectin, WARP and biglycan

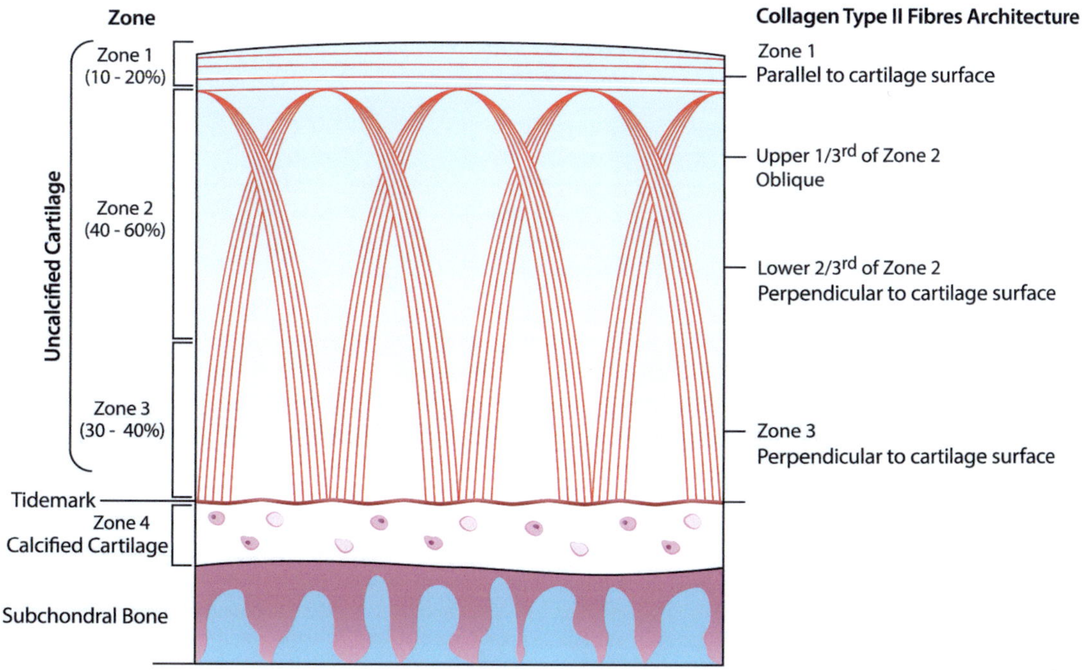

Fig. 1.12 Schematic representation depicting the architectural concept of uncalcified articular cartilage collagen based on the three-dimensional orientation of collagen type II within the various observable zones. The thin collagen fibres at zone 1 are densely packed and aligned parallel to the cartilage surface. Collagen fibres in zone 2 form an oblique transitional network with gothic-like architecture intermediate between the tangential SZ and radial DZ. The thick collagen fibres of zone 3 orient perpendicular to the tidemark. (Schematic created by Dr. Harpal K. Gahunia, and graphic illustration by Danny Aguilar, JD Graphics Solutions, East York, Ontario, Canada)

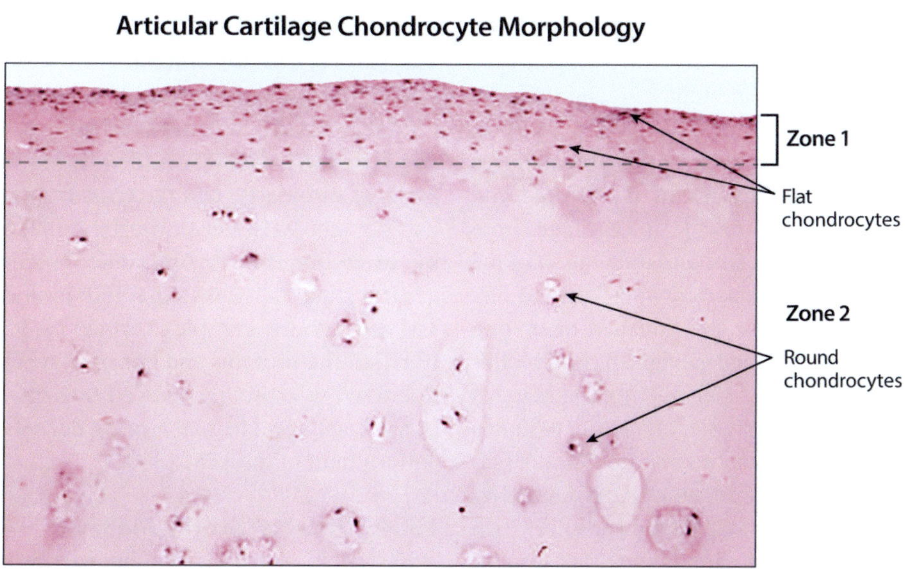

Fig. 1.13 Histological photomicrograph of articular cartilage zone 1 characterized by small ellipsoid chondrocytes with their long axis parallel to the cartilage surface. At a deeper level (zone 2), the chondrocytes are larger, round and more randomly distributed than those in zone 1 (H&E, original magnification: ×5)

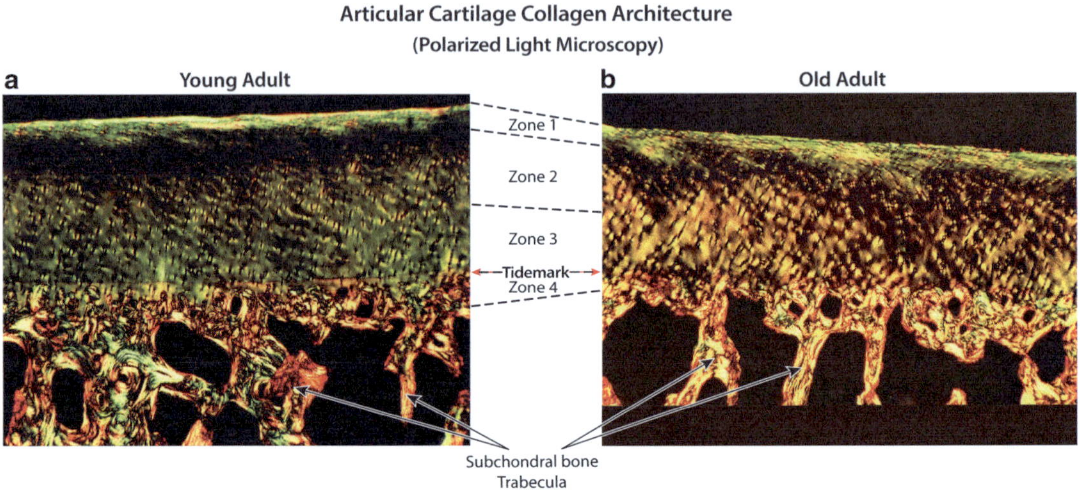

Fig. 1.14 Picrosirius red stained histological sections of knee femoral condyle articular cartilage obtained from a young (**a**) and older (**b**) adult. Polarized light micrograph shows the gothic arcade arrangement of collagen fibre architecture. Note the green layer at the articular surface represents thin collagen fibrils with a preferred orientation parallel with the surface. In young adult, the green colour is mostly maintained throughout the cartilage thickness, whereas in the old adult, a narrow transition zone separates this from the deeper zones (yellow) of thicker collagen fibres that are preferentially oriented perpendicular to the surface and to the subchondral bone. The gothic arcade is relatively better exemplified in old adult, which also shows reduction in the thickness of the various zones (H&E, 5 μm, original magnification ×2.5)

[16, 17, 19, 28, 41, 61, 64, 83, 114, 295, 296, 298–303, 304]. This PCM is surrounded by an outer fibrillar pericellular capsule composed of fibrillar collagen types II, IX and IX, microfibrillar collagen type VI, non-fibrillar collagen type IV, decorin, fibronectin, tenascin and laminin [16–20, 27, 30, 120, 185, 188, 297, 305, 306]. The pericellular capsule surrounds and encloses the PCM and chondrocytes of the middle and deep zones but not of the SZ [19]. Cartilage depth variations in the shape, size and orientation of the chondrons have been reported with flattened discoidal chondrons in the SZ, rounded or oblong chondrons in the MZ and elongated, multicellular chondrons in the DZ [307]. The chondrocytes of the double and multiple chondron columns consisting of three or more chondron units organized in a linear array are typically surrounded by individual pericellular matrix and capsule which suggests that individual chondrocytes are responsible for the formation of their surrounding microenvironment [17]. In addition, the presence of a common capsular sheath around multiple chondron columns suggests cooperative interaction between the chondrocytes of the group.

1.3.4.2 Territorial Matrix

The TM is characterized by abundant PGs, fibronectin and a fine network of fibrillar collagen [19, 308]. The PGs and collagen fibrils are oriented circularly, and the chondrocytes establish contact with the territorial collagen fibrils by extending fine cytoplasmic processes. An in vitro study has shown that IGF is stored in the TM through the complex formed by binding of IGF binding proteins and fibronectin [185, 309]. Polarized microscopy showed that the collagen in the cartilage TM has a more densely packed pattern than in the ITM [310].

1.3.4.3 Interterritorial Matrix

Adjacent to the TM, the interterritorial ECM occupies the space between various territorial matrices. The ITM is the outermost matrix

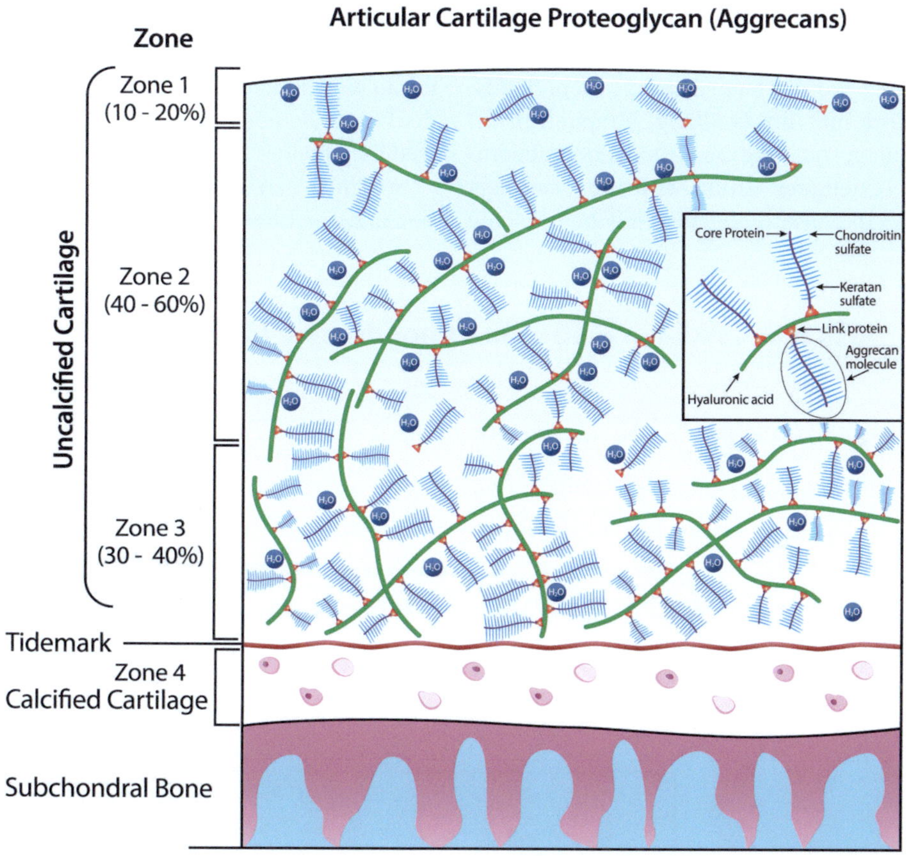

Fig. 1.15 Schematic representation depicting the distribution of proteoglycans and aggrecans within the uncalcified articular cartilage and the associated water molecules. The insert shows link protein which stabilizes the attachment of proteoglycan molecules to the hyaluronic acid. Each proteoglycan monomer consists of a core protein with covalently attached glycosaminoglycan side chains comprising of chondroitin sulfate and keratan sulfate. (Schematic created by Dr. Harpal K. Gahunia, and graphic illustration by Danny Aguilar, JD Graphics Solutions, East York, Ontario, Canada)

compartment surrounding the chondrocytes and constitutes the largest domain of the articular cartilage ECM. The ITM is characterized by collagen fibres that are parallel, longitudinal and interspersed with varying concentrations of aggrecans, versican, PGs, hyaluronan, link proteins and other molecules listed in Table 1.6, depending upon the zone in which the chondrocytes lie [38, 52, 175, 310–313]. The shape and orientation of the chondrocytes and their microenvironment appear to reflect the local collagen architecture of the ITM, which varies significantly with the cartilage depth [307].

1.4 Function of Knee Articular Cartilage

Knee articular cartilage is a dynamic tissue with unique molecular components and 3D architecture that enables it to perform its physiological functions over a lifetime, and under a wide range of loading conditions. Mechanical stress is an important environmental factor in maintaining the differential function of articular cartilage [314]. During daily activities (walking, running, etc.) or specialized activities (e.g. sports), the knees are loaded dynamically, and all its components (articular cartilage, bone, muscles, ligaments, tendons and nerves) participate in transmitting the mechanical loads. Importantly, during knee mobility (walking, jumping, pivoting, kneeling, squatting) the osteochondral component (extending from articular cartilage surface to the base of subchondral bone facing the bone marrow) transmits the compressing, tensile and shear forces from the viscoelastic uncalcified articular cartilage through the tidemark and calcified cartilage to the stiffer mineralized long bone [280, 315].

Articular cartilage provides smooth articulation under variable loads and impaction for very

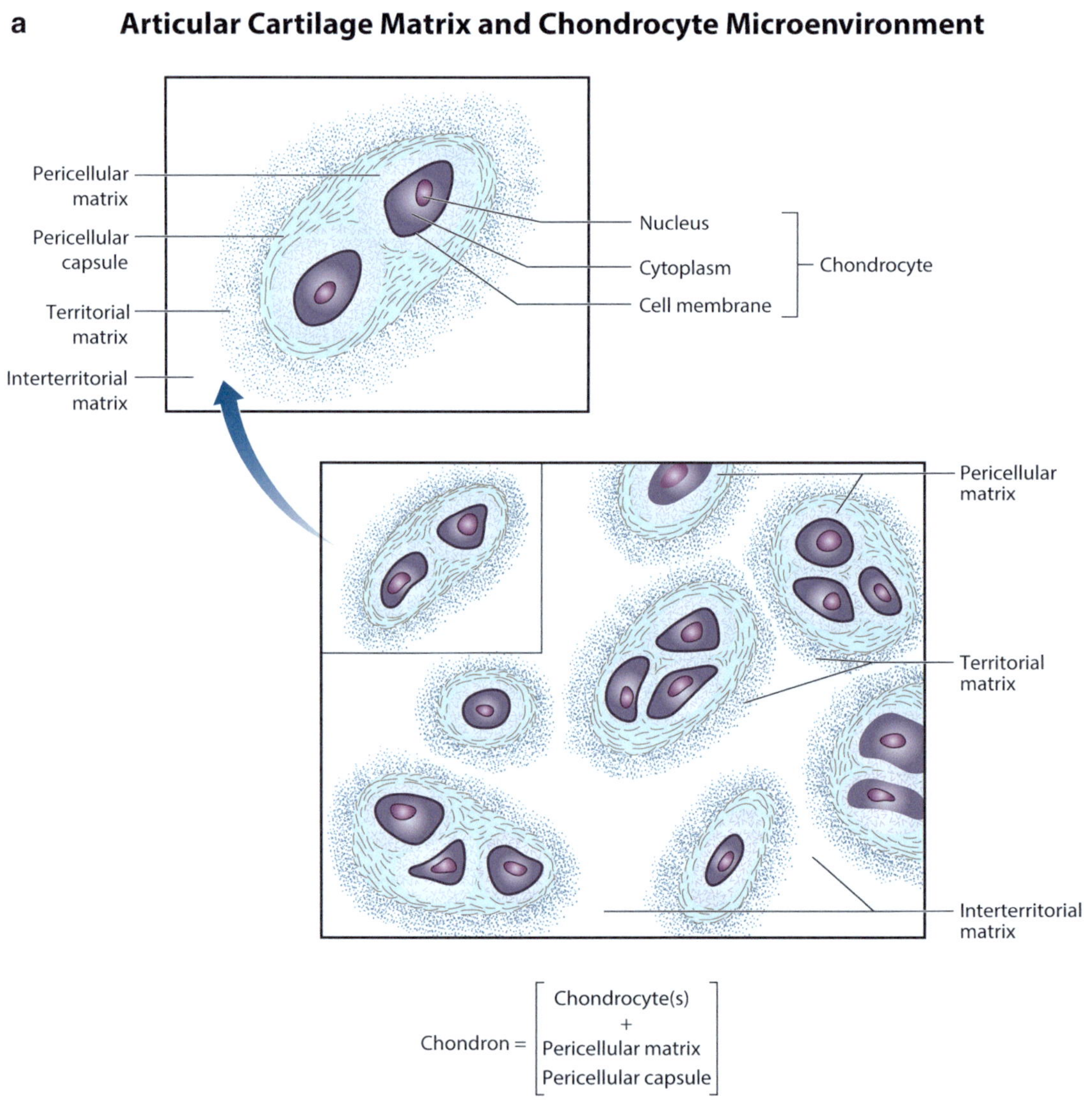

Fig. 1.16 Schematic representation (**a**) depicting the articular cartilage matrix heterogeneity and chondrocyte microenvironment of the zones 2 and 3. The chondrocyte along with its pericellular matrix and capsule constitutes the chondron. Encapsulating the chondron is the territorial matrix. The interterritorial matrix occupies the space between the territorial matrices. (**b**) Haematoxylin- and eosin-stained five-micron histological section showing chondrocyte microenvironment. (Schematic created by Dr. Harpal K. Gahunia, and graphic illustration by Danny Aguilar, JD Graphics Solutions, East York, Ontario, Canada)

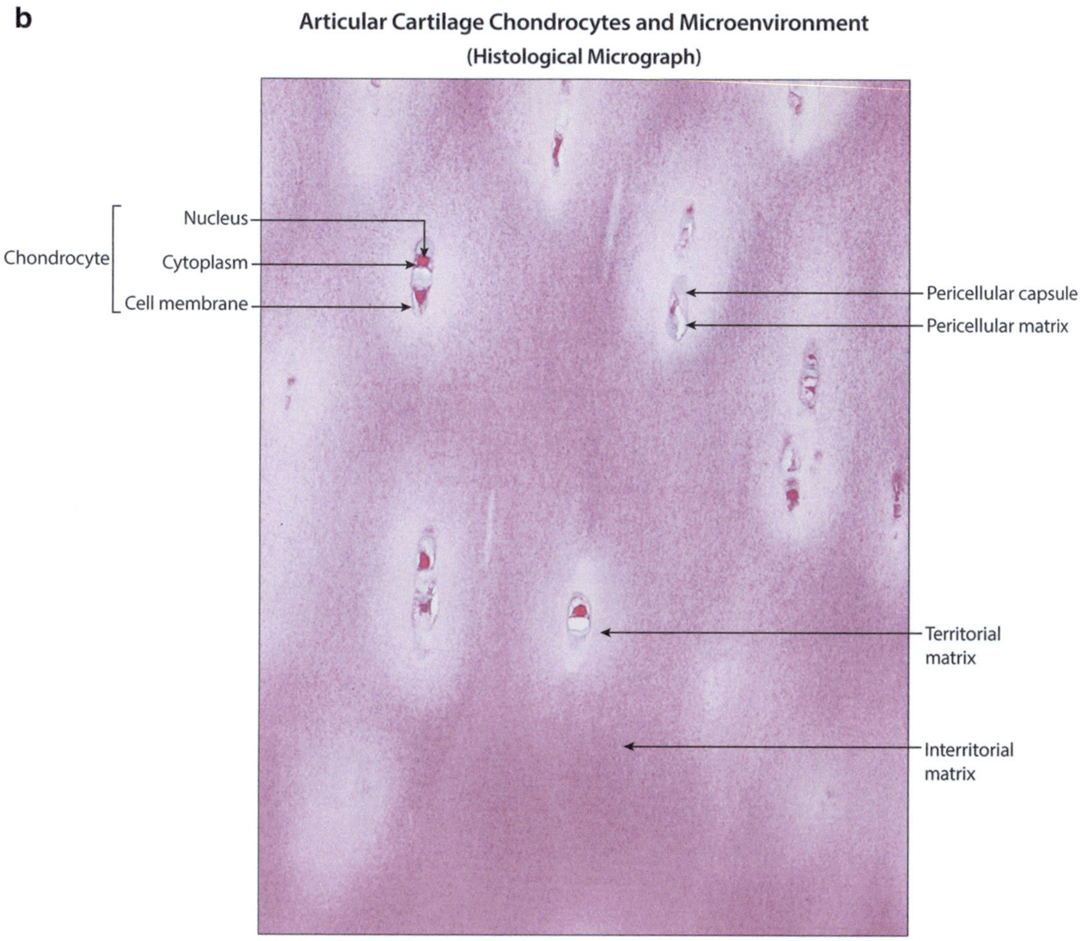

Fig. 1.16 (continued)

long periods of time. Depending on the anatomic site (load-bearing or non-load-bearing site), the cartilage thickness varies significantly across articular surfaces of the same joint. Interestingly, although knee articular cartilage is thin (about 2 to 4 mm in mature cartilage), it is highly resilient with an exceptional ability to distribute variable loads. The normal loading of knees during daily activities causes the articular cartilage to be exposed to high levels of intermittent hydrostatic pressure. The intermittent hydrostatic pressure on articul ar chondrocyte regulates the distribution of cartilage thickness within the joint and maintains a stable articular cartilage by providing an important stimulus for increasing cartilage matrix anabolism [316–318]. Knees that experience high forces and high joint contact pressures often exhibit relatively thicker articular cartilage. However, prolonged period and duration of repetitive high forces may also lead to knee articular cartilage injury and degradation.

1.4.1 Function Related to Structure of Articular Cartilage Components

Articular cartilage consists of several morphologically distinct components that are involved in its attachment to the subchondral bone as well as the formation of an articulating surface and compression-resistant core of the tissue.

Table 1.6 Articular cartilage matrix microenvironment: spatial relationship to chondrocytes

Uncalcified Cartilage Microenvironment	Anatomic Location	Extracellular Molecules	References
		CHONDRON MATRIX	
Pericellular Matrix (PCM)	Surrounds the chondrocytes of the middle and deep zones	Collagen type VI Perlecan Link proteins Integrins Proteoglycan monomer Hyaluronan Chondroitin sulfate Biglycan Chondronectin Glycoproteins WARP	[14, 16, 19, 41, 61, 64, 83, 114, 188, 295-304]
Pericellular Capsule	Encapsulates the pericellular matrix with filamentous and fine fibrillar molecules	Collagen type II Collagen type VI Collagen type IV Collagen type IX Collagen type XI Decorin Fibronectin Tenascin-C Laminin	[17–20, 27, 30, 120, 185, 296, 297, 305, 306]
Territorial Matrix (TM)	Outside of the pericellular zone up to the interterritorial matrix	Collagen type II Collagen type VI Matrillins-1 Matrilin-3 Biglycan Decorin	[17, 19, 20, 185, 296, 297, 305, 309, 310]
Interterritorial Matrix (ITM)	Extracellular matrix between the territorial zones	Collagen type II Collagen type IX Collagen type XI Link proteins Aggrecans Versican Heparan sulfate Decorin Fibromodulin Matrillin-3 Anchorin CII Asporin COMP	[17, 19, 20, 128, 198, 293, 294, 303, 310, 311]

Cartilage fluid plays an important role in decreasing friction and distributing the impact of loading. Cartilage fluid mobility during confined compression is governed by the hydraulic permeability of the macromolecules, primarily PGs, and its interaction with collagen. Due to its superhydrated state and incompressibility of tissue fluid, coupled with the structural organisation of PG and collagen molecules, articular cartilage is able to withstand high compressive forces and the stress of loading. Permeability of lubricating fluid in knee cartilage is dependent on the extent to which it is deformed and decreases as the compressive strain is increased [319, 320]. During loading, the permeability of articular cartilage is low, and this generates large interstitial fluid pressures within the cartilage.

The intrinsic physical properties of collagen fibres and PGs, coupled with the interactions between PG aggregates and collagen fibres, are critical in determining the biomechanical properties of knee cartilage [15, 273, 290, 321–324]. The compressive stiffness of articular cartilage is conferred by the balance between the osmotic swelling generated by fluid molecules bound to the PG/GAG sulfate and carboxylate groups and the tension developed in the collagen network surrounding the PGs, thus providing articular cartilage its resilience (resistance to compression) [153, 154, 292, 323, 325–327]. During tensile loading, PGs intertwined with the collagen network provide a physical restraint on the collagen fibres to effectively prevent sudden extension, fibrillar reorganization and realignment of the collagen network [328]. The PG molecules interact with tissue fluid to provide compressive resistance to cartilage through negative electrostatic repulsion forces and high osmotic pressure [35, 290, 321, 329]. Aggrecans function as molecular organizers of the ECM as these molecules act to immobilize and store growth factors. Importantly, aggrecans have high concentration of negative FCD, and the heavily sulfated GAGs attract fluid molecules that play a critical role in maintaining the compressive properties of articular cartilage. In vitro experiments confirmed that the cartilage hydration property is dependent on the structure and the GAG content of its PGs [330]. The GAGs (namely, CS, KS and DS) provide viscoelastic properties to the cartilage matrix, retain fluid, maintain ECM osmotic pressure and facilitate collagen organization. Also, the CS sulfation motifs are involved in the modulation of signalling gradients responsible for chondrocyte behaviours (such as proliferation, differentiation and matrix turnover) that determine the ECM architecture within the various zones [331].

Collagen fibre content, orientation and amount of intramolecular cross-linking are key determinants of the tensile strength of articular cartilage [152, 259, 332]. Collagen type II provides tensile strength to the articular cartilage ECM and is important in the establishment of temporal and spatial organization with aggrecan, whereas the minor collagens play essential structural roles in the ECM integrity and mechanical properties [104]. Collagen content and orientation have been shown to affect chondrocyte volume and shape changes when exposed to loading [333]. The mechanical characteristics and integrity of the collagen network are important determinants in cell stimulation, and in the control of the matrix maintenance that can modify fluid flow within the articular cartilage and stresses in chondrocytes [334]. Experimental fatigue and tensile testing of articular cartilage to induce microtrauma results in weakening of the interfibril connections which link collagen fibrils in the matrix, subsequently leading to a reduction in tensile strength of the collagen fibres [335]. Often, this weakening of the collagen fibre integrity occurs prior to the visualization of cartilage surface fibrillations.

1.4.2 Function of Articular Cartilage Zones

The articular cartilage zonal composition and 3D architecture heterogeneity are critical for its load-bearing capabilities and are responsible for the superior mechanical response to tension of skeletally immature cartilage when compared to mature cartilage [153, 290, 336]. Due to the variation in cartilage zonal ECM composition, each zone has a different level of osmotic pressure and chondrocytes have zone-specific turnover of ECM in response to changes in osmotic pressure. A recent ex vivo experiment has shown that high osmotic pressure upregulates the transient expression of aggrecan and collagen type II [337]. Also, in response to high osmotic pressure, the SZ chondrocytes significantly upregulate the expression of collagen type-I, whereas the middle- and deep-zone chondrocytes significantly upregulate matrix metalloproteinase-13 (MMP-13). Three-dimensional modelling experiments have demonstrated that the depth-dependent articular cartilage inhomogeneity increased the fluid support to loading in the SZ by simultaneously increasing the fluid pressure and decreasing the compressive effective stress [338]. The FCD of GAG molecules and the collagen fibril orientation of the MZ and DZ are functionally important components during compressive loading (Table 1.7). It has been shown that the tensile strength properties and stiffness of the MZ and

Table 1.7 Biomechanics of adult articular cartilage related to the histologic depth. Collagen fibre concentration, thickness, orientation relative to cartilage surface and their three-dimensional network interactions with entrapped highly sulfated proteoglycans play a critical role in the determination of the mechanical integrity of articular cartilage. The structural and biomechanical properties of knee articular cartilage varies with age

Articular Cartilage	Zones	Extracellular Molecules	Biomechanical Properties	References
Uncalcified Cartilage	*Zone 1* (10 to 20%)	***Surface Layer*** Lubricin, Superficial zone protein, HA, COMP	***Surface Layer*** Boundary lubrication and chondroprotection; Provides high viscocity to minimise friction; Wear resistant; Anchoring of lubricin with COMP facilitates lubrication	[180, 338–340]
		Below Surface Layer Thin collagen type II, other collagens	***Below Surface Layer*** Receive significant frictions from opposing AC; Collagen fibre orientation resist shear stress and carried 20% of the load for all strain rates; Exhibit high collagen fibre deformation under high force and long duration; Maintains tensile strength of cartilage	[323, 325, 338, 341–346]
		PGs, aggreacans, HA	Low permeability barrier to fluid flow during loading; Provides high viscosity; For a given stress, subjected to maximum strain Contributes to elasticity and resiliency to compression during interaction with collagen	
	Zone 2 (40 to 60%)	***Upper 1/3rd*** Collagen type II, Other Collagens	***Upper 1/3rd*** Transition between shear and compression stresses; For a given stress, subjected to moderate strain; Exhibit high collagen fibre deformation during under high force and long duration	[343–347]
		Aggrecans, HA	Compression resistance parallels PG concentration; Contributes to elasticity and resiliency to compression during interaction with collagen	
		Lower 2/3rd Thick collagen type II, Other collagens	***Lower 2/3rd*** *Relative to upper 1/3rd of zone 2:* Decreased tensile strength and stiffness; For a given stress, subjected to lesser strain	[292, 343–345, 348]
		Aggrecan, HA, High fix charge density of GAGs	Interaction of fixed charge density with perpendicular collagen fibres provides higher resistance to compression during loading than upper *1/3rd*	
	Zone 3 (30 to 40%)	Thickest collagen type II; Other collagens	*Relative to zone 2:* Further decreased tensile strength and stiffness; For a given stress, subjected to least strain	[292, 344, 345, 348]
		Aggrecan, HA, high fix charge density of GAGs	Interaction of fixed charge density with perpendicular collagen fibres provide highest resistance to compression during loading within uncalcified AC	

(continued)

Table 1.7 (continued)

Articular Cartilage	Zones	Extracellular Molecules	Biomechanical Properties	References
Tidemark		Mineralization front of collagen types I & II at the base of uncalcified cartilage	Transmit forces from uncalcified to calcified articular cartilage	[278–280, 349]
Calcified Cartilage	***Zone 4***	Mineralised matrix of collagen types I, II, X	Transmits tensile, compressive and shear forces from the viscoelastic uncalcified articular cartilage to subjacent subchondral bone	[280, 349, 350]
Subchondral Bone		Trabecular bone	Transmission of load from AC to knee epiphysis; Responsible for knee axial compressive properties; Large energy absorptive capacity	[351, 352]

AC, *Articular cartilage*; GAG, *Glycosaminoglycans*; COMP, *Cartilage oligomeric matrix protein*

DZ increase in immature cartilage but decline with maturity, whereas the tensile strength properties are comparable in the SZ of both age groups [348].

The SZ plays a critical role in determining the dynamic load-bearing properties of articular cartilage by acting as a low permeability barrier to fluid flow during loading. A recent study showed that due to its viscoelastic nature, during cartilage loading the SZ collagen carries a substantial part of the load under transient conditions [341]. This study suggested that under equilibrium conditions, the swelling pressure generated by the combination of PGs and collagen reinforcement accounts for the cartilage stiffness for more than 90% of the loads carried by articular cartilage [341]. Further, the tangentially oriented collagen fibrils of the SZ function to transfer compressive loads from the directly loaded area of the articular surface to the deeper cartilage zones. It has been shown that cartilage with an intact SZ has superior load-bearing properties compared to cartilage with compromised SZ [353]. The PG concentration increases with depth from the articular surface and the associated compressive resistance parallels this change with increasing depth from the articular surface [344]. As such, the compressive resistance of the DZ is greater than the MZ. Further, for a given stress, the decrease in strain is directly proportional to the cartilage depth from the articular surface [354] (Fig. 1.17).

The collagen fibre thickness, content and orientation in articular cartilage vary from the articular surface of the SZ to the DZ. The articular surface of SZ (composed of parallel, tightly packed, thin bundles of collagen fibres and PGs, such as lubricin) is exposed to significant friction from the opposing articular surface. The horizontal or parallel alignment of the collagen network in the SZ (20%) functions in shearing stress and in maintaining the tensile strength of articular cartilage. High force and long duration loading leads to high deformation of the collagen fibres in the middle and upper deep cartilage zones, along with an increased thickness of the SZ collagen fibres [346]. The MZ with oblique collagen fibres (40–60%) has biomechanical properties designed for shearing and compression stress, whereas the DZ (30%) composed of collagen fibres oriented perpendicular to the articular surface and tidemark can withstand high compression stress. In a 3D collagen fibril-reinforced finite element model of articular cartilage, the depth-related fibre orientation has been shown to depend on the degree of fibre displacement, fluid pressure and velocity for the cases of moderate strain rates

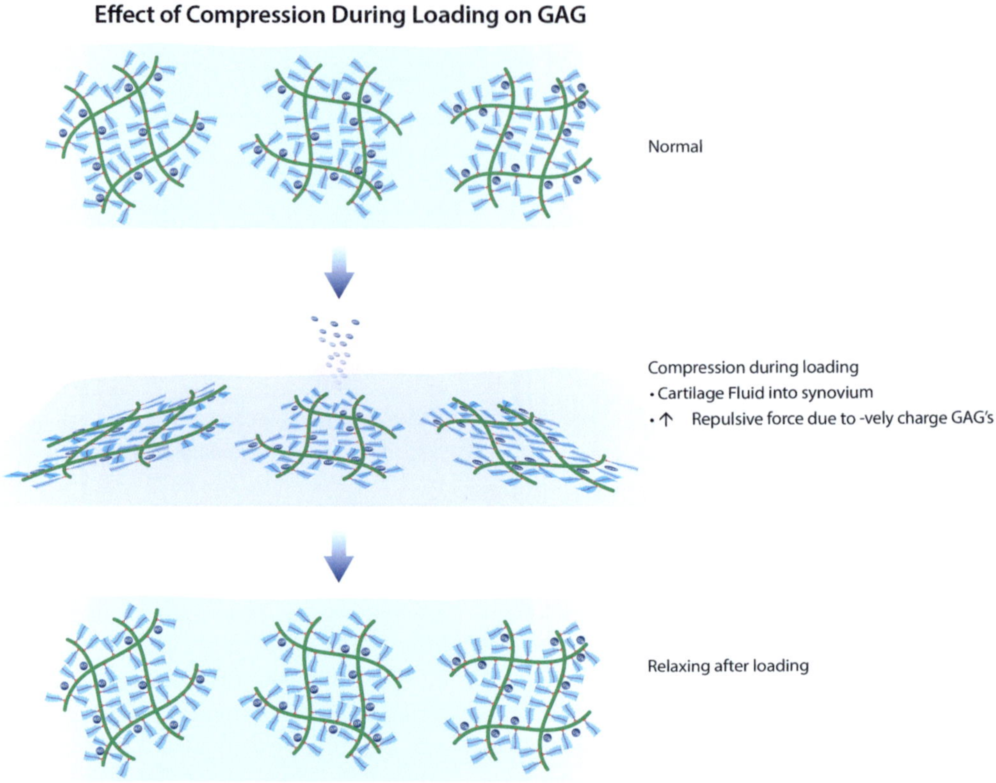

Fig. 1.17 Schematic diagram depicts the effect of compressive loading of the knee on the fixed charge density of proteoglycan's glycosaminoglycan (GAG) side chain. Increase in GAG side chain concentration is associated with increased compressive resistance of deep zone relative to superficial zone. (Schematic courtesy of Dr. Harpal K. Gahunia, and graphic illustration by Danny Aguilar, JD Graphics Solutions, East York, Ontario, Canada)

[345]. Further, the influence of fibre orientation was reported to diminish at static and instantaneous compressions. Disruption of the collagen network of the SZ has been shown to play a critical role in the early signs of knee cartilage OA associated with aging.

The structural integrity between the more compliant uncalcified articular cartilage and the underlying rigid calcified cartilage is achieved by a continuity of collagen fibres across the interface between these two layers [349]. The tidemark and the ZCC serve as an osteochondral interface, which functions as a physical barrier for vascularization and facilitates the pressurization and physiological loading of articular cartilage [278]. The ZCC also functions in distributing the cartilage stress during locomotion and other activities, e.g. sports and exercise [350]. At the cartilage-bone interface, the tensile stress and strain are reduced due to the depth-dependent inhomogeneity [338].

In summary, the biomechanical properties of knee articular cartilage vary from the SZ to the ZCC [11, 342, 355]. The inhomogeneous structural and biochemical distribution of the PGs and collagen fibrils throughout the depth of articular cartilage, and the interstitial fluid zonal variation provide unique depth-dependent mechanical properties during loading, which in turn influence fluid pressurization, local cartilage deformations and compressive stresses [338, 343]. During loading, the zonal PG inhomogeneity also contributes to enhancing the fluid support in the SZ by simultaneously raising the fluid pressure, lowering the compressive effective stress and wear properties of articular cartilage [338, 356]. The SZ chondrocytes and ECM composition,

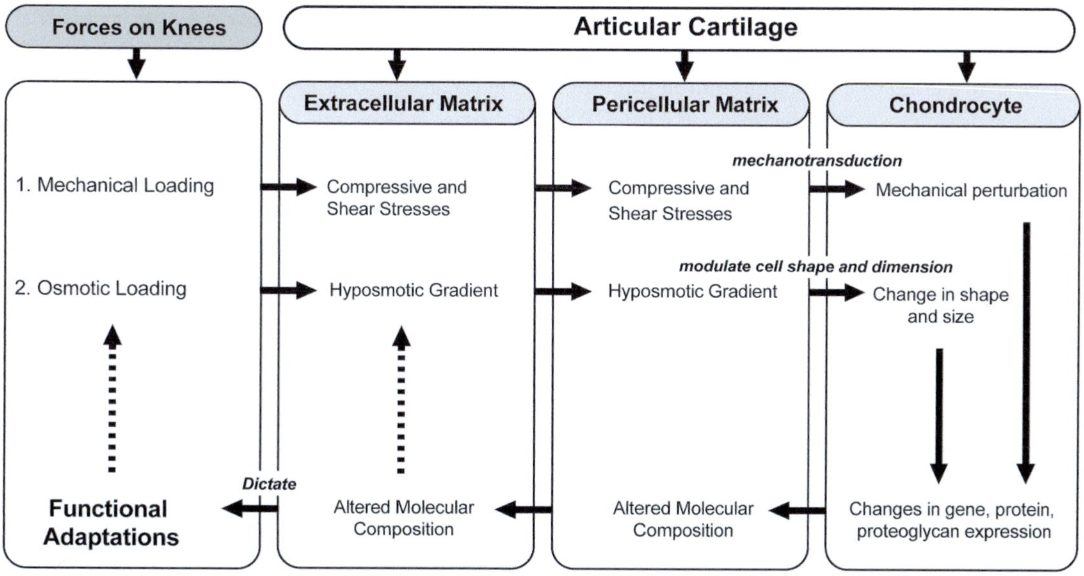

Fig. 1.18 Schematic diagram showing forces on knee articular cartilage. Mechanical and osmotic signals affect the metabolic activity of chondrocytes during cartilage loading. In response to loading, extracellular and pericellular matrix deformation generates chondrocyte signals as well as shape and volume changes (due to osmotic loading and creation of hyposmotic gradient). The consequential changes in gene, protein and proteoglycan expression result in altered molecular composition, which further dictates the functional adaptation of articular cartilage

molecular interactions as well as collagen fibre orientation play a critical role in joint lubrication, energy dissipation and adaptation to changing knee biomechanics [11, 357, 358].

1.4.3 Function of Chondrocytes and Chondrons

Chondrons are the micromechanical and metabolically active functional units of articular cartilage, which mediate the chondrocytic response to physicochemical changes associated with joint loading [13, 116, 359]. Within each zone, the chondrocytes play an important role in maintaining the cartilage homeostasis, and their complex circumferential microenvironment plays a significant role in the chondron mechanics [300, 360–362]. Chondrocytes regulate their metabolic activity (synthetic and degradative) based on the mechanical, electrical and physicochemical signals transmitted during cartilage loading and other environmental factors [7]. In response to loading deformation of the cartilage ECM, in particular the PCM, chondrocytes undergo shape and volume changes, and these properties are attributed both to the structure of the chondrocyte cytoskeleton and the viscoelastic properties of the chondrocyte nucleus [324] (Fig. 1.18).

A unique relationship exists among the biomechanical properties of the chondrocyte, PCM and ECM in different zones of articular cartilage, and the stress–strain environment of the chondrocyte is significantly influenced by its microenvironment [114]. The key structural components of the complex biomechanical microenvironment of chondrons includes the chondrocyte plasma membrane and the molecular components of the PCM and pericellular capsule. The PCM and its capsule have unique physical properties and spatial position to support the chondrocytes and to facilitate the communication between the chondrocytes and molecules of the TM and ITM. The PCM serves as a transducer of biochemical and biomechanical signals to the chondrocyte, and has a significant effect on the flow of cartilage fluid and ions as well as the transport of small molecules to and from the chondrocyte. The PCM has a lower permeability relative to the ECM, which enables the PCM to inhibit fluid flux near the chondrocyte by a factor of 30 [361]. The components of the PCM, specifically collagen type VI, contribute to chondrocyte survival and protection from apoptosis [115]. During compression, the collagen fibrils in the PCM function as a protective capsule to retain the width and volume of the chondrocyte [363]. Using a microstructural model of articular cartilage, the steady-state volume of the flat chondrocytes of the SZ decreased with the increasing pericellular collagen fibril stiffness. In the middle and deep zones, a small increase in the chondrocyte volume was noted with increasing pericellular fibril stiffness. In all the zones, an increase in FCD of the pericellular GAGs was associated with a substantial reduction in the chondrocyte cell volume [359].

Chondrocytes and chondrons have an important influence on the biomechanical microenvironment of the knee joint cartilage degeneration that occurs with aging and disease. A theoretical model to measure the viscoelastic properties of the chondrons as a function of age revealed that the adult and old chondrons generally possessed a thicker PCM with more enclosed cells compared to a young chondron [360]. The young and adult chondrons exhibited the same viscoelastic creep behaviour under a greater applied pressure (1.0–1.1 kPa), but without the deformation observed in the old chondrons. Further, the adult chondrons were stiffer than the young chondrons [360]. Loss of the spatial organization and destruction of the PCM have been reported in the early stage of OA, both in vivo and in vitro [18, 364]. These structural changes to the PCM significantly impact the mechanical microenvironment of the chondrocytes, resulting in almost 66% higher compressive strains, and higher fluid flux near the chondrocytes [361, 364]. In a rabbit model of early post-traumatic OA, after 4 weeks of anterior cruciate ligament transection, altered chondrocyte morphology (significant increase in cell height and decrease in width), decreased cellularity, and a significant decrease in the FCD of the PCM in the SZ of the lateral femoral condyle were noted compared to the cartilage samples obtained from the same site and zones of the control group [365]. These observations could be attributed to the altered biomechanics due to the compromised rotational stability and increased loading, hence high contact forces on the cartilage surface of the affected knee.

1.4.4 Concept of Knee Loading During Walking

The primary function of the knee articular cartilage is to provide a smooth, lubricated surface for articulation, and to facilitate the distribution and dissipation of loads on the opposing joint surfaces with a low frictional coefficient. The functional lifetime of articular cartilage is dependent on minimising friction and wear [366]. In the knee, friction is generated (as opposing forces) when the two contacting articular surfaces (femoro-tibial and petello-femoral) move relative to each other. The frictional coefficient is the measure of the amount of resistance that one cartilage surface exerts on the other. Wear of articular cartilage occurs when asperities, defined as microscopic roughness of cartilage surface, from opposing cartilage surfaces come into contact and deform, resulting in removal of cartilage surface macromolecules, which may eventually lead to the development of frank lesions (fibrillations) as seen in OA cartilage.

Knee loading refers to the force exerted on the weight-bearing compartment of the knee during activity. Walking is the most frequent activity of daily living, and during mobility, the specialized structure and composition of articular cartilage allows the relative movement of opposing cartilage surfaces with minimal friction and wear. The cartilage structural components (primarily collagen fibrils and PGs) interact to constitute the porous fibre-reinforced matrix that supports mechanical stresses applied to cartilage. The intermolecular crosslinks on the surface of the collagen fibres contribute to its tensile strength. However, by themselves, collagen fibres exhibit little resistance (weak) to compression. Formation of aggrecans promotes immobilization of PGs within the collagen meshwork, which in turn adds structural rigidity to the cartilage ECM. When subjected to external loads, the interaction of these macromolecules with the interstitial fluid (80% concentrated in SZ and upper MZ) protects the cartilage against high levels of stress and strain. The movement of cartilage fluid (up to 70% under load) plays an important role in joint lubrication [367].

Although knee articular cartilage is exposed to repetitive mechanical stress, the joint experiences low frictional forces due to the formation of a superhydrated layer of lubricating fluid and molecules on the cartilage surface [367, 368]. Normal physiologic loading is well tolerated, and during severe loading the lubricating monolayer on the cartilage surface and underlying ECM protects the joint by absorbing and dissipating the impact load (high force applied over a short time period). The forces at the joint surface vary from zero to several times body weight (BW). The opposing contact area varies in a complex manner (typically only several square centimetres) and is potentially subjected to high pressure (force/unit area). During level walking and downhill running, the medial tibiofemoral compartment has a greater cartilage contact area when compared to the lateral compartment, which has significantly less cartilage contact area during running versus walking (medial compartment gait cycle affected: 8%-10%; lateral compartment gait cycle affected: 5%-10%) [369]. Further, the compressive strain of normal healthy articular cartilage increases with increased walking speed with maximal strains of 5.0% observed after 60 minutes of walking [370]. Depending on the activity performed, the mechanical measures (such as moments and forces) determined by gait analysis vary. For instance, during level walking, the estimated compressive forces transmitted across the knee range from 2 to 4 times BW; whereas, descending the stairs and walking downhill increases the force to 6 and 8 times BW, respectively. Jumping elevates the load on the knee to 20 times BW [371–374]. A linear relationship between change in BW and change in compressive knee force has been documented [375]. For every pound increase in BW, a fourfold increase in knee compressive forces is transmitted. This ratio of weight gain to joint compressive force is particularly significant as one considers that this additional force is applied with every step. Hence, for every one-pound of weight loss, there is a 4-pound reduction in knee load per step, and assuming there are 1,200 strides/mile, the accumulated reduction in knee load would be more than 4,800 per 1 mile walked [375].

The threshold at which knee articular cartilage mechanical failure occurs is regulated by the prevalent stresses arising in the joint, which in turn is determined by an individual's lifestyle and activities (low versus high level of activity, intensity, duration, etc.) [370, 376]. During the physiological cyclic compressive knee loading, the opposing cartilage surfaces may eventually wear as a consequence of increased fatigue wear mode but not due to adhesive wear mode. This increased fatigue wear mode eventually results in cartilage surface damage in the form of fissures and fibrillation. Application of too high stress and fatigue on the knee has been attributed to the mechanical mechanism of articular cartilage damage.

1.4.5 Role of Articular Cartilage Macromolecules in Joint Biomechanics

Proteoglycans are polyanionic molecule with several long chains of sulfated GAGs (CS and KS) that extend out from the protein core. The carboxyl groups of CS and sulfate groups of KS provide negative FCD to the PGs aggregates, which in turn influence the mechanical and electrical behaviours of articular cartilage [35, 290]. Due to the repulsive forces of these negative charges, the GAG molecules of the aggrecans tend to spread out and occupy a large volume. However, the swelling capability of aggrecans is limited by the collagen molecules [283, 323]. The hydroxyl groups of CS interacts with C=O group of collagen type II of the cartilage ECM, whereas the epitopes representing the aggrecan KS-rich region are associated preferentially near or at collagen fibrils within the PCM and TM of the MZ and DZ [377, 378]. At a compressed stage, such as during locomotion, the mechanical response of cartilage macromolecules is tightly coupled to the fluid flow between the cartilage and joint space as well as the adjacent non-contact area of cartilage (Fig. 1.17). Proportional to the applied load, the fluid flows out of the cartilage through the articular surface into the joint space and through the cartilage at the periphery of the site of compression [319, 379–381]. This results in the close proximity of the negative FCD on the GAG molecules of the aggrecans. As a consequence, the repulsive forces of these negative FCD on the GAG molecules increases the compressive stiffness of articular cartilage. Upon the removal of the compressive load, the fluid from the joint space and adjacent cartilage flows back into the cartilage. As such, during loading of the knee, cartilage fluid mobility involves two processes: firstly, by fluid exudation into the synovial cavity both at the leading edge of the moving contact area and between the opposing cartilage areas, and secondly, the elastic recovery of cartilage that causes the imbibition of the expelled fluid back into the cartilage towards the trailing edge of the contact.

1.4.6 Osmotic Stress and Articular Cartilage Matrix Composition

Cartilage ECM macromolecules and chondrocytes are present in an aqueous, ion rich environment that contributes to the high osmotic pressure present within articular cartilage. Cartilage osmotic pressure is a very important component for absorbing and dissipating mechanical forces, particularly in the equilibrium state [341]. The osmotic pressure fluctuates with load, producing osmotic gradients that result in osmotic stress and consequent feedback loops that affect both chondrocyte function and matrix macromolecular composition (Fig. 1.18). In particular, hypotonic osmolality stimulates chondrocytes to rearrange their intracellular actin, change their shape as well as cell volume and increases the responsiveness of chondrocytes to Ca^{++} ions, resulting in increased synthesis of proteins, PG and GAG macromolecules. In the vicinity of chondrocytes, the amount of osmotic stress within the PCM is regulated by the integrity of collagen type VI within the chondron capsule [113]. Also, osmotic stress during physiologic mechanical loading directly affects the packing of collagen fibrils as well as their relationship to GAGs, thereby affecting capacity of cartilage to absorb mechanical loads. Osmotic PG depletion with age and OA decreases osmotic pressure and tends to decrease osmotic stress. This, in turn, contributes to the decreased capacity of the affected cartilage to regenerate new macromolecules and to respond well to mechanical loads. Further, osmotic stress will vary from matrix domain to domain within cartilage due to the heterogeneity of matrix composition, thereby contributing to the heterogeneity of chondrocyte function.

1.5 Knee Lubrication

The interstitial fluid and lubricating molecules present on the articular surface play an important role in joint lubrication through the formation of a superhydrated layer. The remarkable load-bearing capability of the knee lubrication is reviewed in this section. The characteristics of endogenous lubricants are discussed in depth, followed by the specialized mode of articular cartilage lubrication mechanisms.

1.5.1 Endogenous Lubricants On Articular Cartilage Surface

Healthy knee articular cartilage has a set of unique structural, biochemical and biomechanical properties that provide an efficient load-bearing surface and lubrication mechanisms. Lubrication of articular cartilage within synovial joints entails a complex interaction of several mechanical and molecular factors that are optimized to decreased friction between opposing surfaces of articular cartilage (effecting nearly frictionless motion of joints), and to provide wear protection during loading (static and dynamic) and sliding velocities [272, 321, 382–385]. The molecular factors involved in lubrication include both the lubricating molecules (of the SF and on the cartilage surface) and the constituent molecules of the articular cartilage in the SZ. These molecules collectively play a critical role in maintaining the cartilage surface integrity.

To date, several molecules have been identified that are responsible for the boundary lubrication of articular cartilage surface. These molecules include the homologous protein products of megakaryocyte stimulating factor gene expression (such as lubricin, SZP and PRG4), HA and phospholipids (such as phosphatidylcholine, phosphatidylethanolamine and sphingomyelin) [386–393]. The homologous lubricant molecules have the same primary, secondary and tertiary structure. However, they differ in post-translational O-linked glycosylation [388]. At the physiologic and pathophysiologic concentrations, the lubricating molecules contribute to boundary lubrication and form a protective layer by interacting with and adsorbing to the surface of articular cartilage as a monolayer, both individually or in a complex [368, 385, 394–397].

During physiologic loading on knee articular cartilage, the chondrocytes and ECM (macromolecules and interstitial fluid) of the SZ experience shear forces and friction coefficient that is dependent on the applied load [384]. The molecular structure of biolubricants permits extensive boundary hydration, and this property is conducive to its lubrication performance. An in vitro study demonstrated that the hydrophilic properties of lubricants on the articular surface, along with the fluid content at this layer, play an important role in lubrication [367]. This result was corroborated in an in vitro friction test that found one part of the synovial lubricating glycoprotein was adsorbed to the cartilage surface and that the formation of hydration shells around the polar area of the adsorbed molecule created a thin layer of viscous hydrated surface which aided in reducing the articular cartilage surface shear [398]. To date, several lubricants have been identified, which have been classified under proteins, carbohydrates and fatty acids.

1.5.1.1 Proteins

The human knee protein lubricants, namely, lubricin, PRG4 and SZP, are homologous protein products of megakaryocyte stimulating factor gene expression, encoded by the PRG4 gene [386]. They share a similar protein (primary, secondary and tertiary) structure but differ in post-translational glycosylation with O-linked oligosaccharides being predominant in lubricin and with limited amounts of CS and KS found in SZP [388]. Although of slightly different structure and MWs, these lubricants have been referred to as the same lubricant molecule that is regulated by TGF-β and play a role in lowering the friction properties on the articular cartilage surface [399, 400].

Lubricin a 227 kDa glycoprotein, is synthesized and secreted by the synovial fibroblasts [387]. Lubricin is found in the SF and on the articular cartilage surface of the SZ, which also contains HA and fibronectin [401–403]. Lubricin is relatively more concentrated on the cartilage surface of the anterior aspect of the femoral condyle than the posterior aspect. Lubricin contributes to the lubrication, wear resistance and anti-adhesive properties of cartilage [388, 404–407]. The presence of lubricin on the cartilage surface enables the cartilage to carry loads of normal forces, in particular during mobility, by reducing the friction as it prevents direct surface-to-surface contact and it also maintains the articular cartilage integrity [401, 402]. In vitro experiments corroborated the findings that lubricin reduces friction in cartilage bearings [401]. Under high loads at low relative velocities, lubricin prevents direct contact between surfaces. Lubricin has strong steric-repulsive interactions on collagen surfaces, where it mediates the adhesion and friction forces between the collagen surfaces, hence supporting the hypothesis that lubricin plays an important role in maintaining the structural integrity of the cartilage surface [340]. Several in vitro findings suggest the important role of lubricin in maintaining the structural integrity of the knee articular cartilage by providing a protective layer on the cartilage surface, and most-likely maintaining the contacting surfaces in a sterically repulsive state [340, 397, 408, 409].

In bovine explants, a direct correlation was observed between the coefficient of friction and chondrocyte apoptosis in the SZ of articular cartilage, indicating a direct connection between lubricin, boundary lubrication and chondrocyte survival [410]. Further, less ECM growth and lower compressive properties were exhibited in cartilaginous constructs formed from the SZ chondrocytes compared to the constructs obtained from the MZ chondrocytes [411]. Lubricin provides chondroprotection by dissipating strain energy induced during locomotion and prevents damage to the parallel tangentially aligned collagen type II fibres of the SZ cartilage surface [357, 402, 410, 412, 413]. It is suggested that compression may decrease the vulnerability of articular cartilage to shear-induced damage by lowering the effective strain on individual collagen fibrils [414]. The low frictional stress between two sliding surfaces bearing surfactant monolayers is attributed to the fluid hydration layers, and such hydration forces are thought to be involved in the steric repulsion forces between adherent lubricin layers on apposed cartilage surfaces [402, 415]. In addition to serving as a boundary lubricant, lubricin has been found to prevent hyper-proliferation of synovial cells [404].

Proteoglycan 4, also referred to as PRG4, at the articular cartilage surface and in the SF plays an important role in boundary lubrication. PRG4 is identified as megakaryocyte stimulating factor that is secreted by the chondrocytes of the SZ and synoviocytes of the synovium [392, 406]. The intermolecular disulfide-bonded multimeric structure of PRG4 is responsible for its ability to adsorb to the articular cartilage surface [416]. In vitro expression of PRG4 by subpopulations of chondrocytes from various uncalcified cartilage zones showed that superficial chondrocytes secreted much more PRG4 than the middle- and deep-zone chondrocytes, which expressed little to no PGR4 [406, 417, 418]. Under certain conditions, as suggested in an ex vivo experiment, PRG4 which is normally tightly bound on the cartilage surface can exchange with the PRG4 in SF [419]. Investigation of the mechanical regulation showed that PGR4 expression may be modulated by unconfined, compressive, mechanical forces [420]. Dynamic shear stimulation on PRG4 biosynthesis in cartilage explants demonstrated an increased PRG4 secretion of three to four times and more PRG4 of 345 kDa relative to smaller MW of 315 kDa, as compared with unloaded controls and statically compressed samples [421]. Further, shear stimulation also increased the total number of chondrocytes expressing PRG4 up to the upper MZ. Thus, besides other cartilage matrix constituents, mechanical stimuli upregulate the biosynthesis of PRG4 [420, 421]. Beside its function in reducing shear, controlling adhesion-dependent synovial growth and regulating protein deposition onto the articular cartilage surface, recent findings implicated PGR4 as an inflammatory signalling molecule [422].

Superficial zone protein, also known as SZP, is a heavily glycosylated 345 kDa protein with minimal GAG substitution [406, 423]. SZP accumulates at the articular cartilage-SF interface [386]. SZP exhibits topographical variation across the knee articular surface, and its expression is primarily localized with high concentration at the load-bearing anterior aspect of the femoral condyle [424]. In contrast, significantly less SZP concentration was found on the non-load-bearing cartilage surface at the posterior aspect of the femoral condyle. Further, a decreased coefficient of friction was associated with the enhanced SZP concentration on the load-bearing aspect. SZP is thought to form a nanofilm that functions to reduce friction during mobility and to smoothen asperities on knee articular cartilage [424]. These findings are suggestive of the mechanosensitive nature of SZP expression. Mechanotransduction of SZP occurs via TGF-β signalling [424]. The SZP also serves as a metabolic marker for chondrocytes of the SZ. Direct relationships have been demonstrated between high level of SZP expression, maximum contact pressure and low friction coefficients [399]. Application of shear stress was shown to increase the level of SZP expression and accumulation [424]. Further, platelet-rich plasma has been shown to stimulate both chondrocytes and synoviocytes to significantly increase SZP synthesis and secretion [425].

1.5.1.2 Phospholipids

Phospholipids molecules are organized as spherical bilayer. Each molecule is composed of a hydrophilic head and a hydrophobic tail. Phospholipids such as phosphatidylcholine, phosphatidylethanolamine and sphingomyelin have been identified as constituents of SF and they are also bound to the articular surface [426, 427]. Upon binding with mobile Ca2+, phospholipid becomes active phosphatidylcholine which is adsorbed with the negatively charged PGs on the surface of articular cartilage [427–429]. While most phospholipids are surface active, dipalmitoyl-phosphatidylcholine is particularly active, and is the most abundant form present in SF at 45% [426, 428, 430]. Phosphatidylcholine has better lubricating property to withstand severe loading than phospholipids, thus producing lower frictional resistance [430–432]. In vitro experiments showed that enzymatic degradation of phosphatidylcholine compromises its lubricating quality.

As a boundary lubricant for articular cartilage, surface-active phospholipids (SAPLs) can form a strongly adsorbed layer to provide hydrophobicity to the articular surface and shield asperities from solid-solid contacts [366, 427]. Enzymatic digestion of SAPLs with phospholipase was shown to eliminate the lubricating ability of SF and increases the coefficient of friction [433]. However, other studies that examined the effects of SAPL degradation on the cartilage surface found no effect on the frictional coefficient [434].

1.5.1.3 Glycosaminoglycans

Hyaluronic acid is a non-sulfated GAG without a protein core, which is distributed in human SF with high MW ranging from 27 kDa to 10 MDa [391, 435–437]. HA constitutes long chains of repeating disaccharides, comprised of D-glucuronic acid and N-acetyl D-glucosamine [63]. Experiments using the surface force apparatus suggest that HA serves a chondroprotective role by preventing wear of the articular surface, rather than reducing the coefficient of friction [438, 439].

HA, the major component of the articular cartilage ECM, associates with aggrecan molecules and link protein to form an aggregating complex that provides the compressive and viscoelastic properties of articular cartilage [63, 440]. Within the SF, HA plays a major role in fluid-film lubrication by providing high viscosity to SF through its high MW and concentration (0.1–5 mg/mL) [272, 441, 442]. Separation of HA from SF resulted in a reduction of the fluid viscosity, whereas the boundary lubrication of the treated fluid remained unaffected [443]. Unlike other boundary lubricants, HA does not adsorb to the cartilage surface, but decreased friction in the cartilage-cartilage interface has been reported [409]. HA adjusts SF viscosity and articulating surface lubrication, improves articular cartilage nutrition and mediates cell growth regulation including proliferation, differentiation and migration [444].

1.5.2 Synergy of Molecular Lubricants

The biological lubricants (lubricin, PRG4, SZP, HA, SAPL) play an important role in the boundary lubrication by providing low-friction and low-wear properties to articular cartilage surfaces and are regulated by TGF-β [400, 445]. These lubricants contribute to the boundary lubrication of opposing articular cartilage surfaces, individually and in combination [385]. Under severe joint loading, the combination and concentration of adherent lubricating molecules produces a synergistic effect in reducing the coefficient of friction (i.e. low boundary friction), which results in a low wear rate of the cartilage surface. PRG4 and HA both function as dose-dependent boundary lubricants of cartilage. They also act synergistically through an unknown mechanism. Cartilage boundary lubrication tests using various combinations of HA and PRG4 at physiologic concentrations showed that the reduction of the coefficient of friction was additive [385]. Attachment of COMP with lubricin facilitates lubrication and results in low friction forces [180]. HA forms a complex with the lubricin to form a cross-linked network to effectively eliminate the wear damage to the opposing/shearing surfaces [438]. Under compression, free HA diffuses out of the cartilage into the joint space, but when forming a complex with lubricin, the complex is physically trapped at the cartilage-joint space interface by the increasingly constricted collagen pore network. The mechanically trapped and chemically bound HA-lubricin complex acts as an effective "boundary lubricant", which functions to reduce the friction [438]. Under compressive loading, protein-lipid adsorption occurs on hydrated cartilage surface. Lubricin and HA could have "carrier" functions for the highly insoluble SAPL, while HA has good wetting properties needed to promote hydrodynamic lubrication of articular surface [428]. Although fibronectin strongly interacts with both HA and lubricin, its interaction with lubricin synergistically enhances wear protection of the articular cartilage surface during shear [246]. Recently, an ex-vivo experiment demonstrated the synergy of

HA-lipids in significantly reducing the boundary friction of extrasynovial tendon sliding in its sheath [446].

1.5.3 Deficiency of Molecular Lubricants

Lubrication of knee articular cartilage entails a complex interaction of several mechanical and molecular factors. A layer of lubricating molecules covers the cartilage surface and acts as a boundary lubricant, resulting in decreased friction between opposing surfaces of articular cartilage and effecting nearly frictionless motion of knee [385]. Damage to the articular cartilage surface integrity due to injury and disease causes alterations in the composition, concentration and MW of the lubricant molecules. Consequently, the boundary-lubricating ability of SF may be compromised due to associated changes in the SF pH and characteristics of the lubricant molecules [447–451] (Table 1.8). Damage to the SZ or absence of lubricating molecules often initiates a cascade of mechanical and biological events that can lead to insufficient boundary lubrication and subsequent biomechanical impairment (compromised load-bearing ability and irreversible wear properties), cartilage degradation and progression to disease such as OA and RA [444, 452, 453]. The concentration, composition and MW of the lubricant molecules vary with joint injury, disease (RA versus OA) and stage of OA [444]. Ineffective joint lubrication has been demonstrated to play an important role in the development and progression of knee OA [412]. Early degenerative changes of the articular cartilage SZ have been associated with reduction in the PG content and deviation of the collagen fibril orientation angle compared to the healthy cartilage [453]. These changes affect the lubricating properties of the cartilage surface lubricants, and this impacts the load-bearing properties of articular cartilage by increasing the risk for further ECM degeneration and chondrocyte apoptosis.

In several animal models of OA, the down-regulation of the expression and localization of the lubricants indicated the association between the reduction or loss of these SF and cartilage surface molecules, and OA pathogenesis [405, 454]. In a sheep meniscectomy model, early loss of PRG4 from the cartilage surface has been associated with cartilage degeneration and early onset of OA [455]. In an equine model of acute injury, comparison of SF from injured and control joints for cartilage boundary lubrication function demonstrated that SF from injured joints exhibited poor boundary lubrication properties [456]. SF obtained from joints with acute injury had a lower HA concentration of lower MW forms compared to the control SF, and addition of HA to the deficient equine SF restored its boundary lubrication function [456].

Investigation of the lubricants in disease states showed that, compared with SF from age-matched control individuals, the concentrations of HA and lubricin were lower, whereas those of SAPLs were higher in the SF of OA and RA patients [444]. The HA MW range was lower in the SF of these patients, and the relative distribution of SAPLs as well as the degree of fatty acid saturation and their chain lengths were also altered in OA and RA patients [444]. This result confirmed the presence of different levels, composition and molecular distribution of SF lubricants with joint disease and stage of OA. Decreased concentration of HA in human SF is associated with joint injury and arthritis [447–450]. Investigation on the adsorption of SAPL on the cartilage surface of

Table 1.8 Synovial fluid analysis in different clinical conditions. (Data obtained from Kosinska (2015) [444])

Synovial Fluid Analysis	Normal	Osteoarthritis		Rheumatoid Arthritis
		Early	Late	
pH	7.3	7.8	8.1	6.8
Lubricin (μg/ml)	364	244	152	139
Phospholipids (nmol/ml)	314.2	643.8	758.8	877.7
Hyaluronic Acid (mg/ml)	2.2	1.7	1.9	1.0

OA knees (obtained post-knee replacement) showed that the cartilage surface lubricating layer of SAPL was deficient in these joints [457]. Human SF SAPLs concentration has been reported to decrease following traumatic injury and increase in OA [447, 451].

Decreased PRG4 levels in the SF of OA patients correlated with significantly diminished cartilage boundary-lubricating capacity as compared to normal SF, and improved lubrication function was noted in OA SF with PRG4 supplementation [458]. Using a rabbit knee injury model, the concentration of PRG4 in SF decreased from 280 g/ml to a range of 20 to 100 g/ml at 3-weeks post injury [405]. Post-injury, the loss of boundary-lubricating ability of SF is associated with damage to the articular cartilage ECM, which is attributed to the early-phase inflammatory process [405]. Following anterior cruciate ligament injury, the decreased SF lubricin concentration is associated with an increased level of inflammatory cytokines [459]. These findings suggest that following knee injury, lack of boundary lubrication as a consequence of decreased SF and cartilage surface lubricant concentration may place the articular cartilage at risk of wear-induced damage.

Insufficiency of lubricin due to knee trauma, inflammatory arthritis or genetically mediated lubricin deficiencies have been linked to articular cartilage damage [460–462]. In particular, the SZ and chondrocyte morphology (preservation) have been linked to the critical role played by lubricin. Joints lacking lubricin from SF have shown early wear and higher friction associated with damage to collagen type II of the SZ. Chondrocyte apoptosis are most pronounced among the cells located at the intersection of the tangential and radial collagen fibrils [410]. Chondrocyte cell death may lead to deficient lubricin and SZP production, and focally increase friction on the cartilage surface. Consequently, the friction gradient may lead to decreased capacity to resist impact forces, resulting in the knee articular cartilage SZ fibrillation.

1.5.4 Lubrication Mechanisms (Applicable to Human Knee)

Although knee articular cartilage is exposed to repetitive mechanical stress during various daily (sitting, walking, etc.) and sports-related activities (e.g. running), the SF constituents (mainly glycoproteins and phospholipids) and endogenous lubricants coating the cartilage surface provide very low frictional resistance and high wear resistance to the opposing articular cartilage. Endogenous knee lubricants are viscous, providing protection to the cartilage surface from abrasion and adhesive slide wear. The mechanisms of cartilage-on-cartilage lubrication have been attributed to the boundary lubrication effects and the presence of fluid-film lubrication. The two basic lubrication mechanisms for the lubrication of articular surfaces are the boundary and fluid-film lubrications [366, 463, 464] (Fig. 1.19).

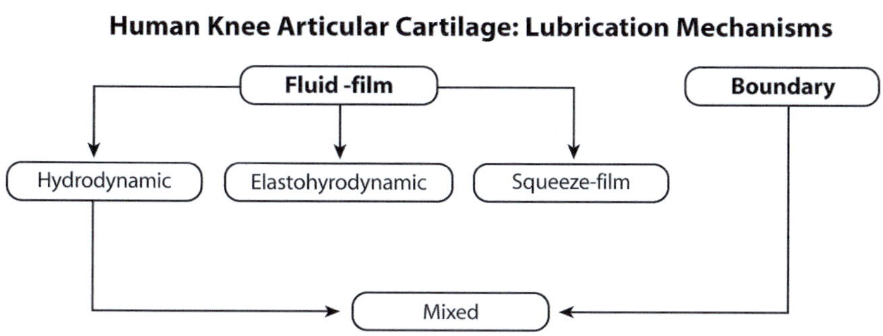

Fig. 1.19 Schematic diagram showing the lubricating mechanisms applicable to human knee articular cartilage

1.5.4.1 Boundary and Contact Lubrication Mechanism

During normal physiologic activity, boundary lubrication functions to protect (via wear reduction) the articular cartilage surface of the knee. However, it is not an effective mechanism under excessive loads [398, 465]. Boundary lubrication occurs when a *lubricant film* is present between the opposing cartilage surfaces, keeping them at a distance, and allowing mobility with a low coefficient of friction. The lubricant component (lipids, carbohydrates or proteins) of the SF that adheres to the articular cartilage surface forms a monolayer, *surface film*, which is the basis of the contact lubrication mechanism [396, 427, 466, 467]. Depending on the MW and concentration of the cartilage surface adhering lubricant, the thickness of the surface film varies, measuring up to 10 nm [468]. The lubricant film between the opposing cartilage surfaces and the biomechanical properties of the macromolecular components of articular cartilage, in particular the SZ and upper MZ, are critical components in the determination of the coefficient of friction [366]. Removal of the adherent molecule from the lubricant film increases the coefficient of friction [469–471].

1.5.4.2 Fluid-Film Lubrication

Fluid-film lubrication involves the presence of a thin film of fluid on the articular surface that provides separation of joint surfaces. The load on the bearing articular cartilage surfaces of the knee in fluid-film lubrication is supported by the pressure in the film. Compared to boundary lubricated surfaces, typically a lower coefficient of friction exists on surfaces lubricated by a fluid film. The low coefficient of friction of the knee suggests that some degree of fluid film lubrication exists. There are two subtypes of the fluid-film lubrication mechanism, the squeeze-film and hydrodynamic lubrication, each of which complements the other and depends on the tissues involved and the load applied to the joint.

Squeeze-Film Lubrication

The squeeze-film lubrication, sufficient to carry high loads for short durations, occurs when the weight-bearing area of the opposing articular cartilage surfaces move perpendicular towards each other, resulting in increased fluid pressure that forces the lower MW components of the lubricant film out. Consequently, an increase in the fluid viscosity due to the increased concentration of HA in the remaining fluid (and possibly ECM of the SZ) facilitates the gliding motion of the opposing articular surface that comes into contact, while assisting to support the load. Thereafter, with load reduction, the hydrodynamic action plays a role decreasing the fluid-film viscosity through the mobility of low MW components into the fluid film between the two opposing surfaces. The value of the load applied on the knee is directly proportional to the value of fluid pressure.

Hydrodynamic Lubrication

The hydrodynamic lubrication, often characterized by conformal surfaces, occurs when two non-parallel opposing surfaces (femoral condyle and tibial plateau) are lubricated by a fluid film that moves tangentially with respect to each other [468, 472]. The viscosity of the lubricant, conformity of the articular surfaces and relative direction of motion of the opposing articular surface generate pressure to maintain a lubricating film between the opposing surfaces [396, 465]. However, when load is applied, the fluid pressure generated by this mechanism is not capable of producing elastic deformation of the cartilage ECM.

1.5.4.3 Elastohydrodynamic Lubrication

The elastohydrodynamic lubrication occurs when the fluid-film pressure between the opposing articular cartilage surfaces causes elastic deformation of the bearing articular cartilage surface, which further influences the pressure developed within the fluid film. During elastohydrodynamic lubrication, the fluid-film formation is strongly affected by lubricant behaviour and the elastic deformation of the opposing articular cartilage surface [431, 473, 474]. The elastic modulus of the load-bearing articular surfaces and the pressure-viscosity coefficient are important features of elastohydrodynamic lubrication. For a given load at the area of contact of load transmission, the elastic distortion of the solid macromolecular component of articular cartilage (in particular, the SZ and upper MZ) provides a flattening geometrical conformity, which in turn increases the size of the contact area that facilitates a thicker lubricating fluid film than can be achieved normally [468]. Coupled with this, due to the high pressure developed within the fluid film, an increase in the viscosity of the lubricant consequently increases the lubricating film thickness. Under physiological loading, articular cartilage has a very small modulus of elasticity and the capability to deform readily. For this lubrication mechanism, the effective elastic modulus of the cartilage macromolecules is added to the parameters during hydrodynamic lubrication [468].

1.5.4.4 Application of Lubrication Mechanisms During "Walk Cycle" Phases

The biomechanical behaviour of the knee (and other synovial joints) is primarily governed by the molecular and fluid characteristics of the articular cartilage and SF. These constituents also play critical roles in joint lubrication when friction force is generated during mobility. Lubrication of the knee depends on several factors as follows: creation of a fluid film (monolayer) over the cartilage surface by lubricating molecules (lubricin); maintenance of a fluid layer between the opposing cartilage surfaces during the elastic deformation of articular cartilage; presence of slight irregularities (asperities) on the articular cartilage surface that trap HA; creation of fluid flow during alternate application and removal of compressive forces; and the movement (squeezing out) of cartilage interstitial fluid into the joint space as loading increases [464]. The tibiofemoral compartment of the knee has a high degree of geometrical conformity. Physiological loading does not damage the joint due to the hydrodynamic action of the lubricating molecules forming a monolayer on the articular cartilage surface.

During the "walk cycle", large normal loads are transmitted from moment to moment across the knee from one bone to another while allowing an efficient relative motion in a direction tangential to the surfaces [463, 464]. Under dynamic gait conditions, the friction coefficient of articular cartilage during swing phase is higher than during stance phase [475]. The load on the knee in a walking cycle of 1 Hz may go up to three times of the BW at heel strike and toe off, while in a vertical drop of 1 meter, the knee may experience up to 25 times BW [476]. After the heel strikes the ground, the joint cartilage plays an important role in dissipating the impact of loading. The elastic deformation of the articular surface occurs upon the activation of the elastohydrodynamic lubrication stage. Depending on the loading conditions and sliding velocity, which is variable during one gate for a typical walk cycle, the profile of the fluid-film lubrication thickness and the pressure developed also varies. The sliding velocity in the knee also varies considerably with time in normal walking. The applied load and sliding velocity are inversely proportional throughout the gait. The "walk cycle" consists of four phases: swing through; heal strike; body weigh transfer and toe-off (Fig. 1.20).

While elastohydrodynamic lubrication is the major mechanism in human knees, they operate with adaptive multimode lubrication. The almost unloaded or minimal loaded state (when the foot is off the ground and the leg swings freely from its posterior to its anterior position) and high sliding velocity phase generate a relatively thicker, full fluid-film lubrication between the opposing cartilage surfaces, referred to as *hydrodynamic lubrication*. Upon loading (when the heel is on the ground and the load on the knee suddenly increases), the velocity is reduced and the lubricant film squeezes out reducing its thickness, referred to as the *squeeze film mechanism*, during which stage a viable lubricant film is maintained. The following phase in the walking cycle (before heel strike and shortly after toe off), when the load on the knee reduces rapidly toward zero and the velocity increases and the lubricating fluid film maintains the separation of the opposing articular surface, is the *elastohydrodynamic lubrication*. Finally, at the toe-off position (when the heel strikes the ground and the toe is leaving the ground), the maximum load state and very low velocity maintain a lubricant film and prevent surface-to-surface contact through a combination of *squeeze film* and *boundary lubrication mechanisms*.

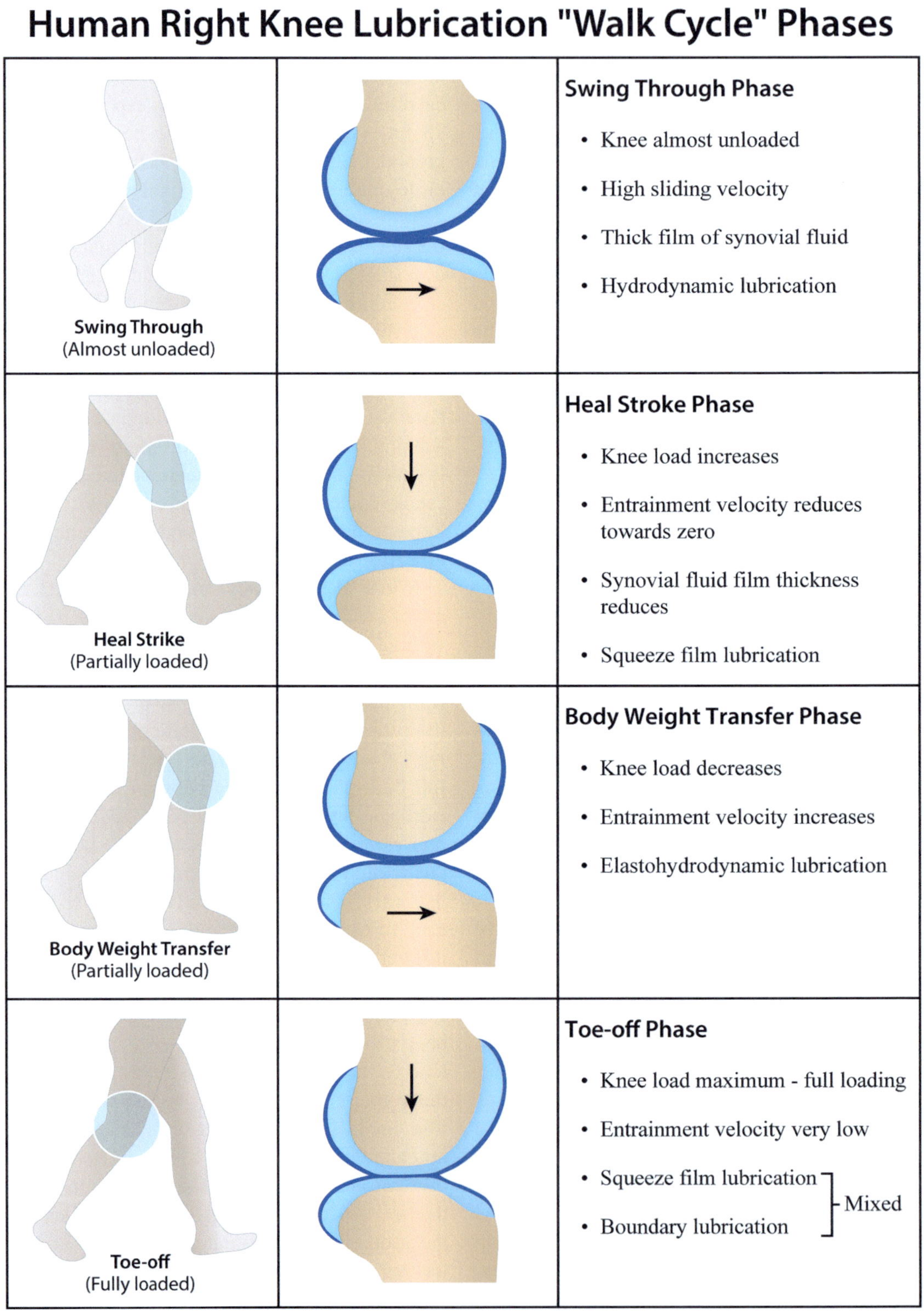

Fig. 1.20 Schematic diagram showing human right knee lubrication during the "Walk Cycle" phases. During "Swing Through" phase minimal load is applied on the knee; whereas, during "Toe-off" phase maximum load is applied. (Courtesy of Dr. Harpal K. Gahunia, and graphic illustration by Danny Aguilar, JD Graphics Solutions, East York, Ontario, Canada)

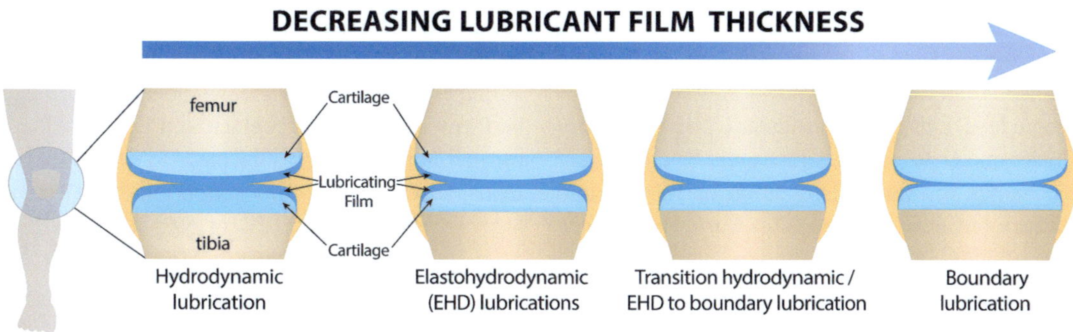

Fig. 1.21 Schematic diagram showing variations in lubricant film thickness in the human knee related to lubrication mechanisms. (Schematic created by Dr. Harpal K Gahunia, and graphic illustration by Danny Aguilar, JD Graphics Solutions, East York Ontario, Canada)

The lubricant film thickness for both static squeeze and the elastohydrodynamic feeding affects the joint conformity, the cartilage surface compliance and the viscosity of the lubricating fluid (Fig. 1.21). Under normal loading conditions, the fluid film is a squeeze film, whereas during sliding or rolling, the elastohydrodynamic film occurs which supplies the squeeze film. The cartilage weeping phenomenon and the boundary lubrication characteristics of joint lubricants on cartilage play secondary roles in healthy knee. During normal compressive loading, due to cyclic loading and unloading on the contact area of cartilage surface, the asperity deformation is elastic and the fatigue strength of asperities is low.

1.5.4.5 Failure of Lubrication Mechanism (Injury, Aging, Disease and Post-Cartilage Repair)

Of all joints, the knee is subjected to significantly high load during walking, running, hiking and sport activities. Normally, the high coefficient of friction between bones is lowered through the presence of articular cartilage and SF, which interact to facilitate a lubrication system. Knee injury (acute or chronic), aging, hereditary disease (lubrication molecule deficiency) and joint disease contribute to the perturbation and impairment to the normal lubrication mechanism. Knee injury that causes depolymerisation of HA complexes contributes to the decreased SF viscosity, which further negatively affects the lubricant-film thickness [458, 471, 477–479]. Often noted in aging and OA articular cartilage are changes that can be explained in terms of failure in lubrication mechanisms. This includes decreased articular cartilage resiliency and loss of structural integrity, in particular at the surface of SZ, which contribute to thinning of the lubricant fluid film and direct cartilage-to-cartilage contact of the two opposing surfaces [383, 480]. Joint friction is elevated and accompanied by accelerated cartilage damage in humans and mice that have genetic deficiency of lubricin. Using ex vivo and in vitro measurements of friction and apoptosis in lubricin-knockout mice, an increase in whole-joint friction and cellular apoptosis was observed when compared with wild-type mice [410]. Further, using the bovine explant system, a direct correlation between coefficient of friction and chondrocyte apoptosis in the SZ of cartilage was observed. This study sheds the light on the relationship between joint mechanics and cartilage deterioration in patients with genetic or acquired deficiency of lubricin. The elastic property of normal, undamaged articular cartilage enables it to deform laterally under excessive load, however this property is reduced in cartilage with compromised ECM due to injury, aging or disease. Further, alterations in the characteristics of lubricant molecules and cartilage integrity may result in abnormally high fluid pressure within the joint and ECM.

Failure of the lubrication mechanism of articular cartilage is also attributed to asperity fatigue. Asperities (in material science) refer to unevenness, roughness or rugged projection of surfaces. When the two macroscopically smooth articular cartilage surface come into contact, asperities at the microscopic level exist on the articular cartilage on very small contact points or surface area, where contact mechanics is exhibited in terms of friction and contact stiffness (Fig. 1.22). Cartilage surface friction and wear originate at these asperity points / areas. The size of an asperity has a very strong effect on the way the two opposing cartilage surfaces behave upon contact, and can contribute to resistance. When subjected to compressive loads, asperities deform through the elastic cartilage surface and the ECM of SZ; hence, further

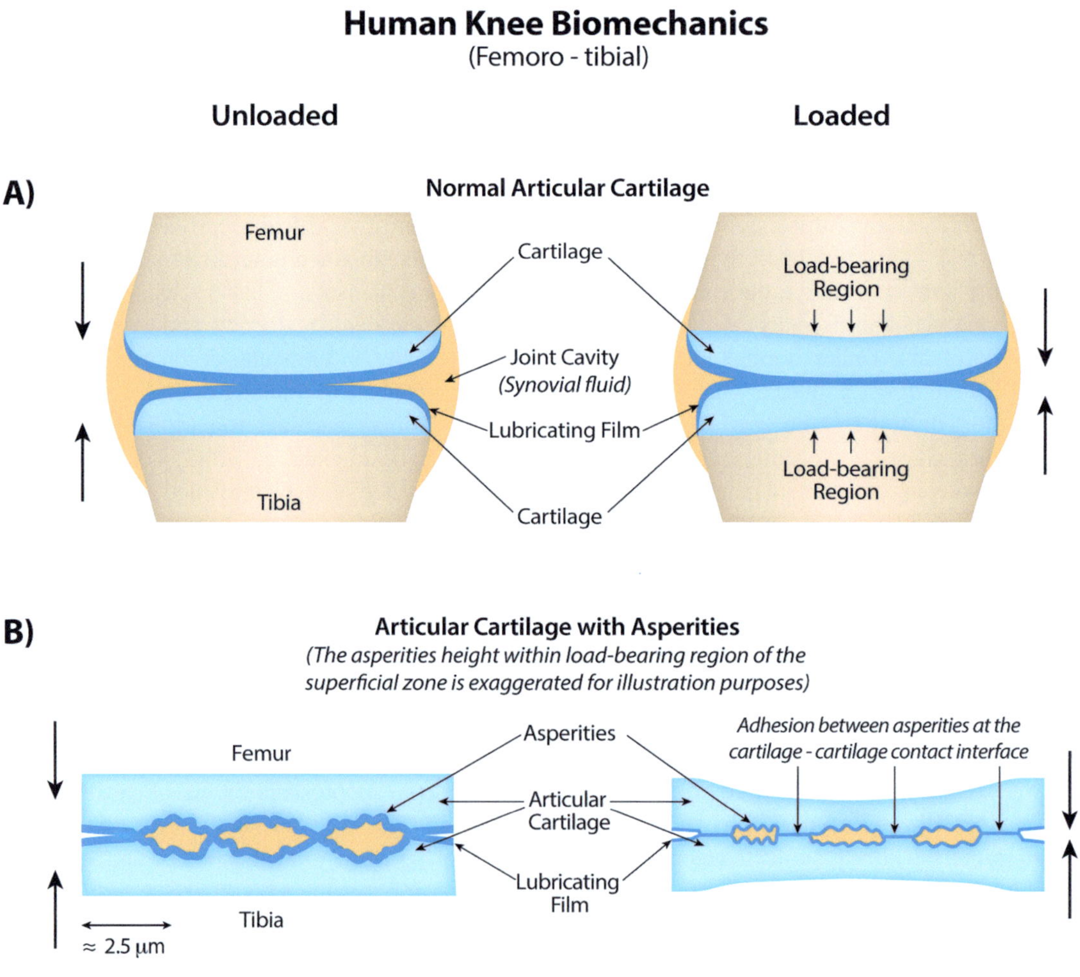

Fig. 1.22 Schematic diagram represents the human femoro-tibial knee during unloaded (left) and loaded (right) state. (**a**) Normal knee with thick articular cartilage and lubricating film during the unloaded state, and compressed cartilage with thinner lubricating film when load is applied. (**b**) Depicts asperities on the opposing articular cartilage at very small contact points or surface areas where friction and contact stiffness occurs within the load-bearing region of the superficial zone. When subjected to repetitive compressive loads, as a result of asperity fatigue at the contact area, the asperities deform through the cartilage surface, and the extracellular matrix of the superficial zone enhances the adhesion between asperities at the cartilage–cartilage contact interface. The thin lubrication film on the cartilage surface asperities area, when damaged, compromises the articular cartilage surface integrity. Subsequent damage to the lubrication film on the cartilage surface asperities area weakens the collagen fibres at the cartilage surface, which can proceed to surface discontinuity lesions (fibrillations) seen in aging or osteoarthritic cartilage. (Schematic created by Dr. Harpal K Gahunia and graphic illustration by Danny Aguilar, JD Graphics Solutions, East York Ontario, Canada)

increasing the contact area between the two opposing surfaces until the contact area sufficiently supports the load. Due to normal fatigue wear, the articular cartilage surface integrity is compromised, and subsequently, the thin lubrication film on the cartilage surface asperity area is damaged. As a consequence of cartilage surface deterioration, the cartilage surface integrity comprising primarily of tightly packed, parallel, tangential collagen fibres become weak, and exhibit decreased modulus of elasticity, decreased tensile strength and decreased wear resistance. Increased stress on the native articular cartilage adjacent to the affected area is also noted. Asperities may precede to frank lesions seen in aging or OA cartilage.

In vitro experiments investigating repeated compressive loads applied to the cartilage surface and repeated tensile loading (fatigue) have shown to decrease the tensile strength of cartilage collagen type II fibrils [335, 481–483]. The decreased tensile strength with repetitive loading at 65 N for 97,200 cycle preceded the surface damage [335]. However, under impulsive loads, the cartilage experiences a large lateral displacement, and this expansion is restrained by the subchondral bone that causes a high shear stress at the cartilage-bone interface.

1.6 Conclusions

Knee articular cartilage plays an essential role in the maintenance of normal synovial joint function by reducing friction, resisting compressive forces associated with mobility and distributing loads. However, the ability of cartilage to perform this function can be compromised by changes in tissue properties that occur with age and as a consequence of cartilage injuries (acute and chronic) and joint diseases such as osteoarthritis and rheumatoid arthritis. Disruption of the collagen network of the superficial zone has been shown to play a critical role in the early signs of knee cartilage osteoarthritis associated with aging. An understanding of articular cartilage structure-function relations is critical to better elucidate both disease processes and treatment strategies to repair or regenerate articular cartilage.

References

1. Kuettner KE, Aydelotte MB, Thonar EJ. Articular cartilage matrix and structure: a minireview. J Rheumatol Suppl. 1991;27:46–8.
2. Ogata K, Whiteside LA. Barrier to material transfer at the bone-cartilage interface: measurement with hydrogen gas in vivo. Clin Orthop Relat Res. 1979:273–6.
3. Visco DM, Van Sickle DC, Hill MA, Kincaid SA. The vascular supply of the chondro-epiphyses of the elbow joint in young swine. J Anat. 1989;163:215–29.
4. Clark JM. The structure of vascular channels in the subchondral plate. J Anat. 1990;171:105–15.
5. Levene C. The patterns of cartilage canals. J Anat. 1964;98:515–38.
6. Ghadially FN. Fine structure of joints. In: Sokoloff L, editor. The joints and synovial fluid. New York: Academic Press; 1978. p. 105–76.
7. Buckwalter JA, Mankin HJ. Articular cartilage: tissue design and chondrocyte-matrix interactions. Instr Course Lect. 1998;47:477–86.
8. van der Kraan PM, Buma P, van Kuppevelt T, van den Berg WB. Interaction of chondrocytes, extracellular matrix and growth factors: relevance for articular cartilage tissue engineering. Osteoarthritis Cartilage. 2002;10:631–7.
9. Hunziker EB, Quinn TM, Hauselmann HJ. Quantitative structural organization of normal adult human articular cartilage. Osteoarthritis Cartilage. 2002;10:564–72.
10. Goyal N, Gupta M, Joshi K. Ultrastructure of chondrocytes in osteoarthritic femoral articular cartilage. Kathmandu Univ Med J (KUMJ). 2013;11:221–5.
11. Quinn TM, Hauselmann HJ, Shintani N, Hunziker EB. Cell and matrix morphology in articular cartilage from adult human knee and ankle joints suggests depth-associated adaptations to biomechanical and anatomical roles. Osteoarthritis Cartilage. 2013;21:1904–12.
12. Poole AR. Cartilage in health and disease. In: OJK MC, Koopman WJ, editors. Arthritis and allied conditions: a textbook of rheumatology. Philadelphia: Lea and Febiger; 1993. p. 279–333.
13. Benninghoff A. Form un Bau der Gelenkknorpel in ihren Beziehungen zur Funktion. II. Der Aufbau des Gelenkknorpels in seinen Bezeihungen zur Funktion. Z Zellforsch Mikrosk Anat. 1925;2:783–862.
14. Poole CA. Articular cartilage chondrons: form, function and failure. J Anat. 1997;191(Pt 1):1–13.
15. Muir H. The chondrocyte, architect of cartilage. Biomechanics, structure, function and molecular biology of cartilage matrix macromolecules. Bioessays. 1995;17:1039–48.
16. Poole CA, Ayad S, Gilbert RT. Chondrons from articular cartilage. V. Immunohistochemical evaluation of type VI collagen organisation in isolated chondrons by light, confocal and electron microscopy. J Cell Sci. 1992;103(Pt 4):1101–10.

17. Poole CA, Ayad S, Schofield JR. Chondrons from articular cartilage: I. Immunolocalization of type VI collagen in the pericellular capsule of isolated canine tibial chondrons. J Cell Sci. 1988;90(Pt 4):635–43.
18. Poole CA, Gilbert RT, Herbage D, Hartmann DJ. Immunolocalization of type IX collagen in normal and spontaneously osteoarthritic canine tibial cartilage and isolated chondrons. Osteoarthritis Cartilage. 1997;5:191–204.
19. Poole CA, Flint MH, Beaumont BW. Morphological and functional interrelationships of articular cartilage matrices. J Anat. 1984;138(Pt 1):113–38.
20. Poole CA, Flint MH, Beaumont BW. Chondrons in cartilage: ultrastructural analysis of the pericellular microenvironment in adult human articular cartilages. J Orthop Res. 1987;5:509–22.
21. Eyre DR, Wu JJ, Apone S. A growing family of collagens in articular cartilage: identification of 5 genetically distinct types. J Rheumatol. 1987;14 Spec No:25–7.
22. Eyre DR. The collagens of articular cartilage. Semin Arthritis Rheum. 1991;21:2–11.
23. Eyre DR, Wu JJ, Woods PE. The cartilage collagens: structural and metabolic studies. J Rheumatol Suppl. 1991;27:49–51.
24. Maroudas A, Bayliss MT, Uchitel-Kaushansky N, Schneiderman R, Gilav E. Aggrecan turnover in human articular cartilage: use of aspartic acid racemization as a marker of molecular age. Arch Biochem Biophys. 1998;350:61–71.
25. Verzijl N, DeGroot J, Thorpe SR, Bank RA, Shaw JN, Lyons TJ, Bijlsma JW, Lafeber FP, Baynes JW, TeKoppele JM. Effect of collagen turnover on the accumulation of advanced glycation end products. J Biol Chem. 2000;275:39027–31.
26. Maroudas A, Palla G, Gilav E. Racemization of aspartic acid in human articular cartilage. Connect Tissue Res. 1992;28:161–9.
27. Glant TT, Hadhazy C, Mikecz K, Sipos A. Appearance and persistence of fibronectin in cartilage. Specific interaction of fibronectin with collagen type II. Histochemistry. 1985;82:149–58.
28. Burton-Wurster N, Horn VJ, Lust G. Immunohistochemical localization of fibronectin and chondronectin in canine articular cartilage. J Histochem Cytochem. 1988;36:581–8.
29. Durr J, Lammi P, Goodman SL, Aigner T, von der Mark K. Identification and immunolocalization of laminin in cartilage. Exp Cell Res. 1996;222:225–33.
30. Kvist AJ, Nystrom A, Hultenby K, Sasaki T, Talts JF, Aspberg A. The major basement membrane components localize to the chondrocyte pericellular matrix–a cartilage basement membrane equivalent? Matrix Biol. 2008;27:22–33.
31. Hyc A, Osiecka-Iwan A, Jozwiak J, Moskalewski S. The morphology and selected biological properties of articular cartilage. Ortop Traumatol Rehabil. 2001;3:151–62.
32. Muller G, Michel A, Altenburg E. COMP (cartilage oligomeric matrix protein) is synthesized in ligament, tendon, meniscus, and articular cartilage. Connect Tissue Res. 1998;39:233–44.
33. Hedbom E, Antonsson P, Hjerpe A, Aeschlimann D, Paulsson M, Rosa-Pimentel E, Sommarin Y, Wendel M, Oldberg A, Heinegard D. Cartilage matrix proteins. An acidic oligomeric protein (COMP) detected only in cartilage. J Biol Chem. 1992;267:6132–6.
34. Roughley PJ, Lee ER. Cartilage proteoglycans: structure and potential functions. Microsc Res Tech. 1994;28:385–97.
35. Han EH, Chen SS, Klisch SM, Sah RL. Contribution of proteoglycan osmotic swelling pressure to the compressive properties of articular cartilage. Biophys J. 2011;101:916–24.
36. Greene GW, Thapa R, Holt SA, Wang X, Garvey CJ, Tabor RF. Structure and property changes in self-assembled lubricin layers induced by calcium ion interactions. Langmuir. 2017;33(10):2559–70.
37. Iozzo RV, Schaefer L. Proteoglycan form and function: a comprehensive nomenclature of proteoglycans. Matrix Biol. 2015;42:11–55.
38. Matsumoto K, Kamiya N, Suwan K, Atsumi F, Shimizu K, Shinomura T, Yamada Y, Kimata K, Watanabe H. Identification and characterization of versican/PG-M aggregates in cartilage. J Biol Chem. 2006;281:18257–63.
39. Kao WW, Funderburgh JL, Xia Y, Liu CY, Conrad GW. Focus on molecules: lumican. Exp Eye Res. 2006;82:3–4.
40. Rodriguez E, Roughley P. Link protein can retard the degradation of hyaluronan in proteoglycan aggregates. Osteoarthritis Cartilage. 2006;14(8):823–9.
41. Iacob S, Cs-Szabo G. Biglycan regulates the expression of EGF receptors through EGF signaling pathways in human articular chondrocytes. Connect Tissue Res. 2010;51:347–58.
42. Roughley PJ. The structure and function of cartilage proteoglycans. Eur Cell Mater. 2006;12:92–101.
43. Sztrolovics RJ, Grover J, Cs-Szabo G, Shi SL, Zhang Y, Mort JS, et al. The characterization of versican and its message in human articular cartilage and intervertebral disc. J Orthop Res. 2002;20(2):257–66.
44. Knudson CB, Knudson W. Cartilage proteoglycans. Semin Cell Dev Biol. 2001;12:69–78.
45. Roughley PJ. Articular cartilage and changes in arthritis: noncollagenous proteins and proteoglycans in the extracellular matrix of cartilage. Arthritis Res. 2001;3:342–7.
46. Poole AR, Rosenberg LC, Reiner A, Ionescu M, Bogoch E, Roughley PJ. Contents and distributions of the proteoglycans decorin and biglycan in normal and osteoarthritic human articular cartilage. J Orthop Res. 1996;14:681–9.
47. Scott JE. Proteodermatan and proteokeratan sulfate (decorin, lumican/fibromodulin) proteins are horseshoe shaped. Implications for their interactions with collagen. Biochemistry. 1996;35:8795–9.

48. Tang LH, Buckwalter JA, Rosenberg LC. Effect of link protein concentration on articular cartilage proteoglycan aggregation. J Orthop Res. 1996;14(2):334–9.
49. SundarRaj N, Fite D, Ledbetter S, Chakravarti S, Hassell JR. Perlecan is a component of cartilage matrix and promotes chondrocyte attachment. J Cell Sci. 1995;108(Pt 7):2663–72.
50. Kahn A, Taitz AD, Pottenger LA, Alberton GM. Effect of link protein and free hyaluronic acid binding region on spacing of proteoglycans in aggregates. J Orthop Res. 1994;12:612–20.
51. Grover J, Roughley PJ. The expression of functional link protein in a baculovirus system: analysis of mutants lacking the A, B and B' domains. Biochem J. 1994;300(Pt 2):317–24.
52. Hedlund H, Mengarelli-Widholm S, Heinegard D, Reinholt FP, Svensson O. Fibromodulin distribution and association with collagen. Matrix Biol. 1994;14:227–32.
53. Bianco P, Fisher LW, Young MF, Termine JD, Robey PG. Expression and localization of the two small proteoglycans biglycan and decorin in developing human skeletal and non-skeletal tissues. J Histochem Cytochem. 1990;38:1549–63.
54. Neame PJ, Choi HU, Rosenberg LC. The primary structure of the core protein of the small, leucine-rich proteoglycan (PG I) from bovine articular cartilage. J Biol Chem. 1989;264:8653–61.
55. Rosenberg LC, Choi HU, Tang LH, Johnson TL, Pal S, Webber C, et al. Isolation of dermatan sulfate proteoglycans from mature bovine articular cartilages. J Biol Chem. 1985;260(10):6304–13.
56. Ryu J, Towle CA, Treadwell BV. Characterisation of human articular cartilage link proteins from normal and osteoarthritic cartilage. Ann Rheum Dis. 1982;41(2):164–7.
57. Roughley PJ, Poole AR, Mort JS. The heterogeneity of link proteins isolated from human articular cartilage proteoglycan aggregates. J Biol Chem. 1982;257(20):11908–14.
58. Oldberg A, Kjellén L, Höök M. Cell-surface heparan sulfate. Isolation and characterization of a proteoglycan from rat liver membranes. J Biol Chem. 1979;254(17):8505–10.
59. Hardingham TE. The role of link-protein in the structure of cartilage proteoglycan aggregates. Biochem J. 1979;177(1):237–47.
60. Ratcliffe A, Mow V. Articular cartilage. In: Comper WD, editor. Extracellular matrix. Amsterdam: Harwood Academic Publishers; 1996. p. S234–302.
61. Melrose J, Smith S, Cake M, Read R, Whitelock J. Perlecan displays variable spatial and temporal immunolocalisation patterns in the articular and growth plate cartilages of the ovine stifle joint. Histochem Cell Biol. 2005;123:561–71.
62. Kiani C, Chen L, Wu YJ, Yee AJ, Yang BB. Structure and function of aggrecan. Cell Res. 2002;12:19–32.
63. Knudson CB, Knudson W. Hyaluronan and CD44: modulators of chondrocyte metabolism. Clin Orthop Relat Res. 2004:S152–62.
64. Knudson CB. Hyaluronan receptor-directed assembly of chondrocyte pericellular matrix. J Cell Biol. 1993;120:825–34.
65. Knudson W, Ishizuka S, Terabe K, Askew EB, Knudson CB. The pericellular hyaluronan of articular chondrocytes. Matrix Biol. 2019;78-79:32–46.
66. Heinegard D. Proteoglycans and more–from molecules to biology. Int J Exp Pathol. 2009;90:575–86.
67. Fosang AJ, Hardingham TE. Isolation of the N-terminal globular protein domains from cartilage proteoglycans. Identification of G2 domain and its lack of interaction with hyaluronate and link protein. Biochem J. 1989;261:801–9.
68. Aspberg A. The different roles of aggrecan interaction domains. J Histochem Cytochem. 2012;60(12):987–96.
69. Yasumoto T, Bird JL, Sugimoto K, Mason RM, Bayliss MT. The G1 domain of aggrecan released from porcine articular cartilage forms stable complexes with hyaluronan/link protein. Rheumatology (Oxford). 2003;42(2):336–42.
70. Kiani C, Lee V, Cao L, Chen L, Wu Y, Zhang Y, et al. Roles of aggrecan domains in biosynthesis, modification by glycosaminoglycans and product secretion. Biochem J. 2001;354(Pt 1):199–207.
71. Watanabe H, Cheung SC, Itano N, Kimata K, Yamada Y. Identification of hyaluronan-binding domains of aggrecan. J Biol Chem. 1997;272(44): 28057–65.
72. Hardingham TE, Fosang AJ. The structure of aggrecan and its turnover in cartilage. J Rheumatol Suppl. 1995;43:86–90.
73. Neame PJ, Barry FP. The link proteins. Experientia. 1993;49:393–402.
74. Aspberg A, Miura R, Bourdoulous S, Shimonaka M, Heinegard D, Schachner M, Ruoslahti E, Yamaguchi Y. The C-type lectin domains of lecticans, a family of aggregating chondroitin sulfate proteoglycans, bind tenascin-R by protein-protein interactions independent of carbohydrate moiety. Proc Natl Acad Sci U S A. 1997;94:10116–21.
75. Kimata K, Oike Y, Tani K, Shinomura T, Yamagata M, Uritani M, et al. A large chondroitin sulfate proteoglycan (PG-M) synthesized before chondrogenesis in the limb bud of chick embryo. J Biol Chem. 1986;261(29):13517–25.
76. Shepard JB, Krug HA, LaFoon BA, Hoffman S, Capehart AA. Versican expression during synovial joint morphogenesis. Int J Biol Sci. 2007;3(6):380–4.
77. Taylor DW, Ahmed N, Parreno J, Lunstrum GP, Gross AE, Diamandis EP, et al. Collagen type XII and versican are present in the early stages of cartilage tissue formation by both redifferentating passaged and primary chondrocytes. Tissue Eng Part A. 2015;21(3–4):683–93.
78. Zimmermann DR, Ruoslahti E. Multiple domains of the large fibroblast proteoglycan, versican. EMBO J. 1989;8(10):2975–81.

79. Matsumoto K, Shionyu M, Go M, Shimizu K, Shinomura T, Kimata K, et al. Distinct interaction of versican/PG-M with hyaluronan and link protein. J Biol Chem. 2003;278(42):41205–12.
80. Lee GM, Johnstone B, Jacobson K, et al. The dynamic structure of the pericellular matrix on living cells. J Cell Biol. 1993;123(6 Pt 2):1899–907.
81. Wight TN. Versican: a versatile extracellular matrix proteoglycan in cell biology. Curr Opin Cell Biol. 2002;14(5):617–23.
82. Timpl R. Proteoglycans of basement membranes. EXS. 1994;70:123–44.
83. Melrose J, Roughley P, Knox S, Smith S, Lord M, Whitelock J. The structure, location, and function of perlecan, a prominent pericellular proteoglycan of fetal, postnatal, and mature hyaline cartilages. J Biol Chem. 2006;281:36905–14.
84. Dreyfuss JL, Regatieri CV, Jarrouge TR, Cavalheiro RP, Sampaio LO, Nader HB. Heparan sulfate proteoglycans: structure, protein interactions and cell signaling. An Acad Bras Cienc. 2009;81:409–29.
85. Scott JE. Proteoglycan-fibrillar collagen interactions. Biochem J. 1988;252:313–23.
86. Scott JE, Glanville RW. Homologous sequences in fibrillar collagens may be proteoglycan binding sites. Biochem Soc Trans. 1993;21:123S.
87. Oldberg A, Antonsson P, Lindblom K, Heinegard D. A collagen-binding 59-kd protein (fibromodulin) is structurally related to the small interstitial proteoglycans PG-S1 and PG-S2 (decorin). EMBO J. 1989;8:2601–4.
88. Noyori K, Takagi T, Jasin HE. Characterization of the macromolecular components of the articular cartilage surface. Rheumatol Int. 1998;18:71–7.
89. Blochberger TC, Cornuet PK, Hassell JR. Isolation and partial characterization of lumican and decorin from adult chicken corneas. A keratan sulfate-containing isoform of decorin is developmentally regulated. J Biol Chem. 1992;267:20613–9.
90. Grover J, Chen XN, Korenberg JR, Roughley PJ. The human lumican gene. Organization, chromosomal location, and expression in articular cartilage. J Biol Chem. 1995;270:21942–9.
91. Melching LI, Roughley PJ. Modulation of keratan sulfate synthesis on lumican by the action of cytokines on human articular chondrocytes. Matrix Biol. 1999;18:381–90.
92. Neame PJ, Sommarin Y, Boynton RE, Heinegard D. The structure of a 38-kDa leucine-rich protein (chondroadherin) isolated from bovine cartilage. J Biol Chem. 1994;269:21547–54.
93. Mansson B, Wenglen C, Morgelin M, Saxne T, Heinegard D. Association of chondroadherin with collagen type II. J Biol Chem. 2001;276:32883–8.
94. Grover J, Chen XN, Korenberg JR, Roughley PJ. The structure and chromosome location of the human chondroadherin gene (CHAD). Genomics. 1997;45:379–85.
95. Haglund L, Tillgren V, Addis L, Wenglen C, Recklies A, Heinegard D. Identification and characterization of the integrin alpha2beta1 binding motif in chondroadherin mediating cell attachment. J Biol Chem. 2011;286:3925–34.
96. Camper L, Heinegard D, Lundgren-Akerlund E. Integrin alpha2beta1 is a receptor for the cartilage matrix protein chondroadherin. J Cell Biol. 1997;138:1159–67.
97. Uitto J, Allan RE, Polak KL. Conversion of type II procollagen to collagen. Extracellular removal of the amino-terminal and carboxy-terminal extensions without a preferential sequence. Eur J Biochem. 1979;99:97–103.
98. Prockop DJ, Kivirikko KI, Tuderman L, Guzman NA. The biosynthesis of collagen and its disorders (first of two parts). N Engl J Med. 1979;301:13–23.
99. Yang C, Notbohm H, Acil Y, Heifeng R, Bierbaum S, Muller PK. In vitro fibrillogenesis of collagen II from pig vitreous humour. Biochem J. 1995;306(Pt 3):871–5.
100. Murdoch AD, Hardingham TE, Eyre DR, Fernandes RJ. The development of a mature collagen network in cartilage from human bone marrow stem cells in Transwell culture. Matrix Biol. 2016;50:16–26.
101. Wu JJ, Eyre DR. Identification of hydroxypyridinium cross-linking sites in type II collagen of bovine articular cartilage. Biochemistry. 1984;23:1850–7.
102. Responte DJ, Natoli RM, Athanasiou KA. Collagens of articular cartilage: structure, function, and importance in tissue engineering. Crit Rev Biomed Eng. 2007;35:363–411.
103. Eyre D. Collagen of articular cartilage. Arthritis Res. 2002;4:30–5.
104. Luo Y, Sinkeviciute D, He Y, Karsdal M, Henrotin Y, Mobasheri A, Onnerfjord P, Bay-Jensen A. The minor collagens in articular cartilage. Protein Cell. 2017;8:560–72.
105. Eyre DR, Apon S, Wu JJ, Ericsson LH, Walsh KA. Collagen type IX: evidence for covalent linkages to type II collagen in cartilage. FEBS Lett. 1987;220:337–41.
106. Cremer MA, Rosloniec EF, Kang AH. The cartilage collagens: a review of their structure, organization, and role in the pathogenesis of experimental arthritis in animals and in human rheumatic disease. J Mol Med (Berl). 1998;76:275–88.
107. Mendler M, Eich-Bender SG, Vaughan L, Winterhalter KH, Bruckner P. Cartilage contains mixed fibrils of collagen types II, IX, and XI. J Cell Biol. 1989;108:191–7.
108. Wu JJ, Lark MW, Chun LE, Eyre DR. Sites of stromelysin cleavage in collagen types II, IX, X, and XI of cartilage. J Biol Chem. 1991;266(9):5625–8.
109. Plumb DA, Ferrara L, Torbica T, Knowles L, Mironov A Jr, Kadler KE, Briggs MD, Boot-Handford RP. Collagen XXVII organises the pericellular matrix in the growth plate. PLoS One. 2011;6:e29422.
110. Hjorten R, Hansen U, Underwood RA, Telfer HE, Fernandes RJ, Krakow D, Sebald E, Wachsmann-Hogiu S, Bruckner P, Jacquet R, Landis WJ, Byers PH, Pace JM. Type XXVII collagen at the transition

of cartilage to bone during skeletogenesis. Bone. 2007;41:535–42.
111. Boot-Handford RP, Tuckwell DS, Plumb DA, Rock CF, Poulsom R. A novel and highly conserved collagen (pro(alpha)1(XXVII)) with a unique expression pattern and unusual molecular characteristics establishes a new clade within the vertebrate fibrillar collagen family. J Biol Chem. 2003;278:31067–77.
112. Pace JM, Corrado M, Missero C, Byers PH. Identification, characterization and expression analysis of a new fibrillar collagen gene, COL27A1. Matrix Biol. 2003;22:3–14.
113. Zelenski NA, Leddy HA, Sanchez-Adams J, Zhang J, Bonaldo P, Liedtke W, Guilak F. Type VI collagen regulates pericellular matrix properties, chondrocyte swelling, and mechanotransduction in mouse articular cartilage. Arthritis Rheumatol. 2015;67:1286–94.
114. Wilusz RE, Sanchez-Adams J, Guilak F. The structure and function of the pericellular matrix of articular cartilage. Matrix Biol. 2014;39:25–32.
115. Peters HC, Otto TJ, Enders JT, Jin W, Moed BR, Zhang Z. The protective role of the pericellular matrix in chondrocyte apoptosis. Tissue Eng Part A. 2011;17:2017–24.
116. Hing WA, Sherwin AF, Poole CA. The influence of the pericellular microenvironment on the chondrocyte response to osmotic challenge. Osteoarthritis Cartilage. 2002;10:297–307.
117. Brown JC, Golbik R, Mann K, Timpl R. Structure and stability of the triple-helical domains of human collagen XIV. Matrix Biol. 1994;14:287–95.
118. Bidanset DJ, Guidry C, Rosenberg LC, Choi HU, Timpl R, Hook M. Binding of the proteoglycan decorin to collagen type VI. J Biol Chem. 1992;267:5250–6.
119. Engel J, Furthmayr H, Odermatt E, von der Mark H, Aumailley M, Fleischmajer R, Timpl R. Structure and macromolecular organization of type VI collagen. Ann N Y Acad Sci. 1985;460:25–37.
120. Foldager CB, Toh WS, Gomoll AH, Olsen BR, Spector M. Distribution of basement membrane molecules, laminin and collagen type IV, in normal and degenerated cartilage tissues. Cartilage. 2014;5:123–32.
121. Johansson C, Butkowski R, Wieslander J. The structural organization of type IV collagen. Identification of three NC1 populations in the glomerular basement membrane. J Biol Chem. 1992;267:24533–7.
122. Parsons P, Gilbert SJ, Vaughan-Thomas A, Sorrell DA, Notman R, Bishop M, Hayes AJ, Mason DJ, Duance VC. Type IX collagen interacts with fibronectin providing an important molecular bridge in articular cartilage. J Biol Chem. 2011;286:34986–97.
123. Budde B, Blumbach K, Ylostalo J, Zaucke F, Ehlen HW, Wagener R, Ala-Kokko L, Paulsson M, Bruckner P, Grassel S. Altered integration of matrilin-3 into cartilage extracellular matrix in the absence of collagen IX. Mol Cell Biol. 2005;25:10465–78.
124. Olsen BR. Collagen IX. Int J Biochem Cell Biol. 1997;29:555–8.
125. Diab M, Wu JJ, Eyre DR. Collagen type IX from human cartilage: a structural profile of intermolecular cross-linking sites. Biochem J. 1996;314(Pt 1):327–32.
126. Ichimura S, Wu JJ, Eyre DR. Two-dimensional peptide mapping of cross-linked type IX collagen in human cartilage. Arch Biochem Biophys. 2000;378(1):33–9. (Move to Collagen IX).
127. Wu JJ, Eyre DR. Cartilage type IX collagen is cross-linked by hydroxypyridinium residues. Biochem Biophys Res Commun. 1984;123:1033–9.
128. Wu JJ, Eyre DR. Covalent interactions of type IX collagen in cartilage. Connect Tissue Res. 1989;20:241–6.
129. Wu JJ, Woods PE, Eyre DR. Identification of cross-linking sites in bovine cartilage type IX collagen reveals an antiparallel type II-type IX molecular relationship and type IX to type IX bonding. J Biol Chem. 1992;267:23007–14.
130. Bruckner P, Mendler M, Steinmann B, Huber S, Winterhalter KH. The structure of human collagen type IX and its organization in fetal and infant cartilage fibrils. J Biol Chem. 1988;263:16911–7.
131. Bruckner P, van der Rest M. Structure and function of cartilage collagens. Microsc Res Tech. 1994;28:378–84.
132. Shen G. The role of type X collagen in facilitating and regulating endochondral ossification of articular cartilage. Orthod Craniofac Res. 2005;8:11–7.
133. Luckman SP, Rees E, Kwan AP. Partial characterization of cell-type X collagen interactions. Biochem J. 2003;372:485–93.
134. Lammi PE, Lammi MJ, Hyttinen MM, Panula H, Kiviranta I, Helminen HJ. Site-specific immunostaining for type X collagen in noncalcified articular cartilage of canine stifle knee joint. Bone. 2002;31:690–6.
135. Rucklidge GJ, Milne G, Robins SP. Collagen type X: a component of the surface of normal human, pig, and rat articular cartilage. Biochem Biophys Res Commun. 1996;224:297–302.
136. Mundlos S, Zabel B. Developmental expression of human cartilage matrix protein. Dev Dyn. 1994;199:241–52.
137. Kirsch T, Pfaffle M. Selective binding of anchorin CII (annexin V) to type II and X collagen and to chondrocalcin (C-propeptide of type II collagen). Implications for anchoring function between matrix vesicles and matrix proteins. FEBS Lett. 1992;310:143–7.
138. Gannon JM, Walker G, Fischer M, Carpenter R, Thompson RC Jr, Oegema TR Jr. Localization of type X collagen in canine growth plate and adult canine articular cartilage. J Orthop Res. 1991;9:485–94.
139. Chiquet M, Birk DE, Bonnemann CG, Koch M. Collagen XII: protecting bone and muscle integrity

by organizing collagen fibrils. Int J Biochem Cell Biol. 2014;53:51–4.
140. Gregory KE, Keene DR, Tufa SF, Lunstrum GP, Morris NP. Developmental distribution of collagen type XII in cartilage: association with articular cartilage and the growth plate. J Bone Miner Res. 2001;16:2005–16.
141. Watt SL, Lunstrum GP, McDonough AM, Keene DR, Burgeson RE, Morris NP. Characterization of collagen types XII and XIV from fetal bovine cartilage. J Biol Chem. 1992;267:20093–9.
142. van der Rest M, Garrone R. Collagen family of proteins. FASEB J. 1991;5:2814–23.
143. Yamagata M, Yamada KM, Yamada SS, Shinomura T, Tanaka H, Nishida Y, Obara M, Kimata K. The complete primary structure of type XII collagen shows a chimeric molecule with reiterated fibronectin type III motifs, von Willebrand factor A motifs, a domain homologous to a noncollagenous region of type IX collagen, and short collagenous domains with an Arg-Gly-Asp site. J Cell Biol. 1991;115:209–21.
144. Giry-Lozinguez C, Aubert-Foucher E, Penin F, Deleage G, Dublet B, van der Rest M. Identification and characterization of a heparin binding site within the NC1 domain of chicken collagen XIV. Matrix Biol. 1998;17:145–9.
145. Aubert-Foucher E, Font B, Eichenberger D, Goldschmidt D, Lethias C, van der Rest M. Purification and characterization of native type XIV collagen. J Biol Chem. 1992;267(22):15759–64.
146. Grassel S, Bauer RJ. Collagen XVI in health and disease. Matrix Biol. 2013;32:64–73.
147. Kassner A, Hansen U, Miosge N, Reinhardt DP, Aigner T, Bruckner-Tuderman L, Bruckner P, Grassel S. Discrete integration of collagen XVI into tissue-specific collagen fibrils or beaded microfibrils. Matrix Biol. 2003;22:131–43.
148. Kassner A, Tiedemann K, Notbohm H, Ludwig T, Morgelin M, Reinhardt DP, Chu ML, Bruckner P, Grassel S. Molecular structure and interaction of recombinant human type XVI collagen. J Mol Biol. 2004;339:835–53.
149. Myers JC, Yang H, D'Ippolito JA, Presente A, Miller MK, Dion AS. The triple-helical region of human type XIX collagen consists of multiple collagenous subdomains and exhibits limited sequence homology to alpha 1(XVI). J Biol Chem. 1994;269:18549–57.
150. Yamaguchi N, Kimura S, McBride OW, Hori H, Yamada Y, Kanamori T, et al. Molecular cloning and partial characterization of a novel collagen chain, alpha 1(XVI), consisting of repetitive collagenous domains and cysteine-containing non-collagenous segments. J Biochem. 1992;112(6):856–63.
151. Koch M, Schulze J, Hansen U, Ashwodt T, Keene DR, Brunken WJ, Burgeson RE, Bruckner P, Bruckner-Tuderman L. A novel marker of tissue junctions, collagen XXII. J Biol Chem. 2004;279:22514–21.
152. Eyre DR, Weis MA, Wu JJ. Articular cartilage collagen: an irreplaceable framework? Eur Cell Mater. 2006;12:57–63.
153. Akizuki S, Mow VC, Muller F, Pita JC, Howell DS, Manicourt DH. Tensile properties of human knee joint cartilage: I. Influence of ionic conditions, weight bearing, and fibrillation on the tensile modulus. J Orthop Res. 1986;4:379–92.
154. Mayne R. Cartilage collagens. What is their function, and are they involved in articular disease? Arthritis Rheum. 1989;32:241–6.
155. Hambach L, Neureiter D, Zeiler G, Kirchner T, Aigner T. Severe disturbance of the distribution and expression of type VI collagen chains in osteoarthritic articular cartilage. Arthritis Rheum. 1998;41:986–96.
156. Dublet B, van der Rest M. Type XIV collagen, a new homotrimeric molecule extracted from fetal bovine skin and tendon, with a triple helical disulfide-bonded domain homologous to type IX and type XII collagens. J Biol Chem. 1991;266:6853–8.
157. Shea MK, Kritchevsky SB, Hsu FC, Nevitt M, Booth SL, Kwoh CK, et al. The association between vitamin K status and knee osteoarthritis features in older adults: the Health, Aging and Body Composition Study. Osteoarthritis Cartilage. 2015;23(3):370–8.
158. Viegas CS, Cavaco S, Neves PL, Ferreira A, João A, Williamson MK, et al. Gla-rich protein is a novel vitamin K-dependent protein present in serum that accumulates at sites of pathological calcifications. Am J Pathol. 2009;175(6):2288–98.
159. Loeser RF. Integrin-mediated attachment of articular chondrocytes to extracellular matrix proteins. Arthritis Rheum. 1993;36:1103–10.
160. Loeser R, Carlson CS, Tulli H, Jerome WG, Miller L, Wallin R. Articular-cartilage matrix gamma-carboxyglutamic acid-containing protein. Characterization and immunolocalization. Biochem J. 1992;282(Pt 1):1–6.
161. Loeser RF Jr, Wallin R. Vitamin K-dependent carboxylation in articular chondrocytes. Connect Tissue Res. 1991;26:135–44.
162. Loeser RF, Wallin R. Cell adhesion to matrix Gla protein and its inhibition by an Arg-Gly-Asp-containing peptide. J Biol Chem. 1992;267:9459–62.
163. Klatt AR, Becker AK, Neacsu CD, Paulsson M, Wagener R. The matrilins: modulators of extracellular matrix assembly. Int J Biochem Cell Biol. 2011;43(3):320–30.
164. Makihira S, Yan W, Ohno S, Kawamoto T, Fujimoto K, Okimura A, et al. Enhancement of cell adhesion and spreading by a cartilage-specific noncollagenous protein, cartilage matrix protein (CMP/Matrilin-1), via integrin alpha1beta1. J Biol Chem. 1999;274(16):11417–23.
165. Argraves WS, Deák F, Sparks KJ, Kiss I, Goetinck PF. Structural features of cartilage matrix protein deduced from cDNA. Proc Natl Acad Sci U S A. 1987;84(2):464–8.
166. Paulsson M, Heinegard D. Noncollagenous cartilage proteins current status of an emerging research field. Coll Relat Res. 1984;4:219–29.
167. Zhang S, Peng J, Guo Y, Javidiparsijani S, Wang G, Wang Y, Liu H, Liu J, Luo J. Matrilin-2 is a widely distributed extracellular matrix protein and a potential

biomarker in the early stage of osteoarthritis in articular cartilage. Biomed Res Int. 2014;2014:986127.
168. Piecha D, Wiberg C, Mörgelin M, Reinhardt DP, Deák F, Maurer P, et al. Matrilin-2 interacts with itself and with other extracellular matrix proteins. Biochem J. 2002;367(Pt 3):715–21.
169. Piecha D, Muratoglu S, Mörgelin M, Hauser N, Studer D, Kiss I, et al. Matrilin-2, a large, oligomeric matrix protein, is expressed by a great variety of cells and forms fibrillar networks. J Biol Chem. 1999;274(19):13353–61.
170. Pullig O, Weseloh G, Klatt AR, Wagener R, Swoboda B. Matrilin-3 in human articular cartilage: increased expression in osteoarthritis. Osteoarthritis Cartilage. 2002;10:253–63.
171. Wagener R, Kobbe B, Paulsson M. Primary structure of matrilin-3, a new member of a family of extracellular matrix proteins related to cartilage matrix protein (matrilin-1) and von Willebrand factor. FEBS Lett. 1997;413(1):129–34.
172. Lucic D, Mollenhauer J, Kilpatrick KE, Cole AA. N-telopeptide of type II collagen interacts with annexin V on human chondrocytes. Connect Tissue Res. 2003;44:225–39.
173. Kurtis MS, Tu BP, Gaya OA, Mollenhauer J, Knudson W, Loeser RF, et al. Mechanisms of chondrocyte adhesion to cartilage: role of beta1-integrins, CD44, and annexin V. J Orthop Res. 2001;19(6):1122–30.
174. Mollenhauer J, Bee JA, Lizarbe MA, von der Mark K. Role of anchorin CII, a 31,000-mol-wt membrane protein, in the interaction of chondrocytes with type II collagen. J Cell Biol. 1984;98:1572–9.
175. Mollenhauer J, Mok MT, King KB, Gupta M, Chubinskaya S, Koepp H, Cole AA. Expression of anchorin CII (cartilage annexin V) in human young, normal adult, and osteoarthritic cartilage. J Histochem Cytochem. 1999;47:209–20.
176. Hendrickx S, Thomas P, Preston BN, Stanton PG, Van Damme MP. Partial characterization of matrix components interacting with cartilage proteoglycans. Arch Biochem Biophys. 2001;390:186–94.
177. Poole AR, Rosenberg LC. Chondrocalcin and the calcification of cartilage. A review. Clin Orthop Relat Res. 1986;208:114–8.
178. Johnson K, Farley D, Hu SI, Terkeltaub R. One of two chondrocyte-expressed isoforms of cartilage intermediate-layer protein functions as an insulin-like growth factor 1 antagonist. Arthritis Rheum. 2003;48:1302–14.
179. Lorenzo P, Bayliss MT, Heinegard D. A novel cartilage protein (CILP) present in the mid-zone of human articular cartilage increases with age. J Biol Chem. 1998;273:23463–8.
180. Raj A, Wang M, Liu C, Ali L, Karlsson NG, Claesson PM, et al. Molecular synergy in biolubrication: the role of cartilage oligomeric matrix protein (COMP) in surface-structuring of lubricin. J Colloid Interface Sci. 2017;495:200–6.
181. Newton G, Weremowicz S, Morton CC, Copeland NG, Gilbert DJ, Jenkins NA, Lawler J. Characterization of human and mouse cartilage oligomeric matrix protein. Genomics. 1994;24:435–9.
182. Connor JR, Dodds RA, Emery JG, Kirkpatrick RB, Rosenberg M, Gowen M. Human cartilage glycoprotein 39 (HCgp-39) mRNA expression in adult and fetal chondrocytes, osteoblasts and osteocytes by in-situ hybridization. Osteoarthritis Cartilage. 2000;8(2):87–95.
183. Harvey S, Weisman M, O'Dell J, Scott T, Krusemeier M, Visor J, Swindlehurst C. Chondrex: new marker of joint disease. Clin Chem. 1998;44:509–16.
184. Hakala BE, White C, Recklies AD. Human cartilage gp-39, a major secretory product of articular chondrocytes and synovial cells, is a mammalian member of a chitinase protein family. J Biol Chem. 1993;268:25803–10.
185. Martin JA, Miller BA, Scherb MB, Lembke LA, Buckwalter JA. Co-localization of insulin-like growth factor binding protein 3 and fibronectin in human articular cartilage. Osteoarthritis Cartilage. 2002;10:556–63.
186. Pfander D, Rahmanzadeh R, Scheller EE. Presence and distribution of collagen II, collagen I, fibronectin, and tenascin in rabbit normal and osteoarthritic cartilage. J Rheumatol. 1999;26:386–94.
187. Piperno M, Reboul P, Hellio le Graverand MP, Peschard M, Annefeld M, Richard M, Vignon E. Osteoarthritic cartilage fibrillation is associated with a decrease in chondrocyte adhesion to fibronectin. Osteoarthritis Cartilage. 1998;6:393–9.
188. Evanko SP, Tammi MI, Tammi RH, Wight TN. Hyaluronan-dependent pericellular matrix. Adv Drug Deliv Rev. 2007;59:1351–65.
189. Ghert MA, Qi WN, Erickson HP, Block JA, Scully SP. Tenascin-C expression and distribution in cultured human chondrocytes and chondrosarcoma cells. J Orthop Res. 2002;20(4):834–41.
190. Savarese JJ, Erickson H, Scully SP. Articular chondrocyte tenascin-C production and assembly into de novo extracellular matrix. J Orthop Res. 1996;14:273–81.
191. Carsons S, Horn VJ. Chondronectin in human synovial fluid. Ann Rheum Dis. 1988;47:797–800.
192. Hewitt AT, Varner HH, Silver MH, Dessau W, Wilkes CM, Martin GR. The isolation and partial characterization of chondronectin, an attachment factor for chondrocytes. J Biol Chem. 1982;257:2330–4.
193. Hewitt AT, Varner HH, Silver MH, Martin GR. The role of chondronectin and cartilage proteoglycan in the attachment of chondrocytes to collagen. Prog Clin Biol Res. 1982;110 Pt B:25–33.
194. Salter DM, Godolphin JL, Gourlay MS. Chondrocyte heterogeneity: immunohistologically defined variation of integrin expression at different sites in human fetal knees. J Histochem Cytochem. 1995;43:447–57.
195. Loeser RF. Chondrocyte integrin expression and function. Biorheology. 2000;37:109–16.

196. Hagg R, Bruckner P, Hedbom E. Cartilage fibrils of mammals are biochemically heterogeneous: differential distribution of decorin and collagen IX. J Cell Biol. 1998;142:285–94.
197. Tondravi MM, Winterbottom N, Haudenschild DR, Goetinck PF. Cartilage matrix protein binds to collagen and plays a role in collagen fibrillogenesis. Prog Clin Biol Res. 1993;383B:515–22.
198. Kuhne SA, Neidhart M, Everson MP, Hantzschel H, Fine PR, Gay S, Hauselmann HJ, Gay RE. Persistent high serum levels of cartilage oligomeric matrix protein in a subgroup of patients with traumatic knee injury. Rheumatol Int. 1998;18:21–5.
199. Cranenburg EC, Koos R, Schurgers LJ, Magdeleyns EJ, Schoonbrood TH, Landewe RB, Brandenburg VM, Bekers O, Vermeer C. Characterisation and potential diagnostic value of circulating matrix Gla protein (MGP) species. Thromb Haemost. 2010;104:811–22.
200. Loeser RF. Modulation of integrin-mediated attachment of chondrocytes to extracellular matrix proteins by cations, retinoic acid, and transforming growth factor beta. Exp Cell Res. 1994;211:17–23.
201. Hauser N, Paulsson M. Native cartilage matrix protein (CMP). A compact trimer of subunits assembled via a coiled-coil alpha-helix. J Biol Chem. 1994;269:25747–53.
202. Zeineldin R, Ekborg S, Baker J. Oligomeric forms of the 148 kDa cartilage matrix protein. Biochem J. 1997;328(Pt 2):665–8.
203. Hauser N, Paulsson M, Heinegard D, Morgelin M. Interaction of cartilage matrix protein with aggrecan. Increased covalent cross-linking with tissue maturation. J Biol Chem. 1996;271:32247–52.
204. Okimura A, Okada Y, Makihira S, Pan H, Yu L, Tanne K, Imai K, Yamada H, Kawamoto T, Noshiro M, Yan W, Kato Y. Enhancement of cartilage matrix protein synthesis in arthritic cartilage. Arthritis Rheum. 1997;40:1029–36.
205. Klatt AR, Nitsche DP, Kobbe B, Morgelin M, Paulsson M, Wagener R. Molecular structure and tissue distribution of matrilin-3, a filament-forming extracellular matrix protein expressed during skeletal development. J Biol Chem. 2000;275:3999–4006.
206. Wu JJ, Eyre DR. Matrilin-3 forms disulfide-linked oligomers with matrilin-1 in bovine epiphyseal cartilage. J Biol Chem. 1998;273:17433–8.
207. Vincourt JB, Etienne S, Grossin L, Cottet J, Bantsimba-Malanda C, Netter P, Mainard D, Libante V, Gillet P, Magdalou J. Matrilin-3 switches from anti- to pro-anabolic upon integration to the extracellular matrix. Matrix Biol. 2012;31:290–8.
208. Kirsch T, Swoboda B, Nah H. Activation of annexin II and V expression, terminal differentiation, mineralization and apoptosis in human osteoarthritic cartilage. Osteoarthritis Cartilage. 2000;8:294–302.
209. Kim HJ, Kirsch T. Collagen/annexin V interactions regulate chondrocyte mineralization. J Biol Chem. 2008;283:10310–7.
210. Ea HK, Monceau V, Camors E, Cohen-Solal M, Charlemagne D, Liote F. Annexin 5 overexpression increased articular chondrocyte apoptosis induced by basic calcium phosphate crystals. Ann Rheum Dis. 2008;67:1617–25.
211. Niyibizi C, Wu JJ, Eyre DR. The carboxypropeptide trimer of type II collagen is a prominent component of immature cartilages and intervertebral-disc tissue. Biochim Biophys Acta. 1987;916:493–9.
212. Van der Rest M, Rosenberg LC, Olsen BR, Poole AR. Chondrocalcin is identical with the C-propeptide of type II procollagen. Biochem J. 1986;237:923–5.
213. Poole AR, Pidoux I, Reiner A, Choi H, Rosenberg LC. The association of a newly discovered protein, called chondrocalcin, with cartilage calcification. Acta Biol Hung. 1984;35:143–9.
214. Neame PJ, Tapp H, Azizan A. Noncollagenous, non-proteoglycan macromolecules of cartilage. Cell Mol Life Sci. 1999;55:1327–40.
215. Bantsimba-Malanda C, Cottet J, Netter P, Dumas D, Mainard D, Magdalou J, Vincourt JB. Chondrocalcin is internalized by chondrocytes and triggers cartilage destruction via an interleukin-1beta-dependent pathway. Matrix Biol. 2013;32:443–51.
216. Hirose J, Masuda I, Ryan LM. Expression of cartilage intermediate layer protein/nucleotide pyrophosphohydrolase parallels the production of extracellular inorganic pyrophosphate in response to growth factors and with aging. Arthritis Rheum. 2000;43:2703–11.
217. Tsuruha J, Masuko-Hongo K, Kato T, Sakata M, Nakamura H, Nishioka K. Implication of cartilage intermediate layer protein in cartilage destruction in subsets of patients with osteoarthritis and rheumatoid arthritis. Arthritis Rheum. 2001;44:838–45.
218. Yamakawa K, Iwasaki H, Masuda I, Ohjimi Y, Honda I, Iyama K, Shono E, Naito M, Kikuchi M. Cartilage intermediate layer protein expression in calcium pyrophosphate dihydrate crystal deposition disease. J Rheumatol. 2002;29:1746–53.
219. Hirose J, Ryan LM, Masuda I. Up-regulated expression of cartilage intermediate-layer protein and ANK in articular hyaline cartilage from patients with calcium pyrophosphate dihydrate crystal deposition disease. Arthritis Rheum. 2002;46:3218–29.
220. Oldberg A, Antonsson P, Lindblom K, Heinegard D. COMP (cartilage oligomeric matrix protein) is structurally related to the thrombospondins. J Biol Chem. 1992;267:22346–50.
221. Flowers SA, Kalamajski S, Ali L, Bjorkman LI, Raj JR, Aspberg A, Karlsson NG, Jin C. Cartilage oligomeric matrix protein forms protein complexes with synovial lubricin via non-covalent and covalent interactions. Osteoarthritis Cartilage. 2017;25:1496–504.
222. Roberts HM, Moore JP, Griffith-McGeever CL, Fortes MB, Thom JM. The effect of vigorous running and cycling on serum COMP, lubricin, and femoral cartilage thickness: a pilot study. Eur J Appl Physiol. 2016;116:1467–77.

223. DiCesare PE, Morgelin M, Carlson CS, Pasumarti S, Paulsson M. Cartilage oligomeric matrix protein: isolation and characterization from human articular cartilage. J Orthop Res. 1995;13:422–8.
224. Rock MJ, Holden P, Horton WA, Cohn DH. Cartilage oligomeric matrix protein promotes cell attachment via two independent mechanisms involving CD47 and alphaVbeta3 integrin. Mol Cell Biochem. 2010;338:215–24.
225. Motaung SC, Di Cesare PE, Reddi AH. Differential response of cartilage oligomeric matrix protein (COMP) to morphogens of bone morphogenetic protein/transforming growth factor-beta family in the surface, middle and deep zones of articular cartilage. J Tissue Eng Regen Med. 2011;5:e87–96.
226. Boeth H, MacMahon A, Poole AR, Buttgereit F, Onnerfjord P, Lorenzo P, Klint C, Pramhed A, Duda GN. Differences in biomarkers of cartilage matrix turnover and their changes over 2 years in adolescent and adult volleyball athletes. J Exp Orthop. 2017;4:7.
227. Cattano NM, Driban JB, Cameron KL, Sitler MR. Impact of physical activity and mechanical loading on biomarkers typically used in osteoarthritis assessment: current concepts and knowledge gaps. Ther Adv Musculoskelet Dis. 2017;9:11–21.
228. Neuman P, Dahlberg LE, Englund M, Struglics A. Concentrations of synovial fluid biomarkers and the prediction of knee osteoarthritis 16 years after anterior cruciate ligament injury. Osteoarthritis Cartilage. 2017;25:492–8.
229. Lorenzo P, Aspberg A, Saxne T, Onnerfjord P. Quantification of cartilage oligomeric matrix protein (COMP) and a COMP neoepitope in synovial fluid of patients with different joint disorders by novel automated assays. Osteoarthritis Cartilage. 2017;25(9):1436–42.
230. Hyldahl RD, Evans A, Kwon S, Ridge ST, Robinson E, Hopkins JT, Seeley MK. Running decreases knee intra-articular cytokine and cartilage oligomeric matrix concentrations: a pilot study. Eur J Appl Physiol. 2016;116:2305–14.
231. Erhart-Hledik JC, Favre J, Asay JL, Smith RL, Giori NJ, Mundermann A, Andriacchi TP. A relationship between mechanically-induced changes in serum cartilage oligomeric matrix protein (COMP) and changes in cartilage thickness after 5 years. Osteoarthritis Cartilage. 2012;20:1309–15.
232. Posey KL, Hecht JT. The role of cartilage oligomeric matrix protein (COMP) in skeletal disease. Curr Drug Targets. 2008;9:869–77.
233. Mundermann A, Dyrby CO, Andriacchi TP, King KB. Serum concentration of cartilage oligomeric matrix protein (COMP) is sensitive to physiological cyclic loading in healthy adults. Osteoarthritis Cartilage. 2005;13:34–8.
234. Kersting UG, Stubendorff JJ, Schmidt MC, Bruggemann GP. Changes in knee cartilage volume and serum COMP concentration after running exercise. Osteoarthritis Cartilage. 2005;13:925–34.
235. Volck B, Ostergaard K, Johansen JS, Garbarsch C, Price PA. The distribution of YKL-40 in osteoarthritic and normal human articular cartilage. Scand J Rheumatol. 1999;28:171–9.
236. Johansen JS, Jensen HS, Price PA. A new biochemical marker for joint injury. Analysis of YKL-40 in serum and synovial fluid. Br J Rheumatol. 1993;32:949–55.
237. Johansen JS, Hvolris J, Hansen M, Backer V, Lorenzen I, Price PA. Serum YKL-40 levels in healthy children and adults. Comparison with serum and synovial fluid levels of YKL-40 in patients with osteoarthritis or trauma of the knee joint. Br J Rheumatol. 1996;35:553–9.
238. Johansen JS, Olee T, Price PA, Hashimoto S, Ochs RL, Lotz M. Regulation of YKL-40 production by human articular chondrocytes. Arthritis Rheum. 2001;44:826–37.
239. De Ceuninck F, Pastoureau P, Bouet F, Bonnet J, Vanhoutte PM. Purification of guinea pig YKL40 and modulation of its secretion by cultured articular chondrocytes. J Cell Biochem. 1998;69:414–24.
240. Rejman JJ, Hurley WL. Isolation and characterization of a novel 39 kilodalton whey protein from bovine mammary secretions collected during the nonlactating period. Biochem Biophys Res Commun. 1988;150:329–34.
241. Zivanovic S, Rackov LP, Vojvodic D, Vucetic D. Human cartilage glycoprotein 39–biomarker of joint damage in knee osteoarthritis. Int Orthop. 2009;33:1165–70.
242. Jacques C, Recklies AD, Levy A, Berenbaum F. HC-gp39 contributes to chondrocyte differentiation by inducing SOX9 and type II collagen expressions. Osteoarthritis Cartilage. 2007;15:138–46.
243. Burton-Wurster N, Butler M, Harter S, Colombo C, Quintavalla J, Swartzendurber D, Arsenis C, Lust G. Presence of fibronectin in articular cartilage in two animal models of osteoarthritis. J Rheumatol. 1986;13:175–82.
244. Burton-Wurster N, Lust G. Fibronectin and water content of articular cartilage explants after partial depletion of proteoglycans. J Orthop Res. 1986;4:437–45.
245. Couchman JR, Austria MR, Woods A. Fibronectin-cell interactions. J Invest Dermatol. 1990;94:7S–14S.
246. Andresen Eguiluz RC, Cook SG, Brown CN, Wu F, Pacifici NJ, Bonassar LJ, Gourdon D. Fibronectin mediates enhanced wear protection of lubricin during shear. Biomacromolecules. 2015;16:2884–94.
247. Mackie EJ, Ramsey S. Expression of tenascin in joint-associated tissues during development and postnatal growth. J Anat. 1996;188(Pt 1):157–65.
248. Varner HH, Horn VJ, Martin GR, Hewitt AT. Chondronectin interactions with proteoglycan. Arch Biochem Biophys. 1986;244:824–30.
249. Pokharna HK, Monnier V, Boja B, Moskowitz RW. Lysyl oxidase and Maillard reaction-mediated crosslinks in aging and osteoarthritic rabbit cartilage. J Orthop Res. 1995;13:13–21.

250. Knott L, Bailey AJ. Collagen cross-links in mineralizing tissues: a review of their chemistry, function, and clinical relevance. Bone. 1998;22:181–7.
251. Frazer WD. The collagen crosslinks pyridinoline and deoxypyridinoline: a review of their biochemistry, physiology, measurement, and clinical applications. J Clin Ligand Assay. 1998;21:102–10.
252. Fujimoto D. Isolation and characterization of a fluorescent material in bovine achilles tendon collagen. Biochem Biophys Res Commun. 1977;76:1124–9.
253. Fujimoto D, Moriguchi T, Ishida T, Hayashi H. The structure of pyridinoline, a collagen crosslink. Biochem Biophys Res Commun. 1978;84:52–7.
254. Fujimoto D. Evidence for natural existence of pyridinoline crosslink in collagen. Biochem Biophys Res Commun. 1980;93:948–53.
255. Fujimoto D, Moriguchi T. Pyridinoline, a nonreducible crosslink of collagen. Quantitative determination, distribution, and isolation of a crosslinked peptide. J Biochem. 1978;83:863–7.
256. Moriguchi T, Fujimoto D. Age-related changes in the content of the collagen crosslink, pyridinoline. J Biochem. 1978;84:933–5.
257. Takahashi M, Kushida K, Hoshino H, Suzuki M, Sano M, Miyamoto S, Inoue T. Concentrations of pyridinoline and deoxypyridinoline in joint tissues from patients with osteoarthritis or rheumatoid arthritis. Ann Rheum Dis. 1996;55:324–7.
258. Takahashi M, Hoshino H, Kushida K, Inoue T. Direct measurement of crosslinks, pyridinoline, deoxypyridinoline, and pentosidine, in the hydrolysate of tissues using high-performance liquid chromatography. Anal Biochem. 1995;232:158–62.
259. Eyre DR, Dickson IR, Van Ness K. Collagen cross-linking in human bone and articular cartilage. Age-related changes in the content of mature hydroxypyridinium residues. Biochem J. 1988;252:495–500.
260. Fujimori E. Cross-linking and fluorescence changes of collagen by glycation and oxidation. Biochim Biophys Acta. 1989;998:105–10.
261. Bailey AJ, Paul RG, Knott L. Mechanisms of maturation and ageing of collagen. Mech Ageing Dev. 1998;106:1–56.
262. Sell DR, Monnier VM. End-stage renal disease and diabetes catalyze the formation of a pentose-derived crosslink from aging human collagen. J Clin Invest. 1990;85:380–4.
263. Grandhee SK, Monnier VM. Mechanism of formation of the Maillard protein cross-link pentosidine. Glucose, fructose, and ascorbate as pentosidine precursors. J Biol Chem. 1991;266:11649–53.
264. Sell DR, Monnier VM. Structure elucidation of a senescence cross-link from human extracellular matrix. Implication of pentoses in the aging process. J Biol Chem. 1989;264:21597–602.
265. Monnier VM. Nonenzymatic glycosylation, the Maillard reaction and the aging process. J Gerontol. 1990;45:B105–11.
266. Bank RA, Bayliss MT, Lafeber FP, Maroudas A, Tekoppele JM. Ageing and zonal variation in post-translational modification of collagen in normal human articular cartilage. The age-related increase in non-enzymatic glycation affects biomechanical properties of cartilage. Biochem J. 1998;330(Pt 1):345–51.
267. van Deemter M, Ponsioen TL, Bank RA, Snabel JM, van der Worp RJ, Hooymans JM, Los LI. Pentosidine accumulates in the aging vitreous body: a gender effect. Exp Eye Res. 2009;88:1043–50.
268. Van der Korst JK, Skoloff L, Miller EJ. Senescent pigmentation of cartilage and degenerative joint disease. Arch Pathol. 1968;86:40–7.
269. Inerot S, Heinegard D, Audell L, Olsson SE. Articular-cartilage proteoglycans in aging and osteoarthritis. Biochem J. 1978;169:143–56.
270. Aydelotte MB, Greenhill RR, Kuettner KE. Differences between sub-populations of cultured bovine articular chondrocytes. II. Proteoglycan metabolism. Connect Tissue Res. 1988;18:223–34.
271. Aydelotte MB, Kuettner KE. Differences between sub-populations of cultured bovine articular chondrocytes. I. Morphology and cartilage matrix production. Connect Tissue Res. 1988;18:205–22.
272. Mow VC, Ratcliffe A, Poole AR. Cartilage and diarthrodial joints as paradigms for hierarchical materials and structures. Biomaterials. 1992;13:67–97.
273. Mow VC, Gu WY, Chen FH. Structure and function of articular cartilage and meniscus. In: Mow VC, Huiskes R, editors. Basic orthopaedic biomechanics and mechano-biology. Philadelphia: Lippincott, Williams & Wilkins; 2003. p. 181–258.
274. Minns RJ, Steven FS. The collagen fibril organization in human articular cartilage. J Anat. 1977;123:437–57.
275. Weiss C, Rosenberg L, Helfet AJ. An ultrastructural study of normal young adult human articular cartilage. J Bone Joint Surg Am. 1968;50:663–74.
276. Jeffery AK, Blunn GW, Archer CW, Bentley G. Three-dimensional collagen architecture in bovine articular cartilage. J Bone Joint Surg. 1991;73:795–801.
277. Xu Y, Pritzker KP, Cruz TF. Characterization of chondrocyte alkaline phosphatase as a potential mediator in the dissolution of calcium pyrophosphate dihydrate crystals. J Rheumatol. 1994;21:912–9.
278. Redler I, Mow VC, Zimny ML, Mansell J. The ultrastructure and biomechanical significance of the tidemark of articular cartilage. Clin Orthop Relat Res. 1975:357–62.
279. Havelka S, Horn V, Spohrova D, Valouch P. The calcified-noncalcified cartilage interface: the tidemark. Acta Biol Hung. 1984;35:271–9.
280. Hoemann CD, Lafantaisie-Favreau CH, Lascau-Coman V, Chen G, Guzman-Morales J. The cartilage-bone interface. J Knee Surg. 2012;25:85–97.
281. Muller-Gerbl M, Schulte E, Putz R. The thickness of the calcified layer of articular cartilage: a function of the load supported? J Anat. 1987;154:103–11.

282. Lyons TJ, McClure SF, Stoddart RW, McClure J. The normal human chondro-osseous junctional region: evidence for contact of uncalcified cartilage with subchondral bone and marrow spaces. BMC Musculoskelet Disord. 2006;7:52.
283. Muir H, Bullough P, Maroudas A. The distribution of collagen in human articular cartilage with some of its physiological implications. J Bone Joint Surg. 1970;52:554–63.
284. de Bont LG, Liem RS, Havinga P, Boering G, van der Korst J. Collagenous network in cartilage of human femoral condyles. A light microscopic and scanning electron microscopic study. Acta Anat. 1986;126:41–7.
285. Clark JM. The organisation of collagen fibrils in the superficial zones of articular cartilage. J Anat. 1990;171:117–30.
286. Hukins DW, Aspden RM, Yarker YE. Fibre reinforcement and mechanical stability in articular cartilage. Eng Med. 1984;13:153–6.
287. Broom ND. Further insights into the structural principles governing the function of articular cartilage. J Anat. 1984;139(Pt 2):275–94.
288. Venn M, Maroudas A. Chemical composition and swelling of normal and osteoarthrotic femoral head cartilage. I. Chemical composition. Ann Rheum Dis. 1977;36:121–9.
289. Maroudas A, Evans H, Almeida L. Cartilage of the hip joint. Topographical variation of glycosaminoglycan content in normal and fibrillated tissue. Ann Rheum Dis. 1973;32:1–9.
290. Maroudas AI. Physicochemical properties of articular cartilage. In: MAR F, editor. Adult articular cartilage. Kent: Pitman Medical; 1979. p. 215–90.
291. Asari A, Miyauchi S, Kuriyama S, Machida A, Kohno K, Uchiyama Y. Localization of hyaluronic acid in human articular cartilage. J Histochem Cytochem. 1994;42:513–22.
292. Maroudas A, Venn M. Chemical composition and swelling of normal and osteoarthrotic femoral head cartilage. II. Swelling. Ann Rheum Dis. 1977;36:399–406.
293. Ratcliffe A, Fryer PR, Hardingham TE. The distribution of aggregating proteoglycans in articular cartilage: comparison of quantitative immunoelectron microscopy with radioimmunoassay and biochemical analysis. J Histochem Cytochem. 1984;32:193–201.
294. Maroudas A, Muir H, Wingham J. The correlation of fixed negative charge with glycosaminoglycan content of human articular cartilage. Biochim Biophys Acta. 1969;177:492–500.
295. Miosge N, Flachsbart K, Goetz W, Schultz W, Kresse H, Herken R. Light and electron microscopical immunohistochemical localization of the small proteoglycan core proteins decorin and biglycan in human knee joint cartilage. Histochem J. 1994;26:939–45.
296. Poole CA. Chondrons: the chondrocyte and its pericellular microenvironment. In: Kuettner KE, Scheyerbach R, Peyron JC, Hascall VC, editors. Articular cartilage and osteoarthritis. London: Raven Press; 1992. p. 201–20.
297. Poole CA, Flint MH, Beaumont BW. Chondrons extracted from canine tibial cartilage: preliminary report on their isolation and structure. J Orthop Res. 1988;6:408–19.
298. Smeriglio P, Dhulipala L, Lai JH, Goodman SB, Dragoo JL, Smith RL, Maloney WJ, Yang F, Bhutani N. Collagen VI enhances cartilage tissue generation by stimulating chondrocyte proliferation. Tissue Eng A. 2015;21:840–9.
299. Allen JM, Bateman JF, Hansen U, Wilson R, Bruckner P, Owens RT, Sasaki T, Timpl R, Fitzgerald J. WARP is a novel multimeric component of the chondrocyte pericellular matrix that interacts with perlecan. J Biol Chem. 2006;281:7341–9.
300. Guilak F, Alexopoulos LG, Upton ML, Youn I, Choi JB, Cao L, Setton LA, Haider MA. The pericellular matrix as a transducer of biomechanical and biochemical signals in articular cartilage. Ann N Y Acad Sci. 2006;1068:498–512.
301. Soder S, Hambach L, Lissner R, Kirchner T, Aigner T. Ultrastructural localization of type VI collagen in normal adult and osteoarthritic human articular cartilage. Osteoarthritis Cartilage. 2002;10:464–70.
302. Winter GM, Poole CA, Ilic MZ, Ross JM, Robinson HC, Handley CJ. Identification of distinct metabolic pools of aggrecan and their relationship to type VI collagen in the chondrons of mature bovine articular cartilage explants. Connect Tissue Res. 1998;37:277–93.
303. Poole CA, Glant TT, Schofield JR. Chondrons from articular cartilage. (IV). Immunolocalization of proteoglycan epitopes in isolated canine tibial chondrons. J Histochem Cytochem. 1991;39:1175–87.
304. Poole CA, Honda T, Skinner SJ, Schofield JR, Hyde KF, Shinkai H. Chondrons from articular cartilage (II): analysis of the glycosaminoglycans in the cellular microenvironment of isolated canine chondrons. Connect Tissue Res. 1990;24: 319–30.
305. Poole CA, Wotton SF, Duance VC. Localization of type IX collagen in chondrons isolated from porcine articular cartilage and rat chondrosarcoma. Histochem J. 1988;20:567–74.
306. Chang J, Poole CA. Confocal analysis of the molecular heterogeneity in the pericellular microenvironment produced by adult canine chondrocytes cultured in agarose gel. Histochem J. 1997;29:515–28.
307. Martin JA, Buckwalter JA. The role of chondrocyte-matrix interactions in maintaining and repairing articular cartilage. Biorheology. 2000;37:129–40.
308. Modis L, Botos A, Kiviranta I, Lukacsko L, Helminen HJ. Differences in submicroscopic structure of the extracellular matrix of canine femoral and tibial condylar articular cartilages as revealed by polarization microscopical analysis. Acta Biol Hung. 1996;47:341–53.

309. Youn I, Choi JB, Cao L, Setton LA, Guilak F. Zonal variations in the three-dimensional morphology of the chondron measured in situ using confocal microscopy. Osteoarthritis Cartilage. 2006;14:889–97.
310. Xia Y, Moody JB, Alhadlaq H, Hu J. Imaging the physical and morphological properties of a multizone young articular cartilage at microscopic resolution. J Magn Reson Imaging. 2003;17:365–74.
311. Poole AR, Pidoux I, Reiner A, Rosenberg L. An immunoelectron microscope study of the organization of proteoglycan monomer, link protein, and collagen in the matrix of articular cartilage. J Cell Biol. 1982;93:921–37.
312. Szirmai JA. Structure of cartilage. In: Engel A, Carsson T, editors. Aging of connective and skeletal tissue. Stockholm: Thule Institute Symposium; 1969. p. 163–84.
313. Mittelstaedt D, Xia Y, Shmelyov A, Casciani N, Bidthanapally A. Quantitative determination of morphological and territorial structures of articular cartilage from both perpendicular and parallel sections by polarized light microscopy. Connect Tissue Res. 2011;52:512–22.
314. Yutani Y, Inui K, Koike T, Yamano Y. Alteration of cartilage specific proteoglycan with non-weight bearing articular cartilage. Osaka City Med J. 1994;40:19–26.
315. Seidenstuecker M, Watrinet J, Bernstein A, Suedkamp NP, Latorre SH, et al. Viscoelasticity and histology of the human cartilage in healthy and degenerated conditions of the knee. J Orthop Surg Res. 2019;14(1):256.
316. Smith RL, Lin J, Trindade MC, Shida J, Kajiyama G, Vu T, et al. Time-dependent effects of intermittent hydrostatic pressure on articular chondrocyte type II collagen and aggrecan mRNA expression. J Rehabil Res Dev. 2000;37(2):153–61.
317. Ikenoue T, Trindade MC, Lee MS, Lin EY, Schurman DJ, Goodman SB, et al. Mechanoregulation of human articular chondrocyte aggrecan and type II collagen expression by intermittent hydrostatic pressure in vitro. J Orthop Res. 2003;21(1):110–6.
318. Hu JC, Athanasiou KA. The effects of intermittent hydrostatic pressure on selfassembled articular cartilage constructs. Tissue Eng. 2006;12(5):1337–44.
319. Mansour JM, Mow VC. The permeability of articular cartilage under compressive strain and at high pressures. J Bone Joint Surg Am. 1976;58:509–16.
320. Fox SAJ, Bedi A, Rodeo SA. The basic science of articular cartilage: structure, composition, and function. Sports Health. 2009;1(6):461–8.
321. Mow VC, Ateshian GA, Spilker RL. Biomechanics of diarthrodial joints: a review of twenty years of progress. J Biomech Eng. 1993;115:460–7.
322. Bleuel J, Zaucke F, Bruggemann GP, Heilig J, Wolter ML, Hamann N, Firner S, Niehoff A. Moderate cyclic tensile strain alters the assembly of cartilage extracellular matrix proteins in vitro. J Biomech Eng. 2015;137:061009.
323. Maroudas AI. Balance between swelling pressure and collagen tension in normal and degenerate cartilage. Nature. 1976;260:808–9.
324. Guilak F. The deformation behavior and viscoelastic properties of chondrocytes in articular cartilage. Biorheology. 2000;37:27–44.
325. Maroudas A. Transport of solutes through cartilage: permeability to large molecules. J Anat. 1976;122:335–47.
326. Maroudas A, Bannon C. Measurement of swelling pressure in cartilage and comparison with the osmotic pressure of constituent proteoglycans. Biorheology. 1981;18:619–32.
327. Maroudas A, Wachtel E, Grushko G, Katz EP, Weinberg P. The effect of osmotic and mechanical pressures on water partitioning in articular cartilage. Biochim Biophys Acta. 1991;1073:285–94.
328. Schmidt MB, Mow VC, Chun LE, Eyre DR. Effects of proteoglycan extraction on the tensile behavior of articular cartilage. J Orthop Res. 1990;8:353–63.
329. Lu XL, Mow VC. Biomechanics of articular cartilage and determination of material properties. Med Sci Sports Exerc. 2008;40:193–9.
330. Wang Q, Yang YY, Niu HJ, Zhang WJ, Feng QJ, Chen WF. An ultrasound study of altered hydration behaviour of proteoglycan-degraded articular cartilage. BMC Musculoskelet Disord. 2013;14:289.
331. Melrose J, Isaacs MD, Smith SM, Hughes CE, Little CB, Caterson B, Hayes AJ. Chondroitin sulphate and heparan sulphate sulphation motifs and their proteoglycans are involved in articular cartilage formation during human foetal knee joint development. Histochem Cell Biol. 2012;138:461–75.
332. Eyre DR. Collagens and cartilage matrix homeostasis. Clin Orthop Relat Res. 2004:S118–22.
333. Turunen SM, Lammi MJ, Saarakkala S, Han SK, Herzog W, Tanska P, Korhonen RK. The effect of collagen degradation on chondrocyte volume and morphology in bovine articular cartilage following a hypotonic challenge. Biomech Model Mechanobiol. 2013;12:417–29.
334. Korhonen RK, Julkunen P, Rieppo J, Lappalainen R, Konttinen YT, Jurvelin JS. Collagen network of articular cartilage modulates fluid flow and mechanical stresses in chondrocyte. Biomech Model Mechanobiol. 2006;5:150–9.
335. McCormack T, Mansour JM. Reduction in tensile strength of cartilage precedes surface damage under repeated compressive loading in vitro. J Biomech. 1998;31:55–61.
336. Schinagl RM, Gurskis D, Chen AC, Sah RL. Depth-dependent confined compression modulus of full-thickness bovine articular cartilage. J Orthop Res. 1997;15:499–506.
337. Takada E, Mizuno S. Reproduction of characteristics of extracellular matrices in specific longitudinal depth zone cartilage within spherical organoids in

response to changes in osmotic pressure. Int J Mol Sci. 2018;19(5):E1507.
338. Dabiri Y, Li LP. Influences of the depth-dependent material inhomogeneity of articular cartilage on the fluid pressurization in the human knee. Med Eng Phys. 2013;35:1591–8.
339. Kienle S, Boettcher K, Wiegleb L, Urban J, Burgkart R, Lieleg O, et al. Comparison of friction and wear of articular cartilage on different length scales. J Biomech. 2015;48(12):3052–8.
340. Chang DP, Guilak F, Jay GD, Zauscher S. Interaction of lubricin with type II collagen surfaces: adsorption, friction, and normal forces. J Biomech. 2014;47:659–66.
341. Quiroga JM, Wilson W, Ito K, van Donkelaar CC. Relative contribution of articular cartilage's constitutive components to load support depending on strain rate. Biomech Model Mechanobiol. 2017;16:151–8.
342. Henak CR, Ross KA, Bonnevie ED, Fortier LA, Cohen I, Kennedy JG, Bonassar LJ. Human talar and femoral cartilage have distinct mechanical properties near the articular surface. J Biomech. 2016;49:3320–7.
343. Halonen KS, Mononen ME, Jurvelin JS, Toyras J, Korhonen RK. Importance of depth-wise distribution of collagen and proteoglycans in articular cartilage–a 3D finite element study of stresses and strains in human knee joint. J Biomech. 2013;46:1184–92.
344. Szarko M, Xia Y. Direct visualisation of the depth-dependent mechanical properties of full-thickness articular cartilage. Open J Orthop. 2012;2. https://doi.org/10.4236/ojo.2012.22007.
345. Li LP, Cheung JT, Herzog W. Three-dimensional fibril-reinforced finite element model of articular cartilage. Med Biol Eng Comput. 2009;47:607–15.
346. Kaab MJ, Ito K, Rahn B, Clark JM, Notzli HP. Effect of mechanical load on articular cartilage collagen structure: a scanning electron-microscopic study. Cells Tissues Organs. 2000;167:106–20.
347. Pierce DM, Ricken T, Holzapfel GA. A hyperelastic biphasic fibre-reinforced model of articular cartilage considering distributed collagen fibre orientations: continuum basis, computational aspects and applications. Comput Methods Biomech Biomed Engin. 2013;16(12):1344–61.
348. Roth V, Mow VC. The intrinsic tensile behavior of the matrix of bovine articular cartilage and its variation with age. J Bone Joint Surg Am. 1980;62:1102–17.
349. Broom ND, Poole CA. A functional-morphological study of the tidemark region of articular cartilage maintained in a non-viable physiological condition. J Anat. 1982;135:65–82.
350. Anderson DD, Brown TD, Radin EL. The influence of basal cartilage calcification on dynamic juxtaarticular stress transmission. Clin Orthop Relat Res. 1993:298–307.
351. Madry H, van Dijk CN, Mueller-Gerbl M. The basic science of the subchondral bone. Knee Surg Sports Traumatol Arthrosc. 2010;18(4):419–33.
352. Hvid I. Mechanical strength of trabecular bone at the knee. Dan Med Bull. 1988;35(4):345–65.
353. Hosseini SM, Wu Y, Ito K, van Donkelaar CC. The importance of superficial collagen fibrils for the function of articular cartilage. Biomech Model Mechanobiol. 2014;13(1):41–51.
354. Komeili A, Abusara Z, Federico S, Herzog W. A compression system for studying depth dependent mechanical properties of articular cartilage under dynamic loading conditions. Med Eng Phys. 2018;60:103–8.
355. Laasanen MS, Toyras J, Korhonen RK, Rieppo J, Saarakkala S, Nieminen MT, Hirvonen J, Jurvelin JS. Biomechanical properties of knee articular cartilage. Biorheology. 2003;40:133–40.
356. Krishnan R, Park S, Eckstein F, Ateshian GA. Inhomogeneous cartilage properties enhance superficial interstitial fluid support and frictional properties, but do not provide a homogeneous state of stress. J Biomech Eng. 2003;125:569–77.
357. Buckley MR, Bonassar LJ, Cohen I. Localization of viscous behavior and shear energy dissipation in articular cartilage under dynamic shear loading. J Biomech Eng. 2013;135:31002.
358. Yusuf KQ, Motta N, Pawlak Z, Oloyede A. A microanalytical study of the surfaces of normal, delipidized, and artificially "resurfaced" articular cartilage. Connect Tissue Res. 2012;53:236–45.
359. Korhonen RK, Herzog W. Depth-dependent analysis of the role of collagen fibrils, fixed charges and fluid in the pericellular matrix of articular cartilage on chondrocyte mechanics. J Biomech. 2008;41:480–5.
360. Duan WP, Sun ZW, Li Q, Li CJ, Wang L, Chen WY, Tickner J, Zheng MH, Wei XC. Normal age-related viscoelastic properties of chondrons and chondrocytes isolated from rabbit knee. Chin Med J. 2012;125:2574–81.
361. Alexopoulos LG, Setton LA, Guilak F. The biomechanical role of the chondrocyte pericellular matrix in articular cartilage. Acta Biomater. 2005;1:317–25.
362. Greco F, Specchia N, Falciglia F, Toesca A, Nori S. Ultrastructural analysis of the adaptation of articular cartilage to mechanical stimulation. Ital J Orthop Traumatol. 1992;18:311–21.
363. Korhonen RK, Julkunen P, Wilson W, Herzog W. Importance of collagen orientation and depth-dependent fixed charge densities of cartilage on mechanical behavior of chondrocytes. J Biomech Eng. 2008;130:021003.
364. Felka T, Rothdiener M, Bast S, Uynuk-Ool T, Zouhair S, Ochs BG, De Zwart P, Stoeckle U, Aicher WK, Hart ML, Shiozawa T, Grodzinsky AJ, Schenke-Layland K, Venkatesan JK, Cucchiarini M, Madry H, Kurz B, Rolauffs B. Loss of spatial organization and destruction of the pericellular matrix in early osteoarthritis in vivo and in a novel in vitro methodology. Osteoarthritis Cartilage. 2016;24:1200–9.

365. Ojanen SP, Finnilä MAJ, Reunamo AE, Ronkainen AP, Mikkonen S, Herzog W, et al. Site-specific glycosaminoglycan content is better maintained in the pericellular matrix than the extracellular matrix in early post-traumatic osteoarthritis. PLoS One. 2018;13(4):e0196203.
366. McNary SM, Athanasiou KA, Reddi AH. Engineering lubrication in articular cartilage. Tissue Eng Part B Rev. 2012;18:88–100.
367. Naka MH, Morita Y, Ikeuchi K. Influence of proteoglycan contents and of tissue hydration on the frictional characteristics of articular cartilage. Proc Inst Mech Eng H. 2005;219:175–82.
368. Charnley J. The lubrication of animal joints. Symp Biomech Inst Mech Eng. 1959;17:12–9.
369. Akpinar B, Thorhauer E, Tashman S, Irrgang JJ, Fu FH, Anderst WJ. Tibiofemoral cartilage contact differences between level walking and downhill running. Orthop J Sports Med. 2019;7(4):2325967119836164.
370. Paranjape CS, Cutcliffe HC, Grambow SC, Utturkar GM, Collins AT, et al. A new stress test for knee joint cartilage. Sci Rep. 2019;9(1):2283.
371. Taylor WR, Heller MO, Bergmann G, Duda GN. Tibio-femoral loading during human gait and stair climbing. J Orthop Res. 2004;22(3):625–32.
372. Kutzner I, Heinlein B, Graichen F, Bender A, Rohlmann A, Halder A, et al. Loading of the knee joint during activities of daily living measured in vivo in five subjects. J Biomech. 2010;43(11):2164–73.
373. Kuster M, Wood GA, Sakurai S, Blatter G. 1994 Nicola Cerulli Young Researchers Award. Downhill walking: a stressful task for the anterior cruciate ligament? A biomechanical study with clinical implications. Knee Surg Sports Traumatol Arthrosc. 1994;2(1):2–7.
374. D'Lima DD, Fregly BJ, Patil S, Steklov N, Colwell CW Jr. Knee joint forces: prediction, measurement, and significance. Proc Inst Mech Eng H. 2012;226(2):95–102.
375. Messier SP, Gutekunst DJ, Davis C, DeVita P. Weight loss reduces knee-joint loads in overweight and obese older adults with knee osteoarthritis. Arthritis Rheum. 2005;52(7):2026–32.
376. Seedhom BB. Conditioning of cartilage during normal activities is an important factor in the development of osteoarthritis. Rheumatology (Oxford). 2006;45:146–9.
377. Tian H, Chen Y, Ding C, Li G. Interaction study in homogeneous collagen/chondroitin sulfate blends by two-dimensional infrared spectroscopy. Carbohydr Polym. 2012;89(2):542–50.
378. Hedlund H, Hedbom E. Heineg rd D, Mengarelli-Widholm S, Reinholt FP, Svensson O. Association of the aggrecan keratan sulfate-rich region with collagen in bovine articular cartilage. J Biol Chem. 1999;274(9):5777–81.
379. Linn FC, Sokoloff L. Movement and composition of interstitial fluid of cartilage. Arthritis Rheum. 1965;8:481–94.
380. Maroudas A, Bullough P, Swanson SA, Freeman MA. The permeability of articular cartilage. J Bone Joint Surg. 1968;50:166–77.
381. Maroudas A, Bullough P. Permeability of articular cartilage. Nature. 1968;219:1260–1.
382. Swanson SAV. Friction, wear and lubrication. In: Freemann MAR, editor. Adult articular cartilage. Tunbridge Wells: Pitman Medical Publishing Co. Ltd; 1979. p. 415–60.
383. Jahn S, Seror J, Klein J. Lubrication of articular cartilage. Annu Rev Biomed Eng. 2016;18:235–58.
384. Chan SM, Neu CP, Komvopoulos K, Reddi AH. Dependence of nanoscale friction and adhesion properties of articular cartilage on contact load. J Biomech. 2011;44:1340–5.
385. Schmidt TA, Gastelum NS, Nguyen QT, Schumacher BL, Sah RL. Boundary lubrication of articular cartilage: role of synovial fluid constituents. Arthritis Rheum. 2007;56:882–91.
386. Flannery CR, Hughes CE, Schumacher BL, Tudor D, Aydelotte MB, Kuettner KE, Caterson B. Articular cartilage superficial zone protein (SZP) is homologous to megakaryocyte stimulating factor precursor and is a multifunctional proteoglycan with potential growth-promoting, cytoprotective, and lubricating properties in cartilage metabolism. Biochem Biophys Res Commun. 1999;254:535–41.
387. Jay GD, Britt DE, Cha CJ. Lubricin is a product of megakaryocyte stimulating factor gene expression by human synovial fibroblasts. J Rheumatol. 2000;27:594–600.
388. Jay GD, Tantravahi U, Britt DE, Barrach HJ, Cha CJ. Homology of lubricin and superficial zone protein (SZP): products of megakaryocyte stimulating factor (MSF) gene expression by human synovial fibroblasts and articular chondrocytes localized to chromosome 1q25. J Orthop Res. 2001;19:677–87.
389. Jay GD. Lubricin and surfacing of articular joints. Curr Opin Orthop. 2004;15:355–9.
390. Rabinowitz JL, Gregg JR, Nixon JE, Schumacher HR. Lipid composition of the tissues of human knee joints. I. Observations in normal joints (articular cartilage, meniscus, ligaments, synovial fluid, synovium, intra-articular fat pad and bone marrow). Clin Orthop Relat Res. 1979:260–5.
391. Fraser JR, Laurent TC, Laurent UB. Hyaluronan: its nature, distribution, functions and turnover. J Intern Med. 1997;242:27–33.
392. Ikegawa S, Sano M, Koshizuka Y, Nakamura Y. Isolation, characterization and mapping of the mouse and human PRG4 (proteoglycan 4) genes. Cytogenet Cell Genet. 2000;90:291–7.
393. Klein TJ, Schumacher BL, Blewis ME, Schmidt TA, Voegtline MS, Thonar EJ, Masuda K, Sah RL. Tailoring secretion of proteoglycan 4 (PRG4) in tissue-engineered cartilage. Tissue Eng. 2006;12:1429–39.
394. Gleghorn JP, Jones AR, Flannery CR, Bonassar LJ. Alteration of articular cartilage frictional prop-

erties by transforming growth factor beta, interleukin-1beta, and oncostatin M. Arthritis Rheum. 2009;60:440–9.
395. Gleghorn JP, Jones AR, Flannery CR, Bonassar LJ. Boundary mode lubrication of articular cartilage by recombinant human lubricin. J Orthop Res. 2009;27:771–7.
396. Daniel M. Boundary cartilage lubrication: review of current concepts. Wien Med Wochenschr. 2014;164:88–94.
397. Zappone B, Ruths M, Greene GW, Jay GD, Israelachvili JN. Adsorption, lubrication, and wear of lubricin on model surfaces: polymer brush-like behavior of a glycoprotein. Biophys J. 2007;92:1693–708.
398. Davis WH, Lee SL, Sokoloff L. A proposed model of boundary lubrication by synovial fluid: structuring of boundary water. J Biomech Eng. 1979;101:185–92.
399. Peng G, McNary SM, Athanasiou KA, Reddi AH. The distribution of superficial zone protein (SZP)/lubricin/PRG4 and boundary mode frictional properties of the bovine diarthrodial joint. J Biomech. 2015;48:3406–12.
400. Cuellar A, Reddi AH. Stimulation of superficial zone protein/lubricin/PRG4 by transforming growth factor-beta in superficial zone articular chondrocytes and modulation by glycosaminoglycans. Tissue Eng A. 2015;21:1973–81.
401. Swann DA, Silver FH, Slayter HS, Stafford W, Shore E. The molecular structure and lubricating activity of lubricin isolated from bovine and human synovial fluids. Biochem J. 1985;225:195–201.
402. Jay GD, Waller KA. The biology of lubricin: near frictionless joint motion. Matrix Biol. 2014;39:17–24.
403. Zea-Aragon Z, Ohtsuki K, Ohnishi M, Ohno S. Immunohistochemical study of the upper surface layer in rat mandibular condylar cartilage. Histol Histopathol. 2004;19:29–36.
404. Rhee DK, Marcelino J, Baker M, Gong Y, Smits P, Lefebvre V, Jay GD, Stewart M, Wang H, Warman ML, Carpten JD. The secreted glycoprotein lubricin protects cartilage surfaces and inhibits synovial cell overgrowth. J Clin Invest. 2005;115:622–31.
405. Elsaid KA, Jay GD, Warman ML, Rhee DK, Chichester CO. Association of articular cartilage degradation and loss of boundary-lubricating ability of synovial fluid following injury and inflammatory arthritis. Arthritis Rheum. 2005;52:1746–55.
406. Schumacher BL, Block JA, Schmid TM, Aydelotte MB, Kuettner KE. A novel proteoglycan synthesized and secreted by chondrocytes of the superficial zone of articular cartilage. Arch Biochem Biophys. 1994;311:144–52.
407. Swann DA, Slayter HS, Silver FH. The molecular structure of lubricating glycoprotein-I, the boundary lubricant for articular cartilage. J Biol Chem. 1981;256:5921–5.
408. Chang DP, Abu-Lail NI, Coles JM, Guilak F, Jay GD, Zauscher S. Friction force microscopy of lubricin and hyaluronic acid between hydrophobic and hydrophilic surfaces. Soft Matter. 2009;5:3438–45.
409. Chang DP, Abu-Lail NI, Guilak F, Jay GD, Zauscher S. Conformational mechanics, adsorption, and normal force interactions of lubricin and hyaluronic acid on model surfaces. Langmuir. 2008;24:1183–93.
410. Waller KA, Zhang LX, Elsaid KA, Fleming BC, arman ML, Jay GD. Role of lubricin and boundary lubrication in the prevention of chondrocyte apoptosis. Proc Natl Acad Sci U S A. 2013;110:5852–7.
411. Klein TJ, Schumacher BL, Schmidt TA, Li KW, Voegtline MS, Masuda K, Thonar EJ, Sah RL. Tissue engineering of stratified articular cartilage from chondrocyte subpopulations. Osteoarthritis Cartilage. 2003;11:595–602.
412. Jay GD, Torres JR, Rhee DK, Helminen HJ, Hytinnen MM, Cha CJ, Elsaid K, Kim KS, Cui Y, Warman ML. Association between friction and wear in diarthrodial joints lacking lubricin. Arthritis Rheum. 2007;56:3662–9.
413. Jay GD, Torres JR, Warman ML, Laderer MC, Breuer KS. The role of lubricin in the mechanical behavior of synovial fluid. Proc Natl Acad Sci U S A. 2007;104:6194–9.
414. Buckley MR, Gleghorn JP, Bonassar LJ, Cohen I. Mapping the depth dependence of shear properties in articular cartilage. J Biomech. 2008;41:2430–7.
415. Briscoe WH, Titmuss S, Tiberg F, Thomas RK, McGillivray DJ, Klein J. Boundary lubrication under water. Nature. 2006;444:191–4.
416. Abubacker S, Ponjevic D, Ham HO, Messersmith PB, Matyas JR, Schmidt TA. Effect of disulfide bonding and multimerization on proteoglycan 4's cartilage boundary lubricating ability and adsorption. Connect Tissue Res. 2016;57:113–23.
417. Schmidt TA, Schumacher BL, Klein TJ, Voegtline MS, Sah RL. Synthesis of proteoglycan 4 by chondrocyte subpopulations in cartilage explants, monolayer cultures, and resurfaced cartilage cultures. Arthritis Rheum. 2004;50:2849–57.
418. Blewis ME, Schumacher BL, Klein TJ, Schmidt TA, Voegtline MS, Sah RL. Microenvironment regulation of PRG4 phenotype of chondrocytes. J Orthop Res. 2007;25:685–95.
419. Nugent-Derfus GE, Chan AH, Schumacher BL, Sah RL. PRG4 exchange between the articular cartilage surface and synovial fluid. J Orthop Res. 2007;25:1269–76.
420. Nugent GE, Schmidt TA, Schumacher BL, Voegtline MS, Bae WC, Jadin KD, Sah RL. Static and dynamic compression regulate cartilage metabolism of PRoteoGlycan 4 (PRG4). Biorheology. 2006;43:191–200.
421. Nugent GE, Aneloski NM, Schmidt TA, Schumacher BL, Voegtline MS, Sah RL. Dynamic shear stimulation of bovine cartilage biosynthesis of proteoglycan 4. Arthritis Rheum. 2006;54:1888–96.

422. Das N, Schmidt TA, Krawetz RJ, Dufour A. Proteoglycan 4: from mere lubricant to regulator of tissue homeostasis and inflammation: does proteoglycan 4 have the ability to buffer the inflammatory response? BioEssays. 2019;41(1):e1800166.
423. Su JL, Schumacher BL, Lindley KM, Soloveychik V, Burkhart W, Triantafillou JA, Kuettner K, Schmid T. Detection of superficial zone protein in human and animal body fluids by cross-species monoclonal antibodies specific to superficial zone protein. Hybridoma. 2001;20:149–57.
424. Neu CP, Khalafi A, Komvopoulos K, Schmid TM, Reddi AH. Mechanotransduction of bovine articular cartilage superficial zone protein by transforming growth factor beta signaling. Arthritis Rheum. 2007;56:3706–14.
425. Sakata R, McNary SM, Miyatake K, Lee CA, Van den Bogaerde JM, Marder RA, Reddi AH. Stimulation of the superficial zone protein and lubrication in the articular cartilage by human platelet-rich plasma. Am J Sports Med. 2015;43:1467–73.
426. Sarma AV, Powell GL, LaBerge M. Phospholipid composition of articular cartilage boundary lubricant. J Orthop Res. 2001;19:671–6.
427. Hills BA, Butler BD. Surfactants identified in synovial fluid and their ability to act as boundary lubricants. Ann Rheum Dis. 1984;43:641–8.
428. Hills BA. Boundary lubrication in vivo. Proc Inst Mech Eng H. 2000;214:83–94.
429. Hills BA. Identity of the joint lubricant. J Rheumatol. 2002;29:200–1.
430. Higaki H, Murakami T, Nakanishi Y, Miura H, Mawatari T, Iwamoto Y. The lubricating ability of biomembrane models with dipalmitoyl phosphatidylcholine and gamma-globulin. Proc Inst Mech Eng H. 1998;212:337–46.
431. Murakami T, Yarimitsu S, Nakashima K, Sakai N, Yamaguchi T, Sawae Y, Suzuki A. Biphasic and boundary lubrication mechanisms in artificial hydrogel cartilage: a review. Proc Inst Mech Eng H. 2015;229:864–78.
432. Murakami T, Sawae Y, Ihara M. Protective mechanism of articular cartilage to severe loading: roles lubricants, cartilage surface layer, extracellular matrix and chondrocyte. JSME Int J. 2003;46:594–603.
433. Schwarz IM, Hills BA. Surface-active phospholipid as the lubricating component of lubricin. Br J Rheumatol. 1998;37:21–6.
434. Chan SM, Neu CP, Duraine G, Komvopoulos K, Reddi AH. Atomic force microscope investigation of the boundary-lubricant layer in articular cartilage. Osteoarthritis Cartilage. 2010;18:956–63.
435. Laurent TC, Laurent UB, Fraser JR. The structure and function of hyaluronan: an overview. Immunol Cell Biol. 1996;74:A1–7.
436. Hui AY, McCarty WJ, Masuda K, Firestein GS, Sah RL. A systems biology approach to synovial joint lubrication in health, injury, and disease. Wiley Interdiscip Rev Syst Biol Med. 2012;4:15–37.
437. Dunn S, Kolomytkin OV, Marino AA. Pathophysiology of osteoarthritis: evidence against the viscoelastic theory. Pathobiology. 2009;76:322–8.
438. Greene GW, Banquy X, Lee DW, Lowrey DD, Yu J, Israelachvili JN. Adaptive mechanically controlled lubrication mechanism found in articular joints. Proc Natl Acad Sci U S A. 2011;108:5255–9.
439. Benz M, Chen N, Israelachvili J. Lubrication and wear properties of grafted polyelectrolytes, hyaluronan and hylan, measured in the surface forces apparatus. J Biomed Mater Res A. 2004;71:6–15.
440. Dicker KT, Gurski LA, Pradhan-Bhatt S, Witt RL, Farach-Carson MC, Jia X. Hyaluronan: a simple polysaccharide with diverse biological functions. Acta Biomater. 2014;10:1558–70.
441. Murano E, Perin D, Khan R, Bergamin M. Hyaluronan: from biomimetic to industrial business strategy. Nat Prod Commun. 2011;6:555–72.
442. Swann DA, Radin EL, Nazimiec M, Weisser PA, Curran N, Lewinnek G. Role of hyaluronic acid in joint lubrication. Ann Rheum Dis. 1974;33:318–26.
443. Radin EL, Swann DA, Weisser PA. Separation of a hyaluronate-free lubricating fraction from synovial fluid. Nature. 1970;228:377–8.
444. Kosinska MK, Ludwig TE, Liebisch G, Zhang R, Siebert HC, Wilhelm J, Kaesser U, Dettmeyer RB, Klein H, Ishaque B, Rickert M, Schmitz G, Schmidt TA, Steinmeyer J. Articular joint lubricants during osteoarthritis and rheumatoid arthritis display altered levels and molecular species. PLoS One. 2015;10:e0125192.
445. Jones AR, Flannery CR. Bioregulation of lubricin expression by growth factors and cytokines. Eur Cell Mater. 2007;13:40–5; discussion 45
446. Lin W, Mashiah R, Seror J, Kadar A, Dolkart O, Pritsch T, et al. Lipid-hyaluronan synergy strongly reduces intrasynovial tissue boundary friction. Acta Biomater. 2019;83:314–21.
447. Mazzucco D, Scott R, Spector M. Composition of joint fluid in patients undergoing total knee replacement and revision arthroplasty: correlation with flow properties. Biomaterials. 2004;25:4433–45.
448. Asari A, Miyauchi S, Sekiguchi T, Machida A, Kuriyama S, Miyazaki K, Namiki O. Hyaluronan, cartilage destruction and hydrarthrosis in traumatic arthritis. Osteoarthritis Cartilage. 1994;2:79–89.
449. Dahl LB, Dahl IM, Engstrom-Laurent A, Granath K. Concentration and molecular weight of sodium hyaluronate in synovial fluid from patients with rheumatoid arthritis and other arthropathies. Ann Rheum Dis. 1985;44:817–22.
450. Watterson JR, Esdaile JM. Viscosupplementation: therapeutic mechanisms and clinical potential in osteoarthritis of the knee. J Am Acad Orthop Surg. 2000;8:277–84.
451. Rabinowitz JL, Gregg JR, Nixon JE. Lipid composition of the tissues of human knee joints. II.

Synovial fluid in trauma. Clin Orthop Relat Res. 1984:292–8.
452. Neu CP, Reddi AH, Komvopoulos K, Schmid TM, Di Cesare PE. Increased friction coefficient and superficial zone protein expression in patients with advanced osteoarthritis. Arthritis Rheum. 2010;62:2680–7.
453. Saarakkala S, Julkunen P, Kiviranta P, Makitalo J, Jurvelin JS, Korhonen RK. Depth-wise progression of osteoarthritis in human articular cartilage: investigation of composition, structure and biomechanics. Osteoarthritis Cartilage. 2010;18:73–81.
454. Elsaid KA, Jay GD, Chichester CO. Reduced expression and proteolytic susceptibility of lubricin/superficial zone protein may explain early elevation in the coefficient of friction in the joints of rats with antigen-induced arthritis. Arthritis Rheum. 2007;56:108–16.
455. Young AA, McLennan S, Smith MM, Smith SM, Cake MA, Read RA, Melrose J, Sonnabend DH, Flannery CR, Little CB. Proteoglycan 4 downregulation in a sheep meniscectomy model of early osteoarthritis. Arthritis Res Ther. 2006;8:R41.
456. Antonacci JM, Schmidt TA, Serventi LA, Cai MZ, Shu YL, Schumacher BL, McIlwraith CW, Sah RL. Effects of equine joint injury on boundary lubrication of articular cartilage by synovial fluid: role of hyaluronan. Arthritis Rheum. 2012;64:2917–26.
457. Hills BA, Monds MK. Deficiency of lubricating surfactant lining the articular surfaces of replaced hips and knees. Br J Rheumatol. 1998;37:143–7.
458. Ludwig TE, McAllister JR, Lun V, Wiley JP, Schmidt TA. Diminished cartilage-lubricating ability of human osteoarthritic synovial fluid deficient in proteoglycan 4: restoration through proteoglycan 4 supplementation. Arthritis Rheum. 2012;64:3963–71.
459. Elsaid KA, Fleming BC, Oksendahl HL, Machan JT, Fadale PD, Hulstyn MJ, Shalvoy R, Jay GD. Decreased lubricin concentrations and markers of joint inflammation in the synovial fluid of patients with anterior cruciate ligament injury. Arthritis Rheum. 2008;58:1707–15.
460. Wanderling C, Liles J, Davis E, Schmitt D, Statz S, Guler N, et al. Levels of matrix-degrading enzymes and lubricin in patients with degenerative joint disease requiring arthroplasty. Clin Appl Thromb Hemost. 2018;24(1):41–6.
461. Galicia K, Thorson C, Banos A, Rondina M, Hopkinson W, Hoppensteadt D, et al. Inflammatory biomarker profiling in total joint arthroplasty and its relevance to circulating levels of lubricin, a novel proteoglycan. Clin Appl Thromb Hemost. 2018;24(6):950–9.
462. Lee Y, Choi J, Hwang NS. Regulation of lubricin for functional cartilage tissue regeneration: a review. Biomater Res. 2018;22:9.
463. Ali AM, Yousif AE. The role of lubrication mechanisms in the knee synovial joints. The 1st regional conference of Eng Sci NUCEJ Spatial ISSUE. 2008;11(3):522–35.
464. Singh N. Synovial joints and lubrication mechanisms. Int J Comput Appl Math (IJCAM). 2017;12(1):29–33.
465. Halling J. In: Halling J, editor. Principles of tribology. London: The MacMillan Press Ltd; 1978.
466. James DF, Fick GM, Baines WD. A mechanism to explain physiological lubrication. J Biomech Eng. 2010;132:071002.
467. Myant CW, Cann P. The effect of transient conditions on synovial fluid protein aggregation lubrication. J Mech Behav Biomed Mater. 2014;34:349–57.
468. Hamrock B. In: Hamrock B, editor. Fundamentals of fluid film lubrication. New York: McGraw-Hill; 1994.
469. Pawlak Z, Urbaniak W, Hagner-Derengowska M, Hagner W. The probable explanation for the low friction of natural joints. Cell Biochem Biophys. 2015;71:1615–21.
470. Lawrence A, Xu X, Bible MD, Calve S, Neu CP, Panitch A. Synthesis and characterization of a lubricin mimic (mLub) to reduce friction and adhesion on the articular cartilage surface. Biomaterials. 2015;73:42–50.
471. Ballard BL, Antonacci JM, Temple-Wong MM, Hui AY, Schumacher BL, Bugbee WD, et al. Effect of tibial plateau fracture on lubrication function and composition of synovial fluid. J Bone Joint Surg Am. 2012;94(10):e64.
472. Pascau A, Guardia B, Puertolas JA, Gomez-Barrena E. Knee model of hydrodynamic lubrication during the gait cycle and the influence of prosthetic joint conformity. J Orthop Sci. 2009;14:68–75.
473. Suciu AN, Iwatsubo T, Matsuda M. Theoretical investigation of an artificial joint with micro-pocket-covered component and biphasic cartilage on the opposite articulating surface. J Biomech Eng. 2003;125:425–33.
474. Dowson D, Jin ZM. Micro-elastohydrodynamic lubrication of synovial joints. Eng Med. 1986;15:63–5.
475. Warnecke D, Meßemer M, de Roy L, Stein S, Gentilini C, et al. Articular cartilage and meniscus reveal higher friction in swing phase than in stance phase under dynamic gait conditions. Sci Rep. 2019;9(1):5785.
476. Wright V, Dowson D. Lubrication and cartilage. J Anat. 1976;121:107–18.
477. McCarty WJ, Cheng JC, Hansen BC, Yamaguchi T, Firestein GS, Masuda K, et al. The biophysical mechanisms of altered hyaluronan concentration in synovial fluid after anterior cruciate ligament transection. Arthritis Rheum. 2012;64(12):3993–4003.
478. Pigman W, Hawkins W, Gramling E, Rizvi S, Holley HL. Factors affecting the viscosity of hyaluronic acid and synovial fluid. Arch Biochem Biophys. 1960;89(2):184–93.

479. Tamer TM. Hyaluronan and synovial joint: function, distribution and healing. Interdiscip Toxicol. 2013;6(3):111–25.
480. Svala E, Jin C, Rüetschi U, Ekman S, Lindahl A, Karlsson NG, et al. Characterisation of lubricin in synovial fluid from horses with osteoarthritis. Equine Vet J. 2017;49(1):116–23.
481. Weightman B. In vitro fatigue testing of articular cartilage. Ann Rheum Dis. 1975;34 (Suppl 2):108–10.
482. Weightman B. Tensile fatigue of human articular cartilage. J Biomech. 1976;9:193–200.
483. Weightman BO, Freeman MA, Swanson SA. Fatigue of articular cartilage. Nature. 1973;244:303–4.

Growth and Development of Articular Cartilage

2

Facundo Las Heras and Harpal K. Gahunia

2.1 Introduction

During embryonic development, external to the early mesodermal limb bud is a specialized region called the apical ectodermal ridge which plays a role in limb bud growth [1]. Within the limb bud, the embryonic mesenchymal stem cells (also called mesenchymal stromal cells, MSCs) migrate to form a vascular-rich myogenic region and an avascular central chondrogenic core surrounded by a perichondrium [2, 3]. MSCs are multipotent stromal cells that can differentiate into a variety of cell types, including osteoblasts, chondroblast, myocytes, and adipocytes [4–6]. The mesenchymal cells in the central core aggregate in the shape of the future bone, which then differentiate into chondroblasts. These chondroblasts secrete extracellular matrix (ECM), and the cartilage model enlarges in length and width through the process of interstitial and appositional growth. Once embedded within its ECM, the chondroblasts are referred to as chondrocytes. With continued growth of this cartilage model, the chondrocytes in its midsection hypertrophy, mature, and deposit insoluble calcium salts. This prenatal event results in chondronecrosis and disintegration of calcified cartilage, followed by vascular invasion and the formation of primary center of ossification (Fig. 2.1). Postnatally, the secondary center of ossification develops within the epiphyses, and cartilage canals extend as branches of the blood vessels to the articular-epiphyseal cartilage complex (AECC) that forms the articulating surface of the growing bone, and the epiphyseal growth plates (GP) [7, 8]. Through the process of endochondral ossification (EO), cartilage is then progressively replaced by bone. In children and adolescents, the epiphysis of the growing bone is capped with AECC, and GP is also formed between the epiphysis and metaphysis. However, with skeletal maturity, the GP eventually gets obliterated, and in adults only the articular cartilage cap of the AECC remains. At skeletal maturity, although the articular cartilage thickness is relatively stabilized, several studies have shown that EO at the cartilage and subchondral interface remains active throughout life and is responsible for the gradual changes in joint shape that occur with aging [9, 10].

During skeletal development and postnatal growth, the biochemical composition of articular cartilages particularly the proteoglycans (PGs),

F. Las Heras, MD, PhD (✉)
Departamento de Anatomia Patologica, Clinica Las Condes, Santiago, Chile

Pathology Department, University of Chile, Santiago, Chile
e-mail: flasheras@clinicalascondes.cl

H. K. Gahunia, MSc, PhD
Orthopaedic Science Consulting Services, Oakville, ON, Canada
e-mail: harpal.gahunia@utoronto.ca

H. K. Gahunia et al. (eds.), *Articular Cartilage of the Knee*,
https://doi.org/10.1007/978-1-4939-7587-7_2

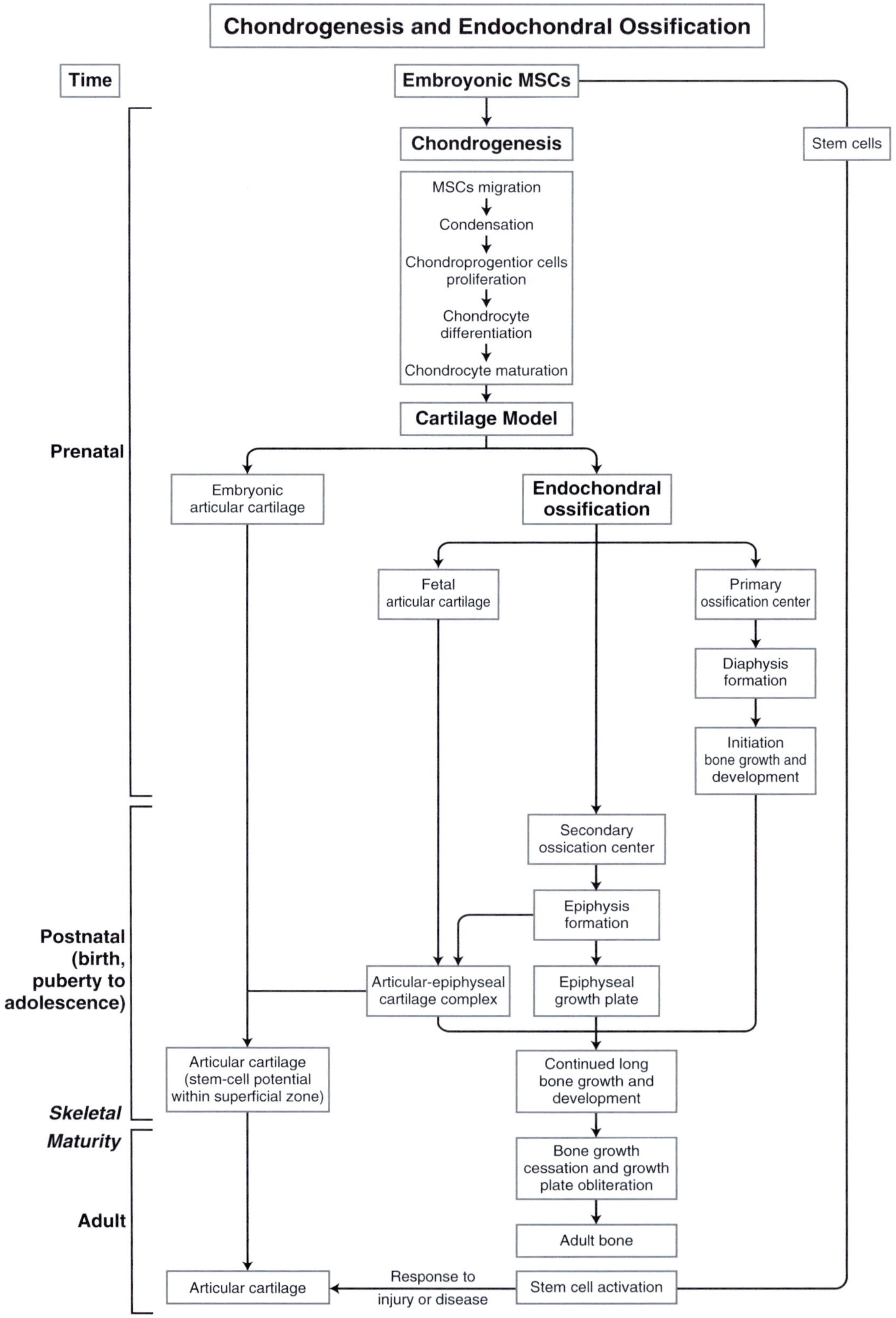

Fig. 2.1 Sequence of cellular and tissue changes during chondrogenesis and endochondral ossification. (Courtesy of Dr. Harpal Gahunia)

collagens, and pyridinoline cross-links per cartilage volume increases [11–14]. From an early stage, mechanical forces strongly influence skeletal morphogenesis, growth, and development [15]. The cartilage superficial zone (SZ) acts as a membrane barrier against substances which invade from the bursa through this cartilage zone [16]. The development period of the SZ coincides with the initiation of weight bearing, which is also thought to further promote cartilage maturation [16]. At different stages of postnatal articular cartilage development and maturation, ex vivo compression of porcine osteochondral core demonstrated that the SZ of articular cartilage undergoes dramatic structural adaptation with growth, which in turn plays a key role in determining the dynamic compressive properties of the articular cartilage [17]. Removal of the SZ negatively impacts the dynamic modulus of the cartilage with the attainment of skeletal maturity.

Investigation of the effects of in vitro mechanical loading on structural proteins composition and mechanical properties of the GP showed that static compression triggers a decrease in PG content and collagen type X in specific zones of the GP [18]. Compared to the control group, a reduction by 40% of PG content was reported in the zone of proliferation. The expression of aggrecan, one of the main PG in the ECM of GP, was reduced by 21% and 17% in the zones of proliferation and hypertrophy (mostly located at the first 30% of hypertrophic zone), respectively. These biochemical changes were associated with decreased GP permeability in the static group. Dynamic mechanical compression did not impact the ECM composition, molecular expression, and biomechanics of the GP.

The objective of this chapter is to review the mechanisms of cartilage morphogenesis, growth, and maturation. We highlight some important growth factors, hormones, signaling molecules, and local regulators that play an important role in chondrogenesis as well as AECC and GP regulation and maturation throughout the process of EO.

2.2 Chondrogenesis

Cartilage, a highly specialized connective tissue of mesenchymal lineage, is often considered an "embryonic" tissue due to its extensive distribution within the fetus, providing templates for skeletal tissue [19]. Cartilage development, a process referred to as chondrogenesis, is one of the earliest morphogenetic steps in skeletogenesis. Chondrogenesis consists of a highly orchestrated series of events involving the commitment, condensation, and differentiation of MSCs to chondrocytes, the synthesis and secretions of cartilaginous matrix by these cells, the formation of cartilage template or anlagen, and, finally, their maturation and replacement by bone [2, 4, 5, 20–29]. Cartilage chondrocytes are solely responsible for generating and maintaining the cartilage ECM and the GPs for the longitudinal bone growth [29].

For simplicity, the process of chondrogenesis can be divided into four phases corresponding to the developmental progression of cartilage genesis that occurs prenatally (Fig. 2.2). These four phases are MSC differentiation to chondroprogenitor cells, cellular migration and condensation, further differentiation of chondroprogenitor cells to chondroblasts/chondrocytes with excretion of ECM, and chondrocyte hypertrophy [31].

2.2.1 Precursor Mesenchymal Stem Cells

The first phase of chondrogenesis is initiated by the differentiation of the prechondrocytic MSCs into chondroprogenitor cells [32]. The prechondrocytic MSCs produce ECM rich in hyaluronan and collagen type I, as well as collagen type IIA containing the exon 2 encoded aminopropeptide found in non-cartilage collagens [33].

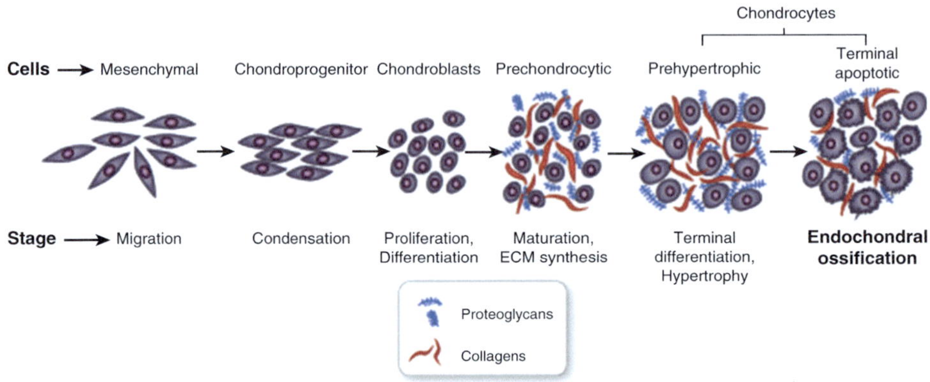

Fig. 2.2 Schematic diagram reflecting the series of cellular changes during chondrogenesis that occurs prenatally. This process is initiated with the precursor mesenchymal stem cell stimulation, followed by cellular condensation and various stages of differentiation of mesenchymal cells to chondrocytes and secretion of extracellular macromolecules. (Schematic created by Dr. Harpal K. Gahunia, and graphic illustration by Danny Aguilar, JD Graphics Solutions, East York, Ontario, Canada)

2.2.2 Mesenchymal Condensation

The second phase of chondrogenesis was first described by Fell [24]. This phase involves cellular interaction, cell shape change, and other events which are necessary to trigger the chondrogenic differentiation of the cells [34]. The transient cellular condensation or aggregation process results in an active movement of the chondroprogenitor MSC, which come into close apposition with one another to form precartilage condensations (Fig. 2.3) [27, 35, 36]. This event favors an increase in cell-cell contacts and interaction through cell-cell adhesion molecules and gap junctions that results in an increase in mesenchymal cell packing within the core of the limb bud (i.e., an increase in cells per unit volume), without an increase in cell proliferation [37, 38].

A change in the cellular morphology from a flattened mesenchymal cell to a rounded chondrocytic cell also plays an important role in this process [39]. In vitro studies have shown increased cytoplasmic collagen type II messenger ribonucleic acid (mRNA) during the condensation stage prior to depositing ECM [40]. Thereafter, a continuous and progressive increase in the cytoplasmic collagen type II mRNA and ECM collagen type II occurs. In parallel, cells peripheral to the condensation differentiate into a fibroblastic cell layer, the perichondrium, surrounding the cartilage core. These peripheral cells in turn differentiate into bone-producing osteoblasts, forming the periosteum [41].

2.2.3 Chondroblast and Chondrocyte Differentiation

Each stage of chondrocyte differentiation is characterized by modifications in cell proliferation and morphology, as well as the nature and amount of ECM macromolecule production. The chondroprogenitor MSCs undergoing chondrogenesis acquire a spherical cell morphology differentiating into the chondroblasts. Subsequently, the chondroblasts proliferate, secrete a cartilage-specific matrix, and further differentiate in chondrocytes to form the cartilage anlagen. The chondrocytes become encased in their ECM, further acquiring a characteristic rounded morphology. The ECM produced and secreted by differentiated chondrocytes maintain and regulate

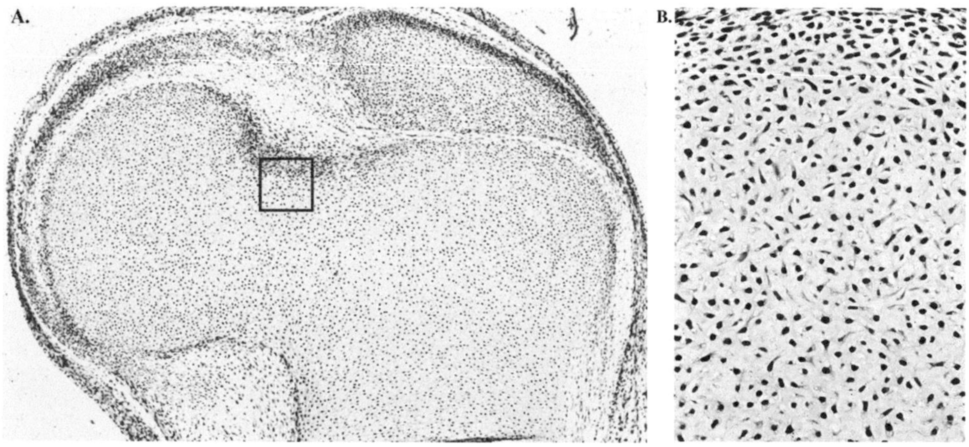

Fig. 2.3 Human fetal cartilage model of the hip femoral head (**a**) showing mesenchymal cell condensation and differentiation to prechondrocytic cells (**b**). Note cell condensation at future articular plate. (H&E, Original magnification, A = x2 and B = x 40)

the chondrocyte phenotype, and it is also essential as a template for the formation of the future bone.

2.2.4 Chondrocyte Hypertrophy

The last phase, chondrocyte hypertrophy, is a central process in chondrogenesis. It includes the progressive differentiation of proliferating matrix assembling chondrocytes to growth-arrested hypertrophic cells [42]. This process is initiated when the most central proliferating chondrocytes within the cartilage anlagen exit the cell cycle and differentiate to hypertrophy. Hypertrophic chondrocytes have increase in cell size and cellular fluid volume by 20 times.

Hypertrophic chondrocytes mineralize their surrounding matrix and eventually undergo apoptosis, while the area of hypertrophic cartilage is invaded by blood vessels, along with osteoclast and osteoblast precursor cells. Collectively, these cells degrade and remodel the cartilage ECM, and osteoblasts adhere to the remnants of the cartilage ECM to form bone tissue in this primary ossification center. The cartilage segments that remain on either side of the primary ossified region are termed the growth plates and are responsible for the longitudinal growth of long bones [19]. In addition to their contribution to bone growth, hypertrophic chondrocytes coordinate multiple aspects of EO through their secreted products [43].

2.2.5 Molecular and Genetic Factors Involved in Chondrogenesis

Several genes and their protein expression pattern the distribution and proliferation of mesenchymal condensations. Figure 2.4 is a schematic diagram showing the key participants involved in chondrogenesis and EO. The key signaling molecules, transcription factors, and gene expressions that are involved through the four stages of chondrogenesis as well as the hypertrophic differentiation are listed in Table 2.1. The differentiation of the prechondrocytic MSCs into chondroprogenitor cells takes place through the action of the transcription factor *SOX9*, which is involved in the progression of these cells through the various phases of chondrocyte differentiation [31, 32]. Fibroblast growth factor (FGF), hedgehog (HH), bone morphogenetic protein (BMP), and the Wnt (Drosophila Wg) pathway coordinate signaling along the three axes of the limb to ensure correct patterning along the dorsoventral

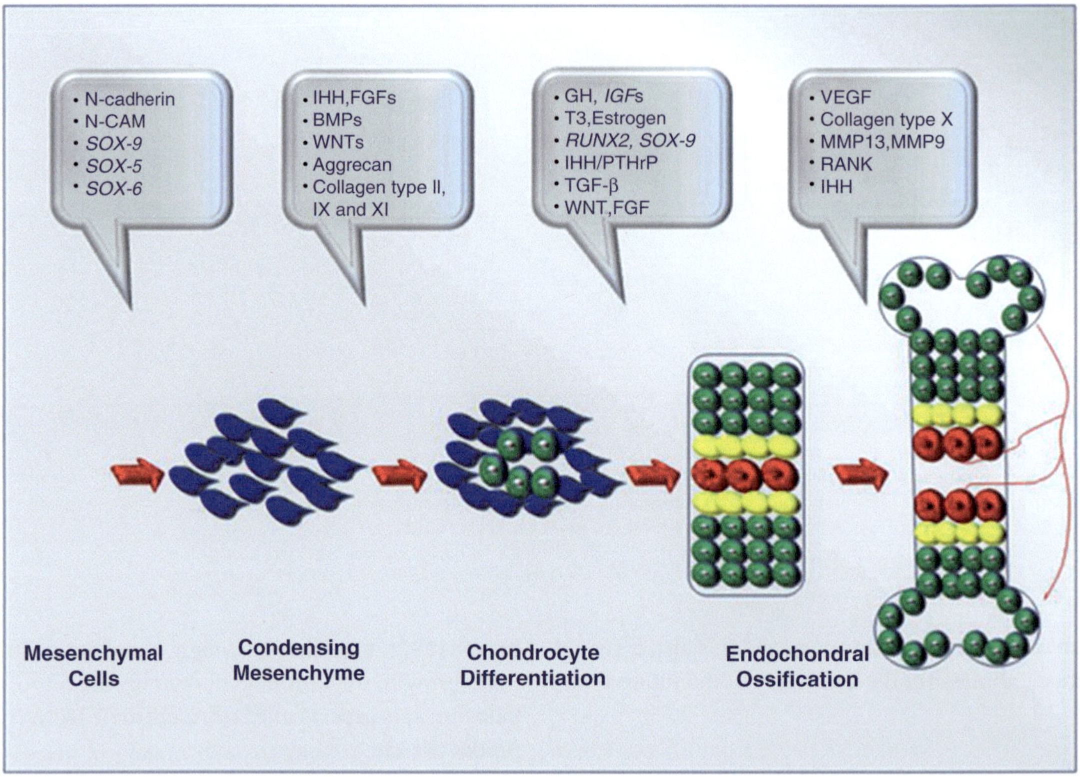

Fig. 2.4 Schematic diagram showing the key signaling molecular factors involved at each stage of chondrogenesis and endochondral ossification (EO). The process of chondrogenesis is initiated with the stimulation of mesenchymal stem cells to differentiate into prechondrocytic cells which migrate and condense to form cartilage template for the formation of long bones. Then the cells differentiate into chondrocytes and start to proliferate. Finally, the process of EO initiates with vascular penetration into the cartilage model forming the primary center of ossification at the diaphyses followed by secondary center of ossifications at the epiphysis of the developing bone. (BMP, bone morphogenetic protein; FGF, fibroblast growth factor; GH, growth hormone; IGF, insulin-like growth factor; IHH, Indian hedgehog homologue; MMP, matrix metalloproteinase; N-CAM, neural cell adhesion molecule; PTHrP, parathyroid hormone–related peptide; RANK, receptor activator of nuclear factor kB; TGF, transforming growth factor; VEGF, vascular endothelial growth factor)

and anteroposterior axes [44]. This is the case for Sonic hedgehog (SHH), a hedgehog member, which plays a pivotal role in development of the digits. The apical ectodermal ridge, on the other hand, expresses genes encoding several different proteins of the FGF family, in addition to BMPs and Wnt signaling molecules [22, 45, 46]. The expression of genes encoding these signaling molecules is mutually regulated, and the proper limb development consists of the cooperative integration of these three axes, including extensive cross talk between numerous signal transduction pathways [37].

The initiation of condensation is associated with increased hyaluronidase activity resulting in progressive decrease in the accumulation of extracellular hyaluronate (HA) [47–49]. The condensation process is also triggered with the involvement of two cell adhesion molecules, N-cadherin and neural cell adhesion molecule (N-CAM), which are Ca^{2+}-dependent and Ca^{2+}-independent cell-cell adhesion molecules, respectively [36, 50, 51]. Transforming growth factor-β (TGF-β), which is among the earliest signals in chondrogenic condensation, stimulates the synthesis of fibronectin, which in turn regulates N-CAM. Syndecan binds to fibronectin and downregulates N-CAM, thereby setting the condensation boundaries [26]. Fibronectin and collagen type I have been implicated in the cell-cell

Table 2.1 Summary of the effect of key signaling molecules, transcription factors, and gene expressions that are involved through the four stages of chondrogenesis as well as terminal differentiation. The important event and associated extracellular matrix molecules for each stage are shown

Chondrogenesis Stage	Cell Type and Important Event	Key Signaling Molecules/Transcription Factors		Extracellular Molecules
		Factors	Function(s)	
Pre-condensation	***Precursor Mesenchymal stem cells***	TGF-β	Regulates proliferation and differentiation of precursor MSCs into prochondrogenic cells; Stimulates fibronectin synthesis	Fibronectin Hyaluronan Collagen type 1
		FGF-2	Mitogen for cells of chondrogenic lineage	
		FGF-8	Mitogen for cells of chondrogenic lineage; Differentiation of precursor MSCs toward chondrogenic lineage	
		SHH	Acts in synergy with FGF-8 to promote prechondrogenic MSC condensation and increases the rate of chondrogenesis	
Condensation	***Mesenchymal stem cells/prochondrogenic cells (aggregation and cell-cell contact)***	TGF-β	Promotes chondrogenic differentiation; Stimulates fibronectin synthesis; Activates expression of Sox9	Fibronectin Hyaluronan Tenascin Versican Perlecan N-cadherin Collagen type 1 Collagen type III Collagen type V
		FGF-2	Mitogen for cells of chondrogenic lineage	
		FGF-8	Mitogen for cells of chondrogenic lineage	
		BMP-7	Maintains chondrogenic potential	
		Perlecan	Induces cell aggregation and condensation	
		N-CAM	Significant adhesive role in cell-cell interactions; Establishes the initial cellular contact	
		N-cadherin	Significant adhesive role in cell-cell interactions	
		SHH	Acts in synergy with FGF-8 to enhance MSC condensation	
		Hyaluronidase	Decreases ECM hyaluronate	
Proliferation and Differentiation	***Chondroprogenitor cells to chondroblasts***	TGF-β	Promotes chondroblast proliferation and differentiation; Activates expression of Sox9	Aggrecan Collagen type 1 Collagen type 1I
		FGF-2	Regulates expression of Sox9	
		FGF-8	Regulates chondroprogenitor cell proliferation and differentiation	
		IGF-1	Promotes chondroblast proliferation	
		BMP-7	Maintains chondrogenic potential; Prevents chondrocyte hypertrophy	
		SOX9	Induces and regulates differentiation of MSCs into chondroprogenitor cells; Responsible for prechondrocyte and chondroblast differentiation	
		SOX9, SOX6, SOX5	Sox9 required for expression of Sox5 and Sox6; Activate and regulate genes for collagen type II and aggrecan	
		Wnt-3	Promotes chondrogenic differentiation; Regulates expression of Sox9	

(continued)

Table 2.1 (continued)

Chondrogenesis Stage	Cell Type and Important Event	Key Signaling Molecules/Transcription Factors		Extracellular Molecules
		Factors	Function(s)	
Differentiation and Maturation	***Chondroblasts maturing to chondrocytes; ECM synthesized***	TGF-β	Promotes chondroblast differentiation; Stabilizes chondrocyte phenotype; Inhibits chondrocyte hypertrophy	Aggrecan CS
		FGF-18	Promotes chondrocyte proliferation and differentiation during initial phase of cartilage development; Enhances ECM production	Link protein COMP
		IGF-1	Promotes chondrocyte proliferation and maturation	Collagen type 1I
		BMP-6	Regulates cartilage growth and differentiation	Collagen type 1X
		BMP-7	Maintains chondrogenic potential; Prevents chondrocyte hypertrophy	Collagen type XI
		IHH	Regulates the rate of cartilage differentiation; Stimulates proliferating chondrocytes to produce PTHrP; Induces expression of various BMPs	
		PTHrP	Stimulates Nkx3.2 to block hypertrophic differentiation; Inhibits expression of IHH; Prevents RUNx2 expression	
		SOX9	Required for co-expression of Sox5 and Sox6; Inhibits chondrocytic hypertrophy; Regulates the expression of the genes Sox5 and Sox6, COLIIα1, COLXIα2 and cartilage link protein; Stimulates synthesis of collagen types II, IX, and XI	
		SOX9, SOX6, SOX5	Co-regulate expression of COLIXα1 and aggrecan; Delays chondrocyte hypertrophy; Suppresses expression of hypertrophic and osteogenic differentiation at the same time	
		Wnt-3, Wnt-5	Promotes chondrogenic differentiation; Delays chondrocyte hypertrophy	
		Wnt-9	Blocks chondrogenic differentiation and chondrocyte hypertrophy	
		RUNx2	Controls chondrocyte maturation	
Maturation to Terminal Differentiation	***Mature chondrocytes to hypertrophic chondrocytes***	FGF-2	Induces chondrocyte hypertrophy; Promotes expression of RUNX2	Aggrecan
		FGF-9	Promotes chondrocyte hypertrophy	COMP
		IGF-1	Increases the size of hypertrophic chondrocytes	Collagen type 1I
		BMP-2, BMP-4	Induces chondrocyte hypertrophy	Collagen type V1
		BMP-6	Contributes to cartilage hypertrophy	Collagen type 1X
		IHH	Stimulates proliferating chondrocytes to produce PTHrP; Induces expression of various BMP's	Collagen type X1
		SOX9	Required for co-expression of Sox5 and Sox6; Regulates the expression of the genes Sox5 and Sox6, COLIIα1, COLXIα2, and cartilage link protein; Stimulates synthesis of collagen types II, IX, and XI	
		SOX6, SOX5	Delays chondrocyte hypertrophy; Upregulates BMP6; Downregulate IHH, FGF-3, and RUNx2	
		Wnt-4, Wnt-8	Blocks chondrogenic differentiation; Promotes chondrocyte hypertrophy	
		PTHrP	Regulates expression and activation of RUNx2	
		RUNx2	Controls chondrocyte maturation	

Terminal Differentiation	***Hypertrophic chondrocytes***	IGF-1	Increases the size of hypertrophic chondrocytes	Collagen type X Alkaline phosphatase Hydroxyapatite Blood vessels
		VEGF	Initiates and promotes angiogenesis by acting on endothelial cells; Induces and regulates blood vessel invasion (neovascularization) into hypertrophic cartilage that results in subsequent bone formation; Acts on osteoclast to stimulate bone resorption; Stimulates EO	
		MMP-9, MMP-13	Degrades ECM collagens and aggrecans	
		ALP	Enzyme essential for mineral deposition	
		IHH	Promotes chondrocyte hypertrophy; Regulates activation and expression of RUNx2	
		RUNx2	Regulates the transcription of hypertrophic markers (collagen type X, MMP-13, VEGF, and IHH)	

MSCs, *Mesenchymal stem cells*; TGF-β, *Transforming growth factor-β*; FGF-2, -3, -8, *Fibroblast growth factor receptor-2, -3, -8*; SHH, *Sonic hedgehog*; BMP, *Bone morphogenetic protein*; N-CAM, *Neural cell adhesion molecule*; GH, *Growth hormone*; IGF, *Insulin-like growth factor*; IHH, *Indian hedgehog homologue*; SOX, *SRY (sex determining region Y)-box transcription factor*; CS, *Chondroitin sulfate*; Wnt, *Wingless-related integration site signaling protein*; RUNx2, *Runt-related transcription factor*; MMP, *Matrix metalloproteinase*; PTHrP, *Parathyroid hormone-related peptide*; VEGF, *Vascular endothelial growth factor*; ALP, *Alkaline phosphatase* interaction, whereas prostaglandin-mediated elevations in cyclic adenosine monophosphate (cAMP) levels regulate chondrogenesis [36, 52–55]. The ECM molecules, which also include tenascins and thrombospondins, including cartilage oligomeric matrix protein (COMP), interact with the cell adhesion molecules to activate intracellular signaling pathways involving focal adhesion kinase and paxillin, to initiate the transition from chondroprogenitor cells to a fully committed chondrocyte [37].

Following cellular condensation, the process of chondroprogenitor cell differentiation to chondrocytes is associated with expression of cartilage-specific genes and initiated with the synthesis of collagen type II. These genes include components of cartilage ECM genes, such as those encoding collagen type II α1 (Col2α1), collagen type IX, collagen type XI, aggrecan, link protein, and COMP [26]. Expression of these genes is regulated at the transcriptional level, spatially and temporally, so that they have different and dynamic expression patterns during chondrogenic differentiation [56]. *SOX9* is a transcriptional activator required for chondrogenesis, whereas *SOX5* and *SOX6* are closely related DNA-binding proteins that critically enhance its function [57]. Cells undergoing chondrogenesis become encased in their ECM, acquire a distinct spherical morphology and initiate expression of the transcription factors *SOX9*, *SOX5*, and *SOX6*. Co-expressed and regulated by *SOX9*, both *SOX5* and *SOX6* play a significant role in activating and regulating the genes encoding the ECM molecules collagen type II and aggrecan [28, 57]. Subsequently, the chondrocytes proliferate and secrete a cartilage-specific matrix to form the cartilage anlagen. This cartilage-specific matrix contains collagen type II, collagen types IX and XI, GLA protein, the large chondroitin sulfate-rich PG, aggrecan, and link protein, while the expression of collagen type I is turned off [56, 58–71].

Collagen type II provides tensile strength to the cartilaginous matrix and is important in the establishment of temporal and spatial organization with other matrix components such as the main PG, aggrecan. Aggrecan is heavily modified by sulfated glycosaminoglycans (GAGs), attracts numerous water molecules, and forms large aggregates in cartilage. Aggrecan and other PGs provide the cushioning capacity of the matrix but also act to immobilize and store growth factors and thereby function as molecular organizers of the ECM and cartilage in general.

Progression through chondrocyte maturation to hypertrophic chondrocytes is repressed by *SOX9* modulation of the Wnt/beta-catenin signaling pathway with beta-catenin degradation or inhibition of beta-catenin transcriptional activity without affecting its stability [24, 72]. In addition, *SOX5* and *SOX6* delay chondrocyte hypertrophy by downregulating Indian hedgehog homologue (IHH) signaling, FGFr3, and RUNx2 and upregulating BMP-6 [57, 73]. Further maturation of chondrocytes is essential for the final remodeling of the cartilage into bone. Chondrocytes achieve this maturation through upregulation of the transcription factor RUNx2, inducing chondrocyte hypertrophy and positive control by BMPs and matrix metalloproteinases (MMPs, also known as matrixins, such as MMP-13) [74]. BMPs play a substantial role in promoting chondrocyte differentiation and maturation [75]. IHH induces the expression of various BMPs, and proliferating chondrocytes react to BMP signals with the upregulation of IHH expression. Another important pathway in chondrocyte development is the Wnt signaling pathway, which is involved in all stages of chondrocyte development.

Chondrocyte hypertrophy is tightly controlled during normal skeletal development by cell-cell signaling and transcription factors [76, 77]. IHH, which is required for endochondral bone formation and synchronizes skeletal angiogenesis with perichondrial maturation, is expressed in prehypertrophic chondrocytes as they enter the hypertrophic phase and begin to downregulate the expression of collagen type II and initiate expression of the hypertrophic chondrocyte markers collagen type X and alkaline phosphatase [26, 78].

The transcription factor RUNx2 plays an important role in the regulation of chondrocyte hypertrophy and associated changes in the ECM [26, 57, 73, 79–81]. In vitro studies demonstrated that the expression and activation of RUNx2 is regulated by parathyroid hormone-related protein (PTHrP) and IHH [82, 83]. Further, through its interaction with TGF signaling via SMADs,

RUNx2 controls chondrocyte maturation [84]. SMADs comprise of a family of structurally similar proteins that are the main intracellular signal transducers for receptors of TGF-β superfamily, which are critically important for regulating cell development and growth. While SMAD3 transduces TGF-β signals, SMAD7 inhibits both TGF-β and BMP signaling [85]. TGF-β is stimulatory in early stages of cartilage formation, but in later stages it inhibits chondrocyte terminal differentiation, and it has been hypothesized that it stabilizes the phenotype of the prehypertrophic chondrocyte [86].

ECM deposited by hypertrophic chondrocytes serves as a template for subsequent bone formation, and these cells also secrete soluble proteins, including vascular endothelial growth factor (VEGF), IHH, and receptor activator of nuclear factor kappa-B (RANK) ligand that control the activities of other cell lineages (endothelial cells, osteoblasts, and osteoclasts, respectively) involved in EO [87]. The proper regulation of chondrocyte hypertrophy is also necessary for maintaining the cartilage lining synovial joint surfaces, as abnormal chondrocyte hypertrophy in articular cartilage is associated with osteoarthritis [88].

2.3 Articular Cartilage Growth: Appositional and Interstitial

The growth of cartilage occurs by two independent mechanisms, both of which can occur simultaneously, namely, appositional growth and interstitial growth. Appositional growth occurs at the chondrogenic level of the perichondrium where new layers of the ECM are formed on the surface of the existing cartilage. This process involves increase of mitotic activity of the surface chondrocytes, thus increasing the thickness of cartilage at the level of the perichondrium. Appositional growth is also responsible for the shape of the cartilage model and for the increase in bone diameter. When vascular infiltration occurs, it triggers the process, whereby the perichondrium of the cartilage model becomes periosteum that in turn initiates the formation of compact bone. Studies with primates revealed significant increase of proliferating cells restricted to the upper half of the articular cartilage, indicating that the majority of growth activity of the developing articular cartilage is occurring in the articular surface regions [89, 90].

Interstitial growth, on the other hand, involves some mitotic division of the existing core chondrocytes and secretion of cartilage ECM components by the daughter chondrocytes, including extracellular GAGs, hyaluronate, collagen, and water. This results in the growth of the matrix surrounding the cells.

2.4 Endochondral Ossification

Endochondral ossification is the complex process that is initiated when the embryonic cartilage model is invaded by blood vessels and infiltrated by bone cell precursors [79, 80]. During prenatal growth, this process occurs first at the center of the cartilaginous model by the formation of the primary center of ossification and diaphyses. Thereafter, during postnatal growth and development, the secondary centers of ossification occur at both ends resulting in the formation of epiphysis [79]. Cartilage canals extend as branches of the blood vessels to the AECC complex that forms the articulating surface of the bone, the epiphyseal center of ossification, and the GP [51]. Figure 2.5 shows the various stages of EO from the formation of cartilage model leading up to the formation of GP.

At birth, the immature AECC is thick and vascular, occupying majority of the epiphysis. With growth and development, the immature cartilage forms a cap over the articulating ends of the epiphyses with the structural features consistent with that of articular cartilage (toward articular surface) and epiphyseal cartilage adjacent to the subchondral bone of the epiphyses (Figs. 2.6a and b). The immature AECC shows five morphologically distinct zones extending from the free articular surface to the subchondral bone as follows: (a) the *zone of articulating cartilage* with characteristic features of a mature cartilage, and the subsequent zones typical of the epiphyseal cartilage consisting of: (b) the *zone of proliferation* with active chondrocytes undergoing mito-

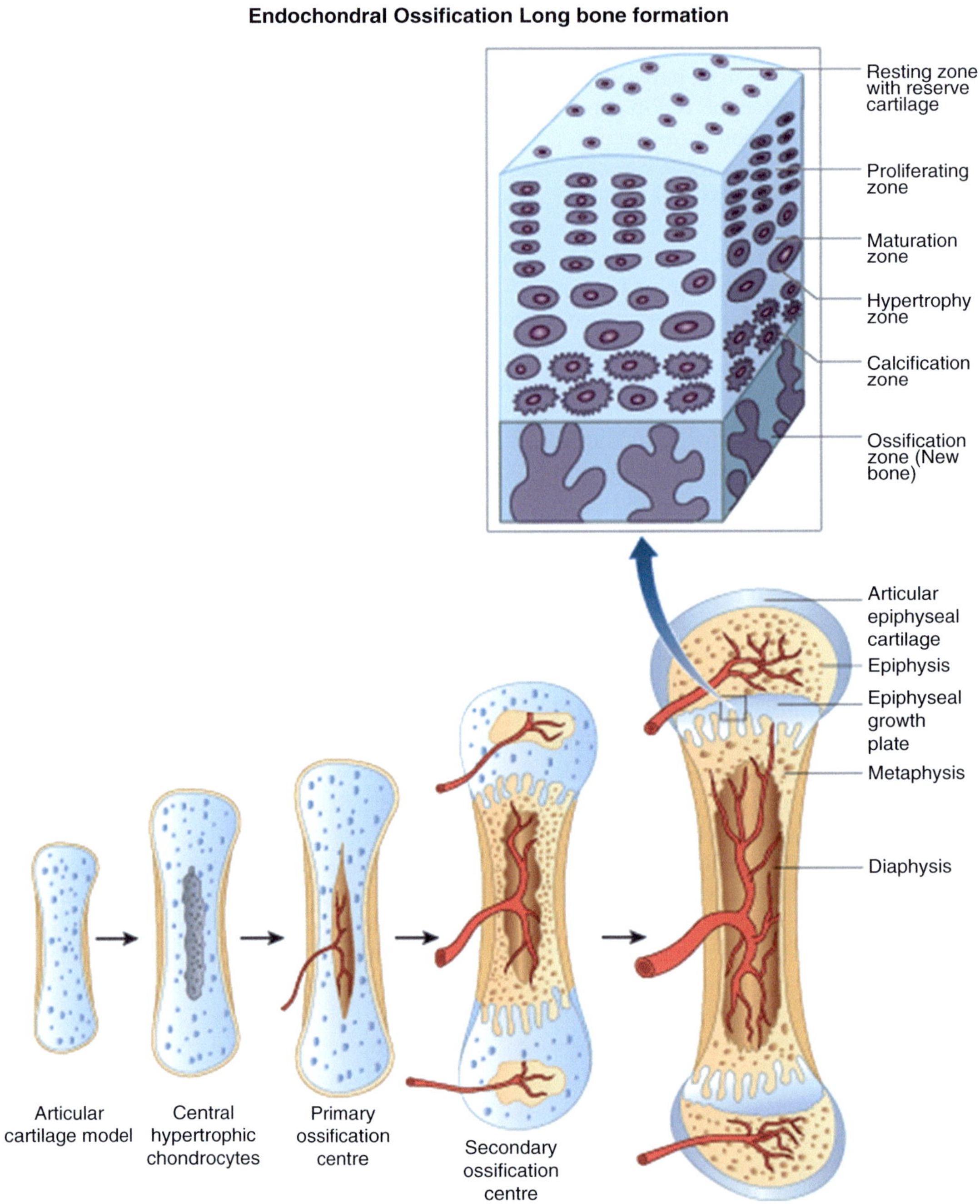

Fig. 2.5 Endochondral ossification from the formation of cartilage model through the development of primary and secondary ossification centers to the formation of epiphyseal (growth) plate as well as articular cartilage at joint surface. (Courtesy of Dr. Harpal K Gahunia)

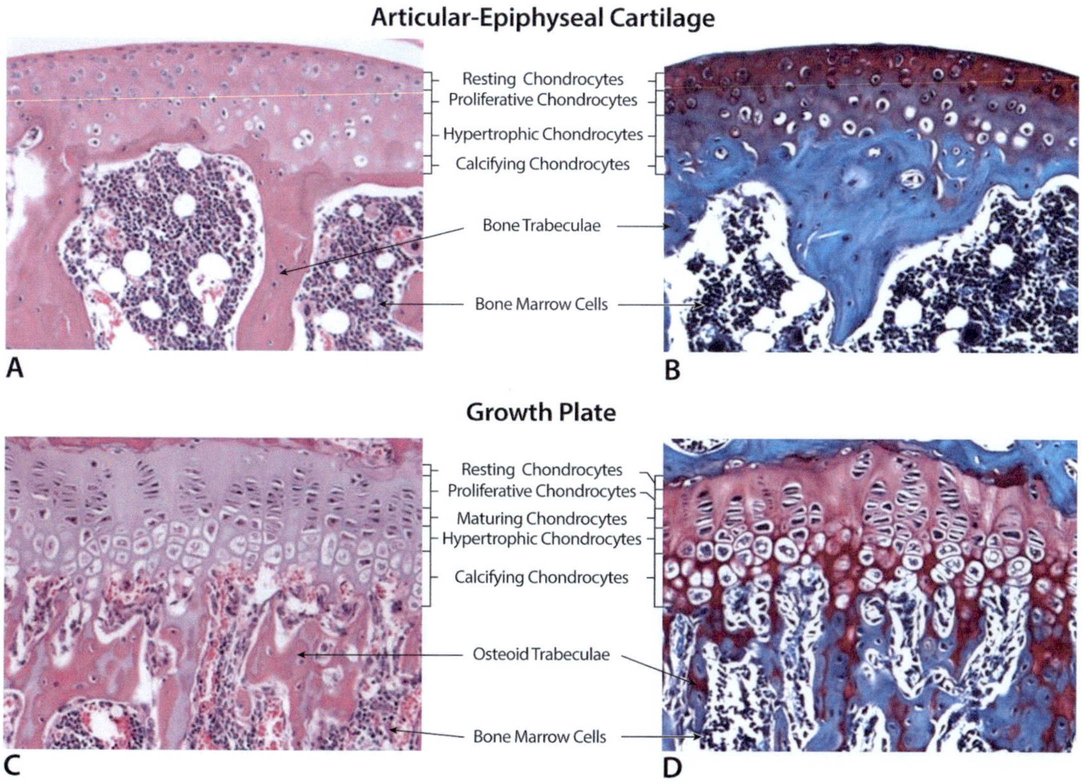

Fig. 2.6 Photographs showing articular-epiphyseal cartilage (**a** and **b**) and the growth plate (**c** and **d**) of a 12-week-old wild-type mouse. Histological sections were stained with hematoxylin and eosin (**a** and **c**) and with Alcian Blue (**b** and **d**). The Alcian Blue stain shows the following structures which are observed during endochondral ossification: cartilage (magenta), calcified cartilage (purple), and bone (blue) (Original magnification, x10)

sis, (c) the *zone of maturation* with enlarged chondrocytes, (d) the *zone of hypertrophy* with hypertrophic chondrocytes that accumulate glycogen and lipid and secretes alkaline phosphatase to the surrounding ECM, and (e) the *zone of calcification* with necrotic chondrocytes and an ECM rich in insoluble salts with traces of bone trabeculae and vascular infiltration. Although longitudinal bone growth primarily occurs at the GP, the AECC that caps the long bone also contributes to its growth [91, 92]. In children, adolescents, and skeletally immature individuals, the GP is a thin layer of growing cartilage between the epiphyseal and metaphyseal bone, one at each distal end of the long bones (Fig. 2.7).

The GP consists of various zones with chondrogenic stem cells and chondrocytes at various stages of differentiation and maturation (Figs. 2.6c and d). The quiescent *zone of resting chondrocytes* is adjacent to the epiphysis and furthest from the ossification front of the metaphysis. These cells replicate at a slow rate and act as stem-like cells that replenish the pool of proliferative chondrocytes [25, 93]. Adjacent is the *zone of proliferation*, where the chondrocytes replicate at a high rate and the resulting daughter cells form a columnar stack along the long axis of the bone (Fig. 2.8). Following proliferation, chondrocytes pass through a transition stage in which they are known as "prehypertrophic"

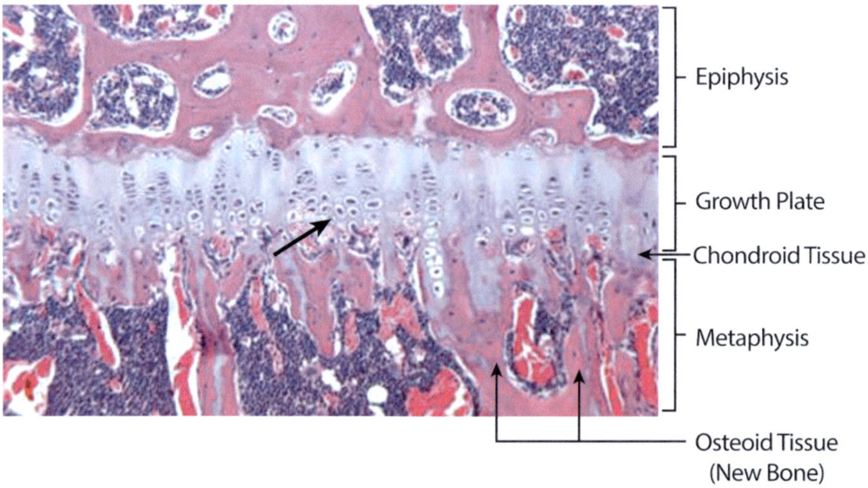

Fig. 2.7 Histological photograph of the distal femur growth plate (maturing) of a 12-week-old wild-type mouse showing the various morphological zones of differentiated chondrocytes. The arrow shows terminally differentiated hypertrophic chondrocytes. Note formation of subepiphyseal bone trabeculae. (H&E, original magnification x10)

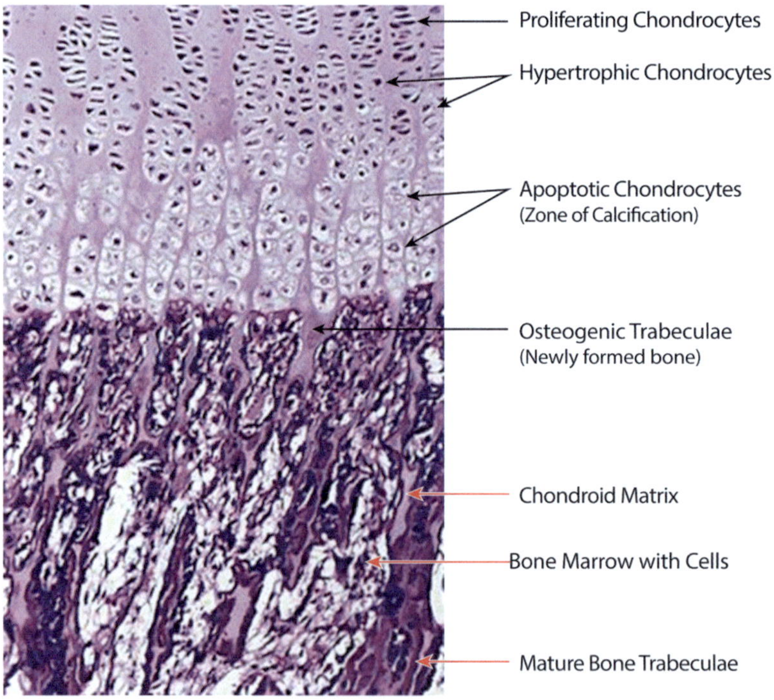

Fig. 2.8 Human, newborn epiphyseal cartilage showing the zone of proliferation, zone of maturation, zone of calcification, and, new bone formation. Note columns of hypertrophic chondrocytes with terminal differentiation. The subjacent columns of chondroid matrix provide the template for new appositional bone formation. (H&E, original magnification x10)

chondrocytes. These cells further increase their height about six- to tenfold in the *zone of hypertrophy* and secrete ECM [79]. Hypertrophic chondrocytes undergo apoptosis shortly before the blood vessels invade the chondrocyte lacunae [94]. Subsequent to vascular invasion and infiltration by bone cell precursors, the cartilagenous matrix begins to calcify at the *zone of calfication* (Figs. 2.9a, b and c). The calcified cartilage invaded by blood vessels, osteoclasts, bone marrow cells, and osteoblasts becomes mineralized and remodels into bone. This area constitutes the *zone of ossification* [79]. The osteoblasts deposit bone on remnants of cartilage matrix [87]. The net effect is that new bone tissue is progressively created at the diaphyses of the growth plate, resulting in bone elongation. A similar phenomenon, albeit at a slower pace, occurs at the AECC capping the long bones.

The GP undergoes structural and functional changes over time. The rate of chondrocyte proliferation reflecting the rate of longitudinal bone growth falls progressively as the GP matures from childhood to skeletally mature adolescence. During this phase, the overall growth plate height and its various zones progressively decrease and eventually fuse when replaced by bone sometime during late puberty [95]. This process involving a decline in both the function and cellularity of the growth plate has been thought to be due to a mechanism intrinsic to the GP rather than hormonal or other systemic mechanisms. Recent evidence suggests that this decline occurs because stem-like cells in the resting zone have a finite proliferative capacity that is gradually exhausted [96, 97].

2.4.1 Molecular and Genetic Factors Involved in Endochondral Ossification

The formation of cartilage and bone is initiated with the migration of undifferentiated MSCs that differentiate and mature into chondrocytes during the embryonic stage of bone development. Postnatally, bone development continues with the maturation of the AECC complex and GP, which is influenced by multiple growth factors and hormones until late puberty when the skeletal maturity is achieved and the GP fuses. Another important contributor to GP regulation is the adjacent perichondrium, which contributes to vascular invasion along with osteogenic cells. Perichondrial cells send signals to chondrocytes via BMPs, FGFs, and Wnt signaling. Also, these perichondrial cells receive signals back from epiphyseal chondrocytes. FGF signaling inhibits chondrocyte proliferation and coordinates the onset of differentiation with chondrocyte growth arrest in the developing GP [98].

Chondrocytes in the zones of proliferation, hypertrophy, and calcification are essential regulators of skeletal development [99, 100]. Changes in chondrocyte morphology and metabolic activity are coordinated with the action of blood vessels, osteoclasts, and osteoblasts. EO is also subjected to the influence of a plethora of ECM molecules and growth/signaling factors, which function to regulate many aspects of EO, including cellular growth and differentiation [101–103]. The major subfamilies of growth factors include TGF-βs and BMPs.

2.4.1.1 Transforming Growth Families-β

During skeletal development, TGF-β has unique functions and acts sequentially to modulate chondrocyte and osteoblast differentiation [104]. Specifically, TGF-β promotes chondrogenesis in cultures of undifferentiated multipotent MSCs but inhibits hypertrophic differentiation of chondrocyte cultures and in cultured mouse long bone rudiments [105]. TGF-βs maintain cartilage homeostasis by preventing inappropriate chondrocyte differentiation [104–106]. TGF-β1, TGF-β2, and TGF-β3 cause arrest in the G1 phase of the cell cycle in many nontransformed cell types in vitro, and they also stimulate matrix production by mesenchymal cells [104]. TGF-βs signal through heteromeric type I and type II receptor serine/threonine. Transgenic mice with a defective TGF-β type II receptor develop progressive skeletal degeneration with the replacement of the articular surfaces by bone and hypertrophic cartilage [105]. Noggin is a

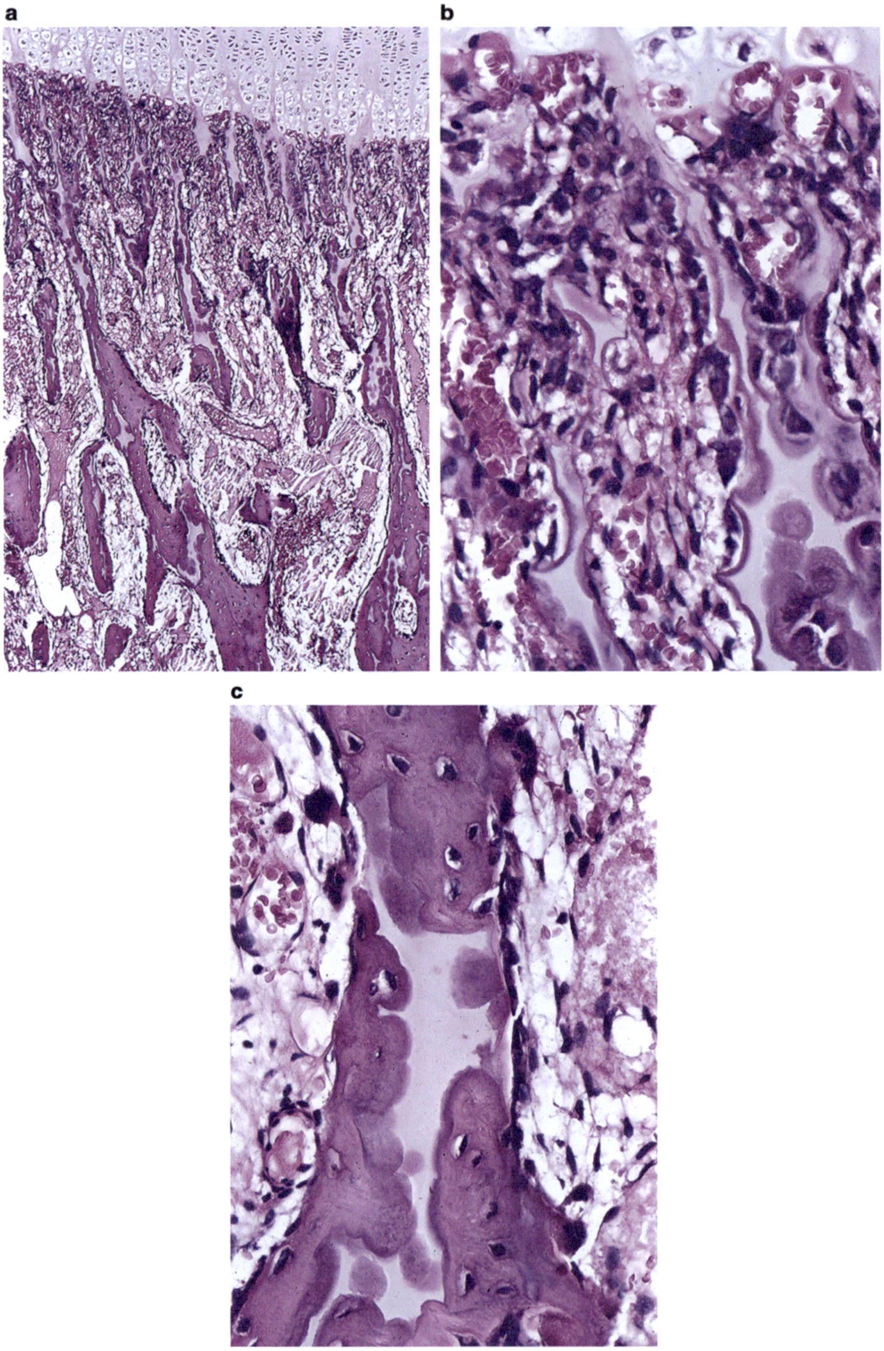

Fig. 2.9 Human newborn epiphyseal cartilage (**a**) showing the zone of maturation with hypertrophic chondrocytes (top) and the subjacent zone of calcification with apoptotic chondrocytes, degraded cartilage matrix, and new bone formation (osteoid tissue). (**b**) Terminal hypertrophic chondrocytes, columns of chondroid matrix, and the replacement of the cartilaginous extracellular matrix by newly formed bone. (**c**) Appositional osteoid tissue formed on chondroid matrix with osteoblasts on the surface and osteocytes embedded within the newly formed bone matrix. Of note is the remnant of the cartilage matrix (light pink stain at the center) of the developing bone trabeculae. (H&E, original magnification: **a** x2, **b** and **c** x20)

protein which in humans is encoded by the NOG gene. Noggin inhibits TGF-β transduction by binding to TGF-β family ligands and preventing them from binding to their corresponding receptors [106].

2.4.1.2 Bone Morphogenetic Proteins

Bone morphogenetic proteins are multifunctional growth factors that belong to the TGF-β superfamily. BMPs are important regulators of growth, differentiation, and morphogenesis during embryology [107–111]. Members of the BMP superfamily regulate multiple aspects of chondrogenesis and act sequentially in regulating specific aspects of EO [112, 113]. BMP signaling leads to compaction of mesenchymal cells, regulating the cell cohesion in condensations and also supports proliferation of chondrocytes in GP [114]. The cartilage interzone expresses both BMPs and their antagonists, such as Noggin, that are thought to interact with and modulated BMP activities. In mice lacking Noggin, cartilage condensations are initiated normally but develop hyperplasia, with unaffected cartilage maturation. Excess BMP activity in the absence of Noggin antagonism increases the recruitment of cells into cartilage, expanding the cartilage at the expense of other tissues, resulting in oversized growth plates and failure to initiate joint formation [106].

BMP-6 has been reported in prehypertrophic and hypertrophic chondrocytes; whereas, BMP-7 was detected in chick sternal prehypertrophic and mouse metatarsal proliferating chondrocytes [113]. However, investigation into the effects of BMP signaling on chondrocyte hypertrophy is poorly understood [115, 116]. Using cultured embryonic upper sternal chondrocytes, it has been suggested that more than one subgroup of BMPs regulate to signal the stimulation of chondrocyte maturation, to increase IHH expression independent of maturational effects, and to partially overcome the inhibitory effects of PTHrP on maturation [117, 118]. Also, results of another study on mice have indicated that Il-10 acts as a stimulator of chondrocyte proliferation and chondrogenic or hypertrophic differentiation via activation of the BMP signaling pathway [119].

2.4.1.3 Wnt Family

Wnt morphogens are secreted signaling proteins that are intrinsically involved in early embryonic development, organogenesis, and tissue homeostasis throughout life [120–123]. The Wnt signaling pathways contribute to diverse cellular activities during cell differentiation, spatial-temporal patterning, and cell motility [124, 125]. In the skeletal system, Wnt signaling is involved in all stages of chondrocyte development, and it stimulates hypertrophic chondrocyte differentiation in the GP [78], whereas deregulation of Wnt signaling is involved in cartilage degeneration [126].

Signaling by the Wnt family of secreted glycolipoproteins via the transcriptional coactivator β-catenin has been recognized as a key regulator of embryonic development and adult homeostasis in bone, cartilage, and joint [127–129]. Developmental regulation of Wnt/β-catenin signals is required for GP assembly, cartilage integrity, and EO [130, 131]. In the presence of Wnt ligands, cytoplasmic β-catenin binds to its receptor and activates Dishevelled type proteins (DVL). DVL isoforms are critical regulatory molecules for chondrocyte proliferation and differentiation [132].

Results from animal studies demonstrate that β-catenin-dependent canonical and β-catenin-independent noncanonical Wnt signaling pathways have multiple roles in the regulation of cartilage development, growth, and maintenance [128]. Activation of the canonical Wnt pathway with β-catenin play important roles in the condensation and differentiation of MSCs, chondrocyte maturation and maintenance of phenotype, hypertrophic chondrocyte maturation during EO, as well as tissue degeneration and regeneration [95, 127, 133]. Wnt/β-catenin signaling inhibits chondrogenesis by preventing differentiation of progenitor cells into chondrocytes. In contrast, noncanonical Wnt signaling is important in columnar organization of GP chondrocytes.

Several studies show that Wnt/β-catenin signaling is active during EO and suggest that β-catenin stimulates chondrocyte maturation [130, 131, 134]. In the GP, once cartilage is formed and the skeletal elements have developed, β-catenin signaling is reestablished where numerous Wnts are expressed and it induces formation of osteoblasts [135].

β-Catenin-dependent signaling is required for progression of EO and growth of axial and appendicular skeletons, while excessive activation of this signaling can cause severe inhibition of initial cartilage formation and GP organization and function in mice. Investigation of the role of canonical Wnt signaling in a mouse model in which the Wnt antagonist secreted frizzled-related protein 1 (sFRP1) was nonfunctional, showed shortened height of the GP, and increased calcification of the hypertrophic zone in the sfrp1-/– mouse, indicating accelerated EO [136]. Wnt/β-catenin signaling is a contributing mechanism for increased chondrocyte hypertrophy and cartilage differentiation. Another study on mice have shown that Wnt signaling may increase bone mass by keeping the osteoblasts in proliferation phase [137].

Overexpression of Wnts 4, 8, and 9, β-catenin, and lymphoid enhancer-binding factor-1 (*LEF*-1) induce collagen type X, alkaline phosphatase, and other genes associated with chondrocyte hypertrophy. Also, overexpression of β-catenin in chondrocytes strongly stimulates the expression of matrix degradation enzymes [138, 139]. Furthermore, activation of β-catenin in mature chondrocytes stimulates hypertrophy, matrix mineralization, and expression of MMP-13 and VEGF, all factors that are present in osteoarthritis [138]. Increased levels of β-catenin have been reported in chondrocytes within areas of degenerative cartilage in osteoarthritic joints [20, 138, 140].

2.4.2 Endocrine Signals

A complex network of endocrine signals governs and regulates the longitudinal growth of the GP through their actions locally on chondrocytes and also indirectly by modulating other endocrine signals in the network. Local effects of hormones are mediated by changes in paracrine factors that control chondrocyte proliferation and differentiation. Growth factors regulate many aspects of EO, including GP cellular growth and differentiation [101, 102]. Growth hormone (GH) and insulin-like growth factors (IGFs) are potent stimulators of longitudinal bone growth. Specifically, GH stimulates local IGF-1 expression and plays a role in the proliferation of the resting zone chondrocytes; whereas, IGF-1 enhances the proliferation of chondrocytes in the resting and proliferative zones and also increases the size of hypertrophic chondrocytes. Thyroid hormone, permissive to chondrocyte proliferation and differentiation, promotes longitudinal growth and maturation with the largest effect seen in the hypertrophic zone. In vitro studies have demonstrated that leptin hormone synergizes with thyroid hormone signaling to promote chondrocyte proliferation and terminal differentiation [141]. Glucocorticoids inhibit chondrocyte proliferation, delay growth plate senescence, and induce chondrocyte apoptosis, hence contributing to the overall inhibition of the longitudinal bone growth. At the zone of proliferation, estrogen inhibits chondrocyte proliferation. As such, estrogen accelerates GP senescence; thus, resulting in its early fusion due to exhaustion of the proliferative capacity of the GP chondrocytes [142]. Androgens have stimulatory effects on chondrocyte proliferation, ECM synthesis, and secretion by the mature chondrocytes, and it also enhances IGF-1 expression. Vitamin D is permissive for normal differentiation and apoptosis of hypertrophic chondrocytes.

Paracrine regulators, PTHrP, and IHH are considered key factors that coordinate EO by regulating chondrocyte proliferation and differentiation as well as osteoblast differentiation [113, 143, 144]. Both factors have been identified in the postnatal human GP and play a role in GP fusion during late puberty [25, 95].

2.4.3 Notch Signals and Smad7

Notch signaling is an evolutionarily conserved pathway downstream of many developmental processes, which is important in cartilage development. Notch signaling suppresses chondrocyte hypertrophy by inhibiting *SOX9* [145]. Notch signaling regulates the onset of chondrocyte maturation in a *SOX9*-dependent manner, while Notch-mediated regulation of terminal chondrocyte maturation likely functions independently of *SOX9* [145].

SMADS are the intracellular mediators of TGF-β signaling. SMAD7 is required for both axial and appendicular skeletal development, and its loss leads to impairment of the cell cycle in chondrocytes and to defects in terminal maturation [146]. SMAD7 is an intracellular inhibitor of BMP and TGF-β signaling, which when overexpressed in chondrocytes can impact chondrogenesis [85]. SMAD7 overexpression in conditional transgenic mice exerts specific functions at multiple stages of chondrocyte differentiation, decreasing proliferation and inhibiting maturation toward hypertrophy. Prechondrocytic cells are capable of differentiating as articular or transient cartilage, depending on exposure to Wnt or BMP signaling, respectively. The spatial organization of the articular cartilage results from a band of Nog-expressing cells, which insulates these proliferating chondrocytes from BMP signaling and allows them to differentiate as articular cartilage under the influence of Wnt signaling emanating from the interzone [110].

2.5 Role of Bone Morphogenetic Proteins and Matrix Metalloproteinases in Articular Cartilage Repair and Degradation

Even though gene expression and protein synthesis can be activated upon injury, articular cartilage has a limited ability of self-repair, and efforts to regenerate articular cartilage are still a work-in-progress. Cartilage genesis, differentiation, and maintenance of homeostasis are finely tuned by a complex network of signaling molecules. A clear understanding of the role and cellular pathways of these signaling molecules and the factors that promote chondrogenesis is important to the development of cell-seeded and non-cell-seeded approaches for cartilage regeneration (Tables 2.1). Refer to Chaps. 16 and 17 for further description of these approaches.

Several BMPs have been implicated in chondrogenic differentiation and/or chondrocyte function. Compared to BMP-2 and BMP-6, the effect of BMP-9 is more significant in inducing chondrogenic differentiation [108]. The use of BMP-9 for chondrogenesis may improve current therapies for regenerative cartilage repair. During cartilage development, various Wnts and their signaling pathway are involved in chondrocyte differentiation and maintenance of articular cartilage [26, 37, 120, 122, 123, 126, 128, 131, 135, 147]. As such, strategies to carefully manipulating this pathway might contribute to improved cartilage regeneration.

Several MMPs, a family of proteases, are expressed during EO, including collagenases (MMP-1 and MMP-13), gelatinases (MMP-2 and MMP-9), stromelysins (MMP-3 and MMP-10), and Membrane type 1 metalloproteinase (MT1-MMP). These proteases are able to cleave a variety of substrates including ECM proteins, extracellular non-ECM proteins, and cell surface proteins. Within the GP, MMP-13, which degrades both fibrillar collagen and aggrecan, is the major collagenase and is selectively expressed by hypertrophic chondrocytes [148]. MMP-13 transcription is controlled by RUNx2, both important participants in the axis "chondrocyte hypertrophy-matrix mineralization" [149]. MMP-9, in contrast to MMP-13, does not cleave native fibrillar collagens, but does cleave denatured collagens and aggrecan. MMP-9 is highly expressed in monocytes, preosteoclasts, and osteoclasts, and is concentrated at sites of cartilage resorption, where vascular invasion occurs [150]. MT1-MMP plays a major role in the ECM remodeling, directly by degrading several of its components and indirectly by activating pro-MMP2. MT1-MMP expression promotes angiogenesis during EO through an up-regulation of VEGF expression.

2.6 Conclusions

Articular cartilage is a dynamic tissue, whose complexity is enhanced by the existence of numerous developmental phases and overlap in phenotypic gene expression with related cell types. In most growing individuals, the complex pattern of cartilage growth regulated by cascades of signaling molecules works seamlessly without fail. However, disruption to the normal balance of synthesis and degradation can lead to variation in the intrinsic characteristics of cartilage matrix. Depending on the extent of the disorder, this can lead to a gradual degeneration of the ECM that is responsible for the genesis of clinically recognizable developmental cartilage diseases. The current knowledge in articular cartilage physiology as well as the growth factors, local regulators, and hormones involved in articular cartilage growth, development, and maturation are described. The objective is to provide a better understanding of the key molecular and genetic participants during the growth and development of articular and epiphyseal cartilage.

Advances in understanding of the age-related morphologic, biochemical, and biomechanical changes in articular cartilage (including growth plate) and their effects on joint homeostasis, the natural healing process after cartilage acute or chronic injury, and improved diagnostic standards for cartilage lesion evaluation make the goal repairing or regenerating a structural, fully functional articular cartilage of the knee a possibility. Ultimately, this may help to develop new strategies for the treatment of knee articular cartilage diseases and growth disorders.

References

1. Solursh M. Ectoderm as a determinant of early tissue pattern in the limb bud. Cell Differ. 1984;15:17–24.
2. Solursh M. Cartilage stem cells: regulation of differentiation. Connect Tissue Res. 1989;20:81–9.
3. Solursh M. Extracellular matrix and cell surface as determinants of connective tissue differentiation. Am J Med Genet. 1989;34:30–4.
4. Grafe I, Alexander S, Peterson JR, Snider TN, Levi B, Lee B, Mishina Y. TGF-β family signaling in mesenchymal differentiation. Cold Spring Harb Perspect Biol. 2018;10(5): pii a022202.
5. Decker RS. Articular cartilage and joint development from emb ryogenesis to adulthood. Semin Cell Dev Biol. 2017;62:50–6.
6. Li Y, Jin D, Xie W, Wen L, Chen W, Xu J, Ding J, Ren D. PPAR-γ and Wnt regulate the differentiation of MSCs into adipocytes and osteoblasts respectively. Curr Stem Cell Res Ther. 2018;13(3): 185–92.
7. Visco DM, Van Sickle DC, Hill MA, Kincaid SA. The vascular supply of the chondro-epiphyses of the elbow joint in young swine. J Anat. 1989;163:215–29.
8. Clark JM. The structure of vascular channels in the subchondral plate. J Anat. 1990;171:105–15.
9. Green WT Jr, Martin GN, Eanes ED, Sokoloff L. Microradiographic study of the calcified layer of articular cartilage. Arch Pathol. 1970;90:151–8.
10. Lane LB, Bullough PG. Age-related changes in the thickness of the calcified zone and the number of tidemarks in adult human articular cartilage. J Bone Joint Surg. 1980;62:372–5.
11. Eyre DR, Dickson IR, Van Ness K. Collagen cross-linking in human bone and articular cartilage. Age-related changes in the content of mature hydroxypyridinium residues. Biochem J. 1988;252:495–500.
12. Pal S, Tang LH, Choi H, Habermann E, Rosenberg L, Roughley P, Poole AR. Structural changes during development in bovine fetal epiphyseal cartilage. Coll Relat Res. 1981;1:151–76.
13. Thonar EJ, Sweet MB. Maturation-related changes in proteoglycans of fetal articular cartilage. Arch Biochem Biophys. 1981;208:535–47.
14. Rux D, Decker RS, Koyama E, Pacifici M. Joints in the appendicular skeleton: developmental mechanisms and evolutionary influences. Curr Top Dev Biol. 2019;133:119–51.
15. Wong M, Carter DR. Mechanical stress and morphogenetic endochondral ossification of the sternum. J Bone Joint Surg Am. 1988;70:992–1000.
16. Takada N, Wada I, Sugimura I, Sakuma E, Maruyama H, Matsui N. A possible barrier function of the articular surface, Kaibogaku zasshi. J Anat. 1999;74:631–7.
17. Gannon AR, Nagel T, Bell AP, Avery NC, Kelly DJ. The changing role of the superficial region in determining the dynamic compressive properties of articular cartilage during postnatal development. Osteoarthritis Cartilage. 2015;23(6):975–84.
18. Kaviani R, Londono I, Parent S, Moldovan F, Villemure I. Changes in growth plate extracellular matrix composition and biomechanics following in vitro static versus dynamic mechanical modulation. J Musculoskelet Neuronal Interact. 2018;18(1):81–91.
19. Woods A, Wang G, Beier F. Regulation of chondrocyte differentiation by the actin cytoskel-

eton and adhesive interactions. J Cell Physiol. 2007;213:1–8.
20. Lories RJ, Corr M, Lane NE. To Wnt or not to Wnt: the bone and joint health dilemma. Nat Rev Rheumatol. 2013;9:328–39.
21. Green JD, Tollemar V, Dougherty M, Yan Z, Yin L, Ye J, Collier Z, Mohammed MK, Haydon RC, Luu HH, Kang R, Lee MJ, Ho SH, He TC, Shi LL, Athiviraham A. Multifaceted signaling regulators of chondrogenesis: implications in cartilage regeneration and tissue engineering. Genes Dis. 2015;2:307–27.
22. Jing J, Hinton RJ, Feng JQ. Bmpr1a signaling in cartilage development and endochondral bone formation. Vitam Horm. 2015;99:273–91.
23. Somoza RA, Welter JF, Correa D, Caplan AI. Chondrogenic differentiation of mesenchymal stem cells: challenges and unfulfilled expectations. Tissue Eng Part B Rev. 2014;20:596–608.
24. Lefebvre V, Dvir-Ginzberg M. SOX9 and the many facets of its regulation in the chondrocyte lineage. Connect Tissue Res. 2016;58(1):2–14.
25. Nilsson O, Marino R, De Luca F, Phillip M, Baron J. Endocrine regulation of the growth plate. Horm Res. 2005;64:157–65.
26. Goldring MB, Tsuchimochi K, Ijiri K. The control of chondrogenesis. J Cell Biochem. 2006;97:33–44.
27. Thorogood PV, Hinchliffe JR. An analysis of the condensation process during chondrogenesis in the embryonic chick hind limb. J Embryol Exp Morphol. 1975;33:581–606.
28. Bi W, Deng JM, Zhang Z, Behringer RR, de Crombrugghe B. Sox9 is required for cartilage formation. Nat Genet. 1999;22:85–9.
29. Gardner OF, Archer CW, Alini M, Stoddart MJ. Chondrogenesis of mesenchymal stem cells for cartilage tissue engineering. Histol Histopathol. 2013;28:23–42.
30. Archer CW, Francis-West P. The chondrocyte. Int J Biochem Cell Biol. 2003;35:401–4.
31. Cole AG. A review of diversity in the evolution and development of cartilage: the search for the origin of the chondrocyte. Eur Cell Mater. 2011;21:122–9.
32. Olsen BR, Reginato AM, Wang W. Bone development. Annu Rev Cell Dev Biol. 2000;16:191–220.
33. Sandell LJ, Nalin AM, Reife RA. Alternative splice form of type II procollagen mRNA (IIA) is predominant in skeletal precursors and non-cartilaginous tissues during early mouse development. Dev Dyn. 1994;199:129–40.
34. Kosher RA. In: Hall BK, editor. The chondroblast and the chondrocyte. New York: Academic Press, Inc; 1983. p. 59–85.
35. Fell HB. The histogenesis of cartilage and bone in the long bones of the embryonic fowl. J Morphol. 1925;40:417–59.
36. Hall BK, Miyake T. All for one and one for all: condensations and the initiation of skeletal development. Bioessays. 2000;22:138–47.
37. DeLise AM, Fischer L, Tuan RS. Cellular interactions and signaling in cartilage development. Osteoarthritis Cartilage. 2000;8:309–34.
38. Janners MY, Searls RL. Changes in rate of cellular proliferation during the differentiation of cartilage and muscle in the mesenchyme of the embryonic chick wing. Dev Biol. 1970;23:136–65.
39. Archer CW, Rooney P, Wolpert L. Cell shape and cartilage differentiation of early chick limb bud cells in culture. Cell Differ. 1982;11:245–51.
40. Ghosh S, Laha M, Mondal S, Sengupta S, Kaplan DL. In vitro model of mesenchymal condensation during chondrogenic development. Biomaterials. 2009;30:6530–40.
41. Erlebacher A, Filvaroff EH, Gitelman SE, Derynck R. Toward a molecular understanding of skeletal development. Cell. 1995;80:371–8.
42. Tchetina EV. Developmental mechanisms in articular cartilage degradation in osteoarthritis. Arthritis. 2011;2011:683970.
43. Chung UI. Essential role of hypertrophic chondrocytes in endochondral bone development. Endocr J. 2004;51:19–24.
44. Tickle C. Molecular basis of vertebrate limb patterning. Am J Med Genet. 2002;112:250–5.
45. Towers M, Tickle C. Generation of pattern and form in the developing limb. Int J Dev Biol. 2009;53:805–12.
46. Niswander L. Pattern formation: old models out on a limb. Nat Rev Genet. 2003;4:133–43.
47. Kosher RA, Savage MP, Walker KH. A gradation of hyaluronate accumulation along the proximodistal axis of the embryonic chick limb bud. J Embryol Exp Morphol. 1981;63:85–98.
48. Toole BP, Okayama M, Orkin RW, Yoshimura M, Muto M, Kaji A. Developmental roles of hyaluronate and chondroitin sulfate proteoglycans. Soc Gen Physiol Ser. 1977;32:139–54.
49. Toole BP, Gross J. The extracellular matrix of the regenerating newt limb: synthesis and removal of hyaluronate prior to differentiation. Dev Biol. 1971;25:57–77.
50. Delise AM, Tuan RS. Analysis of N-cadherin function in limb mesenchymal chondrogenesis in vitro. Dev Dyn. 2002;225:195–204.
51. Tuan RS. Cellular signaling in developmental chondrogenesis: N-cadherin, Wnts, and BMP-2. J Bone Joint Surg Am. 2003;85-A(Suppl 2):137–41.
52. Dessau W, von der Mark H, von der Mark K, Fischer S. Changes in the patterns of collagens and fibronectin during limb-bud chondrogenesis. J Embryol Exp Morphol. 1980;57:51–60.
53. Biddulph DM, Sawyer LM, Smales WP. Chondrogenesis of chick limb mesenchyme in vitro. Effects of prostaglandins on cyclic AMP. Exp Cell Res. 1984;153:270–4.
54. Ballard TA, Biddulph DM. The morphology and hormonal responsiveness of developing skeletal elements in chick limb buds. Am J Anat. 1984;169:221–36.

55. Kosher RA, Walker KH, Ledger PW. Temporal and spatial distribution of fibronectin during development of the embryonic chick limb bud. Cell Differ. 1982;11:217–28.
56. Stirpe NS, Goetinck PF. Gene regulation during cartilage differentiation: temporal and spatial expression of link protein and cartilage matrix protein in the developing limb. Development. 1989;107:23–33.
57. Liu CF, Lefebvre V. The transcription factors SOX9 and SOX5/SOX6 cooperate genome-wide through super-enhancers to drive chondrogenesis. Nucleic Acids Res. 2015;43:8183–203.
58. Kosher RA, Kulyk WM, Gay SW. Collagen gene expression during limb cartilage differentiation. J Cell Biol. 1986;102:1151–6.
59. Kosher RA, Solursh M. Widespread distribution of type II collagen during embryonic chick development. Dev Biol. 1989;131:558–66.
60. Kravis D, Upholt WB. Quantitation of type II procollagen mRNA levels during chick limb cartilage differentiation. Dev Biol. 1985;108:164–72.
61. Nah HD, Rodgers BJ, Kulyk WM, Kream BE, Kosher RA, Upholt WB. In situ hybridization analysis of the expression of the type II collagen gene in the developing chicken limb bud. Coll Relat Res. 1988;8:277–94.
62. Swiderski RE, Solursh M. Localization of type II collagen, long form alpha 1(IX) collagen, and short form alpha 1(IX) collagen transcripts in the developing chick notochord and axial skeleton. Dev Dyn. 1992;194:118–27.
63. Kulyk WM, Coelho CN, Kosher RA. Type IX collagen gene expression during limb cartilage differentiation. Matrix. 1991;11:282–8.
64. Swiderski RE, Solursh M. Differential co-expression of long and short form type IX collagen transcripts during avian limb chondrogenesis in ovo. Development. 1992;115:169–79.
65. Barone LM, Owen TA, Tassinari MS, Bortell R, Stein GS, Lian JB. Developmental expression and hormonal regulation of the rat matrix Gla protein (MGP) gene in chondrogenesis and osteogenesis. J Cell Biochem. 1991;46:351–65.
66. Luo G, D'Souza R, Hogue D, Karsenty G. The matrix Gla protein gene is a marker of the chondrogenesis cell lineage during mouse development. J Bone Miner Res. 1995;10:325–34.
67. Hale JE, Fraser JD, Price PA. The identification of matrix Gla protein in cartilage. J Biol Chem. 1988;263:5820–4.
68. Hascall VC, Oegema TR, Brown M, Caplan AI. Isolation and characterization of proteoglycans from chick limb bud chondrocytes grown in vitro. J Biol Chem. 1976;251:3511–9.
69. Palmoski MJ, Goetinck PF. Synthesis of proteochondroitin sulfate by normal, nanomelic, and 5-bromodeoxyuridine-treated chondrocytes in cell culture. Proc Natl Acad Sci U S A. 1972;69:3385–8.
70. Mallein-Gerin F, Kosher RA, Upholt WB, Tanzer ML. Temporal and spatial analysis of cartilage proteoglycan core protein gene expression during limb development by in situ hybridization. Dev Biol. 1988;126:337–45.
71. Tsonis PA, Walker E. Cell populations synthesizing cartilage proteoglycan core protein in the early chick limb bud. Biochem Biophys Res Commun. 1991;174:688–95.
72. Topol L, Chen W, Song H, Day TF, Yang Y. Sox9 inhibits Wnt signaling by promoting beta-catenin phosphorylation in the nucleus. J Biol Chem. 2009;284:3323–33.
73. Lefebvre V, Smits P. Transcriptional control of chondrocyte fate and differentiation. Birth Defects Res C Embryo Today. 2005;75:200–12.
74. Adams SL, Cohen AJ, Lassova L. Integration of signaling pathways regulating chondrocyte differentiation during endochondral bone formation. J Cell Physiol. 2007;213:635–41.
75. Gamer LW, Pregizer S, Gamer J, Feigenson M, Ionescu A, et al. The role of Bmp2 in the maturation and maintenance of the murine knee joint. J Bone Miner Res. 2018;33(9):1708–17.
76. de Crombrugghe B, Lefebvre V, Nakashima K. Regulatory mechanisms in the pathways of cartilage and bone formation. Curr Opin Cell Biol. 2001;13:721–7.
77. Zelzer E, Olsen BR. The genetic basis for skeletal diseases. Nature. 2003;423:343–8.
78. Las Heras F, Pritzker KP, So A, Tsui HW, Chiu B, Inman RD, Tsui FW. Aberrant chondrocyte hypertrophy and activation of beta-catenin signaling precede joint ankylosis in ank/ank mice. J Rheumatol. 2012;39:583–93.
79. Mackie EJ, Ahmed YA, Tatarczuch L, Chen KS, Mirams M. Endochondral ossification: how cartilage is converted into bone in the developing skeleton. Int J Biochem Cell Biol. 2008;40:46–62.
80. Long F, Ornitz DM. Development of the endochondral skeleton. Cold Spring Harb Perspect Biol. 2013;5:a008334.
81. Catheline SE, Hoak D, Chang M, Ketz JP, Hilton MJ, et al. Chondrocyte-specific RUNX2 overexpression accelerates post-traumatic osteoarthritis progression in adult mice. J Bone Miner Res. 2019;34(9):1676–89.
82. Yoshida CA, Komori T. Role of Runx proteins in chondrogenesis. Crit Rev Eukaryot Gene Expr. 2005;15:243–54.
83. Yoshida CA, Yamamoto H, Fujita T, Furuichi T, Ito K, Inoue K, Yamana K, Zanma A, Takada K, Ito Y, Komori T. Runx2 and Runx3 are essential for chondrocyte maturation, and Runx2 regulates limb growth through induction of Indian hedgehog. Genes Dev. 2004;18:952–63.
84. Leboy P, Grasso-Knight G, D'Angelo M, Volk SW, Lian JV, Drissi H, Stein GS, Adams SL. Smad-Runx interactions during chondrocyte maturation. J Bone Joint Surg Am. 2001;83-A(Suppl 1):S15–22.

85. Iwai T, Murai J, Yoshikawa H, Tsumaki N. Smad7 Inhibits chondrocyte differentiation at multiple steps durin g endochondral bone formation and down-regulates p38 MAPK pathways. J Biol Chem. 2008;283:27154–64.
86. Ballock RT, Heydemann A, Wakefield LM, Flanders KC, Roberts AB, Sporn MB. TGF-beta 1 prevents hypertrophy of epiphyseal chondrocytes: regulation of gene expression for cartilage matrix proteins and metalloproteases. Dev Biol. 1993;158:414–29.
87. Solomon LA, Berube NG, Beier F. Transcriptional regulators of chondrocyte hypertrophy. Birth Defects Res C Embryo Today. 2008;84:123–30.
88. Poole AR. An introduction to the pathophysiology of osteoarthritis. Front Biosci. 1999;4:D662–70.
89. Archer CW, Morrison H, Pitsillides AA. Cellular aspects of the development of diarthrodial joints and articular cartilage. J Anat. 1994;184(Pt 3): 447–56.
90. Hayes AJ, MacPherson S, Morrison H, Dowthwaite G, Archer CW. The development of articular cartilage: evidence for an appositional growth mechanism. Anat Embryol. 2001;203:469–79.
91. Babyn PS, Kim HK, Lemaire C, Gahunia HK, Cross A, DeNanassy J, Pritzker KP. High-resolution magnetic resonance imaging of normal porcine cartilaginous epiphyseal maturation. J Magn Reson Imaging JMRI. 1996;6:172–9.
92. Kim HK, Babyn PS, Harasiewicz KA, Gahunia HK, Pritzker KP, Foster FS. Imaging of immature articular cartilage using ultrasound backscatter microscopy at 50 MHz. J Orthop Res. 1995;13:963–70.
93. Abad V, Meyers JL, Weise M, Gafni RI, Barnes KM, Nilsson O, Bacher JD, Baron J. The role of the resting zone in growth plate chondrogenesis. Endocrinology. 2002;143:1851–7.
94. Farnum CE, Wilsman NJ. Morphologic stages of the terminal hypertrophic chondrocyte of growth plate cartilage. Anat Rec. 1987;219:221–32.
95. Emons J, Chagin AS, Savendahl L, Karperien M, Wit JM. Mechanisms of growth plate maturation and epiphyseal fusion. Horm Res Paediatr. 2011;75:383–91.
96. Weise M, De-Levi S, Barnes KM, Gafni RI, Abad V, Baron J. Effects of estrogen on growth plate senescence and epiphyseal fusion. Proc Natl Acad Sci U S A. 2001;98:6871–6.
97. Gafni RI, Weise M, Robrecht DT, Meyers JL, Barnes KM, De-Levi S, Baron J. Catch-up growth is associated with delayed senescence of the growth plate in rabbits. Pediatr Res. 2001;50:618–23.
98. Dailey L, Laplantine E, Priore R, Basilico C. A network of transcriptional and signaling events is activated by FGF to induce chondrocyte growth arrest and differentiation. J Cell Biol. 2003;161(6):1053–66.
99. Haines RW. The development of joints. J Anat. 1947;81:33–55.
100. Garciadiego-Cazares D, Rosales C, Katoh M, Chimal-Monroy J. Coordination of chondrocyte differentiation and joint formation by alpha5beta1 integrin in the developing appendicular skeleton. Development. 2004;131:4735–42.
101. Ploger F, Seemann P, Schmidt-von Kegler M, Lehmann K, Seidel J, Kjaer KW, Pohl J, Mundlos S. Brachydactyly type A2 associated with a defect in proGDF5 processing. Hum Mol Genet. 2008;17:1222–33.
102. Francis-West PH, Abdelfattah A, Chen P, Allen C, Parish J, Ladher R, Allen S, MacPherson S, Luyten FP, Archer CW. Mechanisms of GDF-5 action during skeletal development. Development. 1999;126:1305–15.
103. Chijimatsu R, Saito T. Mechanisms of synovial joint and articular cartilage development. Cell Mol Life Sci. 2019;76(20):3939–52.
104. Moses HL, Serra R. Regulation of differentiation by TGF-beta. Curr Opin Genet Dev. 1996;6: 581–6.
105. Serra R, Johnson M, Filvaroff EH, LaBorde J, Sheehan DM, Derynck R, Moses HL. Expression of a truncated, kinase-defective TGF-beta type II receptor in mouse skeletal tissue promotes terminal chondrocyte differentiation and osteoarthritis. J Cell Biol. 1997;139:541–52.
106. Brunet LJ, McMahon JA, McMahon AP, Harland RM. Noggin, cartilage morphogenesis, and joint formation in the mammalian skeleton. Science. 1998;280:1455–7.
107. Daans M, Lories RJ, Luyten FP. Dynamic activation of bone morphogenetic protein signaling in collagen-induced arthritis supports their role in joint homeostasis and disease. Arthritis Res Ther. 2008;10:R115.
108. Cheng A, Gustafson AR, Schaner Tooley CE, Zhang M. BMP-9 dependent pathways required for the chondrogenic differentiation of pluripotent stem cells. Differentiation. 2016;92(5):298–305.
109. Drissi H, Gibson JD, Guzzo RM, RH X. Derivation and chondrogenic commitment of human embryonic stem cell-derived mesenchymal progenitors. Methods Mol Biol. 2015;1340:65–78.
110. Ray A, Singh PN, Sohaskey ML, Harland RM, Bandyopadhyay A. Precise spatial restriction of BMP signaling is essential for articular cartilage differentiation. Development. 2015;142: 1169–79.
111. Retting KN, Song B, Yoon BS, Lyons KM. BMP canonical Smad signaling through Smad1 and Smad5 is required for endochondral bone formation. Development. 2009;136:1093–104.
112. Hoffmann A, Gross G. BMP signaling pathways in cartilage and bone formation. Crit Rev Eukaryot Gene Expr. 2001;11:23–45.
113. van der Eerden BC, Karperien M, Wit JM. Systemic and local regulation of the growth plate. Endocr Rev. 2003;24:782–801.
114. Barna M, Niswander L. Visualization of cartilage formation: insight into cellular properties of skeletal progenitors and chondrodysplasia syndromes. Dev Cell. 2007;12:931–41.

115. Grimsrud CD, Romano PR, D'Souza M, Puzas JE, Reynolds PR, Rosier RN, O'Keefe RJ. BMP-6 is an autocrine stimulator of chondrocyte differentiation. J Bone Miner Res. 1999;14:475–82.
116. Minina E, Kreschel C, Naski MC, Ornitz DM, Vortkamp A. Interaction of FGF, Ihh/Pthlh, and BMP signaling integrates chondrocyte proliferation and hypertrophic differentiation. Dev Cell. 2002;3:439–49.
117. Grimsrud CD, Romano PR, D'Souza M, Puzas JE, Schwarz EM, Reynolds PR, Roiser RN, O'Keefe RJ. BMP signaling stimulates chondrocyte maturation and the expression of Indian hedgehog. J Orthop Res. 2001;19:18–25.
118. Yoon BS, Pogue R, Ovchinnikov DA, Yoshii I, Mishina Y, Behringer RR, Lyons KM. BMPs regulate multiple aspects of growth-plate chondrogenesis through opposing actions on FGF pathways. Development. 2006;133:4667–78.
119. Jung YK, Kim GW, Park HR, Lee EJ, Choi JY, Beier F, Han SW. Role of interleukin-10 in endochondral bone formation in mice: anabolic effect via the bone morphogenetic protein/Smad pathway. Arthritis Rheum. 2013;65:3153–64.
120. Malinauskas T, Jones EY. Extracellular modulators of Wnt signalling. Curr Opin Struct Biol. 2014;29:77–84.
121. Kikuchi A, Yamamoto H, Kishida S. Multiplicity of the interactions of Wnt proteins and their receptors. Cell Signal. 2007;19:659–71.
122. Cadigan KM, Liu YI. Wnt signaling: complexity at the surface. J Cell Sci. 2006;119:395–402.
123. Moon RT. Wnt/beta-catenin pathway. Sci STKE. 2005: 2005(271): cm1.
124. Klaus A, Birchmeier W. Wnt signalling and its impact on development and cancer. Nat Rev Cancer. 2008;8:387–98.
125. Chen Y, Alman BA. Wnt pathway, an essential role in bone regeneration. J Cell Biochem. 2009;106:353–62.
126. Ma B, Landman EB, Miclea RL, Wit JM, Robanus-Maandag EC, Post JN, Karperien M. WNT signaling and cartilage: of mice and men. Calcif Tissue Int. 2013;92:399–411.
127. Staines KA, Macrae VE, Farquharson C. Cartilage development and degeneration: a Wnt Wnt situation. Cell Biochem Funct. 2012;30:633–42.
128. Usami Y, Gunawardena AT, Iwamoto M, Enomoto-Iwamoto M. Wnt signaling in cartilage development and diseases: lessons from animal studies. Lab Invest. 2016;96:186–96.
129. Huang Y, Jiang L, Yang H, Wu L, Xu N, et al. Variations of Wnt/β-catenin pathway-related genes in susceptibility to knee osteoarthritis: a three-centre case-control study. J Cell Mol Med. 2019. doi: 10.1111/jcmm.14696. [Epub ahead of print]
130. Tamamura Y, Otani T, Kanatani N, Koyama E, Kitagaki J, Komori T, Yamada Y, Costantini F, Wakisaka S, Pacifici M, Iwamoto M, Enomoto-Iwamoto M. Developmental regulation of Wnt/beta-catenin signals is required for growth plate assembly, cartilage integrity, and endochondral ossification. J Biol Chem. 2005;280:19185–95.
131. Yuan X, Liu H, Huang H, Liu H, Li L, Yang J, Shi W, Liu W, Wu L. The key role of canonical Wnt/beta-catenin signaling in cartilage chondrocytes. Curr Drug Targets. 2016;17:475–84.
132. Zhong N, Gersch RP, Hadjiargyrou M. Wnt signaling activation during bone regeneration and the role of Dishevelled in chondrocyte proliferation and differentiation. Bone. 2006;39:5–16.
133. Hill TP, Spater D, Taketo MM, Birchmeier W, Hartmann C. Canonical Wnt/beta-catenin signaling prevents osteoblasts from differentiating into chondrocytes. Dev Cell. 2005;8:727–38.
134. Dao DY, Yang X, Chen D, Zuscik M, O'Keefe RJ. Axin1 and Axin2 are regulated by TGF- and mediate cross-talk between TGF- and Wnt signaling pathways. Ann N Y Acad Sci. 2007;1116:82–99.
135. Church V, Nohno T, Linker C, Marcelle C, Francis-West P. Wnt regulation of chondrocyte differentiation. J Cell Sci. 2002;115:4809–18.
136. Gaur T, Rich L, Lengner CJ, Hussain S, Trevant B, Ayers D, Stein JL, Bodine PV, Komm BS, Stein GS, Lian JB. Secreted frizzled related protein 1 regulates Wnt signaling for BMP2 induced chondrocyte differentiation. J Cell Physiol. 2006;208:87–96.
137. Bodine PV, Zhao W, Kharode YP, Bex FJ, Lambert AJ, Goad MB, Gaur T, Stein GS, Lian JB, Komm BS. The Wnt antagonist secreted frizzledrelated protein-1 is a negative regulator of trabecular bone formation in adult mice. Mol Endocrinol. 2004;18:1222–37.
138. Corr M. Wnt-beta-catenin signaling in the pathogenesis of osteoarthritis. Nat Clin Pract Rheumatol. 2008;4:550–6.
139. Wu Q, Zhu M, Rosier RN, Zuscik MJ, O'Keefe RJ, Chen D. Beta-catenin, cartilage, and osteoarthritis. Ann N Y Acad Sci. 2010;1192:344–50.
140. Kawaguchi H. Regulation of osteoarthritis development by Wnt-beta-catenin signaling through the endochondral ossification process. J Bone Miner Res. 2009;24:8–11.
141. Wang L, Shao YY, Ballock RT. Leptin synergizes with thyroid hormone signaling in promoting growth plate chondrocyte proliferation and terminal differentiation in vitro. Bone. 2011;48:1022–7.
142. Maeda Y, Nakamura E, Nguyen MT, Suva LJ, Swain FL, Razzaque MS, Mackem S, Lanske B. Indian Hedgehog produced by postnatal chondrocytes is essential for maintaining a growth plate and trabecular bone. Proc Natl Acad Sci U S A. 2007;104:6382–7.
143. van der Eerden BC, Karperien M, Gevers EF, Lowik CW, Wit JM. Expression of Indian hedgehog, parathyroid hormone-related protein, and their receptors in the postnatal growth plate of the

rat: evidence for a locally acting growth restraining feedback loop after birth. J Bone Miner Res. 2000;15:1045–55.
144. Karp SJ, Schipani E, St-Jacques B, Hunzelman J, Kronenberg H, McMahon AP. Indian hedgehog coordinates endochondral bone growth and morphogenesis via parathyroid hormone related-protein-dependent and -independent pathways. Development. 2000;127:543–8.
145. Kohn A, Rutkowski TP, Liu Z, Mirando AJ, Zuscik MJ, O'Keefe RJ, Hilton MJ. Notch signaling controls chondrocyte hypertrophy via indirect regulation of Sox9. Bone Res. 2015;3:15021.
146. Estrada KD, Wang W, Retting KN, Chien CT, Elkhoury FF, Heuchel R, Lyons KM. Smad7 regulates terminal maturation of chondrocytes in the growth plate. Dev Biol. 2013;382:375–84.
147. Dong Y, Drissi H, Chen M, Chen D, Zuscik MJ, Schwarz EM, O'Keefe RJ. Wnt-mediated regulation of chondrocyte maturation: modulation by TGF-beta. J Cell Biochem. 2005;95:1057–68.
148. Cawston TE, Wilson AJ. Understanding the role of tissue degrading enzymes and their inhibitors in development and disease. Best Pract Res Clin Rheumatol. 2006;20:983–1002.
149. Inada M, Wang Y, Byrne MH, Rahman MU, Miyaura C, Lopez-Otin C, Krane SM. Critical roles for collagenase-3 (Mmp-13) in development of growth plate cartilage and in endochondral ossification. Proc Natl Acad Sci U S A. 2004;101:17192–7.
150. Ortega N, Behonick DJ, Werb Z. Matrix remodeling during endochondral ossification. Trends Cell Biol. 2004;4:86–93.

Part II

Aging and Degeneration of Articular Cartilage

3 Articular Cartilage: Homeostasis, Aging and Degeneration

Kenneth P. H. Pritzker and Harpal K. Gahunia

3.1 Introduction

Articular cartilage, formerly considered as an inert material, is a very dynamic and resilient tissue that can maintain functional homeostasis throughout a lifetime. This is remarkable since the joint tissues act synergistically to effectively and efficiently deal with the mechanical loads encountered over a lifetime [1]. The human knee is capable of bearing loads of up to 2.5 times body weight (BW) while walking and more than 12 times BW while running and jumping [2].

Chondrocytes, the key cellular mediators for cartilage homeostasis, normally maintain a functional matrix by modulating extracellular matrix (ECM) synthesis and degradation. The associated balance between proteoglycans (PGs) and integrity of the collagen network is regulated differentially by certain growth factors and varies with age [3]. During prenatal and postnatal growth and maturation, articular cartilage structure, composition and function undergoes continuous change even though the articular chondrocyte phenotype remains conserved and the matrix macromolecular components remain similar. Mature adult articular cartilage ECM is comprised of PGs, collagens and noncollagen proteins and is devoid of blood vessels. In adult, chondrocytes comprise less than 5% of cartilage volume. Chondrocytes embedded within the cartilage matrix survive efficiently in the avascular cartilage matrix and respond to environmental changes. These chondrocytes exist at low oxygen tension, ranging from 10% at the surface to less than 1% in the deep zones [4–6]. In vitro studies have shown that chondrocytes adapt to low oxygen tensions by upregulating hypoxia-inducible factor-1-alpha (HIF-1α) [7, 8].

Chondrocytes are capable of cell division, in particular when cartilage is injured or diseased; however, throughout adult life, without division, these cells can survive and maintain the articular cartilage homeostasis. Chondrocytes have the intrinsic capability to maintain articular cartilage ECM by a balance (homeostatic equilibrium) between the degradation and the synthesis of matrix components with a low-turnover replacement of certain matrix proteins.

Aging, traumatic joint injury (acute or chronic) and joint disease (such as osteoarthritis – OA, rheumatoid arthritis – RA, gout and pseudogout) can initiate and accelerate progressive

K. P. H. Pritzker, MD, FRCPC (✉)
Department of Laboratory Medicine and Pathobiology, Department of Surgery, and Institute of Biomaterials and Biomedical Engineering, University of Toronto, Toronto, ON, Canada

Department of Pathology and Laboratory Medicine, Mount Sinai Hospital, Toronto, ON, Canada
e-mail: kenpritzker@gmail.com

H. K. Gahunia, MSc, PhD
Orthopaedic Science Consulting Services, Oakville, ON, Canada

H. K. Gahunia et al. (eds.), *Articular Cartilage of the Knee*,
https://doi.org/10.1007/978-1-4939-7587-7_3

articular cartilage deterioration in structure and function. With aging and joint disease, the homeostatic equilibrium shifts towards ECM degradation with the matrix having decreased capacity to retain PGs leading to decreased hydration [9].

This chapter reviews the various factors that regulate cartilage homeostasis and highlights the key structural, biochemical and biomechanical changes that occur with aging and cartilage-related joint diseases. Also described are the overlapping and distinguishing features of aging and OA.

3.2 Articular Cartilage Homeostasis

Cartilage homeostasis is maintained in a dynamic mechanical environment, even though metabolic changes in cartilage range on time scales from a fraction of a second (water and ion flow), through hours and days (PG turnover), to years (collagen turnover, chondrocytes). Key features in maintaining cartilage homeostasis include:

1. Elastic resistance to deformation of the cartilage tissue, chondrocytes and chondrons [10, 11]
2. Limited permeability of cartilage matrix to exogenous compounds [12, 13]
3. Presence within cartilage matrix of abundant proteolytic enzyme inhibitors [14, 15]
4. Capacity of chondrocytes to thrive with anaerobic metabolism [8]

The hyaline articular cartilage architecture, described in depth in Chap. 1, is maintained intact throughout life by chondrocytes. Healthy chondrocytes remain in a postmitotic quiescent state throughout life, with their decreasing proliferative potential being attributed to replicative senescence associated with shortened telomere length [9, 16]. Under normal circumstances, chondrocyte turnover is thought to be very low with individual chondrocytes living for decades. Further, chondrocytes beneath the superficial zone (SZ) are present within functional structures called chondrons [17, 18]. Normally, each chondron contains one to two chondrocytes (Fig. 3.1) that are nested within the pericellular matrix (PCM), mostly PG, and are bounded by collagenous matrix that contains collagen types VI and IX and, in deeper zones, collagen type X [18–22]. This architecture has the consequence that the cartilage territorial matrix (TM) composition adjacent to the chondron (typically within 2 chondron diameters) is

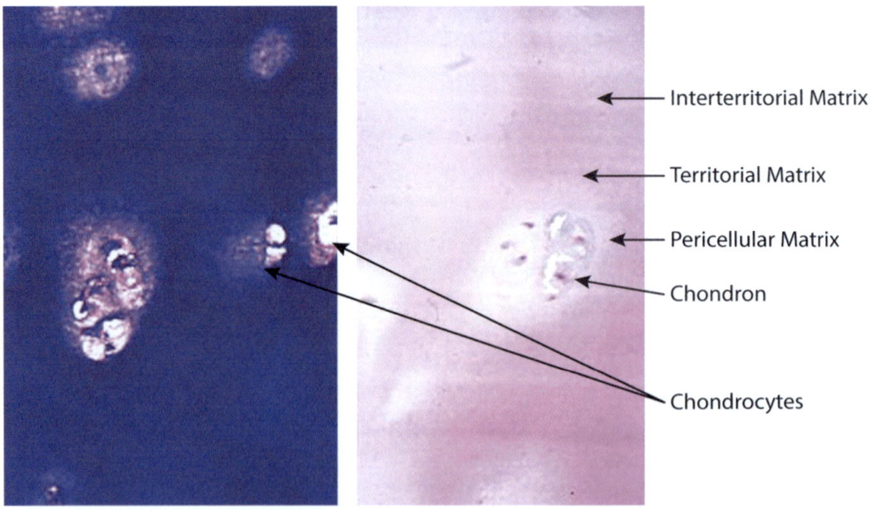

Fig. 3.1 Toluidine blue (left) and hematoxylin and eosin (right) stained photomicrographs obtained from human femoral condyle showing articular cartilage chondrocytes and its specialized microenvironment collectively referred to as chondrons. The articular cartilage is organized into pericellular, territorial and interterritorial matrices, each of which is present at a specific distance from the chondrocyte. (Magnification, 100×)

tightly controlled and more reactive relative to the more distant interterritorial matrix (ITM) that is more stable [23]. An in vitro study showed that the cartilage matrix regenerated by chondrons isolated from the non-damaged site contained more PGs and collagen compared to chondrons isolated from the same site of the contralateral damaged joint [24]. Further, Chondrocytes within chondrons always outperformed bare chondrocytes with increased cartilage matrix production and less collagenase activity, even when isolated from the damaged joints [24]. This study indicated that chondron chondrocytes and their native PCM provides a superior cell source for articular cartilage repair and cell-induced cartilage matrix regeneration. Another study demonstrated that chondrocyte morphology affects the solid but not the fluid microenvironment of the chondrocyte and that maintaining the cell shape is critical for regulating the microenvironment and metabolic activity of the chondrocyte in native articular cartilage [25].

Although embedded within their ECM that also isolates them from each other, chondrocytes are capable of maintaining their ECM under homeostatic conditions (Table 3.1). Due to its avascular nature, chondrocytes rely on facilitated glucose transport via constitutive glucose transporter proteins. The major PG component, aggrecan, is present dissolved within hydrated matrix. The aggrecan core protein has a half-life that ranges from 3 to 24 years, while the aggrecan glycosaminoglycan (GAG) components are synthesized more readily under low-turnover conditions, with most rapid matrix turnover in the pericellular regions [9]. The predominant structural molecule, collagen type II, is arranged in a fibrillar network. If kept in its native state and not subjected to inappropriate degradation, collagen type II has a half-life of more than 100 years [26, 27]. A large number of other noncollagen molecules, including biglycan, decorin, fibromodulin, the matrillins and cartilage oligomeric matrix protein (COMP), are also present in the cartilage ECM.

Over a lifetime, articular cartilage functions as a low-friction, wear-resistant and load-bearing tissue. Because of its compliance, which is attributed to the macromolecular structure and composition, articular cartilage is able to act as a shock absorber and distribute the loads between opposing bones in a synovial joint. Throughout the phase of cartilage growth from prenatal, postnatal, puberty and adolescence to adult, articular cartilage is subjected to and able to adapt to its structure and composition, usually seamlessly to increasing mechanical demands [28–33].

The mechanical response of cartilage is tightly coupled to the flow of fluid through its tissue depth [34]. Further, several studies demonstrated the quantitative correlations between the mechanical properties of articular cartilage and the concentration of tissue water, ions, collagen and negatively charged GAGs [35–38]. The compressive stiffness of cartilage increases as a function of its total GAG content [36, 37, 39]. The compressive moduli of immature cartilage are known to be lower than those of adult cartilage [31]. On the other hand, in addition to the total collagen content, the amount of crosslinking present in the collagen network during growth and maturation has been shown to play an important role in tissue tensile properties [28, 40–42].

3.3 Age-Related Changes in Articular Cartilage

Aging implies changes in mature chondrocytes and cartilage ECM associated with time alone. With aging, cartilage matrix undergoes profound changes in architecture, composition, permeability and biomechanical function [43–45]. In the matrix, this has been attributed to overall accumulation of advanced glycation end products (AGEs) that enhance collagen crosslinking [46]. The accumulation of cartilage matrix proteins in the endoplasmic reticulum and Golgi apparatus of chondrocytes, which have been modified by oxidative stress during aging, may lead to decreased synthesis of cartilage matrix proteins and diminished cell survival [47]. Cartilage injury due to aging or

Table 3.1 Chondron structure reflects cartilage matrix dynamic activity

Articular Cartilage		**Normal** *Homeostasis/ Matrix Maintenance*	**Atrophy/ Senescence**	**Reaction to Injury** **Exogenous** *Inflammation – Synovitis, e.g., Rheumatoid Arthritis*	**Reaction to Injury** **Endogenous** *Mechanical and/or Hyperosmotic Injury, e.g., Osteoarthritis*	**Regeneration**
Chondron Morphology	***Chondron Size***	Normal *Varies with cartilage depth*	↓	↓	↑	↑++
Chondrocytes *Selected Features*	***Chondrocytes/chondron***	1–2	1	1 or absent	1–2+	2+
	Membrane					
	Pseudopodia	Present	↓, absent	↓, absent	↑	↑
	Alkaline phosphatase	Slight	↓, absent	Absent	↑++	↑++
	Cytoplasm					
	Rough endoplasmic reticulum	Present	↓, absent	↓, absent	↑	Present, ↑
	Nucleus	Present	Condensed	Condensed, absent	Enlarged	Mitoses
Extracellular Matrix *Selected Features*	***Pericellular Matrix* (PCM)** Proteoglycan	Present	↓, absent	↓, absent	↑	↑++
	Chondron Capsule					
	Collagens Type VI	Present	Present	↓ Type VI	↑ Type VI	Present
	Type IX	Present	Present	↓ Type IX	↓ Type IX	
	CPPD crystals	Absent	Present	Absent	Absent	Absent
	***Territorial Matrix* (TM)** Proteoglycan	Present ↑ *relative to ITM*	↓, *similar concentration to ITM*	↓, absent *“Lacunar resorption”*	↑ ++ *Relative to ITM*	↑++
	Collagen type I	Absent	Absent	Absent *“Lacunar resorption”* may be present	Present (*microscars*)	Absent
	Lipofuscin	Absent	Present	Absent	Variably present	Absent
	***Interterritorial matrix* (ITM)** Proteoglycan	Present	↓	↓, absent	↑	↑

PCM, *Pericellular matrix*; TM, *Territorial matrix*; ITM, *Interterritorial matrix*; ↓, *Decreased*; ↑, *Increased*; Lacunar resorption represents resorption of both proteoglycan and collagen disease can stimulate chondrocyte replication. Chondrocytes capable of replication can be extracted from cartilage at any age, although extraction of aged chondrocytes from the cartilage matrix is more difficult. This relates to the increased density of chondral proteins and increased chemical bonds amongst the chondral matrix molecules with age.

3.3.1 Homeostatic Imbalance

With aging, the capacity of chondrocytes to maintain cartilage matrix is compromised by focal chondrocyte death and by decreased chondrocyte reactivity (chondrocyte senescence) [48–50]. This focal chondrocyte death is primarily mediated by apoptosis and may be preceded by decreased capacity for autophagy [51–55]. Chondrocyte death by apoptosis is seen primarily in SZ cartilage, suggesting that the cells are affected by exogenous systemic stimuli present in the synovial fluid. Because the effects are focal, cartilage matrix is also affected focally, giving rise to its structural heterogeneity, which in turn accelerates cartilage matrix degeneration related to the heterogeneity of force dissipation at a microstructural level.

Chondrocyte senescence is marked by expression of the senescence-associated enzyme beta-galactosidase and mitochondrial degeneration due to oxidative damage [56, 57]. As well, senescent chondrocytes demonstrate shortened telomeres and have a metabolic profile balanced towards catabolism and proteolysis [58–63]. These changes result in the age-related loss of chondrocyte function [56, 59]. These changes are most likely attributed to decrease in the ability of chondrocytes to maintain and repair the articular cartilage manifested by decreased mitotic and synthetic activity, decreased responsiveness to anabolic growth factors and synthesis of smaller, less uniform aggrecans and less functional link proteins [59]. Aged chondrocytes tend to have increased reactive oxygen species which can be secreted into the matrix causing oxidative injury to matrix components [64–67].

3.3.2 Morphological Changes

Articular cartilage structural failure can result from abnormal mechanical strains on healthy normal cartilage and from the influence of physiological mechanical strains on pathologically impaired cartilage. The articular cartilage architecture is maintained by a mesh of anisotropic collagen type II fibres arranged primarily in a SZ parallel to the joint surface, arching towards deeper zones with fibres oriented perpendicular to the SZ [68, 69]. This architecture originally described using polarized light microscopy by Benninghof is actually a composite of similarly aligned fine collagen fibrils as seen by scanning electron microscopy [70–72]. While not inevitable, when chondrocytes exhibit senescence and apoptosis, the result on chondrocytes is manifested as decreased chondrocyte density. Structural failure of cartilage matrix can be seen as ECM thinning, accompanied by fibrillation as well as focal cleft formation and erosion where applied forces are highest [73].

3.3.3 Biochemical Changes

Proteoglycans are the major noncollagenous matrix component of cartilage. The negatively charged PGs exert their mechanical effects by means of their fixed charge density and high osmotic pressure [39]. Relative to collagen, PG content is maximal in cartilage middle zone (MZ) [74, 75]. These molecules can have rapid turnover. Within 2 days after PG depletion by papain, cartilage PGs can be completely restored [76]. PG depletion diminishes charge density and water content [77]. This indicates that immediately following injury, cartilage is less resistant to compression forces.

With age, decreased size and aggregation of PG aggrecans are noted. Further, the relative concentration of GAGs varies markedly with age. In immature cartilage, there is a preponderance of chondroitin-4-sulfate (C4S) and little keratan sulfate (KS). However, with advancing age there is an appreciable increase in KS content and a corresponding fall in C4S [78]. The C4S chains become shorter, leaving the PGs composed of higher concentration of more acidic KS chains [79–81]. As such, the fixed charge density decreases, which results in decline of the water content and decreased compressive resistance of cartilage. This leads to increased heterogeneity at micro-level boundaries between and within cartilage zones and decreased fibrillar interconnectivity at submicroscopic levels [82]. Decreased fibrillar collagen network interconnectivity leads to decreased capacity to retain PGs. These changes make the cartilage SZ less capable of resisting strain and more vulnerable to damage from impact forces, resulting in visible cartilage surface fibrillation.

With age, the lubrication capacity of the articular cartilage surface decreases. With the reduction in water concentration throughout the cartilage thickness, the ECM is more susceptible to mineralization. This may relate in varying ratio to the decreased hyaluronic acid (HA, also termed hyaluronan) chain length, decreased PGs, decreased availability of lubricin (a glycoprotein) and altered lipids [83–86]. Lipids are present in cartilage ECM, where they participate in lubrication and as nutrients for chondrocytes; whereas, phospholipids present on the surface of articular cartilage have major involvement in the low friction of cartilage [87–91]. Both lipid and lipid peroxides are present in greatest concentration in the SZ of cartilage [92, 93]. Lipid oxidation can lead to oxidative damage in adjacent collagen. Lipid oxidation products, principally lipofuscin, increase in aged cartilage and can be seen macroscopically as the yellow colour in older cartilage [94–96].

With age, in the absence of an active disease such as OA, collagen type II turnover is very low, and the architectural framework of cartilage can remain intact [97]. Age is associated with decreased cartilage collagen birefringence indicating changes in the chemical properties of collagen, which reduce the orderly anisotropy of collagen fibrils [98, 99]. One of the prominent age-related changes in articular cartilage composition involves increased non-enzymatic cross-links by accumulation of Maillard reaction products, which are collectively termed advanced glycation end products, AGEs [100–102]. These reactions result in a variety of fluorescent products including pentosidine cross-links [103]. While the amount of pyridinoline (Pyd) cross-link (an intramolecular covalent cross-link formed between adjacent collagen chains) per collagen remains constant and does not correlate with age, human articular cartilage of various ages revealed that the amount of pentosidine per collagen increases linearly with age and the amount of pentosidine per Pyd increases exponentially during life [104, 105]. This age-associated accumulation of senescent pentosidine cross-links results in stiffer cartilage collagen network which in turn contributes to a more brittle cartilage that is susceptible to fatigue and biomechanical failure [106–108]. Further, increased cross-links, investigated through in vitro glycation of cartilage explants, have shown to variably alter the biomechanical response of chondrocytes in superficial, middle and deeper cartilage zones, thus offering possible insights into how aging could alter cell deformation behaviour in cartilage [109]. Another effect of AGE includes decreased PG synthesis for specific non-cross-linked glycation products such as GA-pyridine to stimulate cell responses through a specific receptor for advanced glycation end products (RAGE), a cell adhesion molecule [108, 110–112]. All these changes have an adverse effect on the cartilage biomechanical properties.

Further, age-related cartilage changes can involve increased noncollagenous protein, interposition of other collagen types such as collagen type I or type III, or cleavage of collagen type II by cathepsin K and other proteolytic enzymes elaborated by senescent chondrocytes [46, 106, 113]. Elaboration of fibrillar collagen types beyond collagen type II is a result of repair following micro-injury [114, 115]. This follows two patterns. First, there is increased collagen in a perichondral distribution reflecting injury and repair involving individual chondrocytes. Second, there is vertical interposition typically of collagen type I fibres between cartilage domains reflecting repair from subchondral articular plate microfractures. As type I and other collagens are less hydrated than collagen type II, this results in matrix compositional heterogeneity with resultant compromise of cartilage mechanical function [116].

Noncollagenous proteins comprise about 50% of cartilage protein [117, 118]. These proteins, elaborated by chondrocytes, are heterogenous and consist in part of enzymes, particularly matrix metalloproteinases (MMPs), lysozyme and alkaline phosphatase, enzyme inhibitors and structural molecules such as fibronectin, link proteins, COMP, cartilage matrix protein (matrillin-1), leucine-rich proteins and collagen precursor products such as C-propeptide of collagen type II [119–121]. With aging, these proteins accumulate in cartilage and contribute to its resistance to repair.

Amyloid, an intercellular substance composed of fibrils and PG, is frequently deposited in aging articular cartilage [122–124]. Amyloid when present is found in both loaded and less loaded cartilage and is unassociated with OA [125, 126]. Cartilage amyloid is associated with matrix domains rich in KS [124]. Amyloid deposited in cartilage is the beta-2 microglobulin type and is thought to be of local origin [127].

3.3.4 Biomechanical Changes

The knee articular cartilage macromolecular architecture as well as biochemical and biomechanical properties are adapted to withstand stresses exposed on it during physiological activities. Compressive resistance is bestowed by the large PG, aggrecan, which is attached to HA polymers via link protein. The collagen network provides the restraining tensile stress that counterbalances the osmotic pressure of the PGs during cartilage mechanical loading [128]. Decreased cartilage matrix permeability, a feature of cartilage aging associated in part with increased matrix noncollagenous protein and oxidized lipid, leads to decreased chondrocyte nutrition and signalling and results in chondrocyte senescence [129, 130]. Further, aging adult articular cartilage matrix exhibits decreased tensile strength and stiffness, decreased viscoelastic properties related to decreased cytoskeletal network, decreased resistance to compressive loads, and increased cartilage sheer modulus [28, 131–135]. Regarding zonal variation, tensile strength and stiffness of the SZ increase with age to reach a maximum value in the third decade; and, thereafter both the tensile strength and stiffness decline markedly with increasing age [28]. On the other hand, tensile strength of cartilage from the deep zone (DZ) decreases continuously with age [28]. These results are likely reflected by changes in the organization of the collagen fibres and collagen crosslinks with age. As a consequence, decreased absorption and spread of mechanical forces within cartilage results in increased forces absorbed focally within the underlying subchondral bone. In turn, this can lead to microfracture of subchondral bone in susceptible individuals (Table 3.2).

3.3.5 Alteration in Signalling Molecules

Articular cartilage is responsive to extrinsic factors that regulate gene expression and protein synthesis in chondrocytes. In the past two decades, numerous in vitro and in vivo studies have confirmed that articular chondrocytes are able to respond to mechanical injury, joint instability due to genetic factors and biological stimuli such as cytokines as well as growth and differentiation factors that contribute to structural changes in the surrounding cartilage matrix [136].

Like other cells, chondrocytes have numerous cell surface receptors for cytokines and chemokines, as well as Toll-like receptors, and can themselves express chemical mediator (such as cytokines, chemokines and adipokines) as a reaction to injury [137]. Unlike other cells, cartilage matrix limits mediator diffusion to paracrine effects on adjacent chondrocytes. Senescent chondrocytes have decreased sensitivity to anabolic growth factors such as insulin-like growth factor 1 (IGF-1) and osteogenic protein-1 (OP-1), an effect similar to that induced by oxidative stress mediators [138]. Expression of transforming growth factor beta (TGF-β) family components, a family which is crucial for the maintenance of healthy articular cartilage, is altered during aging in cartilage. Aging nega-

Table 3.2 Articular cartilage and underlying subchondral bone structure: normal, acute injury, active osteoarthritis, chronic inflammatory arthritis and aging

Articular Cartilage Feature/Zone	Normal	Acute Injury	Osteoarthritis	Chronic Inflammatory Arthritis	Aging
Surface Integrity	Smooth	Smooth	Rough	Smooth with concave profile	Smooth
Superficial Zone	Cells aligned horizontally	Edema above normal surface *(no cells)*	Fibrillation; Fissures; Focal necrotic cells *(no nuclei)*	Extensive necrotic cells; Focal lacunar resorption; ↓ matrix	Atrophic cells; Focal necrosis
Middle Zone	Vertical chondrons 1–2 cells/chondron	Vertical chondrons; (1–2 cells/chondron) ↑ cell size	Fissures; Erosions; (2+ cells/ chondron, *clustering*); Thickened chondron capsule	Some necrotic cells *(otherwise no change in cell architecture from normal)*; ↓ matrix	Atrophic cells Focal necrosis; ↓ matrix
	Slight PCM Limited TM	↑ PCM ↑ TM	Variable PCM ↑ TM+++	PCM not seen TM ↓ PG++	PCM not seen TM ↓ PG+
Deep Zone	Vertical chondrons 1–2 cells/chondron	No change from normal	Fissures; Erosions; Chondrocyte clusters may extend to deep zone;	↓ matrix	↓ matrix
	Slight PCM Limited TM			PCM not seen TM ↓ PG++	TM ↓ PG+
Calcified Cartilage	Chondrons similar to deep cartilage No PCM	No change from normal	↑ and more variable thickness	No change from normal	↓ Thickness
Subchondral Bone	Osteocytes present	Vascular congestion below the bone	Vascular invasion into bone *(and if extensive also invades into calcified cartilage)* ↑ bone remodeling *(osteoclasts, osteoblasts at bone surface)*	Thinner bone *(osteoporosis)* Extensive osteocyte necrosis *(↑ size of osteocyte lacunae and absence of cells)*	Thinner bone *(osteoporosis)* Focal osteocyte necrosis *(↑ size of osteocyte lacunae, and absence of cells)*

PCM, *Pericellular matrix*; TM, *Territorial matrix*; ITM, *Interterritorial matrix*; ↓, *Decreased*; ↑, *Increased*; PG, *Proteoglycan cellular*; *Atrophy* refers to ↓ in cell size *(smaller cells)* caused by loss of subcellular organelles and substances tively affects both the TGF-β - activin receptor-like kinase 5 (ALK5) and bone morphogenetic protein (BMP) with its associated BMP receptor (BMPR) signalling routes, and aged chondrocytes display a lowered pSMAD3-dependent response to TGF-β1 and loss of collagen type 2α1 expression by approximately 256-fold [139].

Experimentally, aged chondrocytes overexpress DNA damage-inducible protein 45β (GADD45β) [140]. FoxO transcription factors play a key role in postnatal cartilage development, maturation and homeostasis and protect against OA-associated cartilage damage [141]. FoxO1 is a gene which encodes a forkhead family transcription factor that regulates cell responses to oxidative stress; whereas, FoxO3 gene functions as a trigger for apoptosis through expression of genes necessary for cell death [141, 142]. Aged chondrocytes express decreased FoxO1 and FoxO3 transcription factors in SZ in matrix regions exposed to maximal weight bearing [141, 143]. Estrogen can delay, attenuate, but not prevent chondrocyte senescence [144]. Similarly, statin can reduce catabolic effects mediated by interleukin (Il)-1β-induced expression of MMP-1 and MMP-13 [145].

3.4 Articular Cartilage Degradation and Related Diseases

Failure in any of the joint components can compromise the normal joint function, which, in turn, may lead to accumulation of damage in other arthrodial structures. Although chondrocyte turnover is thought to be normally very low with individual chondrocytes living for decades, cartilage injury due to aging, trauma or disease can stimulate chondrocyte replication. Cartilage degeneration results in decreased structural, biochemical and biomechanical properties. Accordingly, age-associated decrease in cartilage function can be considered as cartilage degeneration, but diseases such as inflammatory arthritis (IA) and excessive cyclic compressive loading can accelerate cartilage degeneration associated with aging [146–149]. Figures 3.2 and 3.3 illustrate the changes in articular cartilage ECM, chondrons, tidemark and subchondral bone with acute injury, OA, chronic IA and aging.

Degenerative processes involving aberration of cartilage structure are reflected in the breakdown of the normal mechanical function of cartilage. Several factors may lead to the cartilage mechanical breakdown such as direct trauma to the cartilage, obesity, immobilization and excessive repetitive loading of the cartilage. Cartilage shear stresses, particularly within the DZ, increase in response to the thinning of the articular cartilage, and this is associated with tidemark advancement, tidemark reduplication, and thickening of calcified cartilage / subchondral plate [150]. Further, tensile stress may initiate or propagate the splits and cracks observed in diseased cartilage [151, 152]. Also, proteolytic-mediated degradation of cartilage can occur via the action of proteinases or free radicals [153, 154].

Alkaptonuria is a rare inherited genetic disease that is an excellent model for cartilage degeneration related to metabolic products accumulating in collagen and affecting collagen properties [155, 156]. In alkaptonuria, homogentisic acid which is produced from phenylalanine and tyrosine is broken down and accumulates on collagen fibres of connective tissues including articular cartilage rendering the fibres less capable of associating with PGs. This results in brittle cartilage that can break and produce micro shards into the synovial fluid. Over time, a buildup of this substance in the joint leads to arthritis. People with alkaptonuria typically develop arthritis, particularly in the spine and large joints, beginning in the third decade [157]. The associated cartilage matrix dehydration can also lead to calcium pyrophosphate dihydrate (CPPD) crystal deposition.

3.4.1 Gout and Calcium Pyrophosphate Dihydrate Crystal Deposition

A variety of acute and chronic joint disorders are associated with crystal deposits [158, 159]. Endogenous crystals such as monosodium urate, CPPD and basic calcium phosphate (hydroxyap-

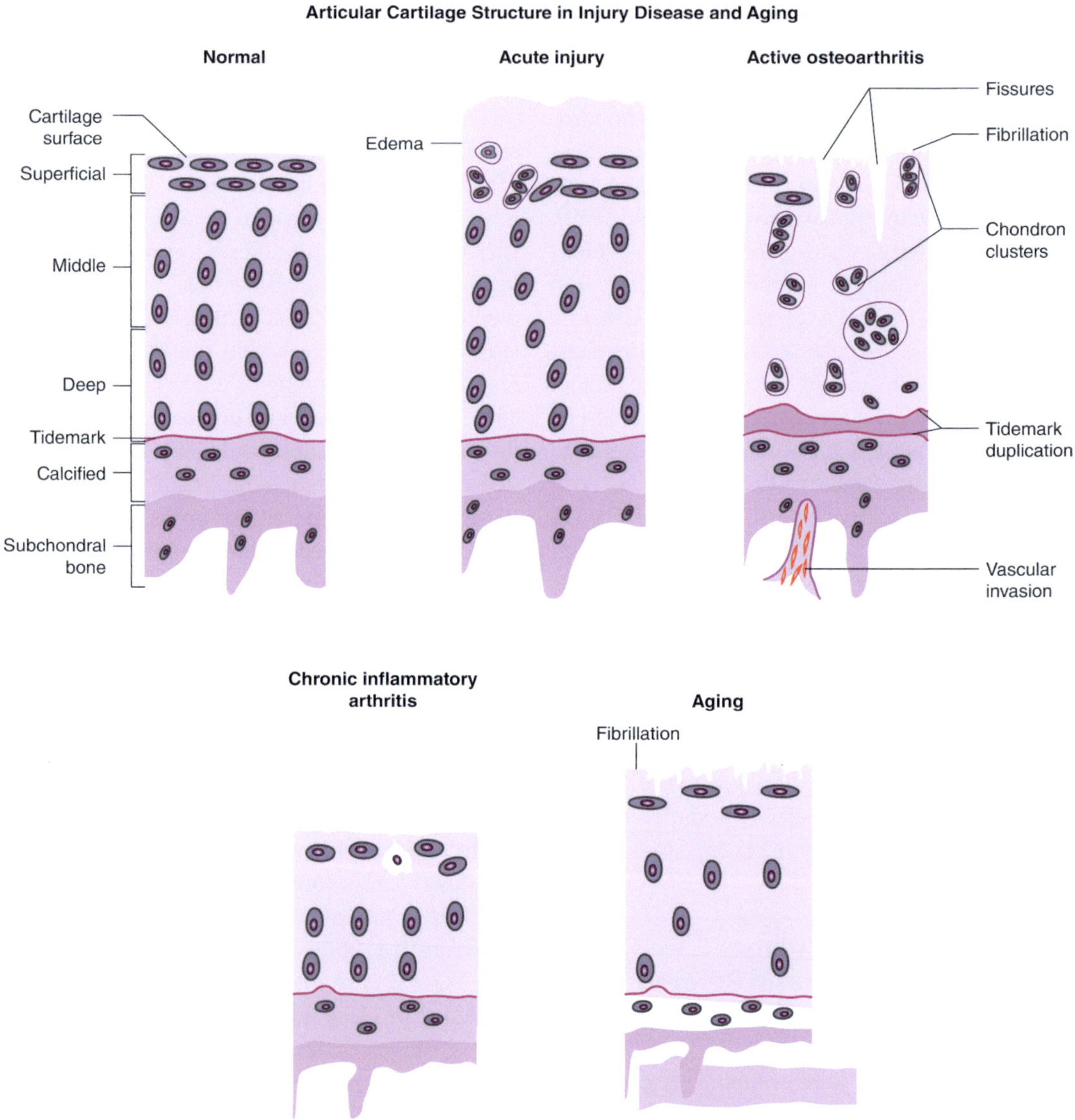

Fig. 3.2 Articular cartilage structure showing changes in extracellular matrix, chondrons, tidemark and subchondral bone with acute injury, osteoarthritis, chronic inflammatory arthritis and aging

atite) have been shown to be pathogenic. These endogenous crystals produce disease by triggering the cascade that results in cytokine-mediated cartilage destruction. The two common crystal arthropathies are gout, caused by urates, and pseudogout, associated with CPPD crystals.

CPPD crystals were first identified in synovial fluid exudates of patients with the pseudogout syndrome. Since their discovery in 1962, it has been recognized that CPPD crystals form within articular tissues and are subsequently shed into the synovial fluid. The most common etiologic association is with aging; by the age of 80 years, CPPD crystal deposits can be found in articular cartilage in 25% of the population [159].

Gout involves urate crystal deposition on the cartilage surface and in the synovial fluid leading to synovial hyperplasia, fibrosis and pannus formation which in turn destroys the underlying articular cartilage. CPPD crystal deposition can occur in tendons, ligaments, synovium and articular cartilage [160–162].

Pathologic calcification of articular cartilage is classified by the type of mineral deposited, most commonly CPPD and less often basic calcium phosphate. Basic calcium phosphate

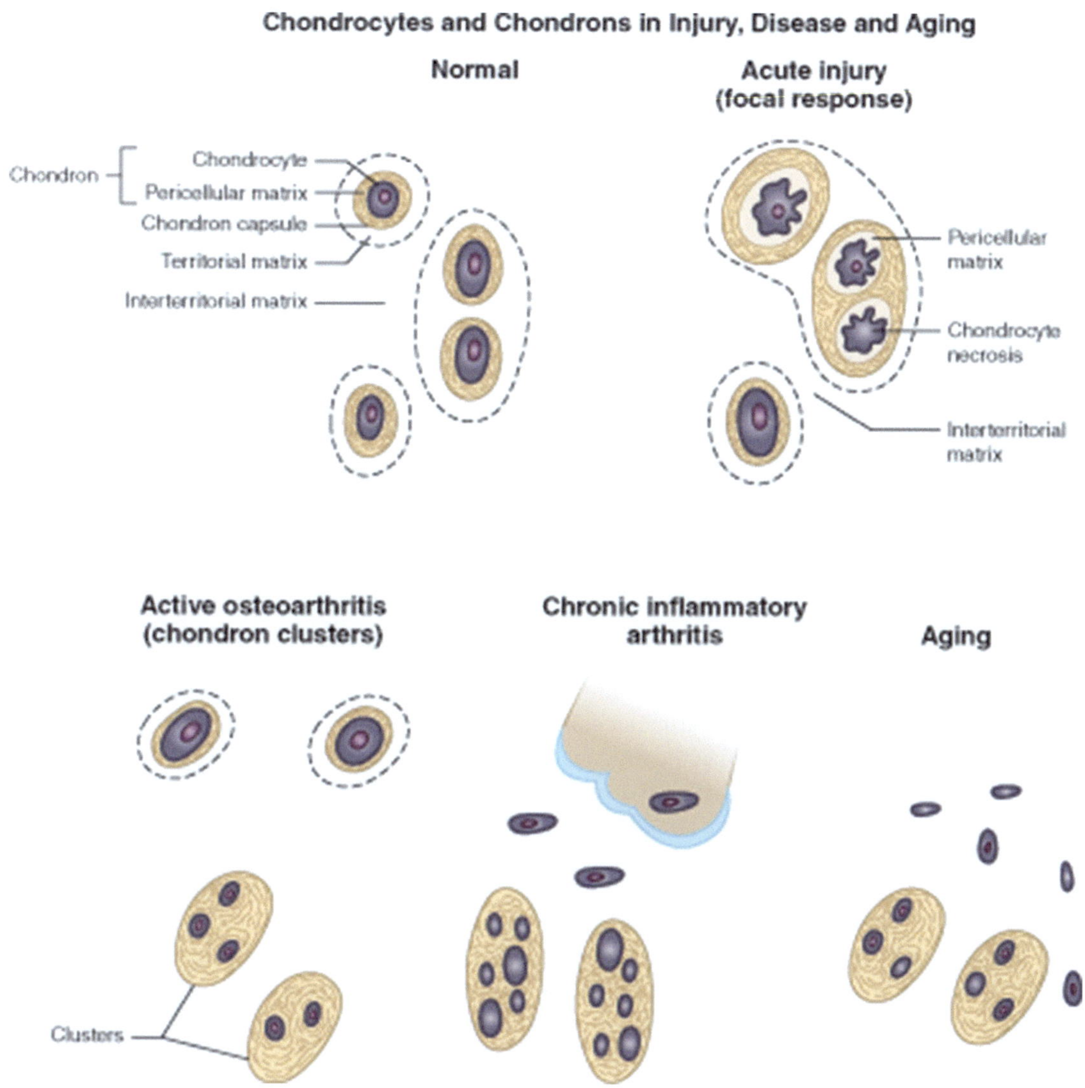

Fig. 3.3 Chondrons and chondrocytes showing changes with acute injury, osteoarthritis, chronic inflammatory arthritis and aging

deposits are associated with joint injury [163, 164]. While CPPD crystal deposits can be associated with familial factors, specific endocrine and metabolic disorders (such as hyperparathyroidism, hypothyroidism, hypomagnesemia, hemochromatosis, alkaptonuria and hypophosphatasia) and previous articular cartilage injury and repair, the most common presentation is that associated with aging [165]. Factors in CPPD pathogenesis include inhibition or deficiency of alkaline phosphatase, which at pH = 7.4 is the dominant pyrophosphatase, and relative cartilage dehydration [158, 166–168]. CPPD deposits in cartilage increase the heterogeneity of tissue mechanics thereby contributing to cartilage degeneration.

3.4.2 Rheumatoid Arthritis

Rheumatoid arthritis is a systemic, chronic inflammatory disorder that mainly affects the joint tissues. The disease onset in RA is usually insidious, with the predominant symptoms being pain, stiffness (especially morning stiffness) and swelling of many joints. Epidemiological studies show that age is the strongest risk factor for the development of RA, and paralleling the global trends in population aging, there is both an increase in the incidence and prevalence of RA [169]. RA is characterized by persistent, extensive synovitis and pannus formation, which ultimately leads to erosions of articular cartilage and marginal subchondral bone [170]. Although RA is of unknown aetiology, autoimmunity plays a pivotal role in its chronicity and progression [171]. The initial pathologic event in RA appears to be injury of synovial microvascular endothelial cells and proliferation / activation of synovial lining macrophages, which in turn send signals to stimulate the superficial chondrocytes to elaborate catabolic enzymes (such as collagenase and stromelysin) into the ECM thereby damaging superficial cartilage.

Although the exact aetiology of RA has not been fully elucidated, a large body of evidence supports a mechanism involving the synergistic interaction between cytokines and other components of synovial fluid that degrades articular cartilage and subchondral bone. Specifically, the presence of two cytokines, namely Il-1 and tumour necrosis factor (TNF), is the main stimuli of cartilage degradation in RA [172–174]. In vitro studies corroborated that cartilage degradation occurs from the stimulatory effect of Il-1 and TNF on chondrocytes to secrete cartilage-degrading MMPs [175, 176]. Inflammatory infiltrates in the subchondral bone, observed in magnetic resonance imaging (MRI) as bone marrow edema (BME), play an important role in the pathogenesis of RA [177]. BME is considered a precursor of rapid disease progression and is observed in 68–75% of patients in early stages of RA [177]. Further, adipose tissue present within the joint is thought to contribute to the pathogenesis of RA through its secretion of adipocytokines and infiltration by inflammatory cells [178–180].

3.4.3 Osteoarthritis

Osteoarthritis is a common, slowly progressive and often debilitating form of degenerative arthritis that results in structural and functional failure of diarthrodial joints that occurs when the dynamic homeostatic equilibrium between the breakdown and repair of joint tissues is overwhelmed [181, 182]. The clinical manifestations of OA include joint pain, stiffness and limitations in activity. The prevalence of clinical OA increases with age [183–185]. While OA is recognized to be heterogenous clinically, OA phenotypes in general [186] and OA phenotypes in particular [187] remain controversial and unresolved. Further, after decades of research, no surrogate markers are available yet in blood or other fluids for reliably detecting or monitoring OA progression [188]. The pathogenesis of OA is thought to be multifactorial, involving environmental factors, such as the influence of occupation, body weight, gait and joint kinematics, trauma, recreational / competitive sports and surgical manipulations as well as genetic factors such as collagen gene mutations [189–193]. Although the lifelong moderate use of normal joints does not increase the risk of OA; nevertheless, high-impact and torsional loads may increase the risk of degeneration of previously normal joints [194].

OA is characterized by an intertwined web of degeneration, regeneration, repair and remodelling of articular cartilage, not just cartilage degeneration [24, 195, 196]. Loss of the normal cartilage homeostasis occurs resulting in imbalance between matrix macromolecule synthesis and degradation [197]. OA is associated with defective integrity of articular cartilage and intra-articular inflammation, in addition to related reactive changes in the underlying trabecular and cortical bone and at the joint margin, in particular the synovium [198–200]. With the progression of OA, the normally whitish-blue translucent cartilage takes on an opaque yellowish appearance on gross observation. An extensively ulcerated area leading to partial or full cartilage thickness erosion follows surface irregularities, due to fissuring and cleft formation. These erosions, which are initially focal, become confluent and progress to large denuded areas, particularly in the load-bearing area [201]. Refer to Chap. 15 for detailed microscopic features of OA.

The mechanism for the onset and progression of OA, though unclear, involves a combination of structural, biochemical and biomechanical factors. Structural failure of articular cartilage could result from abnormal mechanical strains on healthy normal cartilage and from the influence

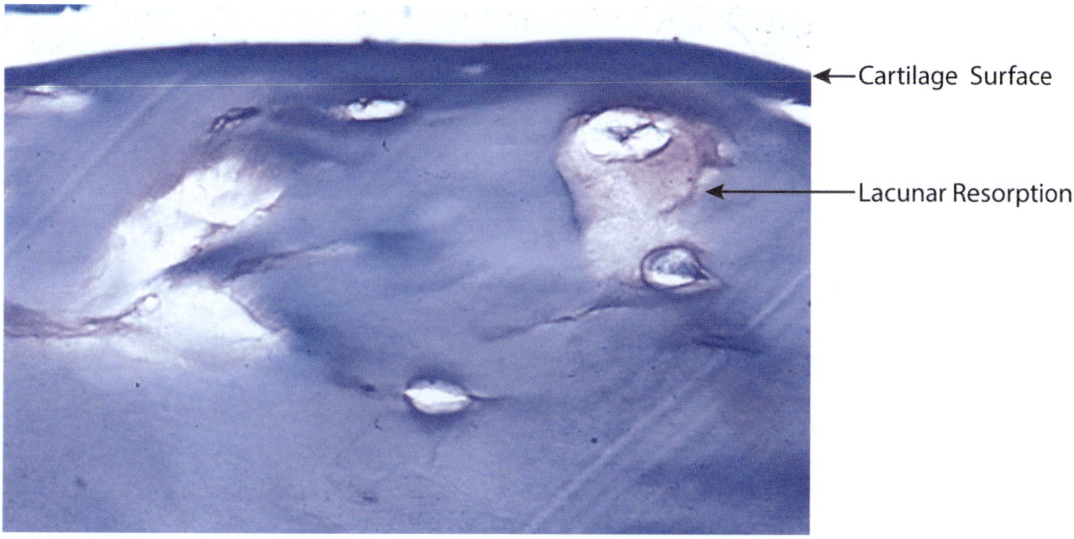

Fig. 3.4 Toluidine blue stained photomicrograph of human articular cartilage showing just underneath the articular surface pale staining matrix lacunar resorption indicating resorption of both proteoglycan and collagen in these regions. (Magnification, 100×)

of physiological mechanical strains on pathologically impaired cartilage. Elevated metabolic activity in human OA cartilage is an early event. Early OA is characterized by episodes of acute cartilage injury as seen by cartilage edema [202–204]. Histologically, although focal lacunar resorptive lesions have been noted in various stages of OA cartilage, there is no evidence of a direct relationship between focal cartilage resorption and OA (Fig. 3.4) [205]. Chondrocyte morphology is altered in OA, and chondrocyte clusters are recognized as a hallmark of OA (Fig. 3.5) [206–208]. Chondrocyte clusters express both catabolic factors (e.g. Il-1β and MMP-13) and anabolic factors (e.g. *SOX9* activation and collagen type II synthesis) indicating the association of several cell signalling pathways and growth factors with chondrocyte clusters [209–212]. Higher incidence of chondron hypertrophy (enlarged) and clustering in OA cartilage compared to normal, aging and injured articular cartilage may initially be due to hydrodynamic swelling, but further increases in size could be due to enhanced anabolic activity resulting in increased matrix deposition (Fig. 3.6). The loss of chondrocyte phenotype stability, and chondrocyte hypertrophy seen in OA articular cartilage are believed to initiate and perpetuate a cascade of events that eventually result in cartilage degeneration; as such, these chondrocytic aberrations are considered as central contributing factors to OA pathogenesis [213, 214].

The microstructural changes of the collagen-PG network at the cartilage surface (rather than its composition change) are responsible for the early increase of hydration [193, 215]. This structural change promotes the deterioration of biomechanical properties of articular cartilage. Though, PG synthesis is markedly increased in OA cartilage compared to normal cartilage, the rate of PG turnover is also increased resulting in an overall reduction in total PG and/or GAG content, which is directly proportional to the OA severity [216]. Also, compared to normal cartilage, the PGs synthesized by OA cartilage chondrocytes are structurally different with shorter GAGs, increased number of PG fragments, decreased size of its subunits with diminished and / or defective aggregation, increased C4S compared to C6S and increased CS/KS ratio. Increased levels of aggrecan, decorin, biglycan, fibromodulin and link protein and increased anchorin CII (annexin V epitopes) and tenascin level have been reported in human OA cartilage (compared to age-matched controls) [217–222]. Further, increased level of pentosi-

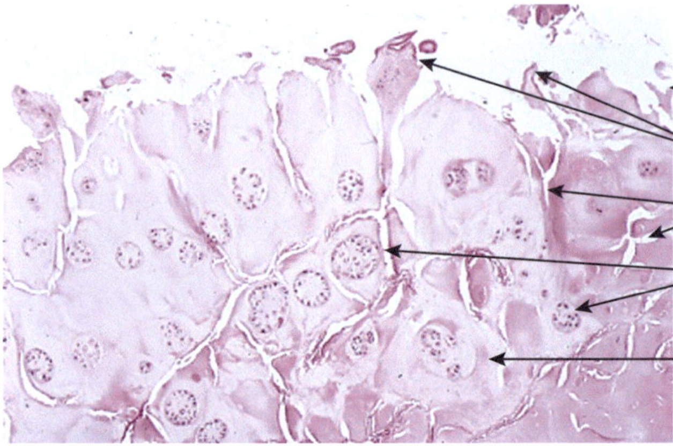

Fig. 3.5 Hematoxylin and eosin stained photomicrograph of a severely osteoarthritic articular cartilage obtained from the femoral condyle illustrating cartilage loss, surface fibrillation and fissures extending from the superficial into middle zone. The cartilage matrix compartments are markedly altered with chondrocytes primarily present in clusters. (Magnification ×10)

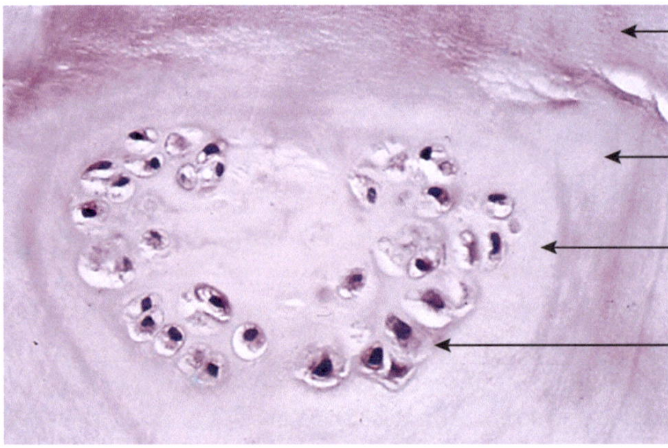

Fig. 3.6 Photomicrograph of a chondrocyte cluster depicting active repair response. Note chondrocyte hyperplasia demonstrating intrinsic proliferative cellular response (chondrocyte regeneration) to cartilage injury. (Magnification ×50)

dine has been documented in the cartilage and body fluids of OA patients [223–225].

Although the total collagen content of OA cartilage varies little, collagen type I, III, VI and X often increase [226–230]. Collagen fibre diameter and orientation may also show considerable variation from normal [231]. A switch to collagen type I synthesis with a decrease in the synthesis of collagen type II is observed in OA cartilage. Under physiological conditions, collagen type II fibrils contain more water than Type I fibrils [116, 232]. Therefore, increased collagen type I and decreased collagen type II could account for decreased water content in severe OA tissue. Studies have shown enhanced deposition of collagen types I and VI and fibronectin in human OA cartilage [233–236]. Also documented is the increased synthesis of collagen type X by OA chondrocytes [21, 237].

Biomechanically, OA cartilage has decreased modulus or stiffness when placed in tension, compression and shear loading, which in turn increases its propensity to swell when compared to healthy cartilage. It is unclear if the initial disruption of the cartilage surface is a direct result of mechanical forces or a product of altered chondrocyte activity. In vitro, early-OA model study of OA-associated structural changes on chondrocyte strains at the macro- (tissue level) and micro- (cellular level) scale showed that micro-scale spatial softening of

PCM and ECM resulted in a 30% increase of chondrocyte shear strain, even without visible structural changes at the macro-scale [238]. This indicates that early OA micromechanical changes at the cellular level may affect chondrocyte activities before macro-scale degradations at the tissue level become apparent. Nevertheless, deterioration of the collagen-PG network appears to be focused at the articular surface. Early signs of OA appear on the cartilage surface as PG depletion, followed by surface irregularity and then fibrillation of the superficial collagen network. Continuous compression of the cartilage diminishes PG synthesis and causes damage of the tissue through necrosis. This further creates an altered stress pattern on joint surfaces eventually leading to frank cartilage structural damage and mechanical failure of articular cartilage. Surface fibrillation and internal collagen damage may both develop after long-term repetitive loading or overloading. An in vitro study demonstrated that bovine osteochondral plugs (2 mm diameter) when compressed at varying loads and duration, the loading magnitude affects the degree of collagen damage [239]. Also, the loading rate on cartilage dominated the location of collagen network damage: low loading rates predominantly damaged superficial collagen, while at high rates, collagen damage occurred at the deeper zones. Early subchondral changes include redistribution of blood supply with marrow hypertension, edema and probably micro-necrosis [240]. Differences in the viscoelastic properties of cartilage, reflected by alterations in the structure and composition of the chondrocyte cytoskeleton, have also been associated with OA [241, 242].

Increased serum concentrations of COMP fragments have been reported for patients with knee OA [243–248]. Reports have suggested [4] that patients with greater serum COMP concentration experience a faster progression of their disease due to increased degradation of their articular cartilage [248, 249]. Refer to Chap. 4 for an in-depth knowledge of the biomarkers in body fluids reflective of knee OA articular cartilage metabolism.

3.5 Aging Versus Osteoarthritis

The relationship of OA to cartilage degeneration and aging is controversial, mostly because different investigators have different perspectives. Whether the changes in aging inevitably progress through an intermediary phase of "degenerated cartilage" to the fibrillated state of OA is unclear. Once believed to be "a disease of the elderly", OA is not primarily a disease of aging as OA can begin shortly after epiphyses are closed and the joint structures including articular cartilage are fully mature [165, 250]. However, OA is often associated with aging due to its chronic nature which often progresses with age and manifestation of the clinical signs and symptoms at the late stage [251, 252]. Although OA is not an inevitable consequence of aging, yet, aging increases the risk of OA [59].

Recent reports of important age-related changes in the function of chondrocytes suggest that age-related changes in articular cartilage can contribute to the development and progression of OA. With aging, chondrocyte senescence decreases capacity to maintain cartilage matrix homeostasis, thereby facilitating cartilage degeneration [61, 73, 253, 254]. Under these circumstances if the residual chondrocytes can stimulate cartilage regenerative or reparative changes, OA often will occur, in particular with advanced chondrocyte senescence.

OA is now regarded as a group of diseases distinct from and superimposed on aging processes. Aging itself may not be a consequence of OA but age-related changes in the function of chondrocytes may contribute for the initiation and progression of the disease. As such, aging is the main risk factor for OA. Aging could alter the matrix composition and accelerate the degradation of the cartilage. Both subchondral bone density and the incidence of OA in joints are known to vary with age in humans [255]. Also documented is the age-related decrease in cell density in all zones of the human femoral condyle articular cartilage, though more markedly in SZ [256]. Vascularity of the zone of calcified cartilage (ZCC, a sign of remodelling) is well developed after 55–65 years of age. Age-related decline in calcified cartilage thickness in human femoral condyles is associated with attenuated number of tidemarks after the sixth decade [257]. These findings suggest that remodelling of the bone appears to cease with increasing age. Reduction in the water content from 70–80% (normal wet weight) to 50–65% (wet weight) accompanies aging process especially in the deeper zone [258].

3.6 Conclusions

Chondrocytes, the sole articular cartilage cellular component, are responsible for maintaining the cartilage homeostasis by regulating a low-turnover state of the cartilage ECM. However, damage to articular cartilage due to aging, acute or chronic injury or cartilage-related diseases shifts the homeostatic equilibrium towards a degenerative or destructive stage. In joint diseases, cartilage homeostasis is disrupted by mechanisms that are driven by combinations of structural, biochemical and biomechanical stimuli that vary according to the disease process.

Chondrocyte senescence associated with aging may limit cartilage adult repair by pharmacologic and tissue engineering methods. Furthermore, these defects may result in progressive articular degeneration and predispose to the development of joint arthropathies. Biological repair techniques (discussed in depth in Chaps. 11, 12, 16, 17 and 18) such as autologous chondrocyte transplantation, osteochondral transplantation (OATS, mosaicplasty) and microfracture are primarily used for surgical treatment. However, although these techniques have shown promising results in younger patients, cartilage repair appears to be less effective with increasing age.

References

1. Gahunia HK, Pritzker KP. Effect of exercise on articular cartilage. Orthop Clin North Am. 2012;43:187–99.
2. Makinejad MD, Abu Osman NA, Abu Bakar Wan Abas W, Bayat M. Preliminary analysis of knee stress in full extension landing. Clinics (Sao Paulo). 2013;68:1180–8.
3. Asanbaeva A, Masuda K, Thonar EJ, Klisch SM, Sah RL. Regulation of immature cartilage growth by IGF-I, TGF-β1, BMP-7, and PDGF-AB: role of metabolic balance between fixed charge and collagen network. Biomech Model Mechanobiol. 2008;7:263–76.
4. Murphy CL, Sambanis A. Effect of oxygen tension on chondrocyte extracellular matrix accumulation. Connect Tissue Res. 2001;42:87–96.
5. Fermor B, Christensen SE, Youn I, Cernanec JM, Davies CM, Weinberg JB. Oxygen, nitric oxide and articular cartilage. Eur Cell Mater. 2007;13:56–65.
6. Schrobback K, Malda J, Crawford RW, Upton Z, Leavesley DI, Klein TJ. Effects of oxygen on zonal marker expression in human articular chondrocytes. Tissue Eng Part A. 2012;18:920–33.
7. Mobasheri A, Richardson S, Mobasheri R, Shakibaei M, Hoyland JA. Hypoxia inducible factor-1 and facilitative glucose transporters GLUT1 and GLUT3: putative molecular components of the oxygen and glucose sensing apparatus in articular chondrocytes. Histol Histopathol. 2005;20:1327–38.
8. Pfander D, Gelse K. Hypoxia and osteoarthritis: how chondrocytes survive hypoxic environments. Curr Opin Rheumatol. 2007;19:457–62.
9. Goldring MB, Marcu KB. Cartilage homeostasis in health and rheumatic diseases. Arthritis Res Ther. 2009;11:224.
10. Guilak F, Jones WR, Ting-Beall HP, Lee GM. The deformation behavior and mechanical properties of chondrocytes in articular cartilage. Osteoarthritis Cartilage. 1999;7:59–70.
11. Knight MM, Ross JM, Sherwin AF, Lee DA, Bader DL, Poole CA. Chondrocyte deformation within mechanically and enzymatically extracted chondrons compressed in agarose. Biochim Biophys Acta. 2001;1526:141–6.
12. Chen SS, Falcovitz YH, Schneiderman R, Maroudas A, Sah RL. Depth-dependent compressive properties of normal aged human femoral head articular cartilage: relationship to fixed charge density. Osteoarthritis Cartilage. 2001;9:561–9.
13. Maroudas A, Bullough P, Swanson SA, Freeman MA. The permeability of articular cartilage. J Bone Joint Surg Br. 1968;50:166–77.
14. Cawston TE, Wilson AJ. Understanding the role of tissue degrading enzymes and their inhibitors in development and disease. Best Pract Res Clin Rheumatol. 2006;20:983–1002.
15. Dancevic CM, McCulloch DR. Current and emerging therapeutic strategies for preventing inflammation and aggrecanase-mediated cartilage destruction in arthritis. Arthritis Res Ther. 2014;16:429.
16. Martin JA, Brown TD, Heiner AD, Buckwalter JA. Chondrocyte senescence, joint loading and osteoarthritis. Clin Orthop Relat Res. 2004;427:S96–103.
17. Poole CA. Articular cartilage chondrons: form, function and failure. J Anat. 1997;191(Pt 1):1–13.
18. Poole CA, Flint MH, Beaumont BW. Chondrons in cartilage: ultrastructural analysis of the pericellular microenvironment in adult human articular cartilages. J Orthop Res. 1987;5:509–22.
19. Chang J, Poole CA. Sequestration of type VI collagen in the pericellular microenvironment of adult chondrocytes cultured in agarose. Osteoarthritis Cartilage. 1996;4:275–85.
20. Poole CA, Wotton SF, Duance VC. Localization of type IX collagen in chondrons isolated from porcine articular cartilage and rat chondrosarcoma. Histochem J. 1988;20:567–74.
21. von der Mark K, Kirsch T, Nerlich A, Kuss A, Weseloh G, Gluckert K, Stoss H. Type X collagen synthesis in human osteoarthritic cartilage. Indication of chondrocyte hypertrophy. Arthritis Rheum. 1992;35:806–11.

22. Wilusz RE, Sanchez-Adams J, Guilak F. The structure and function of the pericellular matrix of articular cartilage. Matrix Biol. 2014;39:25–32.
23. Zhang Z. Chondrons and the pericellular matrix of chondrocytes. Tissue Eng Part B Rev. 2015;21:267–77.
24. Vonk LA, de Windt TS, Kragten AH, Beekhuizen M, Mastbergen SC, Dhert WJ, Lafeber FP, Creemers LB, Saris DB. Enhanced cell-induced articular cartilage regeneration by chondrons; the influence of joint damage and harvest site. Osteoarthritis Cartilage. 2014;22:1910–7.
25. Guo H, Torzilli PA. Shape of chondrocytes within articular cartilage affects the solid but not the fluid microenvironment under unconfined compression. Acta Biomater. 2016;29:170–9.
26. Verzijl N, DeGroot J, Thorpe SR, Bank RA, Shaw JN, Lyons TJ, Bijlsma JW, Lafeber FP, Baynes JW, TeKoppele JM. Effect of collagen turnover on the accumulation of advanced glycation end products. J Biol Chem. 2000;275(50):39027–31.
27. Maroudas A, Palla G, Gilav E. Racemization of aspartic acid in human articular cartilage. Connect Tissue Res. 1992;28(3):161–9.
28. Kempson GE. Relationship between the tensile properties of articular cartilage from the human knee and age. Ann Rheum Dis. 1982;41:508–11.
29. Kempson GE. Mechanical properties of articular cartilage and their relationship to matrix degradation and age. Ann Rheum Dis. 1975;34(Suppl 2):111–3.
30. Kempson GE. Mechanical properties of articular cartilage. J Physiol. 1972;223:23P.
31. Klein TJ, Chaudhry M, Bae WC, Sah RL. Depth-dependent biomechanical and biochemical properties of fetal, newborn, and tissue-engineered articular cartilage. J Biomech. 2007;40:182–90.
32. Chan EF, Harjanto R, Asahara H, Inoue N, Masuda K, Bugbee WD, Firestein GS, Hosalkar HS, Lotz MK, Sah RL. Structural and functional maturation of distal femoral cartilage and bone during postnatal development and growth in humans and mice. Orthop Clin North Am. 2012;43:173–85.
33. Asanbaeva A, Tam J, Schumacher BL, Klisch SM, Masuda K, Sah RL. Articular cartilage tensile integrity: modulation by matrix depletion is maturation-dependent. Arch Biochem Biophys. 2008;474:175–82.
34. Li LP, Cheung JT, Herzog W. Three-dimensional fibril-reinforced finite element model of articular cartilage. Med Biol Eng Comput. 2009;47:607–15.
35. Roth V, Mow VC. The intrinsic tensile behavior of the matrix of bovine articular cartilage and its variation with age. J Bone Joint Surg Am. 1980;62:1102–17.
36. Kempson GE, Spivey CJ, Swanson SA, Freeman MA. Patterns of cartilage stiffness on normal and degenerate human femoral heads. J Biomech. 1971;4:597–609.
37. Kempson GE, Freeman MA, Swanson SA. Tensile properties of articular cartilage. Nature. 1968;220:1127–8.
38. Gottardi R, Hansen U, Raiteri R, Loparic M, Düggelin M, Mathys D, Friederich NF, Bruckner P, Stolz M. Supramolecular organization of collagen fibrils in healthy and osteoarthritic human knee and hip joint cartilage. PLoS One. 2016;11:e0163552.
39. Han EH, Chen SS, Klisch SM, Sah RL. Contribution of proteoglycan osmotic swelling pressure to the compressive properties of articular cartilage. Biophys J. 2011;101:916–24.
40. Broom ND. Further insights into the structural principles governing the function of articular cartilage. J Anat. 1984;139(Pt 2):275–94.
41. Eleswarapu SV, Responte DJ, Athanasiou KA. Tensile properties, collagen content, and crosslinks in connective tissues of the immature knee joint. PLoS One. 2011;6:e26178.
42. Williamson AK, Chen AC, Masuda K, Thonar EJ, Sah RL. Tensile mechanical properties of bovine articular cartilage: variations with growth and relationships to collagen network components. J Orthop Res. 2003;21:872–80.
43. Loeser RF. Molecular mechanisms of cartilage destruction: mechanics, inflammatory mediators, and aging collide. Arthritis Rheum. 2006;54:1357–60.
44. Dudhia J. Aggrecan, aging and assembly in articular cartilage. Cell Mol Life Sci. 2005;62:2241–56.
45. Aigner T, Haag J, Martin J, Buckwalter J. Osteoarthritis: aging of matrix and cells--going for a remedy. Curr Drug Targets. 2007;8:325–31.
46. Verzijl N, Bank RA, TeKoppele JM, DeGroot J. AGEing and osteoarthritis: a different perspective. Curr Opin Rheumatol. 2003;15:616–22.
47. Yang L, Carlson SG, McBurney D, Horton WE Jr. Multiple signals induce endoplasmic reticulum stress in both primary and immortalized chondrocytes resulting in loss of differentiation, impaired cell growth, and apoptosis. J Biol Chem. 2005;280:31156–65.
48. Grogan SP, D'Lima DD. Joint aging and chondrocyte cell death. Int J Clin Rheumatol. 2010;5:199–214.
49. Minguzzi M, Cetrullo S, D'Adamo S, Silvestri Y, Flamigni F, Borzì RM. Emerging players at the intersection of chondrocyte loss of maturational arrest, oxidative stress, senescence and low-grade inflammation in osteoarthritis. Oxid Med Cell Longev. 2018;2018:3075293. doi: 10.1155/2018/3075293.
50. Jeon OH, David N, Campisi J, Elisseeff JH. Senescent cells and osteoarthritis: a painful connection. J Clin Invest. 2018;128(4):1229–37.
51. Blanco FJ, Guitian R, Vazquez-Martul E, de Toro FJ, Galdo F. Osteoarthritis chondrocytes die by apoptosis. A possible pathway for osteoarthritis pathology. Arthritis Rheum. 1998;41:284–9.
52. Aigner T, Hemmel M, Neureiter D, Gebhard PM, Zeiler G, Kirchner T, McKenna L. Apoptotic cell death is not a widespread phenomenon in normal aging and osteoarthritis human articular knee cartilage: a study of proliferation, programmed cell death (apoptosis), and viability of chondrocytes in normal and osteoarthritic human knee cartilage. Arthritis Rheum. 2001;44:1304–12.

53. Chang J, Wang W, Zhang H, Hu Y, Wang M, Yin Z. The dual role of autophagy in chondrocyte responses in the pathogenesis of articular cartilage degeneration in osteoarthritis. Int J Mol Med. 2013;32:1311–8.
54. Carames B, Taniguchi N, Otsuki S, Blanco FJ, Lotz M. Autophagy is a protective mechanism in normal cartilage, and its aging-related loss is linked with cell death and osteoarthritis. Arthritis Rheum. 2010;62:791–801.
55. Carames B, Olmer M, Kiosses WB, Lotz MK. The relationship of autophagy defects to cartilage damage during joint aging in a mouse model. Arthritis Rheum. 2015;67:1568–76.
56. Martin JA, Buckwalter JA. Roles of articular cartilage aging and chondrocyte senescence in the pathogenesis of osteoarthritis. Iowa Orthop J. 2001;21:1–7.
57. Ma CH, Wu CH, Jou IM, Tu YK, Hung CH, et al. PKR promotes oxidative stress and apoptosis of human articular chondrocytes by causing mitochondrial dysfunction through p38 MAPK activation-PKR activation causes apoptosis in human chondrocytes. Antioxidants (Basel). 2019;8(9):E370. doi: 10.3390/antiox8090370.
58. Martin JA, Buckwalter JA. Telomere erosion and senescence in human articular cartilage chondrocytes. J Gerontol A Biol Sci Med Sci. 2001;56A:B172–9.
59. Martin JA, Buckwalter JA. Aging, articular cartilage chondrocyte senescence and osteoarthritis. Biogerontology. 2002;3:257–64.
60. Martin JA, Klingelhutz AJ, Moussavi-Harami F, Buckwalter JA. Effects of oxidative damage and telomerase activity on human articular cartilage chondrocyte senescence. J Gerontol Ser A Biol Sci Med Sci. 2004;59:324–37.
61. Loeser RF. Aging and osteoarthritis: the role of chondrocyte senescence and aging changes in the cartilage matrix. Osteoarthritis Cartilage. 2009;17:971–9.
62. Harbo M, Delaisse JM, Kjaersgaard-Andersen P, Soerensen FB, Koelvraa S, Bendix L. The relationship between ultra-short telomeres, aging of articular cartilage and the development of human hip osteoarthritis. Mech Ageing Dev. 2013;134:367–72.
63. Leong DJ, Sun HB. Events in articular chondrocytes with aging. Curr Osteoporos Rep. 2011;9:196–201.
64. Jallali N, Ridha H, Thrasivoulou C, Underwood C, Butler PE, Cowen T. Vulnerability to ROS-induced cell death in ageing articular cartilage: the role of antioxidant enzyme activity. Osteoarthritis Cartilage. 2005;13:614–22.
65. Bates EJ, Harper GS, Lowther DA, Preston BN. Effect of oxygen-derived reactive species on cartilage proteoglycan-hyaluronate aggregates. Biochem Int. 1984;8:629–37.
66. Bolduc JA, Collins JA, Loeser RF. Reactive oxygen species, aging and articular cartilage homeostasis. Free Radic Biol Med. 2019;132:73–82.
67. Krajewska-Włodarczyk M, Owczarczyk-Saczonek A, Placek W, Osowski A, Wojtkiewicz J. Articular cartilage aging-potential regenerative capacities of cell manipulation and stem cell therapy. Int J Mol Sci. 2018;19(2):E623.
68. Trelstad RL, Kang AH, Igarashi S, Gross J. Isolation of two distinct collagens from chick cartilage. Biochemistry. 1970;9:4993–8.
69. Mayne R. Cartilage collagens. What is their function and are they involved in articular disease? Arthritis Rheum. 1989;32:241–6.
70. Benninghof A. Form und Bau der Gelenkknorpel in ihren Beziehungen zur Function. II. Der Aufbau des Gelenkknorpels in seinen Beziehungen zur Function. Z Zellforsch Mikrosk Anat. 1925;2:783–862.
71. Speer DP, Dahners L. The collagenous architecture of articular cartilage. Clin Orthop Relat Res. 1979;139:267–75.
72. Hwang WS, Li B, Jin LH, Ngo K, Schachar NS, Hughes GNF. Collagen fibril structure of normal aging, and osteoarthritic cartilage. J Pathol. 1992;167:425–33.
73. Lotz M, Loeser RF. Effects of aging on articular cartilage homeostasis. Bone. 2012;51:241–8.
74. Rieppo L, Saarakkala S, Narhi T, Holopainen J, Lammi M, Helminen HJ, Jurvelin JS, Rieppo J. Quantitative analysis of spatial proteoglycan content in articular cartilage with Fourier transform infrared imaging spectroscopy: critical evaluation of analysis methods and specificity of the parameters. Microsc Res Tech. 2010;73:503–12.
75. Yin J, Xia Y, Lu M. Concentration profiles of collagen and proteoglycan in articular cartilage by Fourier transform infrared imaging and principal component regression. Spectrochim Acta Mol Biomol Spectrosc. 2012;88:90–6.
76. Paul PK, O'Byrne E, Blancuzzi V, Wilson D, Gunson D, Douglas FL, Wang JZ, Mezrich RS. Magnetic resonance imaging reflects cartilage proteoglycan degradation in the rabbit knee. Skelet Radiol. 1991;20:31–6.
77. Wang Q, Zheng YP, Niu HJ. Changes in triphasic mechanical properties of proteoglycan-depleted articular cartilage extracted from osmotic swelling behavior monitored using high-frequency ultrasound. Mol Cell Biomech. 2010;7:45–58.
78. Inerot S, Heinegard D, Audell L, Olsson SE. Articular-cartilage proteoglycans in aging and osteoarthritis. Biochem J. 1978;169:143–56.
79. Lauder RM, Huckerby TN, Nieduszynski IA, Plaas AH. Age-related changes in the structure of the keratan sulphate chains attached to fibromodulin isolated from articular cartilage. Biochem J. 1998;330(Pt 2):753–7.
80. Theocharis DA, Kalpaxis DL, Tsiganos CP. Cartilage keratan sulphate: changes in chain length with ageing. Biochim Biophys Acta. 1985;841:131–4.
81. Hopwood JJ, Robinson HC. The structure and composition of cartilage keratan sulphate. Biochem J. 1974;141:517–26.
82. Thambyah A, Zhao JY, Bevill SL, Broom ND. Macro-, micro- and ultrastructural investigation of how degeneration influences the response of cartilage to loading. J Mech Behav Biomed Mater. 2012;5:206–15.

83. Kwiecinski JJ, Dorosz SG, Ludwig TE, Abubacker S, Cowman MK, Schmidt TA. The effect of molecular weight on hyaluronan's cartilage boundary lubricating ability – alone and in combination with proteoglycan 4. Osteoarthritis Cartilage. 2011;19:1356–62.
84. Abubacker S, Ham HO, Messersmith PB, Schmidt TA. Cartilage boundary lubricating ability of aldehyde modified proteoglycan 4 (PRG4-CHO). Osteoarthritis Cartilage. 2013;21:186–9.
85. Oloyede A, Gudimetla P, Chen Y, Crawford R. In vitro reversal of the load-bearing properties of lipid-depleted articular cartilage following exposure to phospholipid surfactant solutions. Clin Biomech (Bristol, Avon). 2008;23:1200–8.
86. Chang DP, Guilak F, Jay GD, Zauscher S. Interaction of lubricin with type II collagen surfaces: adsorption, friction, and normal forces. J Biomech. 2014;47:659–66.
87. Ghadially FN, Meachim G, Collins DH. Extracellular lipid in the matrix of human articular cartilage. Ann Rheum Dis. 1965;24:136–46.
88. Stockwell RA. Lipid in the matrix of ageing articular cartilage. Nature. 1965;207:427–8.
89. Rabinowitz JL, Gregg JR, Nixon JE, Schumacher HR. Lipid composition of the tissues of human knee joints. I. Observations in normal joints (articular cartilage, meniscus, ligaments, synovial fluid, synovium, intra-articular fat pad and bone marrow). Clin Orthop Relat Res. 1979;(143):260–5.
90. Schmidt TA, Gastelum NS, Nguyen QT, Schumacher BL, Sah RL. Boundary lubrication of articular cartilage: role of synovial fluid constituents. Arthritis Rheum. 2007;56:882–91.
91. Sivan S, Schroeder A, Verberne G, Merkher Y, Diminsky D, Priev A, Maroudas A, Halperin G, Nitzan D, Etsion I, Barenholz Y. Liposomes act as effective biolubricants for friction reduction in human synovial joints. Langmuir. 2010;26: 1107–16.
92. Mitrovic DR, Uzan M, Quintero M, Ryckewaert A. Lipid peroxides in human articular cartilage. Rheumatol Int. 1984;5:33–7.
93. Tiku ML, Shah R, Allison GT. Evidence linking chondrocyte lipid peroxidation to cartilage matrix protein degradation. Possible role in cartilage aging and the pathogenesis of osteoarthritis. J Biol Chem. 2000;275:20069–76.
94. Van Der Korst JK, Sokoloff L, Miller EJ. Senescent pigmentation of cartilage and degenerative joint disease. Arch Pathol. 1968;86:40–7.
95. Tsukahara Y, Nasu T. Ceroid-like pigment in age changes of human cartilage. Acta Pathol Jpn. 1974;24:357–69.
96. Van Der Korst JK, Willekens FL, Lansink AG, Henrichs AM. Age-associated glycopeptide pigment in human costal cartilage. Am J Pathol. 1977;89:605–19.
97. Rahmati M, Nalesso G, Mobasheri A, Mozafari M. Aging and osteoarthritis: central role of the extracellular matrix. Ageing Res Rev. 2017;40:20–30.
98. De Campos VB, Vilarta R. Articular cartilage: collagen II-proteoglycans interactions. Availability of reactive groups. Variation in birefringence and differences as compared to collagen I. Acta Histochem. 1988;83:189–205.
99. Panula HE, Hyttinen MM, Arokoski JPA, Langsjo TK, Pelttari A, Kiviranta I, Helminen HJ. Articular cartilage superficial zone collagen birefringence reduced and cartilage thickness increased before surface fibrillation in experimental osteoarthritis. Ann Rheum Dis. 1998;57:237–45.
100. Verzijl N, DeGroot J, Oldehinkel E, Bank RA, Thorpe SR, Baynes JW, Bayliss MT, Bijlsma JW, Lafeber FP, Tekoppele JM. Age-related accumulation of Maillard reaction products in human articular cartilage collagen. Biochem J. 2000;350(Pt 2):381–7.
101. Monnier VM. Nonenzymatic glycosylation, the Maillard reaction and the aging process. J Gerontol. 1990;45:B105–11.
102. Graham L. A comprehensive survey of the acid-stable fluorescent cross-links formed by ribose with basic amino acids, and partial characterization of a novel Maillard cross-link. Biochim Biophys Acta. 1996;1297:9–16.
103. Pokharna HK, Pottenger LA. Nonenzymatic glycation of cartilage proteoglycans: an in vivo and in vitro study. Glycoconj J. 1997;14:917–23.
104. Uchiyama A, Ohishi T, Takahashi M, Kushida K, Inoue T, Fujie M, Horiuchi K. Fluorophores from aging human articular cartilage. J Biochem. 1991;110:714–8.
105. Sell DR, Monnier VM. End-stage renal disease and diabetes catalyze the formation of a pentose-derived crosslink from aging human collagen. J Clin Invest. 1990;85:380–4.
106. Bank RA, Bayliss MT, Lafeber FP, Maroudas A, Tekoppele JM. Ageing and zonal variation in post-translational modification of collagen in normal human articular cartilage. The age-related increase in non-enzymatic glycation affects biomechanical properties of cartilage. Biochem J. 1998;330(Pt 1):345–51.
107. Mow VC. In: Mow VC, Hayes WC, editors. Basic orthopedic biomechanics. 2nd ed. Philadelphia: Lippincott - Raven Press; 1997. p. 113–514.
108. Chen AC, Temple MM, Ng DM, Verzijl N, DeGroot J, TeKoppele JM, Sah RL. Induction of advanced glycation end products and alterations of the tensile properties of articular cartilage. Arthritis Rheum. 2002;46:3212–7.
109. Fick JM, Huttu MR, Lammi MJ, Korhonen RK. In vitro glycation of articular cartilage alters the biomechanical response of chondrocytes in a depth-dependent manner. Osteoarthritis Cartilage. 2014;22:1410–8.
110. DeGroot J, Verzijl N, Bank RA, Lafeber FP, Bijlsma JW, Tekoppele JM. Age-related decrease in proteoglycan synthesis of human articular chondrocytes: the role of nonenzymatic glycation. Arthritis Rheum. 1999;42:1003–9.
111. Hirose J, Yamabe S, Takada K, Okamoto N, Nagai R, Mizuta H. Immunohistochemical distribution of advanced glycation end products (AGEs) in

human osteoarthritic cartilage. Acta Histochem. 2011;113:613–8.

112. Sessa L, Gatti E, Zeni F, Antonelli A, Catucci A, Koch M, Pompilio G, Fritz G, Raucci A, Bianchi ME. The receptor for advanced glycation end-products (RAGE) is only present in mammals, and belongs to a family of cell adhesion molecules (CAMs). PLoS One. 2014;9:e86903.
113. Dejica VM, Mort JS, Laverty S, Antoniou J, Zukor DJ, Tanzer M, Poole AR. Increased type II collagen cleavage by cathepsin K and collagenase activities with aging and osteoarthritis in human articular cartilage. Arthritis Res Ther. 2012;14:R113.
114. Silver FH, Glasgold AI. Cartilage wound healing. An overview. Otolaryngol Clin N Am. 1995;28(5):847–64.
115. Gomoll AH, Minas T. The quality of healing: articular cartilage. Wound Repair Regen. 2014;22(Suppl 1): 30–8.
116. Grynpas MD, Eyre DR, Kirschner DA. Collagen type II differs from type I in native molecular packing. Biochim Biophys Acta. 1980;626:346–55.
117. Chaminade F, Stanescu V, Stanescu R, Maroteaux P, Peyron JG. Noncollagenous proteins in cartilage of normal subjects and patients with degenerative joint disease. A gel electrophoretic study. Arthritis Rheum. 1982;25:1078–83.
118. Roughley PJ. Articular cartilage and changes in arthritis: noncollagenous proteins and proteoglycans in the extracellular matrix of cartilage. Arthritis Res. 2001;3:342–7.
119. Eisenstein R, Kuettner KE, Neapolitan C, Soble LW, Sorgente N. The resistance of certain tissues to invasion. III. Cartilage extracts inhibit the growth of fibroblasts and endothelial cells in culture. Am J Pathol. 1975;81:337–48.
120. Stanescu V, Do TP, Chaminade F, Maroteaux P, Stanescu R. Non-collagenous protein screening in the human chondrodysplasias: link proteins, cartilage oligomeric matrix protein (COMP), and fibromodulin. Am J Med Genet. 1994;51:22–8.
121. Neame PJ, Tapp H, Azizan A. Noncollagenous, non-proteoglycan macromolecules of cartilage. Cell Mol Life Sci. 1999;55:1327–40.
122. Bywaters EG, Dorling J. Amyloid deposits in articular cartilage. Ann Rheum Dis. 1970;29:294–306.
123. Mohr W, Kuhn C, Linke RP, Wessinghage D. Deposition of amyloid of unknown origin in articular cartilage. Virchows Arch B Cell Pathol Incl Mol Pathol. 1991;60(4):259–62.
124. Athanasou NA, West L, Sallie B, Puddle B. Localized amyloid deposition in cartilage is glycosaminoglycans-associated. Histopathology. 1995;26:267–72.
125. Ladefoged C. Amyloid in osteoarthritic hip joints. A pathoanatomical and histological investigation of femoral head cartilage. Acta Orthop Scand. 1982;53:581–6.
126. Ladefoged C, Christensen HE, Sorensen KH. Amyloid in osteoarthritic hip joints. Depositions in cartilage and capsule. Semiquantitative aspects. Acta Orthop Scand. 1982;53:587–90.
127. Westermark P, Benson MD, Buxbaum JN, Cohen AS, Frangione B, Ikeda S, Masters CL, Merlini G, Saraiva MJ, Sipe JD. A primer of amyloid nomenclature. Amyloid. 2007;14:179–83.
128. Maroudas AI. Balance between swelling pressure and collagen tension in normal and degenerate cartilage. Nature. 1976;260:808–9.
129. Stockwell RA, Barnett CH. Changes in permeability of articular cartilage with age. Nature. 1964;201:835–6.
130. Kyriazis AP, Tsaltas TT. Studies in permeability of articular cartilage in New Zealand albino rabbits. The effect of aging, papain, and certain steroid hormones. Am J Pathol. 1971;62:75–85.
131. Duan W, Wei L, Zhang J, Hao Y, Li C, Li H, Li Q, Zhang Q, Chen W, Wei X. Alteration of viscoelastic properties is associated with a change in cytoskeleton components of ageing chondrocytes from rabbit knee articular cartilage. Mol Cell Biomech. 2011;8:253–74.
132. Steklov N, Srivastava A, Sung KL, Chen PC, Lotz MK, D'Lima DD. Aging-related differences in chondrocyte viscoelastic properties. Mol Cell Biomech. 2009;6:113–9.
133. Szarko M, Xia Y. Direct visualisation of the depth dependent mechanical properties of full-thickness articular cartilage. Open J Orthop. 2012; doi. 10.4236/ojo.2012.22007.
134. Chen C, Tambe DT, Deng L, Yang L. Biomechanical properties and mechanobiology of the articular chondrocyte. Am J Physiol Cell Physiol. 2013;305:C1202–8.
135. Peters AE, Akhtar R, Comerford EJ, Bates KT. The effect of ageing and osteoarthritis on the mechanical properties of cartilage and bone in the human knee joint. Sci Rep. 2018;8(1):5931.
136. Goldring MB, Goldring SR. Osteoarthritis. J Cell Physiol. 2007;213:626–34.
137. Houard X, Goldring MB, Berenbaum F. Homeostatic mechanisms in articular cartilage and role of inflammation in osteoarthritis. Curr Rheumatol Rep. 2013;15:375.
138. Loeser RF, Gandhi U, Long DL, Yin W, Chubinskaya S. Aging and oxidative stress reduce the response of human articular chondrocytes to insulin-like growth factor-1 and osteogenic protein-1. Arthritis Rheum. 2014;66:2201–9.
139. van Caam A, Madej W, Thijssen E, Garcia de Vinuesa A, van den Berg W, Goumans MJ, Ten Dijke P, Blaney Davidson E, van der Kraan PM. Expression of TGFβ-family signalling components in ageing cartilage: age-related loss of TGFβ and BMP receptors. Osteoarthritis Cartilage. 2016;24:1235–45.
140. Shimada H, Sakakima H, Tsuchimochi K, Matsuda F, Komiya S, Goldring MB, Ijiri K. Senescence of chondrocytes in aging articular cartilage: GADD45β mediates p21 expression in association with C/EBPβ in senescence-accelerated mice. Pathol Res Pract. 2011;207:225–31.
141. Matsuzaki T, Alvarez-Garcia O, Mokuda S, Nagira K, Olmer M, Gamini R, Miyata K, Akasaki

Y, Su AI, Asahara H, Lotz MK. FoxO transcription factors modulate autophagy and proteoglycan 4 in cartilage homeostasis and osteoarthritis. Sci Transl Med. 2018;10(428):pii eaan0746. doi 10.1126/scitranslmed,aan0746.
142. Akasaki Y, Alvarez-Garcia O, Saito M, Caramés B, Iwamoto Y, Lotz MK. FoxO transcription factors support oxidative stress resistance in human chondrocytes. Arthritis Rheum. 2014;66(12):3349–58.
143. Akasaki Y, Hasegawa A, Saito M, Asahara H, Iwamoto Y, Lotz MK, Dysregulated FOXO. Transcription factors in articular cartilage in aging and osteoarthritis. Osteoarthritis Cartilage. 2014;22:162–70.
144. Breu A, Sprinzing B, Merkl K, Bechmann V, Kujat R, Jenei-Lanzl Z, Prantl L, Angele P. Estrogen reduces cellular aging in human mesenchymal stem cells and chondrocytes. J Orthop Res. 2011;29:1563–71.
145. Yudoh K, Karasawa R. Statin prevents chondrocyte aging and degeneration of articular cartilage in osteoarthritis (OA). Aging (Albany NY). 2010;2:990–8.
146. Henrotin Y, Deby-Dupont G, Deby C, Franchimont P, Emerit I. Active oxygen species, articular inflammation and cartilage damage. EXS. 1992;62:308–22.
147. Schiller J, Fuchs B, Arnhold J, Arnold K. Contribution of reactive oxygen species to cartilage degradation in rheumatic diseases: molecular pathways, diagnosis and potential therapeutic strategies. Curr Med Chem. 2003;10:2123–45.
148. Henrotin YE, Bruckner P, Pujol JP. The role of reactive oxygen species in homeostasis and degradation of cartilage. Osteoarthritis Cartilage. 2003;11:747–55.
149. Tomiyama T, Fukuda K, Yamazaki K, Hashimoto K, Ueda H, Mori S, Hamanishi C. Cyclic compression loaded on cartilage explants enhances the production of reactive oxygen species. J Rheumatol. 2007;34:556–62.
150. Anderson DD, Brown TD, Radin EL. The influence of basal cartilage calcification on dynamic juxtaarticular stress transmission. Clin Orthop Relat Res. 1993;(268):298–307.
151. Kelly PA, O'Connor JJ. Transmission of rapidly applied loads through articular cartilage. Part 1: uncracked cartilage. Proc Insts Mech Eng H. 1996;210:27–37.
152. Kelly PA, O'Connor JJ. Transmission of rapidly applied loads through articular cartilage. Part 2: cracked cartilage. Proc Insts Mech Eng H. 1996;210:39–49.
153. Nguyen Q, Murphy G, Hughes CE, Mort JS, Roughley PJ. Matrix metalloproteinases cleave at two distinct sites on human cartilage link protein. Biochem J. 1993;295(Pt 2):595–8.
154. Roughley PJ, Nguyen Q, Mort JS, Hughes CE, Caterson B. Proteolytic degradation in human articular cartilage: its relationship to stromelysin. Agents Actions Suppl. 1993;39:149–59.
155. Aquaron R. Alkaptonuria: a very rare metabolic disorder. Indian J Biochem Biophys. 2013;50:339–44.
156. Grosicka A, Kucharz EJ. Alkaptonuria. Wiad Lek. 2009;62:197–203.
157. Introne WJ, Gahl WA. In: Pagon RA, Adam MP, Ardinger HH, Wallace SE, Amemiya A, LJH B, Bird TD, Fong CT, Mefford HC, RJH S, Stephens K, editors. Alkaptonuria. Seattle (WA): University of Washington, Seattle; 1993.
158. Pritzker K. Articular pathology of gout, calcium pyrophosphate dihydrate, and basic calcium phosphate crystal deposition arthropathies. In: Terkeltaub R, editor. Gout and other crystal arthropathies. Philadelphia: Elsevier, Saunders; 2012. p. 1–19.
159. Pritzker KP. Calcium pyrophosphate crystal arthropathy: a biomineralization disorder. Hum Pathol. 1986;17:543–5.
160. Ryan LM. Calcium pyrophosphate dihydrate crystal deposition and other crystal deposition diseases. Curr Opin Rheumatol. 1993;5:517–21.
161. Pritzker KP. Crystal deposition in joints: prevalence and relevance for arthritis. J Rheumatol. 2008;35:958–9.
162. Rosenthal AK, McCarty BA, Cheung HS, Ryan LM. A comparison of the effect of transforming growth factor beta 1 on pyrophosphate elaboration from various articular tissues. Arthritis Rheum. 1993;36:539–42.
163. Pritzker KPH, Luk SC. Apatite associated arthropathies: preliminary ultrastructural studies. Scan Electron Microsc. 1976;493–500.
164. Molloy ES, McCarthy GM. Hydroxyapatite deposition disease of the joint. Curr Rheumatol Rep. 2003;5:215–21.
165. Hogan DB, Pritzker KP. Synovial fluid analysis – another look at the mucin clot test. J Rheumatol. 1985;12:242–4.
166. Shinozaki T, Xu Y, Cruz TF, Pritzker KPH. Calcium pyrophosphate dihydrate (CPPD) crystal dissolution by alkaline phosphatase: interaction of alkaline phosphatase on CPPD crystals. J Rheumatol. 1995;22:117–23.
167. So PP, Tsui FW, Vieth R, Tupy JH, Pritzker KP. Inhibition of alkaline phosphatase by cysteine: implications for calcium pyrophosphate dihydrate crystal deposition disease. J Rheumatol. 2007;34:1313–22.
168. Kannampuzha JV, Tupy JH, Pritzker KP. Mercaptopyruvate inhibits tissue-nonspecific alkaline phosphatase and calcium pyrophosphate dihydrate crystal dissolution. J Rheumatol. 2009;36:2758–65.
169. Myasoedova E, Crowson CS, Kremers HM, Therneau TM, Gabriel SE. Is the incidence of rheumatoid arthritis rising? Results from Olmsted County, Minnesota, 1955–2007. Arthritis Rheum. 2010;62:1576–82.
170. Conigliaro P, Chimenti MS, Triggianese P, Sunzini F, Novelli L, Perricone C, Perricone R. Autoantibodies in inflammatory arthritis. Autoimmun Rev. 2016;15:673–83.
171. Harris ED Jr. Rheumatoid arthritis. Pathophysiology and implications for therapy. N Engl J Med. 1990;322:1277–89.

172. Zhou RP, Dai BB, Xie YY, Wu XS, Wang ZS, Li Y, Wang ZQ, Zu SQ, Ge JF, Chen FH. Interleukin-1β and tumor necrosis factor-α augment acidosis-induced rat articular chondrocyte apoptosis via nuclear factor-kappaB-dependent upregulation of ASIC1a channel. Biochim Biophys Acta. 2018;1864(1):162–77.
173. Abramson SB, Amin A. Blocking the effects of IL-1 in rheumatoid arthritis protects bone and cartilage. Rheumatology (Oxford). 2002;41(9):972–80.
174. Malemud CJ. Matrix metalloproteinases and synovial joint pathology. Prog Mol Biol Transl Sci. 2017;148:305–25.
175. Caglič D, Repnik U, Jedeszko C, Kosec G, Miniejew C, Kindermann M, Vasiljeva O, Turk V, Wendt KU, Sloane BF, Goldring MB, Turk B. The proinflammatory cytokines interleukin-1α and tumor necrosis factor α promote the expression and secretion of proteolytically active cathepsin S from human chondrocytes. Biol Chem. 2013;394(2):307–16.
176. Hollander AP, Atkinst RM, Eastwoodt DM, et al. Human cartilage is degraded by rheumatoid arthritis synovial fluid but not by recombinant cytokines in vitro. Clin Exp Immunol. 1991;83:52–7.
177. Ostrowska M, Maśliński W, Prochorec-Sobieszek M, Nieciecki M, Sudoł-Szopińska I. Cartilage and bone damage in rheumatoid arthritis. Reumatologia. 2018;56(2):111–20.
178. Sudoł-Szopińska I, Kontny E, Zaniewicz-Kaniewska K, et al. Role of inflammatory factors and adipose tissue in pathogenesis of rheumatoid arthritis and osteoarthritis. Part I: Rheumatoid adipose tissue. J Ultrason. 2013;13:192–201.
179. Sudoł-Szopińska I, Kontny E, Maśliński W, et al. The pathogenesis of rheumatoid arthritis in radiological studies. Part I: formation of inflammatory infiltrates within the synovial membrane. J Ultrason. 2012;12:202–13.
180. Kontny E, Plebanczyk M, Lisowska B, Olszewska M, Maldyk P, Maslinski W. Comparison of rheumatoid articular adipose and synovial tissue reactivity to proinflammatory stimuli: contribution to adipocytokine network. Ann Rheum Dis. 2012;71(2):262–7.
181. Pritzker KHP. Pathology of osteoarthritis. In: Brandt KD, Doherty M, Lohmander LS, Edition 2nd, editors. Osteoarthritis. Oxford: Oxford University Press; 2003. p. 49–58.
182. Buckwalter JA, Mankin HJ. Articular cartilage: degeneration and osteoarthritis, repair, regeneration, and transplantation. Instr Course Lect. 1998;47:487–504.
183. Buckwalter JA, Mankin HJ, Grodzinsky AJ. Articular cartilage and osteoarthritis. Instr Course Lect. 2005;54:465–80.
184. Lawrence RC, Helmick CG, Arnett FC, Deyo RA, Felson DT, Giannini EH, Heyse SP, Hirsch R, Hochberg MC, Hunder GG, Liang MH, Pillemer SR, Steen VD, Wolfe F. Estimates of the prevalence of arthritis and selected musculoskeletal disorders in the United States. Arthritis Rheum. 1998;41:778–99.
185. Jeon OH, David N, Campisi J, Elisseeff JH. Senescent cells and osteoarthritis: a painful connection. J Clin Invest. 2018;128(4):1229–37.
186. Bierma-Zeinstra SM, van Middelkoop M. Osteoarthritis: in search of phenotypes. Nat Rev Rheumatol. 2017;13:705–6.
187. Deveza LA, Melo L, Yamato TP, Mills K, Ravi V, Hunter DJ. Knee osteoarthritis phenotypes and their relevance for outcomes: a systematic review. Osteoarthritis Cartilage. 2017;25(12):1926–41.
188. Budd E, Nalesso G, Mobasheri A. Extracellular genomic biomarkers of osteoarthritis. Expert Rev Mol Diagn. 2018:18(1):55–74.
189. Nuki G. Osteoarthritis: a problem of joint failure. Z Rheumatol. 1999;58(3):142–7.
190. Varady NH, Grodzinsky AJ. Osteoarthritis year in review 2015: mechanics. Osteoarthritis Cartilage. 2016;24:27–35.
191. Christensen R, Henriksen M, Leeds AR, Gudbergsen H, Christensen P, Sorensen TJ, Bartels EM, Riecke BF, Aaboe J, Frederiksen R, Boesen M, Lohmander LS, Astrup A, Bliddal H. Effect of weight maintenance on symptoms of knee osteoarthritis in obese patients: a twelve-month randomized controlled trial. Arthritis Care Res. 2015;67:640–50.
192. Lee R, Kean WF. Obesity and knee osteoarthritis. Inflammopharmacology. 2012;20:53–8.
193. Jiménez G, Cobo-Molinos J, Antich C, López-Ruiz E. Osteoarthritis: Trauma vs Disease. Adv Exp Med Biol. 2018;1059:63–83.
194. Andriacchi TP, Favre J. The nature of in vivo mechanical signals that influence cartilage health and progression to knee osteoarthritis. Curr Rheumatol Rep. 2014;16:463.
195. Pritzker KP, Gay S, Jimenez SA, Ostergaard K, Pelletier JP, Revell PA, Salter D, van den Berg WB. Osteoarthritis cartilage histopathology: grading and staging. Osteoarthritis Cartilage. 2006;14:13–29.
196. Setton LA, Mow VC, Muller FJ, Pita JC, Howell DS. Altered structure-function relationships for articular cartilage in human osteoarthritis and an experimental canine model. Agents Actions Suppl. 1993;39:27–48.
197. Lohmander LS, Felson DT. Defining the role of molecular markers to monitor disease, intervention, and cartilage breakdown in osteoarthritis. J Rheumatol. 1997;24:782–5.
198. Altman R, Asch E, Bloch D, Bole G, Borenstein D, Brandt K, Christy W, Cooke TD, Greenwald R, Hochberg M, et al. Development of criteria for the classification and reporting of osteoarthritis. Classification of osteoarthritis of the knee. Diagnostic and Therapeutic Criteria Committee of the American Rheumatism Association. Arthritis Rheum. 1986;29:1039–49.
199. Oegema TR Jr, Carpenter RJ, Hofmeister F, Thompson RC Jr. The interaction of the zone of calcified cartilage and subchondral bone in osteoarthritis. Microsc Res Tech. 1997;37:324–32.
200. Vinatier C, Domínguez E, Guicheux J, Caramés B. Role of the inflammation-autophagy-senescence

integrative network in osteoarthritis. Front Physiol. 2018;9:706.
201. Dieppe PA. Recommended methodology for assessing the progression of osteoarthritis of the hip and knee joints. Osteoarthritis Cartilage. 1995;3:73–7.
202. Mankin HJ, Thrasher AZ. Water content and binding in normal and osteoarthritic human cartilage. J Bone Joint Surg Am. 1975;57:76–80.
203. Venn M, Maroudas A. Chemical composition and swelling of normal and osteoarthrotic femoral head cartilage. I. Chemical composition. Ann Rheum Dis. 1977;36:121–9.
204. Maroudas A, Ziv I, Weisman N, Venn M. Studies of hydration and swelling pressure in normal and osteoarthritic cartilage. Biorheology. 1985;22:159–69.
205. Lothe K, Spycher MA, Ruttner JR. Focal lacunar resorption in the articular cartilage of femoral heads. J Bone Joint Surg. 1985;67:543–7.
206. Hashimoto S, Ochs RL, Komiya S, Lotz M. Linkage of chondrocyte apoptosis and cartilage degradation in human osteoarthritis. Arthritis Rheum. 1998;41:1632–8.
207. Mankin HJ, Dorfman H, Lippiello L, Zarins A. Biochemical and metabolic abnormalities in articular cartilage from osteo-arthritic human hips. II. Correlation of morphology with biochemical and metabolic data. J Bone Joint Surg Am. 1971;53:523–37.
208. Mankin HJ, Lippiello L. Biochemical and metabolic abnormalities in articular cartilage from osteo-arthritic human hips. J Bone Joint Surg Am. 1970;52:424–34.
209. Lee GM, Paul TA, Slabaugh M, Kelley SS. The incidence of enlarged chondrons in normal and osteoarthritic human cartilage and their relative matrix density. Osteoarthritis Cartilage. 2000;8:44–52.
210. Lotz MK, Otsuki S, Grogan SP, Sah R, Terkeltaub R, D'Lima D. Cartilage cell clusters. Arthritis Rheum. 2010;62:2206–18.
211. Tetlow LC, Adlam DJ, Woolley DE. Matrix metalloproteinase and proinflammatory cytokine production by chondrocytes of human osteoarthritic cartilage: associations with degenerative changes. Arthritis Rheum. 2001;44:585–94.
212. Sanchez C, Lambert C, Dubuc JE, Bertrand J, Pap T, et al. Syndecan-4 is increased in osteoarthritic knee, but not hip or shoulder, articular hypertrophic chondrocytes. Cartilage. 2019:1947603519870855. doi: 10.1177/1947603519870855. [Epub ahead of print]
213. Singh P, Marcu KB, Goldring MB, Otero M. Phenotypic instability of chondrocytes in osteoarthritis: on a path to hypertrophy. Ann N Y Acad Sci. 2019;1442(1):17–34.
214. Gratal P, Mediero A, Sánchez-Pernaute O, Prieto-Potin I, Lamuedra A, et al. Chondrocyte enlargement is a marker of osteoarthritis severity. Osteoarthritis Cartilage. 2019;27(8):1229–34.
215. Setton LA, Elliott DM, Mow VC. Altered mechanics of cartilage with osteoarthritis: human osteoarthritis and an experimental model of joint degeneration. Osteoarthritis Cartilage. 1999;7:2–14.
216. Maroudas A, Evans H, Almeida L. Cartilage of the hip joint. Topographical variation of glycosaminoglycan content in normal and fibrillated tissue. Ann Rheum Dis. 1973;32:1–9.
217. Cs-Szabo G, Melching LI, Roughley PJ, Glant TT. Changes in messenger RNA and protein levels of proteoglycans and link protein in human osteoarthritic cartilage samples. Arthritis Rheum. 1997;40:1037–45.
218. Barreto G, Soininen A, Ylinen P, Sandelin J, Konttinen YT, Nordstrom DC, Eklund KK. Soluble biglycan: a potential mediator of cartilage degradation in osteoarthritis. Arthritis Res Ther. 2015;17:379.
219. Mort JS, Geng Y, Fisher WD, Roughley PJ. Aggrecan heterogeneity in articular cartilage from patients with osteoarthritis. BMC Musculoskelet Disord. 2016;17:89.
220. Mollenhauer J, Mok MT, King KB, Gupta M, Chubinskaya S, Koepp H, Cole AA. Expression of anchorin CII (cartilage annexin V) in human young, normal adult, and osteoarthritic cartilage. J Histochem Cytochem. 1999;47:209–20.
221. Chevalier X, Groult N, Larget-Piet B, Zardi L, Hornebeck W. Tenascin distribution in articular cartilage from normal subjects and from patients with osteoarthritis and rheumatoid arthritis. Arthritis Rheum. 1994;37:1013–22.
222. Salter DM. Tenascin is increased in cartilage and synovium from arthritic knees. Br J Rheumatol. 1993;32:780–6.
223. Chen JR, Takahashi M, Suzuki M, Kushida K, Miyamoto S, Inoue T. Pentosidine in synovial fluid in osteoarthritis and rheumatoid arthritis: relationship with disease activity in rheumatoid arthritis. J Rheumatol. 1998;25:2440–4.
224. Senolt L, Braun M, Olejarova M, Forejtova S, Gatterova J, Pavelka K. Increased pentosidine, an advanced glycation end product, in serum and synovial fluid from patients with knee osteoarthritis and its relation with cartilage oligomeric matrix protein. Ann Rheum Dis. 2005;64:886–90.
225. Willett TL, Kandel R, De Croos JN, Avery NC, Grynpas MD. Enhanced levels of non-enzymatic glycation and pentosidine crosslinking in spontaneous osteoarthritis progression. Osteoarthritis Cartilage. 2012;20:736–44.
226. Lane JM, Weiss C. Review of articular cartilage collagen research. Arthritis Rheum. 1975;18:553–62.
227. Pullig O, Weseloh G, Swoboda B. Expression of type VI collagen in normal and osteoarthritic human cartilage. Osteoarthritis Cartilage. 1999;7:191–202.
228. Girkontaite I, Frischholz S, Lammi P, Wagner K, Swoboda B, Aigner T. Von der Mark K. Immunolocalization of type X collagen in normal fetal and adult osteoarthritic cartilage with monoclonal antibodies. Matrix Biol. 1996;15:231–8.
229. Aigner T, Bertling W, Stoss H, Weseloh G, von der Mark K. Independent expression of fibril-forming collagens I, II, and III in chondrocytes

of human osteoarthritic cartilage. J Clin Invest. 1993;91:829–37.
230. Aigner T, Reichenberger E, Bertling W, Kirsch T, Stoss H, von der Mark K. Type X collagen expression in osteoarthritic and rheumatoid articular cartilage. Virchows Arch B Cell Pathol Incl Mol Pathol. 1993;63(4):205–11.
231. Weiss C. Ultrastructural characteristics of osteoarthritis. Fed Proc. 1973;32(4):1459–66.
232. Studer D, Chiquet M, Hunziker EB. Evidence for a distinct water-rich layer surrounding collagen fibrils in articular cartilage extracellular matrix. J Struct Biol. 1996;117:81–5.
233. Homandberg GA, Wen C, Hui F. Cartilage damaging activities of fibronectin fragments derived from cartilage and synovial fluid. Osteoarthritis Cartilage. 1998;6:231–44.
234. Jones KL, Brown M, Ali SY, Brown RA. An immunohistochemical study of fibronectin in human osteoarthritic and disease free articular cartilage. Ann Rheum Dis. 1987;46:809–15.
235. Chevalier X. Fibronectin, cartilage, and osteoarthritis. Semin Arthritis Rheum. 1993;22:307–18.
236. Swoboda B, Pullig O, Kladny B, Pfander D, Weseloh G. Collagen type VI content in healthy and arthritis knee joint cartilage. Zeitschrift fur Orthopadie und ihre Grenzgeb. 1999;137:540–4.
237. von der Mark K, Frischholz S, Aigner T, Beier F, Belke J, Erdmann S, Burkhardt H. Upregulation of type X collagen expression in osteoarthritic cartilage. Acta Orthop Scand Suppl. 1995;266:125–9.
238. Khoshgoftar M, Torzilli PA, Maher SA. Influence of the pericellular and extracellular matrix structural properties on chondrocyte mechanics. J Orthop Res. 2018;36(2):721–29.
239. Henao-Murillo L, Ito K, van Donkelaar CC. Collagen damage location in articular cartilage differs if damage is caused by excessive loading magnitude or rate. Ann Biomed Eng. 2018;46(4):605–15.
240. Imhof H, Breitenseher M, Kainberger F, Trattnig S. Degenerative joint disease: cartilage or vascular disease? Skelet Radiol. 1997;26:398–403.
241. Trickey WR, Lee GM, Guilak F. Viscoelastic properties of chondrocytes from normal and osteoarthritic human cartilage. J Orthop Res. 2000;18:891–8.
242. Trickey WR, Vail TP, Guilak F. The role of the cytoskeleton in the viscoelastic properties of human articular chondrocytes. J Orthop Res. 2004;22:131–9.
243. Lai Y, Yu XP, Zhang Y, Tian Q, Song H, Mucignat MT, Perris R, Samuels J, Krasnokutsky S, Attur M, Greenberg JD, Abramson SB, Di Cesare PE, Liu CJ. Enhanced COMP catabolism detected in serum of patients with arthritis and animal disease models through a novel capture ELISA. Osteoarthritis Cartilage. 2012;20:854–62.
244. Verma P, Dalal K. Serum cartilage oligomeric matrix protein (COMP) in knee osteoarthritis: a novel diagnostic and prognostic biomarker. J Orthop Res. 2013;31:999–1006.
245. Song SY, Han YD, Hong SY, Kim K, Yang SS, Min BH, Yoon HC. Chip-based cartilage oligomeric matrix protein detection in serum and synovial fluid for osteoarthritis diagnosis. Anal Biochem. 2012;420:139–46.
246. El-Arman MM, El-Fayoumi G, El-Shal E, El-Boghdady I, El-Ghaweet A. Aggrecan and cartilage oligomeric matrix protein in serum and synovial fluid of patients with knee osteoarthritis. HSS J. 2010;6(2):171–6.
247. Clark AG, Jordan JM, Vilim V, Renner JB, Dragomir AD, Luta G, Kraus VB. Serum cartilage oligomeric matrix protein reflects osteoarthritis presence and severity: the Johnston County Osteoarthritis Project. Arthritis Rheum. 1999;42:2356–64.
248. Hosnijeh FS, Runhaar J, van Meurs JB, Bierma-Zeinstra SM. Biomarkers for osteoarthritis: can they be used for risk assessment? A systematic review. Maturitas. 2015;82:36–49.
249. Neidhart M, Hauser N, Paulsson M, DiCesare PE, Michel BA, Hauselmann HJ. Small fragments of cartilage oligomeric matrix protein in synovial fluid and serum as markers for cartilage degradation. Br J Rheumatol. 1997;36:1151–60.
250. Chateauvert JMD, Grynpas MD, Kessler MJ, Pritzker KPH. Spontaneous osteoarthritis in rhesus macaques. II. Characterization of disease and morphometric studies. J Rheumatol. 1990;17:73–83.
251. Felson DT, Zhang Y, Hannan MT, Naimark A, Weissman BN, Aliabadi P, Levy D. The incidence and natural history of knee osteoarthritis in the elderly. Arthritis Rheum. 1995;38:1500–5.
252. Veronese N, Maggi S, Trevisan C, Noale M, De Rui M, Bolzetta F, Zambon S, Musacchio E, Sartori L, Perissinotto E, Stubbs B, Crepaldi G, Manzato E, Sergi G. Pain increases the risk of developing frailty in older adults with osteoarthritis. Pain Med. 2017;18:414–27.
253. Loeser RF. The effects of aging on the development of osteoarthritis. HSS J. 2012;8:18–9.
254. Varela-Eirin M, Loureiro J, Fonseca E, Corrochano S, Caeiro JR, et al. Cartilage regeneration and ageing: targeting cellular plasticity in osteoarthritis. Ageing Res Rev. 2018;42:56–71.
255. Sokoloff L. Osteoarthritis and aging. In: Sokoloff L, editor. Biology of degenerative joint disease. Chicago: University of Chicago Press, Chicago; 1969. p. 24–7.
256. Mitrovic D, Quintero M, Stankovic A, Ryckewaert A. Cell density of adult human femoral condylar articular cartilage. Joints with normal and fibrillated surfaces. Lab Investig. 1983;49:309–16.
257. Lane LB, Villacin A, Bullough PG. The vascularity and remodelling of subchondrial bone and calcified cartilage in adult human femoral and humeral heads. An age- and stress-related phenomenon. J Bone Joint Surg Br. 1977;59:272–8.
258. Venn MF. Variation of chemical composition with age in human femoral head cartilage. Ann Rheum Dis. 1978;37:168–74.

Articular Cartilage Metabolism: Biochemical Markers and Dynamic Loading

4

Harpal K. Gahunia and Kenneth P. H. Pritzker

4.1 Introduction

Articular cartilage structure is designed to resist compression and redistribute load to the joints over the course of a lifetime. Injury and disease processes involving damage to the knee articular cartilage are reflected directly in acute and chronic changes of cartilage biomechanical function and indirectly in body fluids as biochemical markers. Nonetheless, prognostic biochemical markers are sought to better address prospective pharmacologic and surgical therapies. Many surrogate biomarkers of cartilage metabolism have been evaluated and some markers show promise, but the underlying difficulty has been to relate the short-term changes in markers to longer-term changes in cartilage structure and function. Further, the measured synovial fluid (sf) or plasma (p) concentrations of a cartilage-related marker could arise from either a small volume of cartilage of actively degenerating knee or from a larger cartilage volume which is undergoing structural change more slowly.

Chondrocytes are metabolically active cells that play key roles in extracellular matrix (ECM) remodeling in physiological and pathological conditions. Interactions between chondrocytes and the ECM regulate numerous biological processes important to articular cartilage homeostasis and repair. Changes in chondrocyte metabolism can be triggered by injury, aging, genetic predisposition and metabolic disorders. These are often accompanied by altered gene expression, change in ECM macromolecular components, concentration and/or architecture, decreased articular cartilage thickness, proteolysis, presence of advanced glycation products, and ECM calcification [1–6]. Proteolytic-mediated degradation of cartilage may occur through the action of proteinases or free radicals [7, 8]. However, these processes usually occur on a time scale much longer than the biochemical markers observed in blood.

H. K. Gahunia, MSc, PhD (✉)
Orthopaedic Science Consulting Services, Oakville, ON, Canada
e-mail: harpal.gahunia@utoronto.ca

K. P. H. Pritzker, MD, FRCPC
Department of Laboratory Medicine and Pathobiology, Department of Surgery, and Institute of Biomaterials and Biomedical Engineering, University of Toronto, Toronto, ON, Canada

Department of Pathology and Laboratory Medicine, Mount Sinai Hospital, Toronto, ON, Canada

4.2 Regulation of Articular Cartilage Synthesis

Throughout life, articular cartilage undergoes continual internal remodeling while maintaining its architecture and metabolic homeostasis [9]. During growth and development, matrix synthesis outweighs degradation, whereas in adults, matrix

H. K. Gahunia et al. (eds.), *Articular Cartilage of the Knee*,
https://doi.org/10.1007/978-1-4939-7587-7_4

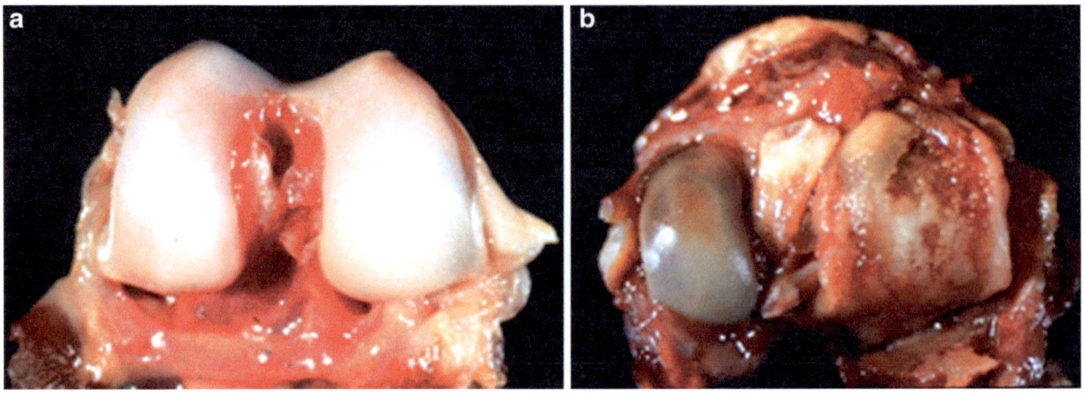

Fig. 4.1 Photomacrographs of the right knee femoral condyles of rhesus macaques. (**a**) Normal articular cartilage of the lateral and medial compartments showing white smooth and glossy articular cartilage surface. (**b**) Osteoarthritic knee shows intact but affected lateral compartment with yellow cartilage; whereas, the medial compartment shows extensive erosion, eburnation and osteophytes

synthesis is decreased and is finely balanced by controlled matrix degradation [10]. However, imbalance in the cartilage homeostasis may induce secretion of the major ECM macromolecular components and release degradative enzymes, such as matrix metalloproteinases (MMPs) including collagenase (MMP-1) and stromelysin (MMP-3). Disruption to the normal balance of synthesis and degradation can alter the intrinsic characteristics and biomechanics of various cartilage zones [1]. This can lead to a gradual degeneration of the ECM that results in the development of clinically recognizable disease(s) [11, 12] (Figs. 4.1a and b).

When articular cartilage is subjected to either an excess of forces (often repetitive) or to biochemical agents, its morphological and functional impairment is associated with a local homeostatic reaction comprising first of chondrocyte proliferation followed by stimulation of proteoglycan (PG) biosynthesis and then collagen formation, either type I or type II, depending on the local ECM environment. This homeostatic reaction was investigated in vitro by using cultures of human chondrocytes [13]. Chondrocyte clusters or clones were formed after 4 days of culture with further proliferation for the first 15 days of culture. This was followed by the release of PGs and collagen type II into the culture medium, which then constituted the ECM of the chondrocyte clusters. In vivo, knee chondral lesions and osteochondral (OC) defects on the articulating surfaces can occur due to homeostatic imbalance as a consequent of traumatic injuries and chronic mechanical overloading or non-loading.

4.3 Biochemical Markers of Articular Cartilage Metabolism in Body Fluids

Biological markers (also referred as biomarkers) are cellular, biochemical or molecular alterations that are measurable in tissues, cells, or body fluids [14]. This definition includes biological characteristics that can be objectively measured and evaluated as an indicator of normal biological processes, pathogenic processes, or pharmacological responses to a therapeutic intervention [15]. In practice, biomarkers include tools and technologies that can aid in understanding the prediction, cause, diagnosis, progression, regression, or outcome of treatment of disease. During normal metabolic processes, cartilage-specific molecules, such as PGs, collagens, and non-collagenous proteins, are continually degraded, releasing fragments of these molecules in the ECM, which then diffuse out of the articular cartilage into the sf. These metabolic products are then carried through the loose connective tissue to the bloodstream. In the circulation, these products are filtered by the kidney either directly or after modification by the liver [16]. These fragments, referred to as *biochemical markers*, produced during cartilage anabolic and catabolic processes, are released into the sf at varying concentrations during both the destructive and repair phases of a pathological process. Since changes can occur in the rate of turnover of the ECM macromolecules during various stages of joint diseases, elevated levels of biochemical markers in the serum can reflect increased synthesis, an increased release due to accelerated tissue catabolism or decreased clearance from serum.

These biological markers are tools for clinical diagnosis and assessing cartilage integrity during injury, aging, and disease [17–27]. Biochemical markers can be used to study growth and development; investigate sports, exercise, or activity-related changes to articular cartilage; detect latent disease; identify disease phenotypes; or monitor pre-existing disease activity and its treatment [28–35]. The most direct measure of knee tissue metabolism is a biochemical assessment of the catabolic or anabolic products of cartilage ECM, synovium, and/or bone found in the body fluids, namely, sf, serum (s), plasma, and/or urine (u) [36–42].

4.3.1 Aggrecan Metabolism Products

Aggrecan has been considered as an excellent marker for articular cartilage damage [39, 43–50]. Biochemical markers in body fluids resulting from articular cartilage aggrecan metabolism are summarized in Table 4.1. The concentration of PG and/or its components in the sf is affected by both disease activity and the stage of disease progression [50, 63, 83]. Using immunochemical and biochemical assays, high concentrations of immunoreactive sulfated glycosaminoglycans (GAGs), keratan sulfate (KS), KS epitope and hyaluronate (also known as hyaluronic acid, HA) as well as aggrecanase and hyaluronidase activities have been reported in the body fluids of patients with post-traumatic knee injury and diseases such as chondromalacia (CM), rheumatoid arthritis (RA), osteoarthritis (OA), pseudogout, gout, and reactive arthritis [19, 51–57, 59–62, 64, 72–77, 84]. Several studies have shown an increase in the cartilage metabolic markers, namely, chondroitin sulfate (C4S and C6S), CS delta disaccharides (Δdi-6S and Δdi-4S), Δdi-6S/Δdi-4S ratio, dermatan sulfate (DS) delta disaccharide (Δdi-DS), and Δdi-HA in the sf of traumatic arthritis, osteonecrosis, RA, and OA patients [63–68]. Aggrecan fragments consisting of alanine-arginine-glycine-serine (ARGS neoepitope) and from the HA binding region (HABR), such as HABR-FVDIPEN (Phe-Val-Asp-Ile-Pro-Glu-Asn) and HABR-FMDIPEN, are released into both articular cartilage and sf by MMP-induced degradation of aggrecan [29, 78–81, 85]. Investigation of the sf concentrations of aggrecan fragments from patients ($N = 385$) with knee injury, OA, or acute calcium pyrophosphate arthritis (also referred as pseudogout) and their relative reactivity with CS 846 epitope (a putative marker of cartilage aggrecan synthesis) showed an increased reactivity of the CS 846 epitope in all the study groups compared with the reference group, with highest reactivity reported in OA patients [45]. Further, upon comparison with other markers of matrix turnover, CS 846 epitope reactivity correlated positively with cartilage oligomeric matrix protein (COMP) and Procollagen II C-Terminal ProPeptide (PIICP). Other studies have also shown an increased reactivity of CS 846 epitope and altered reactivity of CS neoepitopes (3B3-, 3B3+, and 7D4) in patients with knee injury and disease [50, 52–54, 63, 70, 86–88].

4.3.2 Collagen, Crosslinks, and Non-Collagenous Proteins

Several biomarkers identified for assessing articular cartilage turnover are based on the unique metabolism of fibrillar collagens. Biochemical markers derived from collagen fragments of synthesis or breakdown, crosslinks, and non-collagenous protein metabolism are summarized in Table 4.2. Several studies have focused on collagen type II synthesis and degradation to identify biochemical markers to assess the articular carti-

Table 4.1 Knee articular cartilage biochemical markers: aggrecan metabolism detected in body fluid(s) in injury, aging and disease. Body fluids: synovial fluid (sf-), serum (s-), plasma (p-) and urine (u-)

Cartilage Marker (Aggrecan derived)	Marker Reflects	Body Fluid(s)	Marker Level	Reference(s)
Glycosaminoglycans (GAGs)	Proteoglycan metabolism	Synovial fluid; Serum	↑ One-day post injury; ↓ Acute injury (< 2 months); ↑ Chronic injury; ↓ High chondral damage score; ↓ Age; ↑ Gout; ↑ Pseudogout; ↑ Reactive arthritis; ↑ s-RA; ↓ sf-RA; ↓ OA	[17, 51–58]
Keratan Sulfate (KS)	Proteoglycan metabolism	Synovial fluid; Serum	↑ Growth and maturation; ↑ Acute injury (< 2 months); ↓ Chronic injury (high-grade cartilage lesions); ↑ Early (mild) OA; ↑ CM patella	[59–62]
KS Epitope 5D4	Cartilage degradation; KS catabolism	Synovial fluid	↓ Acute injury; ↑ Chronic injury; ↑ Gout; ↑ Pseudogout; ↑ Reactive arthritis; ↓ RA; ↑ Early OA; ↓ Late (severe) OA	[17, 53, 57, 63]
Chondroitin Sulfate (CS) Chondroitin-4-sulfate (C4S) Chondroitin-6-sulfate (C6S)	Proteoglycan metabolism	Synovial fluid	↑ Acute injury; ↓ 30 days post injury; ↑ (C6S) Traumatic arthritis; ↑ Early OA; ↓ Late OA	[50, 64–67]
CS Delta Disaccharides Δdi-6S/Δdi-4S Ratio	Cartilage degradation; CS catabolism	Synovial fluid	↑ Traumatic arthritis; ↓ RA; ↑ Early OA; ↓ Late OA	[51, 63, 66, 68]
CSΔdi-6S	Cartilage degradation; CS catabolism	Synovial fluid	↑ Traumatic arthritis; ↓ RA; ↑ Early OA; ↓ Late OA	[50, 51, 63, 68]
CSΔdi-4S	Cartilage degradation; CS catabolism	Synovial fluid	↑ Traumatic arthritis; ↑ RA; ↓ Late OA	[50, 51, 63, 68]
Aggrecan CS Epitope 846	Aggrecan synthesis; Cartilage turnover	Synovial fluid	↑ Knee injury; ↑ Pseudogout; ↑ RA; ↑ Early OA; ↓ Late OA	[45, 50, 63, 69]
CS Neoepitopes 3B3(−); 3B3(+); 7D4	Cartilage repair	Synovial fluid; Serum	Acute injury,-ve; Chronic injury, +ve; ↓ (3B3) Increasing chondral damage score; ↓ (3B3) Age; ↑ s-RA; ↓ sf-RA; ↑ Early OA; ↓ Late OA	[17, 50, 52–54, 70, 71]
Dermatan Sulfate (DS) Δdi-DS	Proteoglycan metabolism	Synovial fluid	↑ Early OA; ↓ Late OA	[68]
Hyaluronate / Hyaluronic Acid (HA)	Synovium and cartilage metabolism; Inflammation	Synovial fluid; Serum	↓ Age; ↑ RA; ↑ OA and correlate OA severity	[19, 53, 72–76]
Unsaturated Δdi-HA	Synovium and cartilage metabolism; HA catabolism	Synovial fluid	↓ RA	[63]
GAG-rich Core Protein (Large fragments)	Early chondrolysis	Synovial fluid	↑ Reactive arthritis; ↑ calcium pyrophosphate dihydrate (CPPD) crystals; ↑ Juvenile RA; ↑ Early OA	[47, 77]
Aggrecanase-generated Aggrecan Fragment With Alanine-arginine-glycine-serine (ARGS) Neoepitope	Aggrecan degradation	Synovial fluid; Serum; Urine	↑ One-day post injury; ↑ Acute injury; ↓ 48 days post injury; ↑ Late OA; ↑ Acute inflammatory arthritis	[29, 55, 58, 78–82]
Proteoglycan Core Protein β-D-xylosyltransferase	Proteoglycan metabolism	Synovial fluid; Serum	↑ OA; ↑ RA	[20]
Aggrecan Link Protein	Proteoglycan metabolism	Synovial fluid	↓ Acute injury; ↑ Chronic injury; ↑ OA	[17]

RA, *Rheumatoid arthritis*; OA, *Osteoarthritis*; CPPD, *Calcium pyrophosphate dihydrate*

Table 4.2 Knee articular cartilage biochemical markers: collagen and non-collagenous proteins detected in body fluid(s) in injury, aging and disease. Body fluids: synovial fluid (sf-), serum (s-), plasma (p-) and urine (u-)

Cartilage Marker	Marker Reflects	Body Fluid(s)	Marker Level	Reference(s)
		Collagen-Derived Proteins		
Procollagen Type II Carboxy-terminus Propeptide (PIICP)	Collagen synthesis	Synovial fluid; Serum; Urine	↑ Injury; ↑ Traumatic arthritis; ↑ Inflammatory arthritis; ↓ Early (mild) RA; ↑ Late (severe) RA; ↑ Early OA; ↓ Late OA	[45, 50, 63, 64, 89–96]
Procollagen Type II Amino-terminus Propeptide (PIINP)	Collagen synthesis	Synovial fluid; Serum	↓ RA; ↑ Early OA; ↓ Late OA	[97–102]
C-terminal Telopeptide Collagen Type II Fragment (CTX-II)	Collagen degradation	Synovial fluid; Urine	↑ Initial stage of cartilage injury; ↑ OA	[22, 28, 41, 55, 103–107]
Helical Peptide of Collagen Type II (HELIX II)	Collagen degradation	Urine	↑ RA; ↑ OA	[25, 98, 103]
Collagen Type II C-terminal Cleavage Product (C2C epitope)	Collagen degradation	Synovial fluid; Serum; Urine	↑ Initial stage of cartilage injury; ↓ Over time of cartilage injury; ↓ With age in women; ↓ RA; ↑ Early OA	[22, 28, 62, 63, 89, 109–115]
Metalloproteinase-derived Collagen Type II Neoepitope (CIIM or C2M)	Collagen degradation	Serum	↑ RA; ↑ OA	[109, 115–118]
C-terminus Collagen Type X (C-Col10)	Collagen synthesis	Serum	↑ OA	[109, 115]
Collagen Crosslinks *Pyridinoline* (Pyd, Collagen Type II) *Deoxypyridinoline* (Dpyd, Collagen Type I)	Collagen degradation	Synovial fluid; Serum; Urine	↑ Growth and maturation; ↑ Knee effusion; ↑ Skeletal injury; ↑ Repetitive knee usage; ↑ Osteoporosis; ↑ Early RA; ↓ Late RA; ↑ OA	[119–126]
Pentosidine	Cartilage aging	Synovial fluid; Serum; Urine; Plasma	↑ Injury; ↑ Age; ↑ RA; ↑ OA	[73, 125, 127–132]
		Non-collagenous Proteins		
Cartilage Oligomeric Matrix Protein (COMP)	Cartilage turnover; Cartilage degradation	Synovial fluid; Serum	↑ Acute traumatic knee injury; ↑ During mechanical loading exercise and return to baseline 30-min after mechanical loading exercise; ↑ CM patella; ↑ Reactive arthritis; ↑ RA; ↑ Early OA	[41, 133–142]
Uncarboxylated Matrix Gla-Protein (ucMGP, Inactive Form)	Joint inflammation; Mineralization inhibitor	Synovial fluid; Serum	↑ Joint inflammation; ↓ OA progression	[143–145]
Cartilage Matrix Glycoprotein (CMGP)	Cartilage degradation	Synovial fluid; Serum; Plasma	↑ Trauma-related knee arthropathies; ↑ OA	[146, 147]

(continued)

Table 4.2 (continued)

Cartilage Marker	Marker Reflects	Body Fluid(s)	Marker Level	Reference(s)
Human Cartilage Glycoprotein-39 Also Referred as YLK-40	Cartilage turnover; Cartilage degradation; Pro-inflammatory mediator; Angiogenesis	Synovial fluid; Serum	↑ Cartilage injury; ↑ Age > 70 years; ↑ Acute / severe synovial inflammation; ↑ RA; ↑ OA and correlate OA severity	[148–155]
Osteonectin Also Referred as Secreted Protein Acidic and Rich in Cysteine (SPARC) or Basement-membrane Protein-40	Wound healing; Cartilage turnover; Pro-inflammatory mediator	Synovial fluid	↑ Acute injury; ↑ RA; ↑ OA	[58, 156, 157]
Chondronectin	Cartilage degradation	Synovial fluid; Plasma	↑ RA; ↑ OA	[158]
Fibrinogen	Regulate local inflammatory process	Synovial fluid; Plasma	↑ Acute injury; ↑ Inflammatory arthritis; ↑ RA	[159–162]
Tenascin-C (TN-C)	Cartilage degradation; Pro-inflammatory mediator	Synovial fluid; Serum	↓ Cartilage maturation; ↑ Acute cartilage injury; ↑ Acute inflammatory arthritis; ↑ RA; ↑ Moderate and late OA	[123, 126, 163–166]
Lubricin	Lubrication of superficial zone	Synovial fluid; Plasma	↓ Post acute injury (from baseline to follow-up 50 days later); ↓ With increase in inflammatory markers	[55, 167]
Follistatin-like Protein 1 (FSTL1)	Cartilage degradation; Pro-inflammatory mediator	Synovial fluid; Serum	↑ Age; ↑ RA; ↑ Juvenile RA; ↑ OA	[168–170]
Fibulin-3 Peptide 1, 2 (Fib 3-1, Fib 3-2)	Wound repair; Joint inflammation	Serum	↑ OA	[171–173]

lage integrity during health, aging, injury, and disease. Collagen type II is synthesized as procollagen molecules with C- and N-terminal propeptides (referred as PIICP and PIINP, respectively), which are cleaved off during maturation and released into biological fluids as biomarkers of collagen synthesis during injury and disease [45, 50, 63, 64, 89, 95, 97–100]. As the consequence of alternative RNA splicing, N-terminal propeptides of collagen type II procollagen is produced in two forms, one form (IIA – PIIANP) includes and the other form (IIB – PIIBNP) excludes a 69-amino acid cysteine-rich globular domain encoded by exon 2 in PIINP [101]. Patients with knee OA and RA have shown a decrease in s-PIIANP and -PIIBNP [99, 174]. Another marker of synthesis associated with hypertrophic chondrocytes differentiation, C-terminus of collagen type X (C-Col10), showed elevated s-levels in patients with mild/moderate knee OA [109]. In these patients the concentration of C-Col10 strongly correlated with levels of MMP-derived collagen type II neoepitope (CIIM or C2M), a marker of cartilage destruction.

During articular cartilage breakdown, several cleavage fragments of collagen type II degradation have been identified in body fluids [23, 90, 98, 100, 102, 103, 108, 110–112, 175–177]. Cleavage of articular cartilage collagen type II by proteases often occurs pericellularly around chondrocytes at and near the cartilage surface, which subsequently enhances and extends progressively to include the deeper cartilage zones with aging and OA [178]. Among the various collagen type II degradation markers, the C-terminal telopeptide collagen type II fragment (CTX-II) has been extensively investigated [29, 41, 97, 103–107, 111, 179–189]. Among volleyball athletes, an elevated CTX-II level in adolescents compared to adults is thought to reflect increased cartilage turnover in response to higher joint loading [22]. Also, an increased sf and s-CTX-II level have been reported post acute knee injury [55, 107]. Patients with a focal articular cartilage lesion of the knee demonstrated higher levels of u-CTX-II than healthy individuals, which decreased during cartilage healing and rehabilitation [105]. This finding suggests that the CTX-II has the potential for monitoring treatment effects. Elevated u-CTX-II level in OA patients has been reported with a strong correlation with the OA grade and progression [41, 104, 106]. Also, the urinary helical peptide of collagen type II (HELIX II) is associated with the progression of OA and RA [28, 103, 108, 186]. Further, MMP-1 degradation of collagen type II releases a C-terminal cleavage neopeptide (C2C), which can be detected in the sf, serum, and urine. Patients with injured knees and after intense athletic training involving higher knee loading have shown elevated C2C levels [22, 62]. The C2C level is elevated during the acute stage (initial phase) of knee injury which then decreases over time relative to the C2C level of healthy non-injured controls [62, 110, 113, 114]. Higher u-C2C level of patients with mild knee OA compared to the controls has been reported, suggesting a role of C2C as a prognostic marker for patients with early-stage knee OA [28, 89, 115]. In a population-based study involving a patient cohort with symptomatic knee pain, the risk of pre-radiographically defined OA increased with elevated levels of u-C2C, when compared with no OA controls [111]. However, a decrease in C2C level has been associated with aging in women [112]. Another biomarker of collagen type II breakdown, the MMP-derived neoepitope (CIIM or C2M), has shown elevated s-level in patients with knee OA and RA when compared with non-arthritic controls [116, 117].

Pyridinium crosslinks, namely, pyridinoline (Pyd) and deoxypyridinoline (Dpyd), present in the mature insoluble collagen fibrils have been used as biomarkers of bone and cartilage collagen degradation [119–124, 190]. These crosslinks are released in the body fluid as a consequence of collagen breakdown. While Dpyd is a specific marker of collagen type I resorption in bone, Pyd is released from collagen types I and II [120]. Although clinical studies have shown Pyd level in body fluids (sf, serum, and urine) as a marker of bone and cartilage breakdown in joint effusions, RA, OA, and osteoporotic joints; Pyd is not specific to knee disease due to its association with other conditions such as diabetes, breast cancer, osteosarcoma, multiple myeloma, and renal failure [106, 119–124, 190–200].

Glycation is one of the key processes leading to aging of articular cartilage. In vitro glycation through ribose treatment of OC explants has been shown to decrease chondrocyte volume deformation responses in the upper zones compared to control samples. Also, via the transmission of mechanical signals or forces deeper into the cartilage, the chondrocyte volume deformation increased in the deeper zones [201]. This finding along with results of other studies provides insight on how glycation, such as formation of pentosidine crosslinks, can alter the biomechanical responses of chondrocytes in articular cartilage during aging [202–206]. Pentosidine, a fluorescent advanced Maillard/glycosylation crosslink product, is formed by nonenzymatic glycation of PGs and collagens [207–209]. It is detected in articular cartilage and body fluids of patients with knee injury and joint disorders [73, 125, 127–132, 210]. However, extremely high levels of pentosidine have also been detected in the skin and ocular lens as well as in the plasma and urine of patients with diabetes and uremia [210–214]. As such, results pertaining to pentosidine as a biomarker should be interpreted with caution.

Among all non-collagenous and non-aggrecan protein biomarkers, COMP, a constituent of articular cartilage, has been extensively investigated as a biomarker in body fluids reflecting articular cartilage turnover in health as well as cartilage turnover (or degradation) in injury, aging, and disease [179, 215–219]. COMP levels are increased in sf and serum of patients during the acute phase of traumatic knee injury and with elevated symptoms of knee pain without radiological abnormalities as well as during disease activity (CM patella, reactive arthritis, RA, and OA) [41, 133–138, 182, 189, 216–218, 220–224]. An inverse relationship of s-COMP has been reported with bilateral knee cartilage thickness in RA patients and the healthy controls [139]. The knee s-COMP levels have shown to be useful to predict cartilage volume loss, progression of OA, and/or total knee replacement [86, 225]. Further, a reduction in the sf-COMP level has been reported after 30 min of exercise in OA patients, suggesting the utility of COMP biomarker post exercise, repetitive activities, as well as sports (recreational and competitive) [140].

Matrix Gla-protein (MGP), a vitamin K-dependent calcification inhibitor produced by cartilage, has been detected as uncarboxylated MGP (ucMGP, inactive form) in the sf and serum, serving as a joint inflammatory marker [143]. The ucMGP levels in arthritis patients with knee effusions and inflammation have shown lowest s-levels and highest sf-levels compared to the control group and patients with knee effusion but without inflammation [143]. High plasma dephosphorylated-ucMGP, reflective of lower vitamin K status of patients, has been associated with the presence of knee OA features but not progression [144]. Among patients with knee OA, the serum ucMGP levels were significantly lower than that of healthy controls, and the sf ucMGP levels negatively correlated with radiographic OA severity [145].

The cartilage matrix glycoprotein (CMGP), also called chondronectin, specifically mediates the attachment of chondrocytes to collagen type II. CMG have been detected in the knee sf and plasma of RA and OA patients [146, 147, 158, 226]. However, the s-CMG levels were inconsistent in patients with trauma-related, arthroscopically proven focal OA, and the CMG level did not correlate with the severity of arthroscopic or radiologic articular cartilage lesions [146]. CMG in the plasma of OA patients were detected at levels that correlated with but at lower levels than that of sf [147].

Human cartilage glycoprotein-39, also referred as YKL-40, is implicated in tissue injury, remodeling, inflammation, and angiogenesis [148, 149]. Among healthy children and adults (< 70 years), a slight increase in s-YKL-40 was noted with age; but, thereafter (age > 70 years), s-YKL-40 increased significantly [150]. Serum and knee sf-YKL-40 levels have been reported to increase in moderate/severe RA and OA patients compared to the normal adults but not in early-stage of injury or OA [150–152]. Also, the sf-levels of YKL showed significantly higher values than the s-levels [152]. Knee sf-YKL-40 levels have shown a strong association with the serum pro-inflammatory molecules, tumor necrosis factor-α (TNF-α) and interleukin 1-beta (Il-1β), in RA patients as well as sf-levels of MMP-1, MMP-3, Il-6, and Il-17 in OA patients [148, 149, 153]. These studies suggest that YKL-40 and the pro-inflammatory molecules collectively play a dominant role in the RA and OA pathogenesis and activity.

Osteonectin (OSN), also referred as secreted protein acidic and rich in cysteine (SPARC) or basement-membrane protein-40, is an abundant ECM protein. Classified as a marker protein in chondrodifferentiation, SPARC is located in the ECM of hypertrophic chondrocyte zone [227]. Compared to the healthy reference subjects, increased knee sf-SPARC levels are seen in RA and OA patients, with the levels ten-fold higher in the RA than in the OA populations [156]. Significantly high levels of SPARC have also been detected in the sf of injured knees compared to healthy, non-injured knees [58, 157].

The attachment of collagen type II to chondrocytes is mediated by chondronectin, a marker of articular cartilage degradation [228]. Chondronectin levels have shown increased levels in plasma and knee sf of RA and OA patients and positively correlated with sf-fibrinogen levels [158]. Fibrinogen, a prothrombotic protein, was significantly elevated in the plasma (3-weeks post-trauma) and knee sf of patients with history of knee injury/trauma and exudates compared to the plasma and sf-levels obtained from the control group [159, 229]. Also, p-fibrinogen level was elevated in RA patients compared to controls, which showed inverse correlation with clinical measures of RA activity even in RA patients without inflammation or joint effusion [160]. Elevated levels of fibrinogen- and fibronectin-derived endogenous citrullinated peptides have been identified in sf of RA patients [161, 162, 230]. A significantly high level of the fibronectin-aggrecan complex has been identified in sf (aspirated at the time arthroscopic partial meniscectomy) of the affected knee of patients with pain and meniscal tear compared with asymptomatic, pain-free group who underwent knee magnetic resonance imaging (MRI) [231].

The expression of tenascin-C (TN-C), a glycoprotein component of articular cartilage ECM, is seen during growth and development of articular cartilage but markedly reduced during maturation of chondrocytes [163, 232]. In adult articular cartilage, TN-C has the capacity to induce inflammatory mediators and degrade the ECM. In a cross-sectional study, sf obtained from patient knee with articular cartilage lesions showed high correlation coefficient of tenascin and MMP-13 with the Outerbridge and Noyes chondral injury classification (refer to Appendix A) [126]. Relative to the normal knee sf, significantly elevated levels of TN-C in the sf of patients with knee injury, acute inflammatory arthritis, and OA correlated with articular cartilage degradation and inflammation [164]. Compared to the knee sf of non-disease individuals, elevated TN-C levels in the knee sf of RA patients and moderate to severe OA patients as well as elevated s-TN-C in RA patients have been reported [163, 165, 166].

Reduction in the sf lubricating molecule concentration and quality is one of the potential mechanisms for the early lesion to the superficial zone (SZ ie Zone 1) of articular cartilage. Lubricin, a heavily O-glycosylated protein, plays a key role in the boundary lubrication of articular cartilage to provide smooth movement of the opposing articular cartilage surfaces. During locomotion, lubricin provides cartilage with an ability to dissipate strain energy; as such, given the excessive forces that the knee must withstand, a strong adherence of lubricin to the articular cartilage surface of Zone 1 is imperative for boundary lubrication. Reduction in cartilage surface lubricin expression and function, and thus its boundary-lubricating and chondroprotective ability, has been implicated as a contributing factor in the development of OA [233–235]. Lubricin binds with fibronectin and collagen type II on the cartilage surface and is also known to play an anti-inflammatory role in sf [236, 237]. Disulfide bound complexes of lubricin and COMP has been identified in sf of RA and OA patients [238]. A decreased sf-lubricin level is associated with increased levels of inflammatory cytokines (Il-1β, TNF-α, and Il-6) [239].

Follistatin-like glycoprotein 1 (FSTL1, mesenchyme-derived) and fibulin 3 peptide-1 and peptide-2 (Fib 3-1 and -2) are pro-inflammatory mediators which reflect cartilage degradation. SF and s-FSTL1 are significantly elevated in children with systemic onset juvenile RA, adult RA, and OA patients compared to control patients, and the elevated FSTL1 levels are significantly correlated with age and the disease activity/duration [168–170]. Elevated s-FSTL1 levels reported in patients with ulcerative colitis, systemic lupus erythematosus, and systemic sclerosis suggests that FSTL1 does not specifically reflect the integrity of knee articular cartilage [168]. Increased s-level of Fib 3-1 and Fib 3-2 in OA patients compared with normal population correlated with the incidence of radiographic knee OA [171, 172]. The s-Fib 3 level was also associated with the incidence of clinical knee OA among overweight and obese middle-aged female patients [173].

4.3.3 Matrix Metalloproteinases, Cytokines, Adipocytokines, and Growth Factors

The aggrecanases, MMPs, and their inhibitors, cytokines and chemokines, adipocytokines, and growth factors that are present in human body fluids are summarized in Table 4.3. Aggrecanases are ECM proteolytic enzymes that are members of the "disintegrin and metalloproteinases with thrombospondin motifs (ADAMTS) group."

Table 4.3 Knee articular cartilage biochemical markers: matrix metalloproteinases, enzymes, and inhibitors, cytokines and chemokines, adipocytokines and growth factors detected in body fluid(s) during injury, aging and disease. Body fluids: synovial fluid (sf-), serum (s-), plasma (p-) and urine (u-)

Cartilage Marker	Marker Reflects	Body Fluid(s)	Marker Level	Reference(s)
Matrix Metalloproteinases, Enzymes, and Inhibitors				
Aggrecanase	Aggrecan catabolism	Synovial fluid; Serum; Urine	↑ Acute injury; ↑ Inflammatory arthritis; ↑ Pseudogout; ↑ RA; ↑ OA	[39, 44, 46, 48, 80–82, 87, 240]
Collagenase (MMP-1)	Collagen degradation	Synovial fluid; Serum	↑ Acute injury; ↑ Pseudogout; ↑ CM patella; ↑ RA; ↑ Early (mild) OA; ↓ Moderate and late (severe) OA	[60, 87, 110, 241, 242]
Hyaluronidase	Hyaluronic acid catabolism	Synovial fluid, Serum	↑ RA; ↑ OA	[32, 84, 243, 244]
Phospholipase A2	Membrane phospholipid degradation	Synovial fluid, Serum	↑ CM patella; ↑ RA; ↑ OA	[60, 245]
Stromelysin (MMP-3)	Cartilage degradation	Synovial fluid; Serum	↑ Acute injury; ↑ Late CM patella; ↑ Inflammatory arthritis; ↑ RA; ↑ OA	[60, 63, 64, 241, 246–248]
Disintegrin and Metalloproteinase with Thrombospondin Type Motif 4 (ADAMTS-4)	Cartilage degradation	Synovial fluid; Serum	↑ Early OA; Reflect intra-articular environment	[29, 247, 249–251]
Tissue Inhibitor of Metalloproteinases Type I, 2 (TIMP-1, 2)	Cartilage synthesis; Cartilage repair	Synovial fluid; Serum	↑ Injury; ↑ Late CM patella; ↑ RA; ↑ OA progression	[50, 60, 64, 73, 123, 126, 241]
Cytokines and Chemokines				
Interleukins Interleukin 1 (Il-1β) Interleukin 2 (Il-2) Interleukin 4 (Il-4) Interleukin 6 (Il-6) Interleukin 8 (Il-8) Interleukin 13 (Il-13) Interleukin 15 (Il-15) Interleukin 17 (Il-17) Interleukin 18 (Il-18)	Cartilage degradation; Pro-inflammatory	Synovial fluid; Serum; Plasma	↑ Acute injury; ↑ RA; ↑ OA; Positively and significantly associate AC defect	[58, 123, 126, 157, 247, 249, 252–262]
Tumor Necrosis Factor Alpha (TNF-α)	Cartilage degradation; Pro-inflammatory	Synovial fluid; Serum	↑ Age; ↑ Acute injury; ↑ Early RA; ↑ OA	[58, 157, 252, 253, 263–265]
Tumor Necrosis Factor-Receptors (TNF-Rs)	Cartilage degradation; Pro-inflammatory	Synovial fluid; Serum	↑ RA; ↑ OA	[266, 267]
Chemokine (C-C Motif) Ligand 3 (CCL3)	Inflammation mediators	Plasma	↑ Late OA	[29, 259]
Adipocytokines				
Adiponectin	Obesity-related knee inflammation	Serum; Plasma	↑ RA; ↑ Late OA	[29, 262, 268–271]
Apolipoprotein A-I (ApoA-1)	Obesity-related knee inflammation	Synovial fluid; Serum	↑ Inflammatory arthritis; ↑ RA; ↑ OA	[272–274]

(continued)

Table 4.3 (continued)

Cartilage Marker	Marker Reflects	Body Fluid(s)	Marker Level	Reference(s)
Adipsin	Obesity-related knee inflammation	Serum	↑ Cartilage volume loss; ↑ OA	[29, 275]
Leptin	Cartilage degradation; Pro-inflammatory; induce catabolic enzymes	Serum	↑ Age; ↑ Cartilage thinning / volume loss; ↑ OA	[29, 31, 275–279]
Resistin	Cartilage degradation; Pro-inflammatory; Induce catabolic enzymes	Synovial fluid; Serum; Plasma	↑ Acute injury; ↑ OA; Positively and significantly associate AC defect	[31, 260, 278, 280, 281]
Visfatin	Cartilage degradation; Pro-inflammatory; Induce catabolic enzymes	Synovial fluid; Serum; Plasma	↑ RA; ↑ OA	[31, 270, 280, 282–284]
Prostaglandin E2 (PGE2)	Cartilage degradation; Pro-inflammatory	Plasma	↑ OA	[258]
15-hydroxyeicosatetraenoic acid (HETE-15)	Pro-inflammatory	Plasma	↑ OA	[258]
Growth Factors				
Transforming Growth Factor-β (TGF-β)	Cartilage repair; Anti-inflammatory	Synovial fluid; Serum	↑ Gout; ↑ RA; ↑ OA	[262, 285–288]
Vascular Endothelial Growth Factor (VEGF)	Angiogenesis; Cartilage repair	Synovial fluid; Serum; Plasma	↑ Early RA; ↑ OA	[264, 277, 289, 290]
Insulin-like Growth Factor-1 (IGF-β1)	Cartilage repair	Synovial fluid	↑ Early OA	[21]

To date, two forms of aggrecanase exist in humans, aggrecase-1 or ADAMTS-4 and aggrecanase-2 or ADAMTS-5 [78, 291]. While ADAMTS-4 is elevated in the serum of patients with early stage of knee OA, ADAMTS-5 is detected in the moderate and late-stage knee OA. MMPs, also known as matrixins, are a family of calcium-dependent zinc-containing endopeptidases, which in articular cartilage are responsible for the ECM remodeling and functions as key mediators of ECM molecular degradation, including collagens, proteoglycans, and glycoproteins [292–294]. Although aggrecanases and MMPs are the major proteases involved in aggrecan fragmentation, the aggrecanases are more involved than MMPs with the enhanced aggrecan loss associated with OA [47, 240, 295, 296]. The knee sf levels of aggrecanase, MMP-1, MMP-3, MMP-13, and hyaluronidase as well as tissue inhibitor of metalloproteinases type I (TIMP-1) and ECM molecular fragments released into sf, are reported to increase in patients with acute knee injury, inflammatory arthritis, pseudogout, and RA when compared with volunteers with healthy knees [38, 80, 81, 241, 246]. In patients undergoing knee arthroscopy, the intraoperative sf showed a consistent increase in the MMP-3 level compared to asymptomatic knee samples, which directly correlated to increased preoperative baseline data obtained from clinical questionnaires using a visual analog scale (VAS) score [247].

Synovial fluid TIMP-1 levels have been reported to increase in patients with knee injury, OA, and pseudogout compared with controls; and in the injury group, the increase in MMP-1 activity coincided with a decrease in TIMP-1 levels [241]. In a study involving OA patients, knee sf-TIMP-1 levels directly correlated with the levels of MMP-1 and MMP-3, suggesting a link between OA cartilage proteolysis and TIMP concentrations [50]. Also, in the knee sf of late-stage OA patients, the TIMP-1 levels correlated with the aggrecan CS epitope 846 (marker of aggrecan synthesis), whereas, TIMP-2 levels correlated with those of PIICP (marker of collagen synthesis), indicating the link between the production of TIMPs to the synthesis of specific cartilage ECM molecules [50]. In a cohort of OA patients, high s-levels of TIMP, MMP-9, COMP, and pentosidine were detected compared with healthy controls [73].

Hyaluronidase-mediated degradation of HA increases the permeability of articular cartilage and decreases the viscosity of body fluids [243]. In RA patients, s-HA level is higher than the healthy controls, which has been shown to occur as low molecular weight (MW) in all RA patients along with high MW in a few cases [244]. Hyaluronidase activity has shown to be significantly higher in the RA patients compared to OA patients and normal controls, and the activity was lower in RA patients with both low and high HA MW compared to those with only low HA MW [84, 244].

Phospholipase A2 (PLA2) is a calcium-dependent enzyme, which plays a pivotal role in membrane phospholipid degradation by initiating a cascade of events leading to the production of pro-inflammatory prostaglandins [245, 297]. PLA2 is produced in large amounts by both cartilage and synovial membrane, and a high activity of PLA2 has been shown in the sf of OA patients [245]. The lavage sf-level of PLA2 has shown to increase with the severity of CM patella [60]. The synthesis of C-reactive protein (CRP), a key component of the innate immune inflammatory response, is mediated by factors released by macrophages and adipocytes [298, 299]. CRP promotes the secretion of pro-inflammatory cytokines, which in turn increases the inflammatory response in disease of knee [298, 300]. A meta-analysis of 32 studies revealed statistically significant differences in serum CRP levels in patients with OA compared with healthy controls, which is also significantly associated with pain and decreased physical function [301]. Among patients with symptomatic knee OA, the serum ferritin levels significantly correlated with the arthroscopic evaluation of cartilage damage severity, indicating that ferritin may be involved in the progression of cartilage damage [302].

Cytokines are a category of small proteins that are released by cells that function in cell signaling. Although included as a cytokine, in vitro experiments have demonstrated Il-4 is an anabolic, anti-inflammatory, and anti-catabolic cytokine, which is expressed at a significantly low level in OA cartilage [303]. Pro-inflammatory cytokines (Il-1, Il-6, Il-12, Il-15, Il-17, Il-18, and TNF-α) are produced in the synovium and/or cartilage and are released into the circulation (Table 4.3). Levels of these cytokines in the serum and knee sf reflect disease activity and may be associated with increased risk for disease progression [239, 249, 263, 285, 304, 305]. Some of these cytokines (Il-6, Il-8, Il-10, and TNF-α) are elevated in the body fluids of patients post knee injury [58, 157, 306]. With the use of a combination of inflammatory biomarkers, diseases affecting the knee may be differentiated [252, 264] (Fig. 4.2).

A study with inclusion criteria of patients undergoing knee arthroscopy showed a strong positive correlation between the Il-6 and monocyte chemotactic protein 1 (MCP-1) sf-levels, intraoperative International Cartilage Repair Society (ICRS) score, and continued pain at the time of follow-up, and both these sf biomarkers were identified as the strongest predictors of severe cartilage lesions [247]. Patients with knee

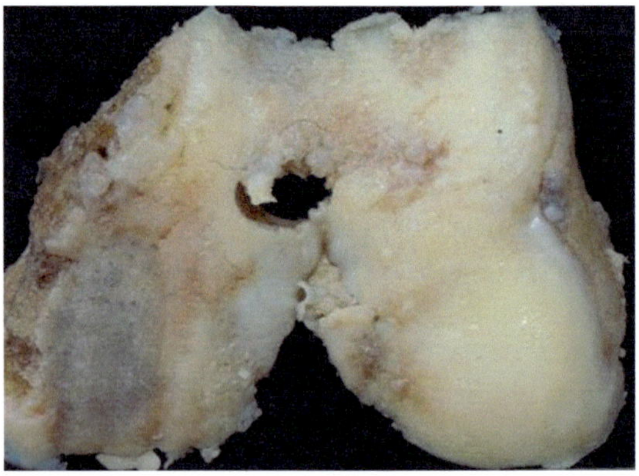

Fig. 4.2 Photomacrograph of human left knee obtained post total knee replacement in a 67-year-old female patient. Note extensive erosion and eburnation on the medial compartment, whereas the articular cartilage of lateral compartment ranges from intact to surface fibrillation

OA who participated in an exercise and nutrition intervention study showed high s-levels of Il-6 which is associated with slower walking speed [266]. Further, this study showed that the significantly high levels of soluble receptors of TNF-α were associated with lower physical function, increased OA symptoms, and worse knee radiographic scores in older obese adults with knee OA [266]. A study with a 3-year follow-up showed elevated s-levels of Il-6 and TNF-α, which is associated with knee articular cartilage loss in the older adults (range 52–78 years) [253].

In a 15-year follow-up study, the s-levels of Il-6 measured at baseline, 5, 8, and 15 years consistently, showed significantly higher levels in individuals radiographically diagnosed with knee OA [254]. A study with a 3-year follow-up showed elevated s-levels of Il-6 and TNF-α, which is associated with knee articular cartilage loss in the older adults (range 52–78 years) [253]. Another study showed that elevated s-Il-6 level is associated with pain in early-stage OA, whereas the varus alignment of the knee is associated with late OA [255]. Serum levels of Il-15 showed an association with the severity of pain in patients with knee OA [256]. Plasma levels of Il-2, Il-4, and Il-6 levels were found to be significantly high in primary knee OA patients compared to controls [257]. Also, both plasma Il-4 and Il-6 levels were positively correlated with the radiographic severity of knee OA. Elevated baseline p-levels of Il-1β and TNF-α in patients with symptomatic knee OA predicted higher risk of radiographic progression of the disease [258]. Another study showed that the p-levels of Il-6, Il-8, resistin, chemokine ligand 3 (CCL3), and CCL4 are significantly associated with the radiographic severity of knee OA [259].

A subfamily of cytokines include chemotactic chemokines, which have the ability to induce direct chemotaxis in nearby responsive cells [307]. Another cytokine class, called adipokines or adipocytokine, are pleiotropic molecules secreted by adipose tissue that exert their actions through endocrine, paracrine, or autocrine mechanisms in a wide spectrum of physiological or pathophysiological processes [280, 308]. Serum adipokines are thought to provide a non-mechanical link between obesity and joint tissue integrity (which may be mediated by bone and cartilage turnover) that subsequently result in changes to the cartilage defects score and cartilage volume loss [309]. However, emerging data suggests that adipokines are involved in the onset and progression of weight-associated cartilage degradative process [308]. Adipokines, such as adiponectin, leptin, and vistafin, act as pro-inflammatory mediators which are involved in the pathophysiology of RA and OA [268, 269]. Using quantitative MRI, the serum levels of adipsin and leptin were associated with knee OA progression, and higher levels of both these adipokines were associated with higher incidence of total knee replacement [275]. Leptin plays a catabolic role in cartilage metabolism via the upregulation of proteolytic enzymes and acts synergistically with other pro-inflammatory stimuli [31, 276, 310, 311]. During acute inflammatory responses, leptin expression is regulated by a wide range of inflammatory mediators such as lipopolysaccharides and cytokines, such as Il-1β, Il-6, and TNF-α, and the leptin production has been positively correlated with body mass index (BMI) and fat mass [312–315]. Leptin, either alone or in synergy with Il-1, significantly induced collagen release from bovine cartilage by upregulating collagenolytic and gelatinolytic activity [316]. In a prospective cohort of randomly selected adults (range: 52–78 years), the s-leptin levels independently and consistently associated with reduced articular cartilage thickness from each of the four compartments of the knee (namely, the lateral and medial femoral condyle and tibial plateau) and patella, indicating the potential role of leptin in articular cartilage thinning [277]. Resistin, a pro-inflammatory mediator and insulin-resistant molecule, has been detected in the sf following knee injury and in patients with knee OA [281]. The sf-resistin level is associated with inflammatory and catabolic factors, indicating its role in articular cartilage injury and the pathogenesis of OA [281]. The s-resistin level is positively associated with knee articular cartilage defects at various compartments (lateral femoral condyle and tibial plateau as well as medial tibial plateau) [260]. Similar to leptin, visfatin also stimulates the expression of pro-inflammatory cytokines and chemokines (Il-1β, Il-6, and TNF-α), vascular endothelial growth factor (VEGF), MMP-2, and MMP-9. The sf-visfatin levels positively correlated with the degradation biomarkers of collagen type II (CTX-II) and aggrecans [282]. The sf-visfatin levels have been shown to be significantly higher in RA patients than in the control group [270, 317]. Also, in severely OA patients requiring total knee arthroplasty (TKA), the sf- and s-visfatin levels were elevated compared to healthy controls [283]. Further among female patients with knee OA and with inflammation, sf-visfatin levels were found to inversely correlate with the clinical severity of OA [278]. Other inflammatory biomarkers, plasma lipid, prostaglandin E2 (PGE2) and 15-hydroxyeicosatetraenoic acid (HETE-15), were reported to be significantly elevated in patients with symptomatic knee OA versus non-OA controls, and these biomarkers identified a subset of these OA patients who are at increased risk of radiographic OA progression [258].

The TGF-β superfamily, such as TGF-β1, plays a crucial role in maintaining homeostasis and repair of both articular cartilage and subchondral bone [318]. Analysis of sf during the various stages of acute gout showed that TGF-β1 level significantly increases from the onset at day 1 to day 7, suggesting the role of TGF-β1 in the resolution of gout [285]. Altered expression and deregulation of TGF-β has been shown to be involved in OA [319–321]. A significant elevation in the s-TGF-β1 levels in the knee of OA patients compared to non-OA controls and a positive correlation of TGF-β1 with the severity of radiographically confirmed OA have been reported [286]. Another signal protein produced by cells, VEGF stimulates the formation of blood vessels [322]. Elevated sf-VEGF level was reported in OA patients with Kellgren-Lawrence (KL) grade 4 compared to those with KL grade 2 and the VEGF level positively correlated with KL grades [279]. Other studies showed that both plasma and sf-VEGF levels positively correlated with the severity of knee OA [289, 323]. VEGF-A, a subtype of VEGF, has been associated with increased MMP activity, which in RA is released at the acute stage in response to TNF-α. The p-VEGF in patients with early-stage RA showed elevated levels compared to healthy controls [290]. Insulin-like growth factor-1 (IGF-1) plays a key role in articular cartilage homeostasis, balancing PG synthesis and breakdown, which has been shown to influence chondrocyte metabolism, by reversing the Il-1-mediated catabolic pathway [324, 325]. The sf-level of IGF in the knee of OA patients has been found to be twice as in normal knee [21].

4.4 Clinical Utility of Biochemical Markers

Biochemical markers of articular cartilage metabolism are increasingly used in both basic and clinical research, for diagnostic, prognostic, and treatment efficacy purposes. In addition, such markers may provide additional information about the various stages of the life cycle of articular cartilage in health, aging, injury, and disease (Table 4.4).

4.4.1 Injury

Knee injury or trauma including sports injuries or repetitive use of the joint is conducive to post-traumatic osteoarthritis (PTOA), in particular if the injury sustained is severe. At the time of injury, PTOA is thought to be initiated by early expression of proteolytic enzymes. To date, several macromolecules and metabolites which act as biomarkers for PTOA have been identified [48, 159]. These injury prognostic body fluid biomarkers are valuable in monitoring and assessing the knee articular cartilage metabolism and health prior to and post knee injury. In an adolescent minipig acute injury model, anterior cruciate ligament (ACL) transaction upregulated MMP-1 gene expression in articular cartilage, synovium, and ligament, whereas MMP-13 expression was suppressed in the articular cartilage but upregulated 100-fold in the synovium and ligament. ADAMTS-4 was upregulated in the synovium and ligament only [110]. Further, in the first 5

Table 4.4 Knee articular cartilage biomarker changes associated with repetitive impact injury, single acute injury, aging, rheumatoid arthritis, and osteoarthritis. Body fluids: synovial fluid (sf-), serum (s-), plasma (p-) and urine (u-). Pericellular matrix (PCM); Extracellular matrix (ECM)

Articular Cartilage	Chondrocyte and Extracellular Matrix Changes	Body Fluid(s)	Key Biomarkers	Reference(s)
Repetitive Impact Injury (Competitive Sports or Long-term Recreational Sports: Mechanical Stress; Strenuous Exercise in Healthy Athletes)	Chondrocyte apoptosis and necrosis; ↑ Cartilage ECM turnover; ↑ Load-induced changes	Synovial fluid; Serum	***Adolescent athletes:*** ↓ s-C2C; ↓ s-CTX-II; ↓ s-PIICP (correlated with clinical scores) ***Adult athletes:*** ↑ Aggrecan; ↑ s-KS; ↓ s-HA; ↑ s-COMP; ↑ s-CILP-2; ↑ s-C2C; ↑ MMP-3; ↑ MMP-9; ↑ sf-Il-1β; ↑ s-Il-6 and -TNF-α (after activity and return to baseline)	[22, 36, 219, 326–332]
Single Acute Injury (Blunt Trauma Episode Often Resulting from Accidents or Sports Injuries)	Anabolic phenotype to regenerate ECM; ↑ Homeostasis, cartilage matrix turnover, and metabolism	Synovial fluid; Serum; Plasma; Urine	↑ sf-GAG and -ARGS when sf aspirated after 1 day post acute injury; ↓ sf-GAG, -ARGS, and -lubricin from baseline to follow-up at 50 days post injury; ↓ sf-3B3(−) and -GAG with ↑ damage score; ↑ s-KS; ↑ sf-CTX-II; ↓ sf-CTX-II with effective treatment; ↑ sf-C2C epitope; ↑ s-C2C epitope; ↑ sf-COMP; ↑ u-CTX; ↓ u-CTX during effective treatment and rehabilitation; ↑ sf-Il-1β, -Il-6, and -Il-8; ↑ sf-TNF-α; ↑ s-leptin; ↑ p-resistin	[31, 54, 55, 58, 59, 105, 107, 113, 114, 157, 183, 333–336]
Aging	Chondrocyte senescence; ↓ Metabolic activity and anabolic responses; ↓ ECM thickness; Enhanced proteolysis; Advanced glycation	Synovial fluid; Serum	↓ s-C2C; ↑ s-pentosidine; ↑ sf-pentosidine; ↑ s-Il-6; ↑ s-TNF-α; ↓ sf-MMP	[5, 112, 202, 203, 253, 254, 337]
Rheumatoid Arthritis	Synovial inflammation; ↓ Chondrocyte metabolism; ↑ MMPs and aggrecanases; ↑ ECM catabolic responses	Synovial fluid; Serum; Urine	↑ u-HELIX-II; ↑ sf-COMP early RA; ↓ sf-COMP late RA; ↑ s-COMP; ↑ s-visfatin early RA; ↑ s-adiponectin early RA (correlate with early radiographic changes); ↑ s-Il-6 (correlate with RA progression); ↑ s-Il-35; ↑ s-TNF-β	[34, 108, 124, 139, 185, 217, 220, 222, 268, 270, 290, 317, 338–340]

(continued)

Table 4.4 (continued)

Articular Cartilage	Chondrocyte and Extracellular Matrix Changes	Body Fluid(s)	Key Biomarkers	Reference(s)
Early / Mild Osteoarthritis	Edema; ↑ Metabolic activity; ↑ Cartilage thickness *Zone 1:* Chondrocyte proliferation and hypertrophy; ↑ Aggrecan and collagen type II degradation *Zone 2 / Zone 3:* ↑ Decorin and aggrecan; ↑ Collagen fibrils formation	Synovial fluid; Serum	↑ s-KS; ↑ sf-IHH; ↑ s-HA; ↑ sf-PIICP with risk factors (obesity, varus alignment); ↑ s-COMP (knee pain without radiological abnormalities) ↑ s-Il-6 and -Il-15 (correlate knee pain); ↑ s-leptin and -resistin	[31, 59, 73, 91, 134, 135, 254, 256, 338]
Moderate / Severe Osteoarthritis	Chondrocyte hypertrophy and clustering; ↓ Metabolic activity; ECM degradation; ↑ Matrillin-1 in PCM and ↑ matrillin-2 in ECM proportional to OA severity	Synovial fluid; Serum; Plasma; Urine	↑ sf-ARGS; ↑ s-ARGS; ↓ s-KS ↑ sf-CTX-II; ↑ sf-COMP; ↑ s-pentosidine; ↑ s-C2C; ↑ s-Fib 3-1; ↑ u-CTX-II (correlate score and progression); ↑ u-C2C; ↑ u-HELIX- II; ↑ sf-CCL2; ↑ sf-VEGF (correlate with radiographic score); ↑ sf-leptin, -resistin, and -visfatin (correlate OA with clinical severity); ↓ sf-ghrelin; ↑ s-visfatin; ↑ s-MMP-9; ↑ s-TIMP; ↑ s-Il-6; ↑ s-TNF-α	[23, 41, 59, 78, 80, 106, 108, 109, 111, 115, 129, 134, 135, 171, 184, 187, 188, 249, 253, 278, 279, 282–284, 289, 341, 342]

days post injury, sf-C2C levels were doubled [110]. This study demonstrated that within the first few days of ACL injury, cells of various knee tissues have the potential to upregulate the genes coding for proteins that degrade articular cartilage ECM.

In a prospective study of patients (age range 18–60 years) with an acute tibial plateau fracture, sf aspirates were obtained from both injured and uninjured knees [48]. Within 24 h post injury, elevated sf-levels of MMP-1, MMP-3, MMP-9, MMP-10, and MMP-12 were reported in injured versus contralateral uninjured knee. The follow-up knee sf aspirate obtained between 3 and 21 days post injury showed elevated MMP-1, MMP-2, MMP-3, MMP-12, MMP-13, and aggrecan fragments compared with the initial aspirate within 24 h post injury [48]. Patients with knee injury have also shown a persistent increase in sf-proMMP-1 and -proMMP-3 as well as an increase in MMP-1 activity, which coincided with a decrease in TIMP levels [241].

Unilateral knee injury is reported to affect the sf concentrations of aggrecan fragments, COMP fragments, MMP-3, and TIMP-1 in the contralateral uninjured knee [216]. Immediate post knee injury evaluation showed increased sf-levels of aggrecan and COMP fragments, MMP-3, and TIMP-1, which were also noted to increase in the contralateral uninjured knee but at a level less than in the injured knee. Subsequently, several days post injury, the level of these markers decreased in the injured knee, although they remained unchanged in the uninjured knee. In the chronic phase, the aggrecan fragment levels in the injured knee decreased to less than that in the uninjured knee. These findings indicate that following unilateral knee injury, changes in articular cartilage metabolism occur both in the injured and contralateral, uninjured knees [216]. Another investigation on males who sustained youth (3 to 10 years prior) sport-related intra-articular knee injury showed increased s-COMP levels compared to uninjured matched controls [343]. Also, the COMP fragmentation patterns were distinct between injured and uninjured participants. Post acute ACL injury, an increase in sf COMP level in the injured knee is noted up to 5 years after injury [335]. These results suggests the utility of COMP and its fragmentation pattern as a marker of cartilage injury.

Although serum concentrations of PG are of limited value due to its rapid clearance from the circulatory and lymphatic systems, the s-KS levels significantly increase at an early stage after traumatic knee injury as well as early-stage knee OA [59]. In a study, the sf-levels of cartilage PG fragments were measured from patients with various post-traumatic knee joint lesions (trauma, cruciate ligament tear with or without meniscus tear, meniscus tear only, and CM patellae) at different durations [43]. Compared to the normal (control) population, patients with post-traumatic cruciate ligament injuries showed elevated sf-PG levels. Of particular note, a slightly to moderately elevated level of sf-PGs persisted for as long as 5–7 years after the initial trauma [43]. Elevated levels of sf-PG or its components in the patients with no apparent degenerative cartilage changes could also represent increased metabolism reflecting ongoing repair after trauma. It appears that high sf-levels of cartilage PG components particularly indicate the active phases of cartilage metabolism or of active matrix depletion.

The increased levels of sf-C2C along with other injury-related biomarkers during the acute phase after knee injury indicate an immediate and sustained local degradation of collagen type II [113]. Acutely injured knees with an OC fracture, particularly fractures with disrupted cortical bone, have higher concentrations of bone markers and cytokines than do knees without an OC fracture [157]. In this study, sf was aspirated in 98 individuals (26% women; mean age, 23 years) 1 day after acute knee injury. Analysis of sulfated GAGs, ARGS-aggrecan, COMP, osteocalcin, SPARC, osteopontin, and pro-inflammatory cytokines, including interleukin Il-1β, Il-6, Il-8, and TNF-α, were adjusted for days between injury and sf aspiration, age at injury, and gender. In the acutely injured knees with an OC fracture and disrupted cortical bone, highly significant levels of SPARC, along with Il-8 and TNF-α, have been identified compared with knees without an OC fracture [157]. In another cross-sectional study, the articular cartilage and bone markers as well as pro-inflammatory cytokine levels in sf (aspirated the same day as the injury and, thereafter, at all subsequent time points) from acutely injured knees with hemarthrosis were investigated [58]. The sf-levels of ARGS, SPARC, and pro-inflammatory cytokines (Il-1β, Il-6, Il-8, and TNF-α) were significantly higher in injured knees compared to the knees of age- and gender-matched healthy reference volunteers. The levels of GAGs and ARGS were significantly higher in knees aspirated later than 1 day post injury, whereas the levels of SPARC and cytokines were higher in knees aspirated the same day as the injury and at all time points thereafter [58]. This result suggests that acute knee injury is associated with an instant local biochemical response to the trauma, which stimulates inflammatory activity and potentially affects both articular cartilage and bone.

At thirty-two days (early-stage) post ACL injury, the sf-lubricin level of injured knee was significantly lower when compared to the contralateral, uninjured knee [239]. At this stage of acute injury, the decreased sf-lubricin level showed a significant inverse relationship with TNF-α, Il-1β, and Il-6. The levels of these pro-inflammatory molecules were significantly higher in sf from recently injured knees compared with those that were chronically injured or uninjured. At 12 months post ACL injury, the lubricin levels were comparable in both the injured and uninjured knee. The release of significant amounts of bone sialoprotein into sf in connection with acute joint trauma may be associated with injury to, and active remodeling of, the calcified cartilage-bone interface and subchondral bone suggesting the utility of bone sialoprotein as a marker of calcified cartilage/subchondral injury and remodeling following joint injury [96].

4.4.2 Aging

The knee tissues (articular cartilage, synovium, ligaments, tendons, menisci) undergo substantial age-related morphological, biochemical, physiological, and biomechanical changes that impact their ability to overcome the effects of mechanical stress, injury, and disease. Age-related imbalances in reactive oxygen species (such as, superoxide, hydrogen peroxide, the reactive nitrogen species nitric oxide, and the nitric oxide derived product peroxynitrite) production relative to the anti-oxidant capacity of chondrocytes have been shown to play a role in cartilage degradation as well as chondrocyte cell death [344]. Aging in articular cartilage adversely affects cartilage biomechanical properties by altering chondrocyte deformation behavior in cartilage and increasing stiffness of both the chondrocytes and ECM [205, 206, 209, 284, 345–348]. Aging also tends to produce some condensation of collagen network without focal increased fibrillar collagen formation. Age-related changes in articular cartilage ECM includes atrophy (reduced cartilage thickness), proteolysis, advanced glycation, and calcification, whereas cellular changes include reduced cell density and focal loss of chondrocytes, senescence, impaired defense mechanism, and decreased anabolic responses [5]. An age-associated decrease in HA concentration and quality (varying HA molecular weight) is reported in the knee sf of non-OA volunteers (23–91 years) and age-matched cadaver knees [75]. In a population-based study, u-CTX-II level strongly correlated with the knee OA severity in older women (> 60 years) [104]. Aging of articular cartilage is associated with altered TGF-β signaling, which has been identified as a causal factor of cartilage degeneration in knee OA [349]. Over a period of 3 years in older adults, the increased s-levels of Il-6 and TNF-α were associated with knee articular cartilage loss and worsening knee pain [253, 350]. During a 15-year follow-up of a cohort of healthy, middle-aged British women, the BMI and s-levels of CRP and Il-6 were consistently and significantly higher in individuals diagnosed as having radiographic knee OA [254]. These results suggest that Il-6 could be a potential therapeutic target to slow down the initiation or progression of diseases such as OA that are related to cartilage metabolic upregulation. In women, s-C2C level has been shown to decrease with age [112].

Pentosidine levels in sf, serum, and urine are used as an established surrogate marker of advanced glycation end products (AGEs) that accumulate in cartilage matrix with increasing age and also detected in patients with knee OA [337]. The accumulation of AGEs reduces chondrocyte-mediated ECM turnover in human articular cartilage [202]. AGEs are known to induce crosslinking of collagens, resulting in cartilage ECM stiffening. In vitro glycation through ribose treatment of OC explants has shown to decrease chondrocyte volume deformation responses in the upper zones, transmit mechanical forces deeper into the tissue, and increase cell deformation responses in the deeper zones [201]. This finding provides insight on how glycation, such as formation of pentosidine crosslinks during aging, can alter chondrocyte deformation behavior and biomechanical responses in articular cartilage.

4.4.3 Disease

In routine clinical practices, early diagnosis, recognition, and therapeutic intervention in knee diseases are the key to halt or slow down the progression of disease. In conjunction with biomarkers, the use of cartilage and knee-specific imaging procedures (ultrasound and MRI) has the potential to identify at-risk patients and those with early disease.

Investigation of the knee lavage concentrations of MMP-1, MMP-3, and TIMP-1 as well as PLA2 of patients with CM patella showed elevated levels in advanced (grade IV) CM compared with controls, and the MMP-1 levels correlated with the severity of CM [60]. While lavage fluid KS concentration was elevated in CM stage I, the s-KS was higher in CM stage IV than in controls [60]. The changes in the release and activity of these marker molecules from serum and sf reflect changes in the metabolism of articular cartilage and synovium in CM. Increased s-levels of COMP have also been reported in CM patients [137].

Increased serum and sf-levels of COMP and YLK-40 have been reported in patients with both inflammatory and degenerative joint disease [134, 139, 153, 154]. These findings suggest that YLK-40 may reflect aspects of joint destruction in addition to inflammation [148]. YLK-40 concentrations were about 2.5-fold greater in the serum of patients with inflammatory or degenerative joint disease compared to healthy adults. The sf-YLK-40 concentrations were 10- to 15-fold higher than in serum suggesting that in the patients with joint disease, most of the YLK-40 found in the serum may be produced in the joint [150–152]. Since collagen type II is essentially unique to cartilage, sf-PIICP levels reflect the synthetic activity of collagen type II of chondrocytes in the diseased joint. MMPs and ADAMTSs have been implicated in the pathology of knee articular cartilage in RA and OA through the action of these enzymes to degrade ECM macromolecules and modulate factors governing cell behavior [294].

4.4.3.1 Rheumatoid Arthritis

Rheumatoid arthritis is a chronic autoimmune disease affecting the knee joint in which chronic inflammation in the synovium is the primary tissue target. The autoimmune process in RA depends on the activation of immune cells, which use intracellular kinases to respond to external stimuli such as cytokines, immune complexes, and antigens [351]. A complex network of cytokines is involved with the inflammatory process and in perpetuation of RA through a positive feedback system to promote a systemic disorder of connective tissues. This inflammatory process is characterized by infiltration of inflammatory cytokines (such as Il-1β and TNF-α) into the joints which in turn stimulates the production of MMPs and aggrecanases (ADAMTSs), both involved in the articular cartilage degradation in RA. The biochemical markers of cytokine-mediated inflammatory processes in RA include the products of the metabolic changes in cartilage and bone. The sf-hyaluronidase activity is elevated in RA patients and has been reported to be significantly higher than the OA group [84]. MMP-3 and TIMP-1 levels in sf are elevated in RA [64]. Increased s-PLA2 levels have been reported in RA patients [352]. MMP-13 collagenase activity cleaves collagen type II; whereas, ADAMTS-1, ADAMTS-4, and ADAMTS-5 have aggrecanase activity which cleaves the aggrecan [87]. Patients with early RA and psoriatic arthritis (PsA) have shown higher sf-TNF-α levels than patients with OA. Further, higher sf-Il-17 levels were seen in PsA than RA patients [252]. Serum adiponectin level is associated with early radiographic RA progression in early RA, independent of RA-confounding factors and metabolic status [268]. Dependent on RA duration, a significantly higher s-visfatin level was found in RA patients with radiographic articular cartilage and synovium lesions compared to patients without lesion [317].

Patients with knee RA have shown decreased s-PIIANP by 35% compared to controls, suggesting decreased collagen type IIA synthesis [353]. Synovial fluid obtained from the knees of 63 RA patients showed reduction in C2C level compared with OA patients and controls [63]. Various studies evaluating COMP levels in patients with early and established RA have shown significant correlation with RA activity [139, 217]. The s-COMP levels have been shown to significantly increase in RA patients compared to the controls, which also correlated significantly with RA activity and duration [139]. An elevated sf-COMP level is reported in the early stage of RA, whereas in advanced stages of RA, the level of COMP decreased. Serum COMP level in RA patients correlated with the age of patients and disease activity score but was found to be independent of the stage of disease, number of painful and swollen joints, duration of morning stiffness, and disease duration [354]. In patients with active RA, a significant association of serum and sf-levels of YKL-40, s-Il-1β and s-TNF-α has been reported [149]. A decreased YLK-40 value from baseline levels in patients treated with disease-modifying antirheumatic drug therapy was found to reflect the clinical improvement observed in responders, whereas the value was maintained or increased in nonresponders [355]. Significantly elevated levels of Pyd were reported in the urine of OA and RA patients, and the Pyd level correlated with disease activity in RA patients [356, 357]. Urinary excretion of collagen crosslinks, expressed as the Pyr/Dpyr ratio, correlates with those in synovial tissue which functions as a marker of collagen degradation [121].

4.4.3.2 Osteoarthritis

Osteoarthritis affects the knee with varying degree of active, progressive degradative and reparative / regenerative changes in the articular cartilage and subchondral bone. The degenerative component include deep cleft formation and branched clefts, whereas the reparative component constitute focal increases in fibrillar collagen (microscars) within the cartilage ECM. These changes are not noted in aging by itself. Metabolic changes may occur early in OA development, long before the appearance of clinical symptoms and morphological changes. The degradation of the perifibrillar adapter proteins (mainly, collagen type IX, decorin, COMP, and matrilin-3), which are important for the stabilization of the collagen network in the cartilage superficial zone, have been thought to be a critical event in early OA [358]. As objectively measureable indicators of the pathophysiology of knee OA, molecular biomarkers have the potential to improve knee OA diagnosis, staging, and prognosis through its ability to evaluate prearthritic articular cartilage metabolic changes and integrity, monitor OA onset and progression, and assess articular cartilage matrix metabolism in drug development [29, 359, 360].

The progression of OA can be described by three stages [28]. The first stage involves disruption of chondrocyte metabolism leading to increased secretion of degradation enzymes, such as collagenases and aggrecanases that initiate the proteolytic breakdown of articular cartilage ECM. This is followed by a release of PG and collagen fragments as breakdown products into the sf, which contributes to articular cartilage surface fibrillations and erosions. The last stage involves the phagocytosis of the breakdown products by synovial cells resulting in synovial inflammation as well as production and secretion of inflammatory cytokines and proteases into the joint space. These pro-inflammatory molecules further enhance the catabolic effect on chondrocyte metabolism by decreasing PG and collagen synthesis and upregulating the degradative proteases. Structural changes in the OA articular cartilage are seen in Figs. 4.3, 4.4, and 4.5.

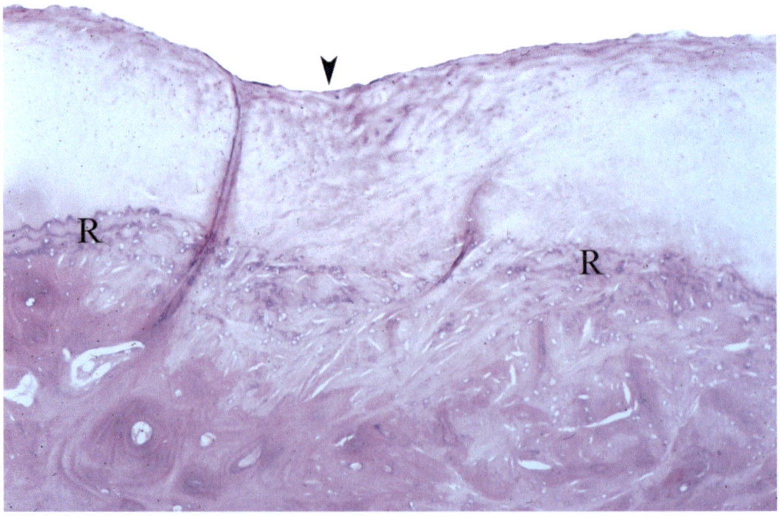

Fig. 4.3 Histological photomicrograph showing mild osteoarthritis of the femoral condyle. Note the disorganization of the articular cartilage extracellular matrix (arrow head), replication of tidemark (R), and subchondral sclerosis seen as thickening of subchondral bone (Toluidine Blue, magnification 5x)

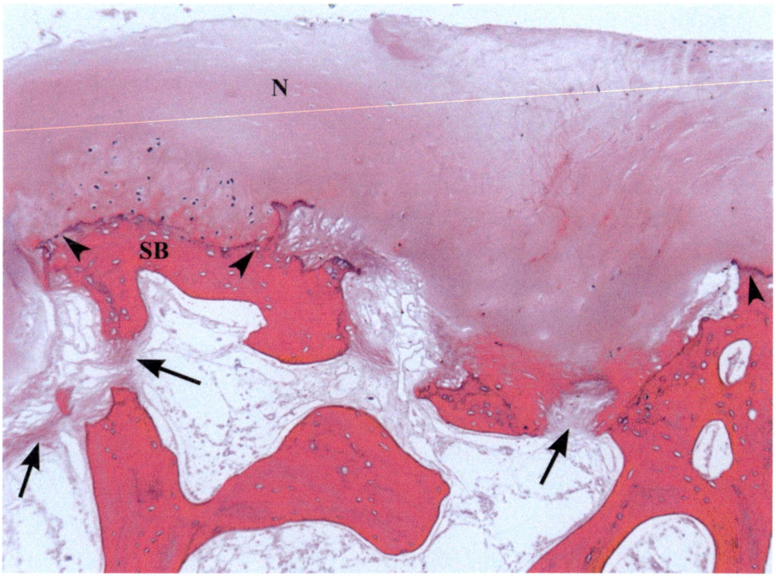

Fig. 4.4 Histological photomicrograph showing moderate osteoarthritis of the femoral condyle. Note the chondrocyte necrosis (N), disorganization of the cartilage extracellular matrix, duplication of tidemark (arrow heads), new bone formation in the subchondral plate, and subjacent reparative soft tissue (arrows) (Hematoxylin and Eosin, magnification 5×)

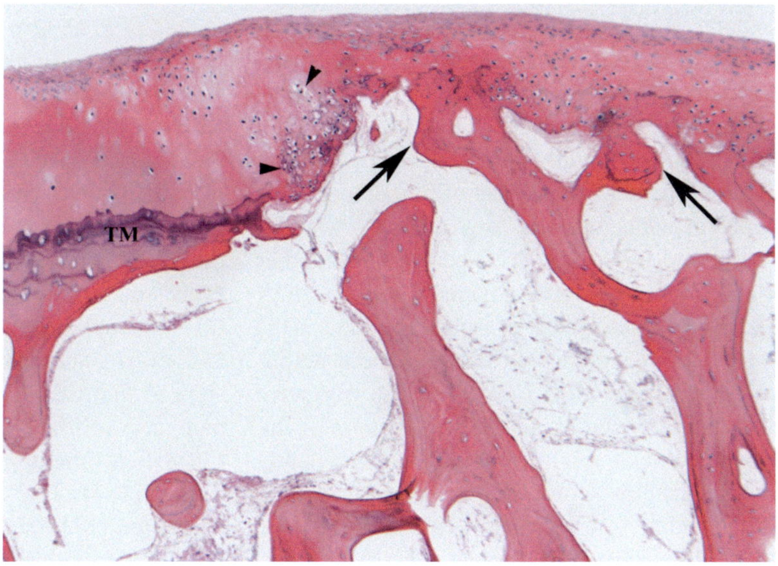

Fig. 4.5 Histological photomicrograph showing severe osteoarthritis of the femoral condyle. Note the thinning of articular cartilage, reparative fibrocartilage (arrowheads), tidemark (TM) reduplication, and osteophytes (arrows) (Hematoxylin and Eosin, magnification 5x)

The biomarkers used to monitor knee OA include five clusters of related markers: *cartilage anabolism markers* (PIICP, PIIANP, HA, epitope 846), *cartilage catabolism markers* (KS, COMP), *inflammation markers* (C-reactive protein, TNF receptor type I and type II, Il-6, eosinophilic cationic protein), *bone markers* (bone sialoprotein, Pyd, Dpyd), and *transforming growth factor-beta* [278, 361, 362].

In 43 patients with knee OA, s-PIIANP was decreased by 53% compared to 88 healthy controls, indicating a marked reduction in collagen type II synthesis [99, 353]. The levels of PIICP were higher in OA and traumatic arthritis than in RA patients [95]. Also, PIICP levels were higher in moderately afflicted OA patients reflecting the chondrocyte synthetic activity of collagen type II in the diseased joint [95]. An increased level of this molecule in the knee correlated well with BMI in primary OA and the degree of cartilage erosion caused by joint instability in traumatic arthritis [64]. C6S and KS were also elevated in

OA and traumatic arthritis joint fluids. The levels of Indian hedgehog homologue (IHH) in articular cartilage and sf-samples were significantly increased in early-stage OA patients compared to normal control [338]. Urinary CTX-II, serum N-terminal telopeptide of collagen type I (s-NTX-I), and s-HA were shown to associate with patients who had both progressive pain and radiographic progression of knee OA [104, 180].

Baseline soluble leptin receptor is associated with reduced levels of PIIANP, an increased cartilage defects score, and increased cartilage volume loss over 2 years in patients with knee OA [225, 309]. Knee OA patients with sarcopenic obesity (obesity with decreased muscle mass) demonstrated significantly higher s-leptin levels than those with non-sarcopenic obesity [363]. In addition, knee OA patients with sarcopenic obesity displayed poor physical performance. Serum samples of obese OA patients have shown much higher acid concentration and oxidative stress agents compared to non-obese OA patients, suggesting that obesity causes oxidative stress and acidosis in obese OA patients [364]. A recent study evaluated the s-levels of adipokines (adiponectin with high and low molecular weight, leptin, and resistin), C2C, and ghrelin together with body composition in patients with knee OA and sex-matched healthy subjects [271]. This study showed significant elevation in total adiponectin level in women with severe OA who were also characterized by a significant excess of fat, compared with the control group. In a study using Lysholm scores and International Knee Documentation Committee (IKDC) subjective scores to evaluate the clinical severity in post-traumatic OA patients, the sf-ghrelin levels of patients with grade-3 OA were significantly decreased compared with grade-2 OA patients [341]. Also, the ghrelin levels were inversely associated with the levels of inflammatory (Il-6 and TNF-α) and degradation (COMP and CTX-II) biomarkers [341]. For patients with symptomatic knee OA, s-levels of resistin were positively and independently associated with cartilage defects and bone marrow lesions, whereas s-Il-17 was significantly associated with both conditions [260]. Further, concentration sf-visfatin has been shown to be significantly greater in patients with knee OA compared to control subjects. Patients with severe knee OA have shown a significant increase in visfatin levels, which also positively correlated with articular cartilage degradation markers of collagen type II (CTX-II) and of aggrecan (AGG1 and AGG2) [282].

Strong evidence in the literature indicates that u-CTX-II and s-COMP are the most consistently associated biomarkers with the presence, incidence, and progression of knee OA [180, 181]. However, one study reported that although u-CTX-II and s-COMP were positively associated with the presence and progression of knee OA, both biomarkers were negatively associated with the incidence of OA [180]. The authors speculated that low levels of cartilage and subchondral bone turnover in the earliest phases of knee OA may explain this latter finding. However, another study reported u-CTX-II as a prognostic marker for knee OA progression with s-COMP level as prognostic marker for incidence of knee OA [181]. The s-COMP levels of patients with confirmed clinical isolated knee OA have been shown to positively correlate with the patient age, BMI, pain score, and Il-1β [135]. Elevated serum and u-levels of COMP and CTX-II are shown to be associated with increased OA severity and body size [184]. Also, this study showed that COMP levels were associated with pain and stiffness but not functioning, while CTX-II elevations were associated with stiffness scores [184]. HA and COMP concentrations were found to be significantly higher in the knee OA patients with early signs of cartilage damage suggesting its utility to predict early cartilage lesions in the knee [365]. However, in another study, the s-HA and -COMP levels were significantly higher in patients with larger amount of effusion and/or synovial proliferation (indicative of inflammatory changes and severe OA) than patients with early-stage OA [366]. It has been shown that TNF receptor type II, COMP, and epitope 846 discriminate OA patients from controls [361]. Further, patients with knee OA showed s-YKL-40 levels that were positively related to symptomatic severity determined using Western Ontario and McMaster Universities Osteoarthritis Index (WOMAC) scores for pain and physical disability as well as OA severity [153, 154]. The risk of pre-radiographic OA (ROA) versus no OA controls increased with elevated u-C2C levels, whereas the risk of ROA versus no OA increased with elevated levels of u-CTX-II and u-C2C, and the risk reduced with elevated s-PIICP levels. Further, this study reported that the ratios of collagen type II degradation markers to collagen synthesis markers were better able to differentiate the stage of OA compared with levels of an individual marker [111]. This finding was corroborated by another study that showed a greater s-level of C2C and PIICP ratio associated with an increased progression of OA [367]. The elevated levels of u-CTX-II in patients with severe knee OA was supported in another study [188].

Aggrecanase cleaved fragments of aggrecan have been detected in the serum and urine of OA patients [82]. Several MMPs, namely, MMP-1, MMP-3, MMP-9, and MMP-13, have been shown to play important roles in the degradation of articular cartilage in OA joints [294]. The decreased sf-MMP-1 levels in OA patients reflected the severity of OA (negative correlation) and perhaps the integrity of the SZ of articular cartilage [242]. Synovial fluid obtained from OA patients undergoing TKA showed significant high levels of Il-1β, MMP-1, and MMP-3 compared to healthy controls [248]. Elevated serum and sf-levels of MMP-1, MMP-3, and MMP-13 have been reported to distinguish knee OA with varying degrees of articular cartilage degradation from healthy knee [248, 265, 368]. Further, at the late-stage knee OA (grade 3 and 4), elevated levels of serum and sf-MMP-13 and -TNF-α as well as sf-PLA2 have also been reported [245, 265]. In this study the elevated MMP-13 levels significantly correlated with the WOMAC scores. However, one study reported a negative correlation between sf-MMP-1 and severity of OA, which may have been caused due to degradation of the various cartilage zones starting from the SZ during the progression of OA [242]. High-activity PLA2 (pro-inflammatory) levels have been reported in the sf of patients with knee OA [245]. At early stages of OA, s-ADAMTS-4 levels are significantly higher compared to intermediate or severe-stage OA and healthy controls, whereas in the intermediate and severe OA patients, the s-levels of ADAMTS-5, MMP-1, and MMP-3 were significantly higher than those in early-stage OA patients and healthy controls [250]. This result suggests s-ADAMTS-4 is a potential indicator for the diagnosis of OA at an early stage. Overall, the combination of biochemical assessment of PG fragments, COMP, and MMPs (MMP-1, MMP-3, and MMP-13) and the balance between MMP-3 and its inhibitor (TIMP) in sf appear to be good indicators of joint tissue damage in the early and later stages of OA. OARSI published a set of recommendations for the use of soluble biomarkers that included knee sf-levels of ADAMTS-4 and aggrecan ARGS neoepitope fragments as well as plasma chemokine (CeC motif) ligand 3 (CCL3) as novel biomarkers of OA [29, 369].

Cytokines (Il-1α, Il-4, Il-6, Il-15, Il-18, and TNF-α) in the plasma and knee sf have been associated with the level of OA severity, whereas baseline Il-18 is linked with the prediction of OA progression [28, 257, 261, 304, 305]. Serum levels of Il-6 and TNF-α have also been associated with the increased prevalence of tibial plateau space narrowing and prediction of knee cartilage volume loss [253]. Among early-stage knee OA patients, elevated levels of s-Il-15 have been reported compared to late-stage OA, which is also associated with the Il-6 levels [305]. Il-18 levels are significantly increased in the plasma, sf, and articular cartilage of patients with primary knee OA patients compared to volunteers, and these elevated levels were positively correlated with radiographic severity [261]. In OA patients, the sf-level of CCL2 was shown to independently and positively associate with self-reported greater pain and physical disability suggesting the utility of this biomarker for assessing symptomatic severity of OA [342]. The elevated serum and sf-CCL 13 levels in patients with knee OA also significantly correlated with the radiographic OA severity evaluated by KL grading system [370]. Chemokine interferon gamma inducible protein 10 (CXCL-10) in plasma and sf have shown to be inversely associated with radiographic knee OA, whereas high levels of sf-CXCL-12 were associated with radiographic severity of OA evaluated using KL grading system [249, 371]. Fractalkine (CX3CL-1) in knee sf and serum has been reported to significantly increase in patients with knee OA, and both levels are significantly associated with the OA severity evaluated by KL grading system and also positively associated with self-evaluated greater pain and physical disability assessed using WOMAC index [372, 373].

Significant increases in serum and sf-pentosidine levels have been reported in patients with OA, which also correlated with increased sf-COMP level [129]. Although aging-associated changes in articular cartilage ECM and chondrocytes are known as important causative factors in OA, a report in human knees has shown an inverse relation between pentosidine and cartilage degradation in late-stage OA [132]. Further, findings in the Hartley guinea pig model of spontaneous knee OA showed that AGEs accumulation due to intra-articular ribose-containing injections did not enhance disease progression [374]. These results suggest that pentosidine is a marker of joint aging but not specifically of knee OA.

4.5 Postsurgery Changes in Knee Synovial Fluid Biochemical Markers

Arthroscopic surgery (AS) of the knee is a minimally invasive surgical procedure which involves examination of the knee structures and sometimes treatment of knee damage. It is performed using an arthroscope, which is inserted into the knee through a small incision to allow lavage to remove abnormalities such as cartilage fragments and calcium crystals, and debridement to surgically remove degenerated cartilage, leaving a stable edge and a smooth articular surface, and to excise osteophytes. Synovial fluid biomarkers have the capacity to reflect the intra-articular environment before surgery and potentially predict postoperative clinical outcomes [247]. KS is found mostly exclusively in articular cartilage, whereas CS and specifically C4S predominate in other knee tissues such as synovium, meniscus, and ligaments [375, 376]. Therefore, increases in s-KS levels in OA patients are primarily attributed to enhanced cartilage degradation in affected knees [377].

In a study, the temporal changes in sf-levels of C4S, C6S, and KS associated with cartilage metabolism were investigated post AS [378]. Fluid from 25 knees (n = 24 patients) was obtained immediately before surgery and after AS at 2, 4, 8, and 12 weeks. The KS level decreased significantly at 2 weeks after AS, whereas C6S, C4S, and total CS levels did not change. Further, a strong, positive correlation was detected between C6S and KS levels at 12 weeks. These results suggest suppressed cartilage metabolism post AS. Two years following AS, seven patients required either total or unicompartmental knee arthroplasties.

Surgical interventions to repair a cartilage lesion can cause increased levels of anabolic and catabolic factors. A study investigated MMP-3 and IGF-I concentrations before autologous chondrocyte transplantation of the knee and after cartilage repair [379]. Synovial fluid samples were collected from 10 patients before and 1 year post the repair procedure. The control group comprised of 15 patients undergoing knee arthroscopy for various symptoms but without apparent cartilage lesions. Before repair procedure, both MMP-3 and IGF-I were higher in patients having cartilage lesions than in control subjects with no cartilage lesions. The elevated levels for both MMP-3 and IGF-1 persisted 1 year post cartilage repair, and arthroscopic evaluation showed the lesions were filled with repair tissue. However, the levels of MMP-3 and IGF-I remained elevated, indicating either graft remodeling or early degeneration [379]. In another study, 49 OA patients with end-stage knee or hip OA who underwent joint replacement surgery showed elevated sf-Il-6 levels (N = 8 patients), indicative of a pro-inflammatory response to postsurgical procedure [380].

Inflammatory cytokines and cartilage degradation biomarkers are elevated at the time of acute knee injury and postoperatively. These biomarkers can be elevated in the sf several years after reconstruction of the anterior cruciate ligament (ACL), indicating an ongoing homeostatic imbalance between ECM destruction and repair. This suggests that patients who sustain ACL rupture are at increased risk to develop post-traumatic arthritis (PTA) in the injured knee whether the ACL is reconstructed or treated nonoperatively. One mechanism for PTA may be an inflammatory degradative process initiated on the acute injury that is sustained for some period of time independent of whether adequate joint stability is restored. In a cohort of 11 patients who had undergone ACL reconstruction 8 years earlier, knee sf was aspirated from the operated knee and the contralateral nonoperated knee to evaluate levels of inflammatory cytokines and cartilage degradative markers [381]. At follow-up, the patients underwent bilateral weight-bearing radiographs and bilateral MRIs of their knees. The sf concentrations of Il-1β, Il-6, TNF-α, GAGs, ARGS-aggrecan, or COMP did not show significant differences between the operated and the contralateral knee. However, significant radiographically visible OA lesions were observed in the operated knees compared with the contralateral knees. MRIs revealed that all grafts and all contralateral ACLs were intact and confirmed that there was significantly more meniscal and cartilage damage in the operated knees than the contralateral knees. The limitation of this study is the lack of baseline levels of the biomarkers used post the repair procedure for comparison. Further, unilateral knee injury is reported to affect the sf concentrations of several biomarkers in the contralateral uninjured knee of the same patient [216]. This might explain the reason why even though there were significant OA changes, meniscal and cartilage damage in the operated knee, as seen on weight-bearing radiographs and MRI, there were no significant differences in biomarker levels between the nonoperated and the ACL-reconstructed knee.

These studies highlight the clinical utility of biomarkers in assessing the structural integrity and cartilage metabolism of injured and reparative tissue before and after cartilage repair procedure as well as at follow-up.

4.6 Limitations of Cartilage Biochemical Markers

Identification of appropriate biological markers for disease activity in OA or other types of arthritis is a challenging and complex endeavor. While some limitations may be related to the assay itself, type of assay, and reproducibility of the technique used, others may be related to environmental conditions such as food intake, physical activity, and circadian rhythms [172]. All these conditions must be verified before the use of an assay in clinical study. Further, analysis of the level of articular cartilage-specific biochemical markers should be taken into consideration and be adjusted for several confounding factors such as age, gender, BMI, and bone status for markers of bone turnover. The presence of other knee tissue lesions or disease as well as presence of severe kidney or liver disease could distort the interpretation of a biomarker value.

To date, several markers have been used in clinical and animal studies either by themselves or in combination. However, only a few studies specify the stage (severity level) of the disease. Lack of the specification of the stage of disease can result in the misinterpretation of data because the level of joint markers could vary depending on the stage of the disease. Although markers of knee articular cartilage degradation have been evaluated, the clinical utility of these markers can be limited due to the anatomic location of the degradation which could either arise from a focal area of cartilage with severe degradation or from a larger area with very mild degradation.

Several factors including variations in the immunochemical reactivity, the possible presence of degradation fragments of non cartilage tissues in serum, and the dependence of vitamin K status for adequate enzymatic carboxylation may complicate the result interpretation of biochemical markers of articular cartilage. During the early-stage of cartilage lesions in disease, sensitive serum or urinary indices for cartilage metabolism and, importantly, development of more specific markers are required to identify and differentiate articular cartilage reparative response and cartilage remodeling.

Several PG cleavage products and enzyme activities reflect formation as well as degradation of cartilage. Clinical studies have demonstrated that the concentration of s-KS epitope and -HA are on average higher in OA patients than in normal group [377, 382, 383]. The increased level of KS was associated with cartilage destruction or response to acute injury. However, the overlap between healthy and diseased individuals was almost complete [18]. The large range of normal values and small, if any, changes with disease combine to make a single observation of little diagnostic use. For example, the values in the upper range of normal may reflect high metabolic turnover or could actually reflect degenerative joint disease. Substantial interindividual variability was observed in the increase of KS level, which was consistently higher in the OA patients. KS is also present in the aorta and cornea; therefore, it is not a cartilage-specific molecule. Further, increased s-KS levels did not reflect the cartilage histological changes. Some animal studies also indicate that s-KS is not a reliable marker for the activity of OA [384]. Although HA has been documented among the best candidates as markers for cartilage metabolism, HA is more a marker of synovial membrane hyperplasia and hyperactivity rather than that of cartilage per se. Thus, determining the concentrations of s-KS epitope and -HA as reliable markers for the diagnostic test for OA cartilage damage seems to be presently of limited value.

In OA patients, COMP is modified only in the presence of substantial and sustained local overproduction. Also, neither plasma nor serum levels of CMG have been found to reflect the extent of cartilage degradation. YLK-40 has been identified in human synovial fibroblasts, and YLK-40 mRNA is expressed strongly in chondrocytes and liver. YLK-40 is weakly expressed in the brain, kidney, and placenta and in small amounts in the heart, lungs, skeletal muscle, pancreas, mononuclear cells, and skin fibroblasts. Although an increased serum and sf-YLK-40 level in patients with OA has been reported, suggesting that YLK-40 may be a useful marker for assessing articular cartilage degradation, it is not cartilage specific.

Assessment of the urinary and sf concentrations of Pyd crosslinks in RA and OA patients showed that u-Pyd and Dpyd levels were significantly greater in RA than in OA patients [124]. The sf from both groups showed only relatively small amounts of Pyd. This is indicative of either a flaw in the experimental design or in the tissue processing, or alternatively it could support the hypothesis of an extraskeletal origin of Pyd in chronic joint diseases. Although Pyd crosslinks have been extensively used as markers of bone resorption, inconsistency in the published results question their utility as bone-specific resorption markers. Crosslink levels in knee articular cartilage of partially meniscectomized rabbits were compared with those occurring during aging. The total Pyd content did not change with age or OA, a result which does not corroborate the previous findings. The total pentosidine concentration, as expected, increased significantly with age but remained constant with OA [207]. Although the Pyd/Dpyd ratio is used as a marker to distinguish between destruction of cartilage and bone collagen, the usefulness of Pyd/Dpyd ratio is questionable based on a study that reported a discrepancy in this ratio in urine and serum samples of 38 RA patients [120]. A correlation between serum and u-level was demonstrable for Pyd, but not for Dpyd. Since bone metabolizes at a higher rate than articular cartilage, crosslink levels from urine or serum samples generally reflect bone metabolism. Further, a great variability between the urinary crosslinks and the clinical activity has been reported [198]. Pyd and Dpyd are products of collagen turnover from the bone, cartilage, tendon, and ligament. It is difficult to distinguish between Pyd and Dpyd of collagen type I (mostly bone derived) and collagen type II (cartilage specific). Pyd levels but not the Dpyd were significantly elevated in the patients with active inflammatory disease and strongly correlated with the inflammatory activity. An accurate quantitative marker of bone and cartilage breakdown should be used as a tool for monitoring disease activity in OA, RA, and possibly in other joint diseases.

In view of the above concerns, what values do current biochemical markers have for clinical utility? For individuals, selected markers can be used as indices of response to either cartilage or bone disease-modifying strategies. These markers tend to change more rapidly than imaging and so can be useful for monitoring therapy.

A biochemical marker, which primarily reflects cartilage metabolism, would be useful for assessing the stage of disease and in evaluating new therapeutic regimens. An ideal cartilage biochemical marker should be sensitive to change in cartilage structure and/or biochemistry and would reflect disease progression over time. To obtain accurate and reliable results, levels of the marker should be correlated with the severity of the joint disease. Tissue sample or tissue fluid sample, and the sensitivity and accuracy of technique used for processing plays a crucial role in the result outcome. For example, extensive analytical preparation of urine samples could lead to substantial loss of the marker hence inconsistency in the results.

An ideal set of biological markers would distinguish and measure arthritis activity and progression. Most importantly, an ideal biomarker would be sensitive and specific to identify the early-stage of joint disease. To date, an ideal marker for cartilage metabolism and destruction is still not available. Currently available biochemical markers for the detection of degradation processes of cartilage are largely non-specific. Further studies should be directed toward defining the biological and pathological profiles that are capable of distinguishing cartilage lesions from those of bone and synovium. Also these studies should be able to separate cartilage catabolic from anabolic activity as well as determine and/or monitor the extent and stage of the cartilaginous lesions.

4.7 Biochemical Markers During Dynamic Loading

The unique biological and mechanical properties of articular cartilage depend on its complex 3D architecture and the interactions of its biochemical constituents, mainly water, electrolytes, collagen, and PGs as well as the interactions between the ECM molecules and the chondrocytes [9, 385, 386]. Biomarker response to knee loading assesses function as a measure of holistic joint health. Post knee injury, gradual return to physical activity enables the joint tissue to adapt to load, and biomarker responses to physical activity may be monitored to determine appropriate level of loading for return to activity. In response to several activities, changes in sf bone and cartilage biomarkers occur, and are influenced by variables such as body weight, load, and duration of activity [326]. Within the normal physiologic range of pressure, the cartilage matrix is intrinsically incompressible when loaded [387]. Studies using OA induced animal models reported that the physiological level of mechanical loading regulates and effectively manages increases in cartilage chondrocyte endoplasmic reticulum stress and autophagy, which in turn has the potential to delay the onset of OA and to mitigate OA symptoms [388, 389]. While mild/moderate mechanical loading is necessary for maintaining healthy knee articular cartilage and subchondral bone, abnormal physiological knee loading, including disuse and overuse, increases the risk of cartilage injury, degeneration and OA [390–392]. Mechanical impact force can induce simple fibrillations (no branching) in aging or OA cartilage, which often extends deep to superficial cartilage as clefts. The mechanical changes of degenerated human cartilage include decreased stiffness in compression, tension, and shear, as well as increased permeability to fluid flow [393, 394]. In vitro experiments have shown that both static and dynamic compressive stress decreases PG biosynthesis (range 25–85%), and this inhibition is proportional to the applied stress but independent of loading time [395].

Mechanical forces have great influence on the synthesis and rate of turnover of articular cartilage molecules [396, 397]. The chondrocyte interactions with ECM are one of the key events in the mechanotransduction of chondrocytes [9, 398]. Several in vitro studies using cartilage or OC explants investigated the effects of load magnitude, frequency, and duration on the macromolecular biosynthesis, loss, and structural deformation as well as chondrocyte viability

[399–401]. Regular cyclic loading of the joint enhances PG synthesis and augments cartilage stiffness. The results from these studies confirm that an increased duration and intensity of loading stimulated the inhibition of PG biosynthesis, while PG loss is only modulated by increasing the magnitude and duration of loading.

In response to physical activities and knee loading, investigation of the changes in the levels of key biomarkers in the body fluids could provide an important information regarding patients with knees that are failing to adapt to a given loading stimulus. In an in vitro experiment, the enhanced expression of COMP was found to be sensitive to long-term cyclic compression of calf articular cartilage explants [402]. In young healthy adults, load-induced increases in sCOMP was reported with increasing ambulatory load magnitude, indicating a dose-response relationship between ambulatory load magnitude and load-induced changes in sCOMP [403]. During physical exercise as well as recreational and competitive sports, an increased s-COMP level is associated with acute effects on the deformational behavior of knee articular cartilage, which may be attributed to the impact of loading [327, 328, 404]. Also, among patients with medial compartment knee OA, an increase in s-COMP levels by the mechanical stimulus of daily 30-min walking activity revealed thinning of articular cartilage at a 5-year follow-up (visualized with MRI), suggesting the utility of COMP as a mechano-sensitive biomarker [219]. However, one must appreciate that the compromised integrity of OA articular cartilage relative to a healthy articular cartilage may have contributed to the observed cartilage thinning.

Depending on the local mechanical demands on the healthy knee articular cartilage, MMPs play an important role in regulating the cartilage homeostasis. In response to mechanical pressure, loading of healthy articular cartilage reduced MMP-1 and MMP-3 synthesis [405]. However, this homeostatic regulation is compromised in injured and diseased cartilage, which results in increased sf-MMP-1, MMP-2, and Il-β [60, 241, 248].

Thinning of articular cartilage increases the cartilage shear stresses, particularly within the deep zone (DZ), and this is associated with tidemark advancement and reduplication, thickening of the zone of calcified cartilage (ZCC), and subchondral bone sclerosis. These events are associated with the attempt of articular cartilage and bone to repair in response to the injury. Furthermore, tensile stress occurs at the articular surface and in regions close to the cartilage-bone interface [406]. This stress on cartilage surface may initiate the fibrillation and fissures noted in diseased articular cartilage [407]. The sf-PIICP levels from 65 patients radiologically diagnosed with primary early OA of the knee correlated with mechanical risk factors, namely, obesity (BMI) and varus alignment (lateral femorotibial angle) [91]. This finding was confirmed by another study that reported PIICP evaluation is sensitive in the evaluation of risk factors of OA, which includes obesity and joint instability [64]. This finding suggests that altered mechanical stress due to obesity and varus alignment enhanced the chondrocytic synthesis of collagen type II. A study demonstrated that in vivo loading during walking, which is consistent with cartilage water exudation and an increase in sf-PG concentration, correlated with decreased MRI T1rho relaxation times, which corroborated in-vitro experiments as well [408, 409]. These findings suggest that combining cartilage MR imaging and sf biomarkers can provide a noninvasive tool for characterizing changes in the biochemical and biomechanical environment of the joint.

4.7.1 Superficial Zone Molecules

The process of chondrolysis releases COMP, which was detected in the cartilage SZ. In an ex-vivo experiment, mature bovine cartilage explants were cyclically loaded at 0.5 Hz with 1 and 5 MPa for 1, 6, and 24 h to evaluate cell viability and ECM integrity [410]. Mechanical cyclic loading caused chondrocyte death and PG loss within 6 h starting from the articular surface and increasing in cartilage depth with loading time. A decrease in the 7D4 epitope (native CS) in the SZ of cartilage loaded for longer than 1 h was noted; but, in the DZ, an increase in the 7D4 epitope was noted at the pericellular matrix (PCM) surrounding the chondrocytes [410]. The degraded/abnormal C4S neoepitope appeared only in cartilage loaded under the most severe condition (5 MPa, 24 h). The elevation of MMP-3 was co-localized with fragmented collagen (COL2 -3/4 m) at the SZ in explants loaded with 1 and 5 MPa for 24 h [410]. Following chondronecrosis due to excessive loading, the increase in MMP-3 levels can induce PG depletion and ECM degradation in mechanically injured articular cartilage.

4.7.2 Running

Regular exercise protects against degenerative joint disorders. In a study involving 33 healthy athletes, the level of biomarkers was measured from the sf (aggrecan, MMP-3, TIMP-1, and PIICP) and serum (aggrecan, hyaluronan, and KS) at 24 h before and 30–60 min after running (9 athletes ran on a treadmill for 60 mins and 16 ran on road for 80 min) or playing soccer (8 played the game for 90 mins) [329]. For comparison, sf and serum samples were obtained from a reference group of 28 patients with knee pain but without evidence of joint pathology or injury. All biomarkers measured from the joint fluid samples showed an increasing trend with exercise. Further, all markers except MMP-3 showed lower concentrations in athletes at rest compared to the reference group. The concentration of s-KS from runners before exercise was significantly higher than in both the soccer and reference groups and further increased after exercise [329]. The increased levels of biomarkers after exercise appear to reflect an effect of mechanical loading in combination with a possible high turnover rate of body cartilage matrix in these individuals.

Articular cartilage turnover and load-induced biochemical changes were assessed by evaluating cartilage biomarker levels in serum in a cohort of volunteers (n = 36) participating in multistage ultramarathon running [36]. Blood samples were collected before and at four time points (approximately equal distance) during the 4486-km multistage marathon. Significant elevation in s-COMP, -MMP-9, and -MMP-3 levels were noted throughout the multistage ultramarathon and changes in MMP-3 level positively correlated with those of COMP level [36]. Elevated s-COMP levels among multistage ultramarathon runners indicate COMP turnover in response to extreme running [36]. Further, the association between elevated s-COMP and load-induced increase in MMP-3 suggested the possibility of MMP-3 involvement in the degradation of COMP.

The effect of running on knee intra-articular and circulating markers of inflammation and cartilage turnover was investigated in six healthy recreational runners [404]. Each participant completed a running (30 min) and control (unloaded for 30 min) session in a counterbalanced order. Serum and sf samples were taken before and after each session. The control condition did not change cytokine concentrations. A trend for decreasing Il-15 concentration was noted from pre- to post-run. A decreased s-COMP and an increased sf-COMP was seen in the control condition, while the run state induced an increase in s-COMP and a decrease in sf-COMP. Also, the pre- to post-intervention changes in serum and sf-COMP were inversely related. These results suggest that running decreases knee intra-articular pro-inflammatory cytokine concentration and facilitates the movement of COMP from the joint space to the serum.

4.7.3 Exercise

As a marker of cartilage degradation, COMP is the most frequently investigated biomarker in studies pertaining to response to load and physical activity. In response to physical exercise, acute effects on the deformational behavior of articular cartilage and temporary dose-dependent increase in the concentration of COMP that gradually returns to baseline level are known [326,

327]. The adequate amount and impact of physical exercise to stimulate the functional behavior of articular cartilage was investigated in 44 healthy males (age range 21–32 years) [327]. Their physical-fitness levels were recorded, and serum samples were collected before, immediately after, and half an hour after a 30-min walking exercise at a self-selected pace. Each participant was then assigned for a 12-week duration to one of the following activity groups: running, cycling, swimming, or control. Pre-test measurements showed a significant elevation of s-COMP levels by 5–10% in all groups after 30 min of walking activity, which was also elevated in all post-test groups except running, suggesting that running decreases the deformational effect of walking activity [327]. This finding was confirmed by another study, which aimed to identify walking and running mechanics that are associated with acute changes in s-COMP due to ambulation in 18 healthy volunteers (age range 21–25 years) [411]. The study design included instrumented treadmill on three separate days with each day corresponding to a different ambulation speed: slow (preferred walking speed), medium (+50% of slow), and fast (+100% of slow). Serum samples were collected at pre-, post-, 30-min post-, and 60-min post-ambulation. Serum COMP increased 29%, 18%, and 5% immediately post-ambulation for the fast, medium, and slow sessions showing that elevated s-COMP concentration correlated with increased ambulation speed. Elevated s-COMP levels corresponded to increased load [330, 412]. Self-selected walking on a treadmill with unadjusted body weight caused a 10% increase in COMP, whereas the same walking task with a weighted vest increased COMP concentrations by 22% [412]. Increased intensities, such as walking on an incline, significantly elevated COMP concentration levels in comparison with a walking on a level surface. To investigate the effect of inclined, uphill walk (loading activity) on the serum biomarkers level, healthy participants ($N = 82$) were divided into the experimental ($N = 58$) and control ($N = 24$) groups [330]. While participants of control group walked for 14 km on a horizontal pathway, the participants of experimental group walked for the same distance on an inclined (5.97^{0}) pathway. Serum was collected prior to, immediately after, and 24-h post walking. Immediately after the walk, the s-COMP level of the experimental group was significantly higher than that of the control group demonstrating the association of additional loading on articular cartilage with elevated COMP levels [330].

4.7.4 Sports: Recreational and Competitive

Healthy articular cartilage and joints are essential to maintain athletic performance and general activities. In the maturing athlete, numerous factors affect the knee mechanical function ranging from chondrocyte survival and metabolism, structural composition, age-related changes for joint homeostasis, repetitive knee injury to genetic/epigenetic factors governing articular cartilage, synovium, and other joint tissues. These mature athletes face challenges in maintaining healthy cartilage and joint function due to inevitable age-related changes to articular cartilage biology, morphology, and physiology [413]. The age-related change that impacts the athlete's performance includes chondrocyte necrosis and a decline in its metabolic response, alterations to matrix and synovial tissue composition, and dysregulation of intrinsic reparative responses [413].

Longitudinal changes in biomarkers of knee articular cartilage turnover and their association with patient-rated outcomes over 2 years were investigated in 37 volleyball athletes [22]. Eighteen adolescents (age range: 15–16 years) were in a 2-year intensive volleyball training program and 19 adults (age range 41–50 years) were recreational volleyball players. Among the adolescents, 13 were skeletally immature with open growth plates at baseline, and all but one adolescent had closed growth plates at follow-up as revealed by MRI. Blood and serum samples were taken at baseline and 2-year follow-up. Subjects completed the IKDC Subjective Knee Form and the 36-Item Short-Form Health Survey (SF-36) at baseline. At baseline all adolescents had greater levels of the cartilage degradation-based biomarkers, 45 mer collagenase peptide of collagen type II (C2C-HUSA ELISA kit), and CTX-II than adults.

Baseline open adolescents showed decreased C2C-HUSA, PIICP (collagen synthesis marker), and CTX-II, while adults showed increased cartilage intermediate layer protein 2 (CILP-2) and C2C-HUSA. In adolescents, IKDC scores correlated with PIICP changes, and in adults SF-36 Physical Component Scores correlated with COMP changes. Elevated levels of C2C-HUSA and CTX-II in adolescents compared to adults may reflect increased cartilage turnover in response to higher knee loading. Further, PIICP and COMP positively correlated with the subjective patient outcomes, suggesting the benefit of using these markers in assessing mechanical loading-induced cartilage changes, their associated symptoms, and risk of OA in athletes [22].

A study investigated the longitudinal effect of intense, continuous physical activity on s-COMP levels and patient-reported outcomes (PRO) values in 29 National Collegiate Athletic Association soccer athletes (18 men, 11 women; age range 18–21 years) without a history of severe knee injury at the study phase over the duration of the spring soccer season [328]. The athletes participated in pre-, mid-, and post-season data collection sessions and completed PROs (Lysholm, and IKDC scores) before serum collection at each session. A significant elevation in COMP level was seen at mid- and post-season compared to pre-season as athletes reported (PROs) an increased level of function over time. In a comparable outcome study, s-COMP levels were measured weekly in a group of six female collegiate soccer athletes over the duration of a spring soccer season and 2 weeks following the conclusion of the season [414]. Eleven serum samples were collected on separate occasions: 1 week prior to the start of the season (baseline), once a week during the 8-week season, and once a week for 2 weeks following the conclusion of the season. Minutes of participation were documented following all spring soccer activities for each week. Higher s-COMP levels were reported when the athletes' participation in soccer-related activities was higher. This suggests an association between increased cartilage turnover and increased in physical activity.

Running a marathon causes strenuous joint loading. In a 10-week marathon training program, blood samples were collected from 45 runners of varying BMI and running experience before and after a 10-week marathon training program as well as before, immediately, and 24 h after each marathon race [331]. Serum biomarker concentrations (COMP, TNF-α, Il-6, and high-sensitivity CRP), BMI, and marathon finishing time were measured. BMI did not affect changes in biomarker concentrations, and differences in marathon finishing time explained the variability in changes in s-COMP and -hsCRP during the 24 h recovery after the marathon race. As such, slower marathon finishing time but not a higher BMI modulated increases in pro-inflammatory markers or cartilage markers following a marathon race.

The effect of running a marathon (mean time 3 h) on the levels of adipokines and biomarker indices of cartilage metabolism was investigated in 46 male marathoners [415]. Blood samples were obtained before and after a marathon run to measure levels of MMP-3, COMP, and YKL-40 and plasma concentrations of pro-inflammatory adipokines, namely, adiponectin, leptin, and resistin. Running a marathon more than doubled the MMP-3 levels and increased YKL-40 levels by 56% but had variable effect on COMP and negatively correlated with marathon time. The faster the marathon was run, the greater was the increase in MMP-3 levels. Further, an elevated level of resistin and adiponectin was noted, while leptin levels remained unchanged. The marathon-induced changes in resistin levels positively associated with the changes in MMP-3 and YKL-40, and the pre-marathon resistin levels correlated positively with the marathon-induced change in YKL-40 [415]. These results show the utility of the biomarkers used to study the impact of running a marathon on cartilage metabolism and degradation.

In another study, sixty college student athletes undergoing high-intensity training for diverse types of aerobic sports (crew, cross-country running, and swimming) and 16 non-athlete undergraduate controls participated in a cross-sectional study to investigate the effect of skeletal stresses on cartilage and bone metabolism of athletes involved with aerobic sports training [416]. Urine samples were collected for crosslinked

N-telopeptide (NTx) (bone resorption marker) and CTX-II (cartilage degradation marker). Athletes in training in the three sports revealed significant differences in the markers. NTx and CTX-II showed significant differences between groups before and after adjusting for BMI. NTx was highest in the rowers and was higher in rowers and runners than in swimmers or controls. CTX-II was significantly higher in runners than in crew, swimmers, or controls, when BMI was not adjusted. This study suggests the utility of NTx and CTX-II to reflect differences in skeletal stresses associated with individual strenuous training during various sports and the effect of these stresses on articular cartilage and bone metabolism.

Several factors are involved in the articular cartilage mechanical breakdown including direct lesion to the cartilage structure due to sports or accidental trauma, obesity, excessive repetitive loading of the cartilage, and/or joint immobilization. Although sports activity, without traumatic injury, does not appear to be a risk factor for the cartilage degradation in the normal joint, such activity may have adverse consequences for an abnormal joint in the long-term because it may eventually lead to and even accelerate degradation of articular cartilage. Often resulting from accidents or sports knee injuries, blunt trauma of articular cartilage is associated with local inflammatory reactions and represents a major risk factor for development of post-traumatic OA [333, 385, 417]. Several inflammatory and cartilage biomarkers have been identified in sf soon after trauma [43, 59, 157, 216].

4.8 Conclusions

Biomarkers can be helpful in assessing the status of knee articular cartilage such as homeostasis, injury, and degradation due to disease; however, their use and interpretation require caution and are often far from straightforward. While blood, urine, and synovial fluid analytes as surrogate biomarkers for articular cartilage function currently enjoy limited clinical utility, the need for these markers continues to propel considerable investigative activity. Among the many variables affecting cartilage biomarker levels is the biodynamic load history in the individual. The several avenues toward improving cartilage biomarker clinical utility include more precise definition of cartilage disorders, e.g., osteoarthritis phenotyping, better understanding of analyte metabolism, biomarker assessment under conditions of active load, and algorithms incorporating biodynamic load considerations.

References

1. Goldring MB, Marcu KB. Cartilage homeostasis in health and rheumatic diseases. Arthritis Res Ther. 2009;11:224.
2. Houard X, Goldring MB, Berenbaum F. Homeostatic mechanisms in articular cartilage and role of inflammation in osteoarthritis. Curr Rheumatol Rep. 2013;15:375.
3. Longobardi L, Li T, Tagliafierro L, Temple JD, Willcockson HH, Ye P, Esposito A, Xu F, Spagnoli A. Synovial joints: from development to homeostasis. Curr Osteoporos Rep. 2015;13:41–51.
4. Lories RJ. Joint homeostasis, restoration, and remodeling in osteoarthritis. Best Pract Res Clin Rheumatol. 2008;22:209–20.
5. Lotz M, Loeser RF. Effects of aging on articular cartilage homeostasis. Bone. 2012;51:241–8.
6. Lotz MK, Carames B. Autophagy and cartilage homeostasis mechanisms in joint health, aging and OA. Nat Rev Rheumatol. 2011;7:579–87.
7. Roughley PJ, Nguyen Q, Mort JS, Hughes CE, Caterson B. Proteolytic degradation in human articular cartilage: its relationship to stromelysin. Agents Actions Suppl. 1993;39:149–59.
8. Cicek E. Hydrogen peroxide induced oxidative damage on mechanical properties of the articular cartilage. Acta Biol Hung. 2017;68(4):368–75.
9. Buckwalter JA, Mankin HJ. Articular cartilage: tissue design and chondrocyte-matrix interactions. Instr Course Lect. 1998;47:477–86.
10. Buckwalter JA, Rosenberg LA, Hunziker EB. Articular cartilage and knee joint function: basic science and arthroscopy. New York: Raven Press; 1990.
11. Poole AR, Rizkalla G, Ionescu M, Reiner A, Brooks E, Rorabeck C, Bourne R, Bogoch E. Osteoarthritis in the human knee: a dynamic process of cartilage matrix degradation, synthesis and reorganization. Agents Actions Suppl. 1993;39:3–13.
12. Venn M, Maroudas A. Chemical composition and swelling of normal and osteoarthrotic femoral head cartilage. I. Chemical composition. Ann Rheum Dis. 1977;36:121–9.

13. Franchimont P, Bassleer C, Henrotin Y. Effects of hormones and drugs on cartilage repair. J Rheumatol Suppl. 1989;18:5–9.
14. Hulka BS. Overview of biological markers. In: Hulka BS, Griffith JD, Wilcosky TC, editors. Biological markers in epidemiology. New York: Oxford University Press; 1990. p. 3–15.
15. Naylor S. Biomarkers: current perspectives and future prospects. Expert Rev Mol Diagn. 2003;3(5):525–9.
16. Lohmander LS. Markers of cartilage metabolism in arthrosis. A review. Acta Orthop Scand. 1991;62:623–32.
17. Ratcliffe A, Grelsamer RP, Kiernan H, Saed-Nejad F, Visco D. High levels of aggrecan aggregate components are present in synovial fluids from human knee joints with chronic injury or osteoarthrosis. Acta Orthop Scand Suppl. 1995;266:111–5.
18. Ratcliffe A, Seibel MJ. Biochemical markers of osteoarthritis. Curr Opin Rheumatol. 1990;2:770–6.
19. Chevalier X. Is a biological marker for osteoarthritis within reach? Rev Rhum Engl Ed. 1997;64:562–77.
20. Kleesiek K, Reinards R, Okusi J, Wolf B, Greiling H. UDP-D-xylose: proteoglycan core protein beta-D-xylosyltransferase: a new marker of cartilage destruction in chronic joint diseases. J Clin Chem Clin Biochem. 1987;25:473–81.
21. Schneiderman R, Rosenberg N, Hiss J, Lee P, Liu F, Hintz RL, Maroudas A. Concentration and size distribution of insulin-like growth factor-I in human normal and osteoarthritic synovial fluid and cartilage. Arch Biochem Biophys. 1995;324:173–88.
22. Boeth H, MacMahon A, Poole AR, Buttgereit F, Onnerfjord P, Lorenzo P, Klint C, Pramhed A, Duda GN. Differences in biomarkers of cartilage matrix turnover and their changes over 2 years in adolescent and adult volleyball athletes. J Exp Orthop. 2017;4:7.
23. Garvican ER, Vaughan-Thomas A, Innes JF, Clegg PD. Biomarkers of cartilage turnover. Part 1: markers of collagen degradation and synthesis. Vet J. 2010;185(1):36–42.
24. Garvican ER, Vaughan-Thomas A, Clegg PD, Innes JF. Biomarkers of cartilage turnover. Part 2: non-collagenous markers. Vet J. 2010b;185(1):43–9.
25. Carlson AK, Rawle RA, Wallace CW, Brooks EG, Adams E, et al. Characterization of synovial fluid metabolomic phenotypes of cartilage morphological changes associated with osteoarthritis. Osteoarthritis Cartilage. 2019;27(8):1174–84.
26. Carlson AK, Rawle RA, Wallace CW, Adams E, Greenwood MC, et al. Global metabolomic profiling of human synovial fluid for rheumatoid arthritis biomarkers. Clin Exp Rheumatol. 2019;37(3):393–99.
27. Carlson AK, Rawle RA, Adams E, Greenwood MC, Bothner B, et al. Application of global metabolomic profiling of synovial fluid for osteoarthritis biomarkers. Biochem Biophys Res Commun. 2018;499(2):182–88.
28. Nguyen LT, Sharma AR, Chakraborty C, Saibaba B, Ahn ME, Lee SS. Review of prospects of biological fluid biomarkers in osteoarthritis. Int J Mol Sci. 2017;18:E601.
29. Mobasheri A, Bay-Jensen AC, van Spil WE, Larkin J, Levesque MC. Osteoarthritis year in review 2016: biomarkers (biochemical markers). Osteoarthritis Cartilage. 2017;25:199–208.
30. Legrand CB, Lambert CJ, Comblain FV, Sanchez C, Henrotin YE. Review of soluble biomarkers of osteoarthritis: lessons from animal models. Cartilage. 2017;8:211–33.
31. Kluzek S, Arden NK, Newton J. Adipokines as potential prognostic biomarkers in patients with acute knee injury. Biomarkers. 2015;20:519–25.
32. Hsueh MF, Onnerfjord P, Kraus VB. Biomarkers and proteomic analysis of osteoarthritis. Matrix Biol. 2014;39:56–66.
33. Patra D, Sandell LJ. Evolving biomarkers in osteoarthritis. J Knee Surg. 2011;24:241–9.
34. Karsdal MA, Woodworth T, Henriksen K, Maksymowych WP, Genant H, Vergnaud P, Christiansen C, Schubert T, Qvist P, Schett G, Platt A, Bay-Jensen AC. Biochemical markers of ongoing joint damage in rheumatoid arthritis – current and future applications, limitations and opportunities. Arthritis Res Ther. 2011;13:215.
35. Gahunia HK, Lough A, Vieth R, Pritzker K. A cartilage derived novel compound DDP (2,6-dimethyldifuro-8-pyrone): isolation, purification, and identification. J Rheumatol. 2002;29(1):147–53.
36. Mündermann A, Klenk C, Billich C, Nüesch C, Pagenstert G, Schmidt-Trucksäss A, Schütz U. Changes in cartilage biomarker levels during a transcontinental multistage footrace over 4486 km. Am J Sports Med. 2017;45(11):2630–6.
37. Wasilko SM, Tourville TW, DeSarno MJ, Slauterbeck JR, Johnson RJ, Struglics A, Beynnon BD. Relationship between synovial fluid biomarkers of articular cartilage metabolism and the patient's perspective of outcome depends on the severity of articular cartilage damage following ACL trauma. J Orthop Res. 2016;34:820–7.
38. Lohmander LS, Hoerrner LA, Lark MW. Metalloproteinases, tissue inhibitor, and proteoglycan fragments in knee synovial fluid in human osteoarthritis. Arthritis Rheum. 1993;36:181–9.
39. Lohmander LS. The release of aggrecan fragments into synovial fluid after joint injury and in osteoarthritis. J Rheumatol Suppl. 1995;43:75–7.
40. Lohmander LS, Lark MW, Dahlberg L, Walakovits LA, Roos H. Cartilage matrix metabolism in osteoarthritis: markers in synovial fluid, serum, and urine. Clin Biochem. 1992;25:167–74.
41. Lotz M, Martel-Pelletier J, Christiansen C, Brandi ML, Bruyere O, Chapurlat R, Collette J, Cooper C, Giacovelli G, Kanis JA, Karsdal MA, Kraus V, Lems WF, Meulenbelt I, Pelletier JP, Raynauld JP, Reiter-Niesert S, Rizzoli R, Sandell LJ, Van Spil WE, Reginster JY. Value of biomarkers in osteoar-

thritis: current status and perspectives. Ann Rheum Dis. 2013;72:1756–63.

42. Gahunia HK, Vieth R, Pritzker K. Novel fluorescent compound (DDP) in calf, rabbit, and human articular cartilage and synovial fluid. J Rheumatol. 2002;29(1):154–60.
43. Lohmander LS, Dahlberg L, Ryd L, Heinegard D. Increased levels of proteoglycan fragments in knee joint fluid after injury. Arthritis Rheum. 1989;32:1434–42.
44. Lohmander LS, Hoerrner LA, Dahlberg L, Roos H, Bjornsson S, Lark MW. Stromelysin, tissue inhibitor of metalloproteinases and proteoglycan fragments in human knee joint fluid after injury. J Rheumatol. 1993;20:1362–8.
45. Lohmander LS, Ionescu M, Jugessur H, Poole AR. Changes in joint cartilage aggrecan after knee injury and in osteoarthritis. Arthritis Rheum. 1999;42:534–44.
46. Lohmander LS, Neame PJ, Sandy JD. The structure of aggrecan fragments in human synovial fluid. Evidence that aggrecanase mediates cartilage degradation in inflammatory joint disease, joint injury, and osteoarthritis. Arthritis Rheum. 1993;36:1214–22.
47. Mort JS, Geng Y, Fisher WD, Roughley PJ. Aggrecan heterogeneity in articular cartilage from patients with osteoarthritis. BMC Musculoskelet Disord. 2016;17:89.
48. Haller JM, Swearingen CA, Partridge D, McFadden M, Thirunavukkarasu K, Higgins TF. Intraarticular matrix metalloproteinases and aggrecan degradation are elevated after articular fracture. Clin Orthop Relat Res. 2015;473:3280–8.
49. Thonar EJ, Manicourt DM, Williams J, Lenz ME, Sweet MB, Schnitzer TJ, Otten L, Glant T, Kuettner KE. Circulating keratan sulfate: a marker of cartilage proteoglycan catabolism in osteoarthritis. J Rheumatol Suppl. 1991;27:24–6.
50. Ishiguro N, Ito T, Ito H, Iwata H, Jugessur H, Ionescu M, Poole AR. Relationship of matrix metalloproteinases and their inhibitors to cartilage proteoglycan and collagen turnover: analyses of synovial fluid from patients with osteoarthritis. Arthritis Rheum. 1999;42:129–36.
51. Sharif M, Osborne DJ, Meadows K, Woodhouse SM, Colvin EM, Shepstone L, Dieppe PA. The relevance of chondroitin and keratan sulphate markers in normal and arthritic synovial fluid. Br J Rheumatol. 1996;35:951–7.
52. Bautch JC, Clayton MK, Chu Q, Johnson KA. Synovial fluid chondroitin sulphate epitopes 3B3 and 7D4, and glycosaminoglycan in human knee osteoarthritis after exercise. Ann Rheum Dis. 2000;59:887–91.
53. Belcher C, Yaqub R, Fawthrop F, Bayliss M, Doherty M. Synovial fluid chondroitin and keratan sulphate epitopes, glycosaminoglycans, and hyaluronan in arthritic and normal knees. Ann Rheum Dis. 1997;56:299–307.
54. Bello AE, Garrett WE Jr, Wang H, Lohnes J, DeLong E, Caterson B, Kraus VB. Comparison of synovial fluid cartilage marker concentrations and chondral damage assessed arthroscopically in acute knee injury. Osteoarthritis Cartilage. 1997;5:419–26.
55. Catterall JB, Stabler TV, Flannery CR, Kraus VB. Changes in serum and synovial fluid biomarkers after acute injury (NCT00332254). Arthritis Res Ther. 2010;12:R229.
56. Gyorgy B, Tothfalusi L, Nagy G, Pasztoi M, Geher P, Lorinc Z, Polgar A, Rojkovich B, Ujfalussy I, Poor G, Pocza P, Wiener Z, Misjak P, Koncz A, Falus A, Buzas EI. Natural autoantibodies reactive with glycosaminoglycans in rheumatoid arthritis. Arthritis Res Ther. 2008;10:R110.
57. Ratcliffe A, Doherty M, Maini RN, Hardingham TE. Increased concentrations of proteoglycan components in the synovial fluids of patients with acute but not chronic joint disease. Ann Rheum Dis. 1988;47:826–32.
58. Sward P, Frobell R, Englund M, Roos H, Struglics A. Cartilage and bone markers and inflammatory cytokines are increased in synovial fluid in the acute phase of knee injury (hemarthrosis) – a cross-sectional analysis. Osteoarthritis Cartilage. 2012;20:1302–8.
59. Wakitani S, Nawata M, Kawaguchi A, Okabe T, Takaoka K, Tsuchiya T, Nakaoka R, Masuda H, Miyazaki K. Serum keratan sulfate is a promising marker of early articular cartilage breakdown. Rheumatology (Oxford). 2007;46:1652–6.
60. Vaatainen U, Lohmander LS, Thonar E, Hongisto T, Agren U, Ronkko S, Jaroma H, Kosma VM, Tammi M, Kiviranta I. Markers of cartilage and synovial metabolism in joint fluid and serum of patients with chondromalacia of the patella. Osteoarthritis Cartilage. 1998;6:115–24.
61. Thonar EJ, Pachman LM, Lenz ME, Hayford J, Lynch P, Kuettner KE. Age related changes in the concentration of serum keratan sulphate in children. J Clin Chem Clin Biochem. 1988;26:57–63.
62. Yoshida H, Kojima T, Kurokouchi K, Takahashi S, Hanamura H, Kojima M, Poole AR, Ishiguro N. Relationship between pre-radiographic cartilage damage following anterior cruciate ligament injury and biomarkers of cartilage turnover in clinical practice: a cross-sectional observational study. Osteoarthritis Cartilage. 2013;21:831–8.
63. Ishiguro N, Ito T, Oguchi T, Kojima T, Iwata H, Ionescu M, Poole AR. Relationships of matrix metalloproteinases and their inhibitors to cartilage proteoglycan and collagen turnover and inflammation as revealed by analyses of synovial fluids from patients with rheumatoid arthritis. Arthritis Rheum. 2001;44:2503–11.
64. Shinmei M, Kobayashi T, Yoshihara Y, Samura A. Significance of the levels of carboxy terminal type II procollagen peptide, chondroitin sulfate isomers, tissue inhibitor of metalloproteinases, and metallo-

proteinases in osteoarthritis joint fluid. J Rheumatol Suppl. 1995;43:78–81.
65. Uesaka S, Nakayama Y, Shirai Y, Yoshihara K. Serum and synovial fluid levels of chondroitin sulfate in patients with osteoarthritis of the knee joint. J Nippon Med Sch. 2001;68(2):165–70.
66. Uesaka S, Nakayama Y, Yoshihara K, Ito H. Significance of chondroitin sulfate isomers in the synovial fluid of osteoarthritis patients. J Orthop Sci. 2002;7(2):232–7.
67. Yoshihara Y, Yamada H, Miyauchi S, Ito K, Samura A, Shinmei M. Levels of chondroitin 4-sulfate, chondroitin 6-sulfate and carboxy-terminal type II procollagen peptide in knee synovial fluid after injury to the anterior cruciate ligament. Ryumachi. 1996;36(5):734–40.
68. Momohara S, Okada N, Ikari K, Mizuno S, Okamoto H. Dermatan sulfate in the synovial fluid of patients with knee osteoarthritis. Mod Rheumatol. 2007;17(4):301–5.
69. Matyas JR, Atley L, Ionescu M, Eyre DR, Poole AR. Analysis of cartilage biomarkers in the early phases of canine experimental osteoarthritis. Arthritis Rheum. 2004;50(2):543–52.
70. Chan SS, Kent GN, Will RK. A sensitive assay for the measurement of serum chondroitin sulfate 3B3(−) epitope levels in human rheumatic diseases. Clin Exp Rheumatol. 2001;19:533–40.
71. Ratcliffe A, Shurety W, Caterson B. The quantitation of a native chondroitin sulfate epitope in synovial fluid lavages and articular cartilage from canine experimental osteoarthritis and disuse atrophy. Arthritis Rheum. 1993;36(4):543–51.
72. Bastick AN, Belo JN, Runhaar J, Bierma-Zeinstra SM. What are the prognostic factors for radiographic progression of knee osteoarthritis? A meta-analysis. Clin Orthop Relat Res. 2015;473:2969–89.
73. Pavelka K, Forejtova S, Olejarova M, Gatterova J, Senolt L, Spacek P, Braun M, Hulejova M, Stovickova J, Pavelkova A. Hyaluronic acid levels may have predictive value for the progression of knee osteoarthritis. Osteoarthritis Cartilage. 2004;12:277–83.
74. Pothacharoen P, Teekachunhatean S, Louthrenoo W, Yingsung W, Ong-Chai S, Hardingham T, Kongtawelert P. Raised chondroitin sulfate epitopes and hyaluronan in serum from rheumatoid arthritis and osteoarthritis patients. Osteoarthritis Cartilage. 2006;14:299–301.
75. Temple-Wong MM, Ren S, Quach P, Hansen BC, Chen AC, Hasegawa A, D'Lima DD, Koziol J, Masuda K, Lotz MK, Sah RL. Hyaluronan concentration and size distribution in human knee synovial fluid: variations with age and cartilage degeneration. Arthritis Res Ther. 2016;18:18.
76. Turan Y, Bal S, Gurgan A, Topac H, Koseoglu M. Serum hyaluronan levels in patients with knee osteoarthritis. Clin Rheumatol. 2007;26:1293–8.
77. Saxne T, Heinegard D, Wollheim FA. Cartilage proteoglycans in synovial fluid and serum in patients with inflammatory joint disease. Relation to systemic treatment. Arthritis Rheum. 1987;30:972–9.
78. Germaschewski FM, Matheny CJ, Larkin J, Liu F, Thomas LR, Saunders JS, Sully K, Whittall C, Boyle Y, Peters G, Graham NM. Quantitation OF ARGS aggrecan fragments in synovial fluid, serum and urine from osteoarthritis patients. Osteoarthritis Cartilage. 2014;22:690–7.
79. Larsson S, Englund M, Struglics A, Lohmander LS. Association between synovial fluid levels of aggrecan ARGS fragments and radiographic progression in knee osteoarthritis. Arthritis Res Ther. 2010;12:R230.
80. Larsson S, Lohmander LS, Struglics A. Synovial fluid level of aggrecan ARGS fragments is a more sensitive marker of joint disease than glycosaminoglycan or aggrecan levels: a cross-sectional study. Arthritis Res Ther. 2009;11:R92.
81. Struglics A, Hansson M, Lohmander LS. Human aggrecanase generated synovial fluid fragment levels are elevated directly after knee injuries due to proteolysis both in the inter globular and chondroitin sulfate domains. Osteoarthritis Cartilage. 2011;19:1047–57.
82. Swearingen CA, Carpenter JW, Siegel R, Brittain IJ, Dotzlaf J, Durham TB, Toth JL, Laska DA, Marimuthu J, Liu C, Brown DP, Carter QL, Wiley MR, Duffin KL, Mitchell PG, Thirunavukkarasu K. Development of a novel clinical biomarker assay to detect and quantify aggrecanase-generated aggrecan fragments in human synovial fluid, serum and urine. Osteoarthritis Cartilage. 2010;18:1150–8.
83. Hao D, Li M, Wu Z, Duan Y, Li D, Qiu G. Synovial fluid level of adiponectin correlated with levels of aggrecan degradation markers in osteoarthritis. Rheumatol Int. 2011;31:1433–7.
84. Nagaya H, Ymagata T, Ymagata S, Iyoda K, Ito H, Hasegawa Y, Iwata H. Examination of synovial fluid and serum hyaluronidase activity as a joint marker in rheumatoid arthritis and osteoarthritis patients (by zymography). Ann Rheum Dis. 1999;58:186–8.
85. Olszewski JM, Moore VL, McDonnell J, Williams H, Saphos CA, Green BG, Knight WB, Chapman KT, Hagmann WK, Dorn CP, Hale JJ, Mumford RA. Proteoglycan-degrading activity of human stromelysin-1 and leukocyte elastase in rabbit joints. Quantitation of proteoglycan and a stromelysin-induced HABR fragment of aggrecan in synovial fluid and cartilage. Connect Tissue Res. 1996;33:291–9.
86. Hunter DJ, Li J, LaValley M, Bauer DC, Nevitt M, DeGroot J, Poole R, Eyre D, Guermazi A, Gale D, Felson DT. Cartilage markers and their association with cartilage loss on magnetic resonance imaging in knee osteoarthritis: the Boston Osteoarthritis Knee Study. Arthritis Res Ther. 2007;9:R108.
87. Ishiguro N. Cartilage degradation in rheumatoid arthritis. Clin Calcium. 2009;19(3):347–54.

88. Ishiguro N, Kojima T, Poole AR. Mechanism of cartilage destruction in osteoarthritis. Nagoya J Med Sci. 2002;65:73–84.
89. Elsaid KA, Chichester CO. Review: collagen markers in early arthritic diseases. Clin Chim Acta. 2006;365:68–77.
90. Fraser A, Fearon U, Billinghurst RC, Ionescu M, Reece R, Barwick T, Emery P, Poole AR, Veale DJ. Turnover of type II collagen and aggrecan in cartilage matrix at the onset of inflammatory arthritis in humans: relationship to mediators of systemic and local inflammation. Arthritis Rheum. 2003;48:3085–95.
91. Kobayashi T, Yoshihara Y, Yamada H, Fujikawa K. Procollagen IIC-peptide as a marker for assessing mechanical risk factors of knee osteoarthritis: effect of obesity and varus alignment. Ann Rheum Dis. 2000;59:982–4.
92. Lohmander LS, Yoshihara Y, Roos H, Kobayashi T, Yamada H, Shinmei M. Procollagen II C-propeptide in joint fluid: changes in concentration with age, time after knee injury, and osteoarthritis. J Rheumatol. 1996;23:1765–9.
93. Mullan RH, Matthews C, Bresnihan B, FitzGerald O, King L, Poole AR, Fearon U, Veale DJ. Early changes in serum type II collagen biomarkers predict radiographic progression at one year in inflammatory arthritis patients after biologic therapy. Arthritis Rheum. 2007;56:2919–28.
94. Prince HE. Biomarkers for diagnosing and monitoring autoimmune diseases. Biomarkers. 2005;10(Suppl 1):S44–9.
95. Shinmei M, Ito K, Matsuyama S, Yoshihara Y, Matsuzawa K. Joint fluid carboxy-terminal type II procollagen peptide as a marker of cartilage collagen biosynthesis. Osteoarthritis Cartilage. 1993;1:121–8.
96. Lohmander LS, Saxne T, Heinegard D. Increased concentrations of bone sialoprotein in joint fluid after knee injury. Ann Rheum Dis. 1996;55:622–6.
97. Garnero P, Ayral X, Rousseau JC, Christgau S, Sandell LJ, Dougados M, Delmas PD. Uncoupling of type II collagen synthesis and degradation predicts progression of joint damage in patients with knee osteoarthritis. Arthritis Rheum. 2002;46:2613–24.
98. Kraus VB, Hargrove DE, Hunter DJ, Renner JB, Jordan JM. Establishment of reference intervals for osteoarthritis-related soluble biomarkers: the FNIH/OARSI OA Biomarkers Consortium. Ann Rheum Dis. 2017;76:179–85.
99. Rousseau JC, Zhu Y, Miossec P, Vignon E, Sandell LJ, Garnero P, Delmas PD. Serum levels of type IIA procollagen amino terminal propeptide (PIIANP) are decreased in patients with knee osteoarthritis and rheumatoid arthritis. Osteoarthritis Cartilage. 2004;12:440–7.
100. Sharif M, Kirwan J, Charni N, Sandell LJ, Whittles C, Garnero P. A 5-yr longitudinal study of type IIA collagen synthesis and total type II collagen degradation in patients with knee osteoarthritis – association with disease progression. Rheumatology (Oxford). 2007;46:938–43.
101. Rousseau JC, Sandell LJ, Delmas PD, Garnero P. Development and clinical application in arthritis of a new immunoassay for serum type IIA procollagen NH2 propeptide. Methods Mol Med. 2004;101:25–37.
102. Rousseau J, Garnero P. Biological markers in osteoarthritis. Bone. 2012;51:265–77.
103. Charni-Ben Tabassi N, Desmarais S, Bay-Jensen AC, Delaisse JM, Percival MD, Garnero P. The type II collagen fragments helix-II and CTX-II reveal different enzymatic pathways of human cartilage collagen degradation. Osteoarthritis Cartilage. 2008;16:1183–91.
104. Tanishi N, Yamagiwa H, Hayami T, Mera H, Koga Y, Omori G, Endo N. Usefulness of urinary CTX-II and NTX-I in evaluating radiological knee osteoarthritis: the Matsudai knee osteoarthritis survey. J Orthop Sci. 2014;19:429–36.
105. Rotterud JH, Reinholt FP, Beckstrom KJ, Risberg MA, Aroen A. Relationship between CTX-II and patient characteristics, patient-reported outcome, muscle strength, and rehabilitation in patients with a focal cartilage lesion of the knee: a prospective exploratory cohort study of 48 patients. BMC Musculoskelet Disord. 2014;15:99.
106. Jordan KM, Syddall HE, Garnero P, Gineyts E, Dennison EM, Sayer AA, Delmas PD, Cooper C, Arden NK. Urinary CTX-II and glucosyl-galactosyl-pyridinoline are associated with the presence and severity of radiographic knee osteoarthritis in men. Ann Rheum Dis. 2006;65:871–7.
107. Lohmander LS, Atley LM, Pietka TA, Eyre DR. The release of crosslinked peptides from type II collagen into human synovial fluid is increased soon after joint injury and in osteoarthritis. Arthritis Rheum. 2003;48:3130–9.
108. Charni N, Juillet F, Garnero P. Urinary type II collagen helical peptide (HELIX-II) as a new biochemical marker of cartilage degradation in patients with osteoarthritis and rheumatoid arthritis. Arthritis Rheum. 2005;52:1081–90.
109. He Y, Siebuhr AS, Brandt-Hansen NU, Wang J, Su D, Zheng Q, Simonsen O, Petersen KK, Arendt-Nielsen L, Eskehave T, Hoeck HC, Karsdal MA, Bay-Jensen AC. Type X collagen levels are elevated in serum from human osteoarthritis patients and associated with biomarkers of cartilage degradation and inflammation. BMC Musculoskelet Disord. 2014;15:309.
110. Haslauer CM, Elsaid KA, Fleming BC, Proffen BL, Johnson VM, Murray MM. Loss of extracellular matrix from articular cartilage is mediated by the synovium and ligament after anterior cruciate ligament injury. Osteoarthritis Cartilage. 2013;21:1950–7.
111. Cibere J, Zhang H, Garnero P, Poole AR, Lobanok T, Saxne T, Kraus VB, Way A, Thorne A, Wong H, Singer J, Kopec J, Guermazi A, Peterfy C, Nicolaou

S, Munk PL, Esdaile JM. Association of biomarkers with pre-radiographically defined and radiographically defined knee osteoarthritis in a population-based study. Arthritis Rheum. 2009;60:1372–80.
112. Kojima T, Kojima M, Noda K, Ishiguro N, Poole AR. Influences of menopause, aging, and gender on the cleavage of type II collagen in cartilage in relationship to bone turnover. Menopause. 2008;15(1):133–7.
113. Kumahashi N, Sward P, Larsson S, Lohmander LS, Frobell R, Struglics A. Type II collagen C2C epitope in human synovial fluid and serum after knee injury – associations with molecular and structural markers of injury. Osteoarthritis Cartilage. 2015;23:1506–12.
114. Svoboda SJ, Harvey TM, Owens BD, Brechue WF, Tarwater PM, Cameron KL. Changes in serum biomarkers of cartilage turnover after anterior cruciate ligament injury. Am J Sports Med. 2013;41:2108–16.
115. He G, Chen X, Zhang G, Lin H, Li R, Wu X. Detection of urine C2C and trace element level in patients with knee osteoarthritis. Cell Biochem Biophys. 2014;70:475–9.
116. Bay-Jensen AC, Liu Q, Byrjalsen I, Li Y, Wang J, Pedersen C, Leeming DJ, Dam EB, Zheng Q, Qvist P, Karsdal MA. Enzyme-linked immunosorbent assay (ELISAs) for metalloproteinase derived type II collagen neoepitope, CIIM – increased serum CIIM in subjects with severe radiographic osteoarthritis. Clin Biochem. 2011;44:423–9.
117. Egsgaard LL, Eskehave TN, Bay-Jensen AC, Hoeck HC, Arendt-Nielsen L. Identifying specific profiles in patients with different degrees of painful knee osteoarthritis based on serological biochemical and mechanistic pain biomarkers: a diagnostic approach based on cluster analysis. Pain. 2015;156:96–107.
118. Poole AR, Ionescu M, Fitzcharles MA, Billinghurst RC. The assessment of cartilage degradation in vivo: development of an immunoassay for the measurement in body fluids of type II collagen cleaved by collagenases. J Immunol Methods. 2004;294(1–2):145–53.
119. Furumitsu Y, Inaba M, Yukioka K, Yukioka M, Kumeda Y, Azuma Y, Ohta T, Ochi T, Nishizawa Y, Morii H. Levels of serum and synovial fluid pyridinium crosslinks in patients with rheumatoid arthritis. J Rheumatol. 2000;27:64–70.
120. Hein G, Franke S, Muller A, Braunig E, Eidner T, Stein G. The determination of pyridinium crosslinks in urine and serum as a possible marker of cartilage degradation in rheumatoid arthritis. Clin Rheumatol. 1997;16:167–72.
121. Kaufmann J, Mueller A, Voigt A, Carl HD, Gursche A, Zacher J, Stein G, Hein G. Hydroxypyridinium collagen crosslinks in serum, urine, synovial fluid and synovial tissue in patients with rheumatoid arthritis compared with osteoarthritis. Rheumatology (Oxford). 2003;42:314–20.
122. Ricard-Blum S, Chevalier X, Grimaud JA, Larget-Piet B, Uebelhart D. Detectable levels of pyridinoline are present in synovial fluid from various patients with knee effusion: preliminary results. Eur J Clin Invest. 1995;25:438–41.
123. Schmidt-Rohlfing B, Thomsen M, Niedhart C, Wirtz DC, Schneider U. Correlation of bone and cartilage markers in the synovial fluid with the degree of osteoarthritis. Rheumatol Int. 2002;21:193–9.
124. Sinigaglia L, Varenna M, Binelli L, Bartucci F, Arrigoni M, Ferrara R, Abbiati G. Urinary and synovial pyridinium crosslink concentrations in patients with rheumatoid arthritis and osteoarthritis. Ann Rheum Dis. 1995;54:144–7.
125. Spacek P, Adam M. Pentosidine in osteoarthritis: HPLC determination in body fluids and in tissues. Rheumatol Int. 2006;26:923–7.
126. Schmidt-Rohlfing B, Gavenis K, Kippels M, Schneider U. New potential markers for cartilage degradation of the knee joint. Scand J Rheumatol. 2002;31:151–7.
127. Chen JR, Takahashi M, Suzuki M, Kushida K, Miyamoto S, Inoue T. Pentosidine in synovial fluid in osteoarthritis and rheumatoid arthritis: relationship with disease activity in rheumatoid arthritis. J Rheumatol. 1998;25:2440–4.
128. Miyata T, Ishiguro N, Yasuda Y, Ito T, Nangaku M, Iwata H, Kurokawa K. Increased pentosidine, an advanced glycation end product, in plasma and synovial fluid from patients with rheumatoid arthritis and its relation with inflammatory markers. Biochem Biophys Res Commun. 1998;244:45–9.
129. Senolt L, Braun M, Olejarova M, Forejtova S, Gatterova J, Pavelka K. Increased pentosidine, an advanced glycation end product, in serum and synovial fluid from patients with knee osteoarthritis and its relation with cartilage oligomeric matrix protein. Ann Rheum Dis. 2005;64(6):886–90.
130. Senolt L, Braun M, Vencovsky J, Sedova L, Pavelka K. Advanced glycation end-product pentosidine is not a relevant marker of disease activity in patients with rheumatoid arthritis. Physiol Res. 2007;56:771–7.
131. Takahashi M, Suzuki M, Kushida K, Miyamoto S, Inoue T. Relationship between pentosidine levels in serum and urine and activity in rheumatoid arthritis. Br J Rheumatol. 1997;36:637–42.
132. Vos PA, Mastbergen SC, Huisman AM, de Boer TN, DeGroot J, Polak AA, Lafeber FP. In end stage osteoarthritis, cartilage tissue pentosidine levels are inversely related to parameters of cartilage damage. Osteoarthritis Cartilage. 2012;20:233–40.
133. Lohmander LS, Saxne T, Heinegard DK. Release of cartilage oligomeric matrix protein (COMP) into joint fluid after knee injury and in osteoarthritis. Ann Rheum Dis. 1994;53:8–13.
134. Fernandes FA, Pucinelli ML, da Silva NP, Feldman D. Serum cartilage oligomeric matrix protein (COMP) levels in knee osteoarthritis in a Brazilian population: clinical and radiological correlation. Scand J Rheumatol. 2007;36:211–5.
135. Verma P, Dalal K. Serum cartilage oligomeric matrix protein (COMP) in knee osteoarthritis: a novel diag-

nostic and prognostic biomarker. J Orthop Res. 2013;31:999–1006.
136. Sharif M, Granell R, Johansen J, Clarke S, Elson C, Kirwan JR. Serum cartilage oligomeric matrix protein and other biomarker profiles in tibiofemoral and patellofemoral osteoarthritis of the knee. Rheumatology (Oxford). 2006;45:522–6.
137. Murphy E, FitzGerald O, Saxne T, Bresnihan B. Increased serum cartilage oligomeric matrix protein levels and decreased patellar bone mineral density in patients with chondromalacia patellae. Ann Rheum Dis. 2002;61:981–5.
138. Kuhne SA, Neidhart M, Everson MP, Hantzschel H, Fine PR, Gay S, Hauselmann HJ, Gay RE. Persistent high serum levels of cartilage oligomeric matrix protein in a subgroup of patients with traumatic knee injury. Rheumatol Int. 1998;18:21–5.
139. Sakthiswary R, Rajalingam S, Hussein H, Sridharan R, Asrul AW. Cartilage oligomeric matrix protein (COMP) in rheumatoid arthritis and its correlation with sonographic knee cartilage thickness and disease activity. Clin Rheumatol. 2017;36(12):2683–8.
140. Helmark IC, Petersen MC, Christensen HE, Kjaer M, Langberg H. Moderate loading of the human osteoarthritic knee joint leads to lowering of intraarticular cartilage oligomeric matrix protein. Rheumatol Int. 2012;32:1009–14.
141. Roberts HM, Moore JP, Thom JM. The effect of aerobic walking and lower body resistance exercise on serum COMP and hyaluronan, in both males and females. Eur J Appl Physiol. 2018;118(6):1095–105.
142. Roberts HM, Moore JP, Griffith-McGeever CL, Fortes MB, Thom JM. The effect of vigorous running and cycling on serum COMP, lubricin, and femoral cartilage thickness: a pilot study. Eur J Appl Physiol. 2016;116(8):1467–77.
143. Silaghi CN, Fodor D, Cristea V, Craciun AM. Synovial and serum levels of uncarboxylated matrix Gla-protein (ucMGP) in patients with arthritis. Clin Chem Lab Med. 2011;50:125–8.
144. Shea MK, Kritchevsky SB, Hsu FC, Nevitt M, Booth SL, Kwoh CK, McAlindon TE, Vermeer C, Drummen N, Harris TB, Womack C, Loeser RF, Health ABCS. The association between vitamin K status and knee osteoarthritis features in older adults: the health, aging and body composition study. Osteoarthritis Cartilage. 2015;23:370–8.
145. Bing W, Feng L. Attenuate synovial fluid uncarboxylated matrix Gla-protein (ucMGP) concentrations are linked with radiographic progression in knee psteoarthritis. Adv Clin Exp Med. 2015;24:1013–7.
146. Fife RS. Cartilage matrix glycoprotein as a possible marker of osteoarthritis. J Rheumatol Suppl. 1991;27:30–1.
147. Fife RS, Rachow JW, Ryan LM. Synovial fluid and plasma levels of cartilage matrix glycoprotein in arthritis. Calcif Tissue Int. 1994;55(2):100–2.
148. Vaananen T, Koskinen A, Paukkeri EL, Hamalainen M, Moilanen T, Moilanen E, Vuolteenaho K. YKL-40 as a novel factor associated with inflammation and catabolic mechanisms in osteoarthritic joints. Mediators Inflamm. 2014;2014:215140.
149. Kazakova MH, Batalov AZ, Mateva NG, Kolarov ZG, Sarafian VS. YKL-40 and cytokines – a new diagnostic constellation in rheumatoid arthritis? Folia Med. 2017;59:37–42.
150. Johansen JS, Hvolris J, Hansen M, Backer V, Lorenzen I, Price PA. Serum YKL-40 levels in healthy children and adults. Comparison with serum and synovial fluid levels of YKL-40 in patients with osteoarthritis or trauma of the knee joint. Br J Rheumatol. 1996;35:553–9.
151. Volck B, Johansen JS, Stoltenberg M, Garbarsch C, Price PA, Ostergaard M, Ostergaard K, Lovgreen-Nielsen P, Sonne-Holm S, Lorenzen I. Studies on YKL-40 in knee joints of patients with rheumatoid arthritis and osteoarthritis. Involvement of YKL-40 in the joint pathology. Osteoarthritis Cartilage. 2001;9:203–14.
152. Johansen JS, Jensen HS, Price PA. A new biochemical marker for joint injury. Analysis of YKL-40 in serum and synovial fluid. Br J Rheumatol. 1993;32:949–55.
153. Guan J, Liu Z, Li F, Feng JS, Wang HJ, Chu JG, Song YZ, Xie L, Ding LB. Increased synovial fluid YKL-40 levels are linked with symptomatic severity in knee osteoarthritis patients. Clin Lab. 2015;61:991–7.
154. Huang K, Wu LD. YKL-40: a potential biomarker for osteoarthritis. J Int Med Res. 2009;37:18–24.
155. Karalilova R, Kazakova M, Batalov A, Sarafian V. Correlation between protein YKL-40 and ultrasonographic findings in active knee osteoarthritis. Med Ultrason. 2018;1(1):57–63.
156. Nakamura S, Kamihagi K, Satakeda H, Katayama M, Pan H, Okamoto H, Noshiro M, Takahashi K, Yoshihara Y, Shimmei M, Okada Y, Kato Y. Enhancement of SPARC (osteonectin) synthesis in arthritic cartilage. Increased levels in synovial fluids from patients with rheumatoid arthritis and regulation by growth factors and cytokines in chondrocyte cultures. Arthritis Rheum. 1996;39:539–51.
157. Sward P, Struglics A, Englund M, Roos HP, Frobell RB. Soft tissue knee injury with concomitant osteochondral fracture is associated with higher degree of acute joint inflammation. Am J Sports Med. 2014;42:1096–102.
158. Carsons S, Horn VJ. Chondronectin in human synovial fluid. Ann Rheum Dis. 1988;47:797–800.
159. Golightly YM, Adams SB, Kraus VB. In: Olson SG, editor. Biomarkers of PTA. Boston, MA: Springer; 2015. p. 317–30.
160. Rooney T, Scherzer R, Shigenaga JK, Graf J, Imboden JB, Grunfeld C. Levels of plasma fibrinogen are elevated in well-controlled rheumatoid arthritis. Rheumatology (Oxford). 2011;50:1458–65.
161. Raijmakers R, van Beers JJ, El-Azzouny M, Visser NF, Bozic B, Pruijn GJ, Heck AJ. Elevated lev-

els of fibrinogen-derived endogenous citrullinated peptides in synovial fluid of rheumatoid arthritis patients. Arthritis Res Ther. 2012;14:R114.
162. Senolt L, Grassi W, Szodoray P. Laboratory biomarkers or imaging in the diagnostics of rheumatoid arthritis? BMC Med. 2014;12:49.
163. Hasegawa M, Yoshida T, Sudo A. Role of tenascin-C in articular cartilage. Mod Rheumatol. 2017:1–6.
164. Chockalingam PS, Glasson SS, Lohmander LS. Tenascin-C levels in synovial fluid are elevated after injury to the human and canine joint and correlate with markers of inflammation and matrix degradation. Osteoarthritis Cartilage. 2013;21:339–45.
165. Hasegawa M, Nakoshi Y, Muraki M, Sudo A, Kinoshita N, Yoshida T, Uchida A. Expression of large tenascin-C splice variants in synovial fluid of patients with rheumatoid arthritis. J Orthop Res. 2007;25:563–8.
166. Hasegawa M, Hirata H, Sudo A, Kato K, Kawase D, Kinoshita N, Yoshida T, Uchida A. Tenascin-C concentration in synovial fluid correlates with radiographic progression of knee osteoarthritis. J Rheumatol. 2004;31:2021–6.
167. Galicia K, Thorson C, Banos A, Rondina M, Hopkinson W, Hoppensteadt D, Fareed J. Inflammatory biomarker profiling in total joint arthroplasty and its relevance to circulating levels of lubricin, a novel proteoglycan. Clin Appl Thromb Hemost. 2018;24(6):950–9.
168. Li D, Wang Y, Xu N, Wei Q, Wu M, Li X, Zheng P, Sun S, Jin Y, Zhang G, Liao R, Zhang P. Follistatin-like protein 1 is elevated in systemic autoimmune diseases and correlated with disease activity in patients with rheumatoid arthritis. Arthritis Res Ther. 2011;13:R17.
169. Wang Y, Li D, Xu N, Tao W, Zhu R, Sun R, Fan W, Zhang P, Dong T, Yu L. Follistatin-like protein 1: a serum biochemical marker reflecting the severity of joint damage in patients with osteoarthritis. Arthritis Res Ther. 2011;13:R193.
170. Wilson DC, Marinov AD, Blair HC, Bushnell DS, Thompson SD, Chaly Y, Hirsch R. Follistatin-like protein 1 is a mesenchyme-derived inflammatory protein and may represent a biomarker for systemic-onset juvenile rheumatoid arthritis. Arthritis Rheum. 2010;62:2510–6.
171. Henrotin Y, Gharbi M, Mazzucchelli G, Dubuc JE, De Pauw E, Deberg M. Fibulin 3 peptides Fib3-1 and Fib3-2 are potential biomarkers of osteoarthritis. Arthritis Rheum. 2012;64:2260–7.
172. Henrotin Y, Sanchez C, Bay-Jensen AC, Mobasheri A. Osteoarthritis biomarkers derived from cartilage extracellular matrix: current status and future perspectives. Ann Phys Rehabil Med. 2016;59:145–8.
173. Runhaar J, Sanchez C, Taralla S, Henrotin Y, Bierma-Zeinstra SM. Fibulin-3 fragments are prognostic biomarkers of osteoarthritis incidence in overweight and obese women. Osteoarthritis Cartilage. 2016;24:672–8.
174. Luo Y, He Y, Reker D, Gudmann NS, Henriksen K, Simonsen O, Ladel C, Michaelis M, Mobasheri A, Karsdal M, Bay-Jensen AC. A novel high sensitivity type II collagen blood-based biomarker, PRO-C2, for assessment of cartilage formation. Int J Mol Sci. 2018;19(11). pii: E3485.
175. Deberg MA, Labasse AH, Collette J, Seidel L, Reginster JY, Henrotin YE. One-year increase of Coll 2-1, a new marker of type II collagen degradation, in urine is highly predictive of radiological OA progression. Osteoarthritis Cartilage. 2005;13:1059–65.
176. Garnero P, Delmas PD. Biomarkers in osteoarthritis. Curr Opin Rheumatol. 2003;15:641–6.
177. Poole AR, Kobayashi M, Yasuda T, Laverty S, Mwale F, Kojima T, Sakai T, Wahl C, El-Maadawy S, Webb G, Tchetina E, Wu W. Type II collagen degradation and its regulation in articular cartilage in osteoarthritis. Ann Rheum Dis. 2002;61(Suppl 2):ii78–81.
178. Dejica VM, Mort JS, Laverty S, Antoniou J, Zukor DJ, Tanzer M, Poole AR. Increased type II collagen cleavage by cathepsin K and collagenase activities with aging and osteoarthritis in human articular cartilage. Arthritis Res Ther. 2012;14:R113.
179. Bay-Jensen AC, Reker D, Kjelgaard-Petersen CF, Mobasheri A, Karsdal MA, Ladel C, Henrotin Y, Thudium CS. Osteoarthritis year in review 2015: soluble biomarkers and the BIPED criteria. Osteoarthritis Cartilage. 2016;24:9–20.
180. Van Spil WE, Welsing PM, Bierma-Zeinstra SM, Bijlsma JW, Roorda LD, Cats HA, Lafeber FP. The ability of systemic biochemical markers to reflect presence, incidence, and progression of early-stage radiographic knee and hip osteoarthritis: data from CHECK. Osteoarthritis Cartilage. 2015;23:1388–97.
181. Hosnijeh FS, Runhaar J, van Meurs JB, Bierma-Zeinstra SM. Biomarkers for osteoarthritis: can they be used for risk assessment? A systematic review. Maturitas. 2015;82:36–49.
182. Kumm J, Tamm A, Lintrop M, Tamm A. The value of cartilage biomarkers in progressive knee osteoarthritis: cross-sectional and 6-year follow-up study in middle-aged subjects. Rheumatol Int. 2013;33:903–11.
183. Streich NA, Zimmermann D, Schmitt H, Bode G. Biochemical markers in the diagnosis of chondral defects following anterior cruciate ligament insufficiency. Int Orthop. 2011;35:1633–7.
184. Sowers MF, Karvonen-Gutierrez CA, Yosef M, Jannausch M, Jiang Y, Garnero P, Jacobson J. Longitudinal changes of serum COMP and urinary CTX-II predict X-ray defined knee osteoarthritis severity and stiffness in women. Osteoarthritis Cartilage. 2009;17:1609–14.
185. Dam EB, Byrjalsen I, Karsdal MA, Qvist P, Christiansen C. Increased urinary excretion of C-telopeptides of type II collagen (CTX-II) predicts cartilage loss over 21 months by MRI. Osteoarthritis Cartilage. 2009;17:384–9.

186. Bay-Jensen AC, Andersen TL, Charni-Ben Tabassi N, Kristensen PW, Kjaersgaard-Andersen P, Sandell L, Garnero P, Delaisse JM. Biochemical markers of type II collagen breakdown and synthesis are positioned at specific sites in human osteoarthritic knee cartilage. Osteoarthritis Cartilage. 2008;16:615–23.
187. Meulenbelt I, Kloppenburg M, Kroon HM, Houwing-Duistermaat JJ, Garnero P, Hellio Le Graverand MP, Degroot J, Slagboom PE. Urinary CTX-II levels are associated with radiographic subtypes of osteoarthritis in hip, knee, hand, and facet joints in subject with familial osteoarthritis at multiple sites: the GARP study. Ann Rheum Dis. 2006;65:360–5.
188. Jung M, Christgau S, Lukoschek M, Henriksen D, Richter W. Increased urinary concentration of collagen type II C-telopeptide fragments in patients with osteoarthritis. Pathobiology. 2004;71:70–6.
189. Garnero P, Piperno M, Gineyts E, Christgau S, Delmas PD, Vignon E. Cross sectional evaluation of biochemical markers of bone, cartilage, and synovial tissue metabolism in patients with knee osteoarthritis: relations with disease activity and joint damage. Ann Rheum Dis. 2001;60:619–26.
190. Takahashi M, Kushida K, Hoshino H, Suzuki M, Sano M, Miyamoto S, Inoue T. Concentrations of pyridinoline and deoxypyridinoline in joint tissues from patients with osteoarthritis or rheumatoid arthritis. Ann Rheum Dis. 1996;55:324–7.
191. Behre A, Janott J, Pfohl M, Schatz H, Pfeiffer A. Clinical value of urinary pyridinium crosslinks as osteoporosis markers: evaluation of a population survey of vertebral osteoporosis. Med Klin (Munich). 2001;96:378–82.
192. Cloos C, Wahl P, Hasslacher C, Traber L, Kistner M, Jurkuhn K, Schmidt-Gayk H. Urinary glycosylated, free and total pyridinoline and free and total deoxypyridinoline in diabetes mellitus. Clin Endocrinol (Oxf). 1998;48:317–23.
193. Coleman RE, Houston S, James I, Rodger A, Rubens RD, Leonard RC, Ford J. Preliminary results of the use of urinary excretion of pyridinium crosslinks for monitoring metastatic bone disease. Br J Cancer. 1992;65:766–8.
194. Ferrari S, Zolezzi C, Pratelli L, Fasano MC, Bacci G. Urinary excretion of pyridinium cross-links and serum osteocalcin levels in patients with primary high-grade osteosarcoma. Calcif Tissue Int. 2003;73:1–4.
195. Fledelius C, Riis BJ, Overgaard K, Christiansen C. The diagnostic validity of urinary free pyridinolines to identify women at risk of osteoporosis. Calcif Tissue Int. 1994;54:381–4.
196. Gough AK, Peel NF, Eastell R, Holder RL, Lilley J, Emery P. Excretion of pyridinium crosslinks correlates with disease activity and appendicular bone loss in early rheumatoid arthritis. Ann Rheum Dis. 1994;53:14–7.
197. Ibrahim S, Mojiminiyi S, Barron JL. High-performance liquid chromatographic determination of pyridinium crosslinks in serum, urine and dialysate of patients in chronic renal failure. Ann Clin Biochem. 1996;33(Pt 1):31–5.
198. MacDonald AG, McHenry P, Robins SP, Reid DM. Relationship of urinary pyridinium crosslinks to disease extent and activity in osteoarthritis. Br J Rheumatol. 1994;33:16–9.
199. Marowska J, Kobylinska M, Lukaszkiewicz J, Talajko A, Rymkiewicz-Kluczynska B, Lorenc RS. Pyridinium crosslinks of collagen as a marker of bone resorption rates in children and adolescents: normal values and clinical application. Bone. 1996;19:669–77.
200. Seibel MJ, Duncan A, Robins SP. Urinary hydroxy-pyridinium crosslinks provide indices of cartilage and bone involvement in arthritic diseases. J Rheumatol. 1989;16:964–70.
201. Fick JM, Huttu MR, Lammi MJ, Korhonen RK. In vitro glycation of articular cartilage alters the biomechanical response of chondrocytes in a depth-dependent manner. Osteoarthritis Cartilage. 2014;22:1410–8.
202. DeGroot J, Verzijl N, Jacobs KM, Budde M, Bank RA, Bijlsma JW, TeKoppele JM, Lafeber FP. Accumulation of advanced glycation end-products reduces chondrocyte-mediated extracellular matrix turnover in human articular cartilage. Osteoarthritis Cartilage. 2001;9:720–6.
203. DeGroot J, Verzijl N, Wenting-Van Wijk MJ, Bank RA, Lafeber FP, Bijlsma JW, TeKoppele JM. Age-related decrease in susceptibility of human articular cartilage to matrix metalloproteinase-mediated degradation: the role of advanced glycation end products. Arthritis Rheum. 2001;44:2562–71.
204. Verzijl N, DeGroot J, Bank RA, Bayliss MT, Bijlsma JW, Lafeber FP, Maroudas A, TeKoppele JM. Age-related accumulation of the advanced glycation endproduct pentosidine in human articular cartilage aggrecan: the use of pentosidine levels as a quantitative measure of protein turnover. Matrix Biol. 2001;20:409–17.
205. Verzijl N, DeGroot J, Ben ZC, Brau-Benjamin O, Maroudas A, Bank RA, Mizrahi J, Schalkwijk CG, Thorpe SR, Baynes JW, Bijlsma JW, Lafeber FP, TeKoppele JM. Crosslinking by advanced glycation end products increases the stiffness of the collagen network in human articular cartilage: a possible mechanism through which age is a risk factor for osteoarthritis. Arthritis Rheum. 2002;46:114–23.
206. Verzijl N, DeGroot J, Thorpe SR, Bank RA, Shaw JN, Lyons TJ, Bijlsma JW, Lafeber FP, Baynes JW, TeKoppele JM. Effect of collagen turnover on the accumulation of advanced glycation end products. J Biol Chem. 2000;275:39027–31.

207. Pokharna HK, Monnier V, Boja B, Moskowitz RW. Lysyl oxidase and Maillard reaction-mediated crosslinks in aging and osteoarthritic rabbit cartilage. J Orthop Res. 1995;13:13–21.
208. Pokharna HK, Pottenger LA. Nonenzymatic glycation of cartilage proteoglycans: an in vivo and in vitro study. Glycoconj J. 1997;14:917–23.
209. Verzijl N, DeGroot J, Oldehinkel E, Bank RA, Thorpe SR, Baynes JW, Bayliss MT, Bijlsma JW, Lafeber FP, Tekoppele JM. Age-related accumulation of Maillard reaction products in human articular cartilage collagen. Biochem J. 2000;350 Pt 2:381–7.
210. Vos PA, DeGroot J, Huisman AM, Oostveen JC, Marijnissen AC, Bijlsma JW, van El B, Zuurmond AM, Lafeber FP. Skin and urine pentosidine weakly correlate with joint damage in a cohort of patients with early signs of osteoarthritis (CHECK). Osteoarthritis Cartilage. 2010;18:1329–36.
211. Odetti P, Fogarty J, Sell DR, Monnier VM. Chromatographic quantitation of plasma and erythrocyte pentosidine in diabetic and uremic subjects. Diabetes. 1992;41:153–9.
212. Requena JR, Price DL, Thorpe SR, Baynes JW. Measurement of pentosidine in biological samples. Methods Mol Med. 2000;38:209–17.
213. Sell DR, Lapolla A, Odetti P, Fogarty J, Monnier VM. Pentosidine formation in skin correlates with severity of complications in individuals with long-standing IDDM. Diabetes. 1992;41:1286–92.
214. Miyata T, van Ypersele de Strihou C, Kurokawa K, Baynes JW. Alterations in nonenzymatic biochemistry in uremia: origin and significance of "carbonyl stress" in long-term uremic complications. Kidney Int. 1999;55:389–99.
215. Bleasel JF, Poole AR, Heinegard D, Saxne T, Holderbaum D, Ionescu M, Jones P, Moskowitz RW. Changes in serum cartilage marker levels indicate altered cartilage metabolism in families with the osteoarthritis-related type II collagen gene COL2A1 mutation. Arthritis Rheum. 1999;42:39–45.
216. Dahlberg L, Roos H, Saxne T, Heinegard D, Lark MW, Hoerrner LA, Lohmander LS. Cartilage metabolism in the injured and uninjured knee of the same patient. Ann Rheum Dis. 1994;53:823–7.
217. El Defrawy AO, Gheita TA, Raslan HM, El Ansary MM, El Awar AH. Serum and synovial cartilage oligomeric matrix protein levels in early and established rheumatoid arthritis. Z Rheumatol. 2016;75:917–23.
218. El-Arman MM, El-Fayoumi G, El-Shal E, El-Boghdady I, El-Ghaweet A. Aggrecan and cartilage oligomeric matrix protein in serum and synovial fluid of patients with knee osteoarthritis. HSS J. 2010;6:171–6.
219. Erhart-Hledik JC, Favre J, Asay JL, Smith RL, Giori NJ, Mundermann A, Andriacchi TP. A relationship between mechanically-induced changes in serum cartilage oligomeric matrix protein (COMP) and changes in cartilage thickness after 5 years. Osteoarthritis Cartilage. 2012;20:1309–15.
220. Momohara S, Yamanaka H, Holledge MM, Mizumura T, Ikari K, Okada N, Kamatani N, Tomatsu T. Cartilage oligomeric matrix protein in serum and synovial fluid of rheumatoid arthritis: potential use as a marker for joint cartilage damage. Mod Rheumatol. 2004;14:356–60.
221. Morozzi G, Fabbroni M, Bellisai F, Pucci G, Galeazzi M. Cartilage oligomeric matrix protein level in rheumatic diseases: potential use as a marker for measuring articular cartilage damage and/or the therapeutic efficacy of treatments. Ann N Y Acad Sci. 2007;1108:398–407.
222. Neidhart M, Hauser N, Paulsson M, DiCesare PE, Michel BA, Hauselmann HJ. Small fragments of cartilage oligomeric matrix protein in synovial fluid and serum as markers for cartilage degradation. Br J Rheumatol. 1997;36:1151–60.
223. Posey KL, Hecht JT. The role of cartilage oligomeric matrix protein (COMP) in skeletal disease. Curr Drug Targets. 2008;9:869–77.
224. Saxne T, Heinegard D. Cartilage oligomeric matrix protein: a novel marker of cartilage turnover detectable in synovial fluid and blood. Br J Rheumatol. 1992;31:583–91.
225. Berry PA, Maciewicz RA, Wluka AE, Downey-Jones MD, Forbes A, Hellawell CJ, Cicuttini FM. Relationship of serum markers of cartilage metabolism to imaging and clinical outcome measures of knee joint structure. Ann Rheum Dis. 2010;69:1816–22.
226. Fife RS. Identification of cartilage matrix glycoprotein in synovial fluid in human osteoarthritis. Arthritis Rheum. 1988;31:553–6.
227. Haas DW, Holick MF. Enhanced osteonectin expression in the chondroid matrix of the unloaded mandibular condyle. Calcif Tissue Int. 1996;59:200–6.
228. Hewitt AT, Varner HH, Silver MH, Martin GR. The role of chondronectin and cartilage proteoglycan in the attachment of chondrocytes to collagen. Prog Clin Biol Res. 1982;110 Pt B:25–33.
229. Rosc D, Powierza W, Zastawna E, Drewniak W, Michalski A, Kotschy M. Post-traumatic plasminogenesis in intraarticular exudate in the knee joint. Med Sci Monit. 2002;8:CR371–8.
230. Tabushi Y, Nakanishi T, Takeuchi T, Nakajima M, Ueda K, Kotani T, Makino S, Shimizu A, Hanafusa T, Takubo T. Detection of citrullinated proteins in synovial fluids derived from patients with rheumatoid arthritis by proteomics-based analysis. Ann Clin Biochem. 2008;45:413–7.
231. Scuderi GJ, Golish SR, Cook FF, Cuellar JM, Bowser RP, Hanna LS. Identification of a novel fibronectin-aggrecan complex in the synovial fluid of knees with painful meniscal injury. J Bone Joint Surg Am. 2011;93:336–40.

232. Nakoshi Y, Hasegawa M, Akeda K, Iino T, Sudo A, Yoshida T, Uchida A. Distribution and role of tenascin-C in human osteoarthritic cartilage. J Orthop Sci. 2010;15:666–73.
233. Musumeci G, Trovato FM, Loreto C, Leonardi R, Szychlinska MA, Castorina S, Mobasheri A. Lubricin expression in human osteoarthritic knee meniscus and synovial fluid: a morphological, immunohistochemical and biochemical study. Acta Histochem. 2014;116:965–72.
234. Jones AR, Gleghorn JP, Hughes CE, Fitz LJ, Zollner R, Wainwright SD, Caterson B, Morris EA, Bonassar LJ, Flannery CR. Binding and localization of recombinant lubricin to articular cartilage surfaces. J Orthop Res. 2007;25:283–92.
235. Jay GD, Torres JR, Warman ML, Laderer MC, Breuer KS. The role of lubricin in the mechanical behavior of synovial fluid. Proc Natl Acad Sci U S A. 2007;104:6194–9.
236. Flowers SA, Zieba A, Ornros J, Jin C, Rolfson O, Bjorkman LI, Eisler T, Kalamajski S, Kamali-Moghaddam M, Karlsson NG. Lubricin binds cartilage proteins, cartilage oligomeric matrix protein, fibronectin and collagen II at the cartilage surface. Sci Rep. 2017;7:13149.
237. Alquraini A, Garguilo S, D'Souza G, Zhang LX, Schmidt TA, Jay GD, Elsaid KA. The interaction of lubricin/proteoglycan 4 (PRG4) with toll-like receptors 2 and 4: an anti-inflammatory role of PRG4 in synovial fluid. Arthritis Res Ther. 2015;17:353.
238. Flowers SA, Kalamajski S, Ali L, Bjorkman LI, Raj JR, Aspberg A, Karlsson NG, Jin C. Cartilage oligomeric matrix protein forms protein complexes with synovial lubricin via non-covalent and covalent interactions. Osteoarthritis Cartilage. 2017;25:1496–504.
239. Elsaid KA, Fleming BC, Oksendahl HL, Machan JT, Fadale PD, Hulstyn MJ, Shalvoy R, Jay GD. Decreased lubricin concentrations and markers of joint inflammation in the synovial fluid of patients with anterior cruciate ligament injury. Arthritis Rheum. 2008;58:1707–15.
240. Charni-Ben Tabassi N, Garnero P. Monitoring cartilage turnover. Curr Rheumatol Rep. 2007;9:16–24.
241. Tchetverikov I, Lohmander LS, Verzijl N, Huizinga TW, TeKoppele JM, Hanemaaijer R, DeGroot J. MMP protein and activity levels in synovial fluid from patients with joint injury, inflammatory arthritis, and osteoarthritis. Ann Rheum Dis. 2005;64:694–8.
242. Rubenhagen R, Schuttrumpf JP, Sturmer KM, Frosch KH. Interleukin-7 levels in synovial fluid increase with age and MMP-1 levels decrease with progression of osteoarthritis. Acta Orthop. 2012;83:59–64.
243. Girish KS, Kemparaju K. The magic glue hyaluronan and its eraser hyaluronidase: a biological overview. Life Sci. 2007;80:1921–43.
244. Sasaki Y, Uzuki M, Nohmi K, Kitagawa H, Kamataki A, Komagamine M, Murakami K, Sawai T. Quantitative measurement of serum hyaluronic acid molecular weight in rheumatoid arthritis patients and the role of hyaluronidase. Int J Rheum Dis. 2011;14:313–9.
245. Pruzanski W, Bogoch E, Wloch M, Vadas P. The role of phospholipase A2 in the physiopathology of osteoarthritis. J Rheumatol Suppl. 1991;27:117–9.
246. Ribbens C, Andre B, Kaye O, Kaiser MJ, Bonnet V, Jaspar JM, de Groote D, Franchimont N, Malaise MG. Synovial fluid matrix metalloproteinase-3 levels are increased in inflammatory arthritides whether erosive or not. Rheumatology (Oxford). 2000;39:1357–65.
247. Cuellar VG, Cuellar JM, Kirsch T, Strauss EJ. Correlation of synovial fluid biomarkers with cartilage pathology and associated outcomes in knee arthroscopy. Arthroscopy. 2016;32:475–85.
248. Sauerschnig M, Stolberg-Stolberg J, Schulze A, Salzmann GM, Perka C, Dynybil CJ. Diverse expression of selected cytokines and proteinases in synovial fluid obtained from osteoarthritic and healthy human knee joints. Eur J Med Res. 2014;19:65.
249. Daghestani HN, Kraus VB. Inflammatory biomarkers in osteoarthritis. Osteoarthritis Cartilage. 2015;23:1890–6.
250. Li W, Du C, Wang H, Zhang C. Increased serum ADAMTS-4 in knee osteoarthritis: a potential indicator for the diagnosis of osteoarthritis in early stages. Genet Mol Res. 2014;13:9642–9.
251. Roberts S, Evans H, Wright K, et al. ADAMTS-4 activity in synovial fluid as a biomarker of inflammation and effusion. Osteoarthritis Cartilage. 2015;23(9):1622–6.
252. Altobelli E, Angeletti PM, Piccolo D, De Angelis R. Synovial fluid and serum concentrations of inflammatory markers in rheumatoid arthritis, psoriatic arthritis and osteoarthitis: a systematic review. Curr Rheumatol Rev. 2017. https://doi.org/10.2174/1573397113666170427125918.
253. Stannus O, Jones G, Cicuttini F, Parameswaran V, Quinn S, Burgess J, Ding C. Circulating levels of IL-6 and TNF-alpha are associated with knee radiographic osteoarthritis and knee cartilage loss in older adults. Osteoarthritis Cartilage. 2010;18:1441–7.
254. Livshits G, Zhai G, Hart DJ, Kato BS, Wang H, Williams FM, Spector TD. Interleukin-6 is a significant predictor of radiographic knee osteoarthritis: The Chingford Study. Arthritis Rheum. 2009;60:2037–45.
255. Shimura Y, Kurosawa H, Sugawara Y, Tsuchiya M, Sawa M, Kaneko H, Futami I, Liu L, Sadatsuki R, Hada S, Iwase Y, Kaneko K, Ishijima M. The factors associated with pain severity in patients with knee osteoarthritis vary according to the radiographic disease severity: a cross-sectional study. Osteoarthritis Cartilage. 2013;21:1179–84.
256. Sun JM, Sun LZ, Liu J, BH S, Shi L. Serum interleukin-15 levels are associated with severity of pain

in patients with knee osteoarthritis. Dis Markers. 2013;35:203–6.
257. Mabey T, Honsawek S, Tanavalee A, Yuktanandana P, Wilairatana V, Poovorawan Y. Plasma and synovial fluid inflammatory cytokine profiles in primary knee osteoarthritis. Biomarkers. 2016;21:639–44.
258. Attur M, Krasnokutsky S, Statnikov A, Samuels J, Li Z, Friese O, Hellio Le Graverand-Gastineau MP, Rybak L, Kraus VB, Jordan JM, Aliferis CF, Abramson SB. Low-grade inflammation in symptomatic knee osteoarthritis: prognostic value of inflammatory plasma lipids and peripheral blood leukocyte biomarkers. Arthritis Rheumatol. 2015;67:2905–15.
259. Zhao XY, Yang ZB, Zhang ZJ, Zhang ZQ, Kang Y, Huang GX, Wang SW, Huang H, Liao WM. CCL3 serves as a potential plasma biomarker in knee degeneration (osteoarthritis). Osteoarthritis Cartilage. 2015;23:1405–11.
260. Wang K, Xu J, Cai J, Zheng S, Yang X, Ding C. Serum levels of resistin and interleukin-17 are associated with increased cartilage defects and bone marrow lesions in patients with knee osteoarthritis. Mod Rheumatol. 2017;27:339–44.
261. Wang Y, Xu D, Long L, Deng X, Tao R, Huang G. Correlation between plasma, synovial fluid and articular cartilage Interleukin-18 with radiographic severity in 33 patients with osteoarthritis of the knee. Clin Exp Med. 2014;14:297–304.
262. Gross JB, Guillaume C, Gégout-Pottie P, et al. Synovial fluid levels of adipokines in osteoarthritis: association with local factors of inflammation and cartilage maintenance. Biomed Mater Eng. 2014;24(1 Suppl):17–25.
263. Imamura M, Ezquerro F, Marcon Alfieri F, Vilas Boas L, Tozetto-Mendoza TR, Chen J, Ozcakar L, Arendt-Nielsen L, Rizzo Battistella L. Serum levels of proinflammatory cytokines in painful knee osteoarthritis and sensitization. Int J Inflamm. 2015;2015:329792.
264. Ding J, Niu X, Su Y, Li X. Expression of synovial fluid biomarkers in patients with knee osteoarthritis and meniscus injury. Exp Ther Med. 2017;14:1609–13.
265. Ozler K, Aktas E, Atay C, Yilmaz B, Arikan M, Gungor S. Serum and knee synovial fluid matrixmetalloproteinase-13 and tumor necrosis factor-alpha levels in patients with late stage osteoarthritis. Acta Orthop Traumatol Turc. 2016;50:670–3.
266. Penninx BW, Abbas H, Ambrosius W, Nicklas BJ, Davis C, Messier SP, Pahor M. Inflammatory markers and physical function among older adults with knee osteoarthritis. J Rheumatol. 2004;31:2027–31.
267. Vaiopoulos G, Boki K, Kapsimali V, Coulocheri S, Papadaki HA, Eliopoulos GD. Hemoglobin levels correlate with serum soluble CD23 and TNF-Rs concentrations in patients with rheumatoid arthritis. Haematologia (Budap). 1998;29(2):89–99.
268. Meyer M, Sellam J, Fellahi S, Kotti S, Bastard JP, Meyer O, Liote F, Simon T, Capeau J, Berenbaum F. Serum level of adiponectin is a surrogate independent biomarker of radiographic disease progression in early rheumatoid arthritis: results from the ESPOIR cohort. Arthritis Res Ther. 2013;15:R210.
269. Koskinen A, Juslin S, Nieminen R, Moilanen T, Vuolteenaho K, Moilanen E. Adiponectin associates with markers of cartilage degradation in osteoarthritis and induces production of proinflammatory and catabolic factors through mitogen-activated protein kinase pathways. Arthritis Res Ther. 2011;13:R184.
270. Lee YH, Bae SC. Circulating adiponectin and visfatin levels in rheumatoid arthritis and their correlation with disease activity: a meta-analysis. Int J Rheum Dis. 2018;21(3):664–72.
271. Toussirot E, Michel F, Bereau M, Dehecq B, Gaugler B, Wendling D, Grandclement E, Saas P, Dumoulin G. Serum adipokines, adipose tissue measurements and metabolic parameters in patients with advanced radiographic knee osteoarthritis. Clin Rheumatol. 2017;36(11):2531–9.
272. Oliviero F, Sfriso P, Baldo G, Dayer JM, Giunco S, Scanu A, et al. Apolipoprotein A-I and cholesterol in synovial fluid of patients with rheumatoid arthritis, psoriatic arthritis and osteoarthritis. Clin Exp Rheumatol. 2009;27(1):79–83.
273. de Seny D, Cobraiville G, Charlier E, Neuville S, Lutteri L, Le Goff C, Malaise D, Malaise O, Chapelle JP, Relic B, Malaise MG. Apolipoprotein-A1 as a damage-associated molecular patterns protein in osteoarthritis: ex vivo and in vitro proinflammatory properties. PLoS One. 2015;10(4):e0122904.
274. Oliviero F, Lo Nigro A, Bernardi D, Giunco S, Baldo G, Scanu A, Sfriso P, Ramonda R, Plebani M, Punzi L. A comparative study of serum and synovial fluid lipoprotein levels in patients with various arthritides. Clin Chim Acta. 2012;413(1–2):303–7.
275. Martel-Pelletier J, Raynauld JP, Dorais M, Abram F, Pelletier JP. The levels of the adipokines adipsin and leptin are associated with knee osteoarthritis progression as assessed by MRI and incidence of total knee replacement in symptomatic osteoarthritis patients: a post hoc analysis. Rheumatology (Oxford). 2016;55:680–8.
276. Terlain B, Presle N, Pottie P, Mainard D, Netter P. Leptin: a link between obesity and osteoarthritis? Bull Acad Natl Med. 2006;190:1421–35; discussion 1435–1427, 1475–1427.
277. Stannus OP, Cao Y, Antony B, Blizzard L, Cicuttini F, Jones G, Ding C. Cross-sectional and longitudinal associations between circulating leptin and knee cartilage thickness in older adults. Ann Rheum Dis. 2015;74:82–8.
278. Calvet J, Orellana C, Gratacos J, Berenguer-Llergo A, Caixas A, Chillaron JJ, Pedro-Botet J, Garcia-Manrique M, Navarro N, Larrosa M. Synovial fluid

adipokines are associated with clinical severity in knee osteoarthritis: a cross-sectional study in female patients with joint effusion. Arthritis Res Ther. 2016;18:207.
279. Kim HR, Lee JH, Kim KW, Kim BM, Lee SH. The relationship between synovial fluid VEGF and serum leptin with ultrasonographic findings in knee osteoarthritis. Int J Rheum Dis. 2016;19:233–40.
280. Azamar-Llamas D, Hernandez-Molina G, Ramos-Avalos B, Furuzawa-Carballeda J. Adipokine contribution to the pathogenesis of osteoarthritis. Mediators Inflamm. 2017;2017:5468023.
281. Koskinen A, Vuolteenaho K, Moilanen T, Moilanen E. Resistin as a factor in osteoarthritis: synovial fluid resistin concentrations correlate positively with interleukin 6 and matrix metalloproteinases MMP-1 and MMP-3. Scand J Rheumatol. 2014;43:249–53.
282. Duan Y, Hao D, Li M, Wu Z, Li D, Yang X, Qiu G. Increased synovial fluid visfatin is positively linked to cartilage degradation biomarkers in osteoarthritis. Rheumatol Int. 2012;32:985–90.
283. Chen WP, Bao JP, Feng J, PF H, Shi ZL, LD W. Increased serum concentrations of visfatin and its production by different joint tissues in patients with osteoarthritis. Clin Chem Lab Med. 2010;48:1141–5.
284. Duan WP, Sun ZW, Li Q, Li CJ, Wang L, Chen WY, Tickner J, Zheng MH, Wei XC. Normal age-related viscoelastic properties of chondrons and chondrocytes isolated from rabbit knee. Chin Med J (Engl). 2012;125:2574–81.
285. Scanu A, Oliviero F, Ramonda R, Frallonardo P, Dayer JM, Punzi L. Cytokine levels in human synovial fluid during the different stages of acute gout: role of transforming growth factor beta1 in the resolution phase. Ann Rheum Dis. 2012;71:621–4.
286. He J, Cao W, Azeem I, Zhao Q, Shao Z. Transforming growth factor Beta1 being considered a novel biomarker in knee osteoarthritis. Clin Chim Acta. 2017;472:96–101.
287. Chen YH, Hsieh SC, Chen WY, Li KJ, Wu CH, Wu PC, Tsai CY, Yu CL. Spontaneous resolution of acute gouty arthritis is associated with rapid induction of the anti-inflammatory factors TGFβ1, IL-10 and soluble TNF receptors and the intracellular cytokine negative regulators CIS and SOCS3. Ann Rheum Dis. 2011;70(9):1655–63.
288. Zhang GM, Zhang GM, Gu B. Serum transforming growth factor beta1 level for knee osteoarthritis diagnosis. Clin Chim Acta. 2017;474:136.
289. Saetan N, Honsawek S, Tanavalee A, Yuktanandana P, Meknavin S, Ngarmukos S, Tanpowpong T, Parkpian V. Relationship of plasma and synovial fluid vascular endothelial growth factor with radiographic severity in primary knee osteoarthritis. Int Orthop. 2014;38:1099–104.
290. Knudsen LS, Klarlund M, Skjodt H, Jensen T, Ostergaard M, Jensen KE, Hansen MS, Hetland ML, Nielsen HJ, Johansen JS. Biomarkers of inflammation in patients with unclassified polyarthritis and early rheumatoid arthritis. Relationship to disease activity and radiographic outcome. J Rheumatol. 2008;35:1277–87.
291. Flannery CR, Zeng W, Corcoran C, Collins-Racie LA, Chockalingam PS, Hebert T, Mackie SA, McDonagh T, Crawford TK, Tomkinson KN, LaVallie ER, Morris EA. Autocatalytic cleavage of ADAMTS-4 (Aggrecanase-1) reveals multiple glycosaminoglycan-binding sites. J Biol Chem. 2002;277:42775–80.
292. Verma RP, Hansch C. Matrix metalloproteinases (MMPs): chemical-biological functions and (Q) SARs. Bioorg Med Chem. 2007;15:2223–68.
293. Clark IM, Parker AE. Metalloproteinases: their role in arthritis and potential as therapeutic targets. Expert Opin Ther Targets. 2003;7:19–34.
294. Murphy G, Nagase H. Reappraising metalloproteinases in rheumatoid arthritis and osteoarthritis: destruction or repair? Nat Clin Pract Rheumatol. 2008;4:128–35.
295. Sandy JD, Verscharen C. Analysis of aggrecan in human knee cartilage and synovial fluid indicates that aggrecanase (ADAMTS) activity is responsible for the catabolic turnover and loss of whole aggrecan whereas other protease activity is required for C-terminal processing in vivo. Biochem J. 2001;358:615–26.
296. Struglics A, Hansson M. MMP proteolysis of the human extracellular matrix protein aggrecan is mainly a process of normal turnover. Biochem J. 2012;446:213–23.
297. Bomalaski JS, Fallon M, Turner RA, Crooke ST, Meunier PC, Clark MA. Identification and isolation of a phospholipase A2 activating protein in human rheumatoid arthritis synovial fluid: induction of eicosanoid synthesis and an inflammatory response in joints injected in vivo. J Lab Clin Med. 1990;116:814–25.
298. Du Clos TW, Mold C. C-reactive protein: an activator of innate immunity and a modulator of adaptive immunity. Immunol Res. 2004;30:261–77.
299. Peisajovich A, Marnell L, Mold C, Du Clos TW. C-reactive protein at the interface between innate immunity and inflammation. Expert Rev Clin Immunol. 2008;4:379–90.
300. Marnell L, Mold C, Du Clos TW. C-reactive protein: ligands, receptors and role in inflammation. Clin Immunol. 2005;117:104–11.
301. Jin X, Beguerie JR, Zhang W, Blizzard L, Otahal P, Jones G, Ding C. Circulating C reactive protein in osteoarthritis: a systematic review and meta-analysis. Ann Rheum Dis. 2015;74:703–10.
302. Nugzar O, Zandman-Goddard G, Oz H, Lakstein D, Feldbrin Z, et al. The role of ferritin and adiponectin as predictors of cartilage damage assessed by arthroscopy in patients with symptomatic knee osteoarthritis. Best Pract Res Clin Rheumatol. 2018;32(5):662–68.
303. Assirelli E, Pulsatelli L, Dolzani P, Platano D, Olivotto E, Filardo G, Trisolino G, Facchini A, Borzi RM, Meliconi R. Human osteoarthritic car-

tilage shows reduced in vivo expression of IL-4, a chondroprotective cytokine that differentially modulates IL-1beta-stimulated production of chemokines and matrix-degrading enzymes in vitro. PLoS One. 2014;9:e96925.

304. Larsson S, Englund M, Struglics A, Lohmander LS. Interleukin-6 and tumor necrosis factor alpha in synovial fluid are associated with progression of radiographic knee osteoarthritis in subjects with previous meniscectomy. Osteoarthritis Cartilage. 2015;23:1906–14.

305. Scanzello CR, Umoh E, Pessler F, Diaz-Torne C, Miles T, Dicarlo E, Potter HG, Mandl L, Marx R, Rodeo S, Goldring SR, Crow MK. Local cytokine profiles in knee osteoarthritis: elevated synovial fluid interleukin-15 differentiates early from end-stage disease. Osteoarthritis Cartilage. 2009;17:1040–8.

306. Struglics A, Larsson S, Kumahashi N, Frobell R, Lohmander LS. Changes in cytokines and aggrecan ARGS neoepitope in synovial fluid and serum and in C-terminal crosslinking telopeptide of type II collagen and N-terminal crosslinking telopeptide of type I collagen in urine over five years after anterior cruciate ligament rupture: an exploratory analysis in the knee anterior cruciate ligament, nonsurgical versus surgical treatment trial. Arthritis Rheumatol. 2015;67:1816–25.

307. Borzi RM, Mazzetti I, Marcu KB, Facchini A. Chemokines in cartilage degradation. Clin Orthop Relat Res. 2004:S53–61.

308. Dozio E, Corsi MM, Ruscica M, Passafaro L, Steffani L, Banfi G, Magni P. Adipokine actions on cartilage homeostasis. Adv Clin Chem. 2011;55:61–79.

309. Berry PA, Jones SW, Cicuttini FM, Wluka AE, Maciewicz RA. Temporal relationship between serum adipokines, biomarkers of bone and cartilage turnover, and cartilage volume loss in a population with clinical knee osteoarthritis. Arthritis Rheum. 2011;63:700–7.

310. King LK, Henneicke H, Seibel MJ, March L, Anandacoomarasmy A. Association of adipokines and joint biomarkers with cartilage-modifying effects of weight loss in obese subjects. Osteoarthritis Cartilage. 2015;23:397–404.

311. Gegout PP, Francin PJ, Mainard D, Presle N. Adipokines in osteoarthritis: friends or foes of cartilage homeostasis? Joint Bone Spine. 2008;75:669–71.

312. Faggioni R, Fantuzzi G, Fuller J, Dinarello CA, Feingold KR, Grunfeld C. IL-1 beta mediates leptin induction during inflammation. Am J Physiol. 1998;274:R204–8.

313. Neumann E, Junker S, Schett G, Frommer K, Muller-Ladner U. Adipokines in bone disease. Nat Rev Rheumatol. 2016;12:296–302.

314. Vuolteenaho K, Koskinen A, Kukkonen M, Nieminen R, Paivarinta U, Moilanen T, Moilanen E. Leptin enhances synthesis of proinflammatory mediators in human osteoarthritic cartilage – mediator role of NO in leptin-induced PGE2, IL-6, and IL-8 production. Mediators Inflamm. 2009;2009:345838.

315. Junker S, Frommer KW, Krumbholz G, Tsiklauri L, Gerstberger R, Rehart S, et al. Expression of adipokines in osteoarthritis osteophytes and their effect on osteoblasts. Matrix Biol. 2017;62:75–91.

316. Hui W, Litherland GJ, Elias MS, Kitson GI, Cawston TE, Rowan AD, Young DA. Leptin produced by joint white adipose tissue induces cartilage degradation via upregulation and activation of matrix metalloproteinases. Ann Rheum Dis. 2012;71:455–62.

317. Mirfeizi Z, Noubakht Z, Rezaie AE, Jokar MH, Sarabi ZS. Plasma levels of leptin and visfatin in rheumatoid arthritis patients; is there any relationship with joint damage? Iranian J Basic Med Sci. 2014;17:662–6.

318. Zhen G, Cao X. Targeting TGFbeta signaling in subchondral bone and articular cartilage homeostasis. Trends Pharmacol Sci. 2014;35:227–36.

319. Finnson KW, Chi Y, Bou-Gharios G, Leask A, Philip A. TGF-b signaling in cartilage homeostasis and osteoarthritis. Front Biosci (Schol Ed). 2012;4:251–68.

320. Pujol JP, Chadjichristos C, Legendre F, Bauge C, Beauchef G, Andriamanalijaona R, Galera P, Boumediene K. Interleukin-1 and transforming growth factor-beta 1 as crucial factors in osteoarthritic cartilage metabolism. Connect Tissue Res. 2008;49:293–7.

321. Pelletier JP, Roughley PJ, DiBattista JA, McCollum R, Martel-Pelletier J. Are cytokines involved in osteoarthritic pathophysiology? Semin Arthritis Rheum. 1991;20:12–25.

322. Vadalà G, Russo F, Musumeci M, Giacalone A, Papalia R, et al. Targeting VEGF-A in cartilage repair and regeneration: state of the art and perspectives. J Biol Regul Homeost Agents. 2018;32(6 Suppl. 1):217–24.

323. Mabey T, Honsawek S, Saetan N, Poovorawan Y, Tanavalee A, Yuktanandana P. Angiogenic cytokine expression profiles in plasma and synovial fluid of primary knee osteoarthritis. Int Orthop. 2014;38:1885–92.

324. Schmidt MB, Chen EH, Lynch SE. A review of the effects of insulin-like growth factor and platelet derived growth factor on in vivo cartilage healing and repair. Osteoarthritis Cartilage. 2006;14:403–12.

325. Wang J, Elewaut D, Veys EM, Verbruggen G. Insulin-like growth factor 1-induced interleukin-1 receptor II overrides the activity of interleukin-1 and controls the homeostasis of the extracellular matrix of cartilage. Arthritis Rheum. 2003;48:1281–91.

326. Cattano NM, Driban JB, Cameron KL, Sitler MR. Impact of physical activity and mechanical loading on biomarkers typically used in osteoarthritis assessment: current concepts and knowledge gaps. Ther Adv Musculoskelet Dis. 2017;9:11–21.

327. Celik O, Salci Y, Ak E, Kalaci A, Korkusuz F. Serum cartilage oligomeric matrix protein accumulation

decreases significantly after 12 weeks of running but not swimming and cycling training – a randomised controlled trial. Knee. 2013;20:19–25.
328. Hoch JM, Mattacola CG, Bush HM, Medina McKeon JM, Hewett TE, Lattermann C. Longitudinal documentation of serum cartilage oligomeric matrix protein and patient-reported outcomes in collegiate soccer athletes over the course of an athletic season. Am J Sports Med. 2012;40:2583–9.
329. Roos H, Dahlberg L, Hoerrner LA, Lark MW, Thonar EJ, Shinmei M, Lindqvist U, Lohmander LS. Markers of cartilage matrix metabolism in human joint fluid and serum: the effect of exercise. Osteoarthritis Cartilage. 1995;3:7–14.
330. Pruksakorn D, Tirankgura P, Luevitoonvechkij S, Chamnongkich S, Sugandhavesa N, Leerapun T, Pothacharoen P. Changes in the serum cartilage biomarker levels of healthy adults in response to an uphill walk. Singapore Med J. 2013;54:702–8.
331. Mundermann A, Geurts J, Hugle T, Nickel T, Schmidt-Trucksass A, Halle M, Hanssen H. Marathon performance but not BMI affects post-marathon pro-inflammatory and cartilage biomarkers. J Sports Sci. 2017;35:711–8.
332. Carbone A, Rodeo S. Review of current understanding of post-traumatic osteoarthritis resulting from sports injuries. J Orthop Res. 2017;35(3):397–405.
333. Hogrefe C, Joos H, Maheswaran V, Durselen L, Ignatius A, Brenner RE. Single impact cartilage trauma and TNF-alpha: interactive effects do not increase early cell death and indicate the need for bi−/multidirectional therapeutic approaches. Int J Mol Med. 2012;30:1225–32.
334. Palmieri-Smith RM, Wojtys EM, Potter HG. Early cartilage changes after anterior cruciate ligament injury: evaluation with imaging and serum biomarkers - a pilot study. Arthroscopy. 2016;32(7):1309–18.
335. Struglics A, Larsson S, Pramhed A, Frobell R, Swärd P. Changes in synovial fluid and serum concentrations of cartilage oligomeric matrix protein over 5 years after anterior cruciate ligament rupture: an exploratory analysis in the KANON trial. Osteoarthritis Cartilage. 2018;26(10):1351–8.
336. Wei S-T, Sun Y-H, Zong S-H, Xiang Y-B. Serum levels of IL-6 and TNF -α may correlate with activity and severity of rheumatoid arthritis. Med Sci Monit. 2015;21:4030–8.
337. Saudek DM, Kay J. Advanced glycation endproducts and osteoarthritis. Curr Rheumatol Rep. 2003;5:33–40.
338. Zhang C, Wei X, Chen C, Cao K, Li Y, Jiao Q, Ding J, Zhou J, Fleming BC, Chen Q, Shang X, Wei L. Indian hedgehog in synovial fluid is a novel marker for early cartilage lesions in human knee joint. Int J Mol Sci. 2014;15:7250–65.
339. Senolt L, Sumova B, Jandova R, Hulejova H, Mann H, Pavelka K, et al. Interleukin 35 synovial fluid levels are associated with disease activity of rheumatoid arthritis. PLoS One. 2015;10(7):e0132674.
340. Sglunda O, Mann H, Hulejova H, Kuklova M, Pecha O, Plestilova L, et al. Decreased circulating visfatin is associated with improved disease activity in early rheumatoid arthritis: data from the PERAC cohort. PLoS One. 2014;9(7):e103495.
341. Zou YC, Chen LH, Ye YL, Yang GG, Mao Z, Liu DD, Chen JQ, Chen JJ, Liu G. Attenuated synovial fluid ghrelin levels are linked with cartilage damage, meniscus injury, and clinical symptoms in patients with knee anterior cruciate ligament deficiency. Discov Med. 2016;22:325–35.
342. Li L, Jiang BE. Serum and synovial fluid chemokine ligand 2/monocyte chemoattractant protein 1 concentrations correlates with symptomatic severity in patients with knee osteoarthritis. Ann Clin Biochem. 2015;52:276–82.
343. Laudon J, Whittaker JL, Ren G, Jaremko JL, Emery CA, Krawetz RJ. Serum cartilage oligomeric matrix protein (COMP) expression in individuals who sustained a youth sport-related intra-articular knee injury 3-10 years previously and uninjured matched controls. Osteoarthritis Cartilage. 2018; pii: S1063-4584(18)31482-1. https://doi.org/10.1016/j.joca.2018.09.011.
344. Bolduc JA, Collins JA, Loeser RF. Reactive oxygen species, aging and articular cartilage homeostasis. Free Radic Biol Med. 2018; pii: S0891-5849(18)31500-4. https://doi.org/10.1016/j.freeradbiomed.2018.08.038.
345. Bank RA, Bayliss MT, Lafeber FP, Maroudas A, Tekoppele JM. Ageing and zonal variation in post-translational modification of collagen in normal human articular cartilage. The age-related increase in non-enzymatic glycation affects biomechanical properties of cartilage. Biochem J. 1998;330(Pt 1):345–51.
346. Chen AC, Temple MM, Ng DM, Verzijl N, DeGroot J, TeKoppele JM, Sah RL. Induction of advanced glycation end products and alterations of the tensile properties of articular cartilage. Arthritis Rheum. 2002;46:3212–7.
347. Matsushita T, Tanaka T. Aging and homeostasis. Aging of articular cartilage and chondrocytes. Clin Calcium. 2017;27:933–9.
348. Rahmati M, Nalesso G, Mobasheri A, Mozafari M. Aging and osteoarthritis: central role of the extracellular matrix. Ageing Res Rev. 2017;40:20–30.
349. van der Kraan PM. Age-related alterations in TGF beta signaling as a causal factor of cartilage degeneration in osteoarthritis. Biomed Mater Eng. 2014;24:75–80.
350. Stannus OP, Jones G, Blizzard L, Cicuttini FM, Ding C. Associations between serum levels of inflammatory markers and change in knee pain over 5 years in older adults: a prospective cohort study. Ann Rheum Dis. 2013;72:535–40.
351. Chimenti MS, Triggianese P, Conigliaro P, Candi E, Melino G, Perricone R. The interplay between inflammation and metabolism in rheumatoid arthritis. Cell Death Dis. 2015;6:e1887.

352. Pruzanski W, Keystone EC, Sternby B, Bombardier C, Snow KM, Vadas P. Serum phospholipase A2 correlates with disease activity in rheumatoid arthritis. J Rheumatol. 1988;15:1351–5.
353. Martel-Pelletier J, Raynauld JP, Mineau F, Abram F, Paiement P, Delorme P, Pelletier JP. Levels of serum biomarkers from a two-year multicentre trial are associated with treatment response on knee osteoarthritis cartilage loss as assessed by magnetic resonance imaging: an exploratory study. Arthritis Res Ther. 2017;19:169.
354. Wislowska M, Jablonska B. Serum cartilage oligomeric matrix protein (COMP) in rheumatoid arthritis and knee osteoarthritis. Clin Rheumatol. 2005;24:278–84.
355. Harvey S, Weisman M, O'Dell J, Scott T, Krusemeier M, Visor J, Swindlehurst C. Chondrex: new marker of joint disease. Clin Chem. 1998;44:509–16.
356. Robins SP, Stewart P, Astbury C, Bird HA. Measurement of the cross linking compound, pyridinoline, in urine as an index of collagen degradation in joint disease. Ann Rheum Dis. 1986;45:969–73.
357. Black D, Marabani M, Sturrock RD, Robins SP. Urinary excretion of the hydroxypyridinium cross links of collagen in patients with rheumatoid arthritis. Ann Rheum Dis. 1989;48:641–4.
358. Firner S, Zaucke F, Michael J, Dargel J, Schiwy-Bochat KH, Heilig J, et al. Extracellular distribution of collagen II and Perifibrillar adapter proteins in healthy and osteoarthritic human knee joint cartilage. J Histochem Cytochem. 2017;65(10):593–606.
359. Sanchez C, Bay-Jensen AC, Pap T, Dvir-Ginzberg M, Quasnichka H, Barrett-Jolley R, Mobasheri A, Henrotin Y. Chondrocyte secretome: a source of novel insights and exploratory biomarkers of osteoarthritis. Osteoarthritis Cartilage. 2017;25:1199–209.
360. Mobasheri A, van Spil WE, Budd E, Uzieliene I, Bernotiene E, Bay-Jensen AC, et al. Molecular taxonomy of osteoarthritis for patient stratification, di sease management and drug development: biochemical markers associated with emerging clinical phenotypes and molecular endotypes. Curr Opin Rheumatol. 2019;31(1):80–9.
361. Otterness IG, Swindell AC, Zimmerer RO, Poole AR, Ionescu M, Weiner E. An analysis of 14 molecular markers for monitoring osteoarthritis: segregation of the markers into clusters and distinguishing osteoarthritis at baseline. Osteoarthritis Cartilage. 2000;8:180–5.
362. Azukizawa M, Ito H, Hamamoto Y, Fujii T, Morita Y, et al. The effects of well-rounded exercise program on systemic biomarkers related to cartilage metabolism. Cartilage. 2019;10(4):451–58.
363. Manoy P, Anomasiri W, Yuktanandana P, Tanavalee A, Ngarmukos S, Tanpowpong T, Honsawek S. Elevated serum leptin levels are associated with low vitamin D, sarcopenic obesity, poor muscle strength, and physical performance in knee osteoarthritis. Biomarkers. 2017:1–8.
364. Senol O, Gundogdu G, Gundogdu K, Miloglu FD. Investigation of the relationships between knee osteoarthritis and obesity via untargeted metabolomics analysis. Clin Rheumatol. 2019;38(5):1351–60.
365. Jiao Q, Wei L, Chen C, Li P, Wang X, Li Y, Guo L, Zhang C, Wei X. Cartilage oligomeric matrix protein and hyaluronic acid are sensitive serum biomarkers for early cartilage lesions in the knee joint. Biomarkers. 2016;21:146–51.
366. Jung YO, Do JH, Kang HJ, Yoo SA, Yoon CH, Kim HA, Cho CS, Kim WU. Correlation of sonographic severity with biochemical markers of synovium and cartilage in knee osteoarthritis patients. Clin Exp Rheumatol. 2006;24:253–9.
367. Cahue S, Sharma L, Dunlop D, Ionescu M, Song J, Lobanok T, King L, Poole AR. The ratio of type II collagen breakdown to synthesis and its relationship with the progression of knee osteoarthritis. Osteoarthritis Cartilage. 2007;15:819–23.
368. Hwang IY, Youm YS, Cho SD, Choi SW, Bae MH, et al. Synovial fluid levels of TWEAK and matrix metalloproteinase 1 in patients with osteoarthritis, and associations with disease severity. J Orthop Surg (Hong Kong). 2018;26(1):2309499018760112.
369. Mobasheri A, Bay-Jensen AC, Gualillo O, Larkin J, Levesque MC, et al. Soluble biochemical markers of osteoarthritis: are we close to using them in clinical practice? Best Pract Res Clin Rheumatol. 2017;31(5):705–20.
370. Gao F, Tian J, Pan H, Gao J, Yao M. Association of CCL13 levels in serum and synovial fluid with the radiographic severity of knee osteoarthritis. J Investig Med. 2015;63:545–7.
371. Xu Q, Sun XC, Shang XP, Jiang HS. Association of CXCL12 levels in synovial fluid with the radiographic severity of knee osteoarthritis. J Invest Med. 2012;60:898–901.
372. Huo LW, Ye YL, Wang GW, Ye YG. Fractalkine (CX3CL1): a biomarker reflecting symptomatic severity in patients with knee osteoarthritis. J Investig Med. 2015;63:626–31.
373. Zou Y, Li Y, Lu L, Lin Y, Liang W, Su Z, Wang X, Yang H, Wang J, Yu C, Huo L, Ye Y. Correlation of fractalkine concentrations in serum and synovial fluid with the radiographic severity of knee osteoarthritis. Ann Clin Biochem. 2013;50:571–5.
374. Willett TL, Kandel R, De Croos JN, Avery NC, Grynpas MD. Enhanced levels of non-enzymatic glycation and pentosidine crosslinking in spontaneous osteoarthritis progression. Osteoarthritis Cartilage. 2012;20:736–44.
375. Michelacci YM, Mourão PA, Laredo J, Dietrich CP. Chondroitin sulfates and proteoglycans from normal and arthrosic human cartilage. Connect Tissue Res. 1979;7:29–36.
376. Bayliss MT, Davidson C, Woodhouse SM, Osborne DJ. Chondroitin sulphation in human joint tissues varies with age, zone and topography. Acta Orthop Scand Suppl. 1995;266:22–5.

377. Thonar EJ, Schnitzer TJ, Kuettner KE. Quantification of keratan sulfate in blood as a marker of cartilage catabolism. J Rheumatol. 1987;14 Spec No:23–4.
378. Nakajima A, Nakagawa K, Aoki Y, Sonobe M, Shibata Y, Yamazaki M, Murakami M. Changes in synovial fluid biochemical markers following arthroscopic surgery in patients with knee osteoarthritis. Rheumatol Int. 2013;33:209–14.
379. Vasara AI, Konttinen YT, Peterson L, Lindahl A, Kiviranta I. Persisting high levels of synovial fluid markers after cartilage repair: a pilot study. Clin Orthop Relat Res. 2009;467:267–72.
380. Doss F, Menard J, Hauschild M, Kreutzer HJ, Mittlmeier T, Muller-Steinhardt M, Muller B. Elevated IL-6 levels in the synovial fluid of osteoarthritis patients stem from plasma cells. Scand J Rheumatol. 2007;36:136–9.
381. Ahlen M, Roshani L, Liden M, Struglics A, Rostgard-Christensen L, Kartus J. Inflammatory cytokines and biomarkers of cartilage metabolism 8 years after anterior cruciate ligament reconstruction: results from operated and contralateral knees. Am J Sports Med. 2015;43:1460–6.
382. Sweet MB, Coelho A, Schnitzler CM, Schnitzer TJ, Lenz ME, Jakim I, Kuettner KE, Thonar EJ. Serum keratan sulfate levels in osteoarthritis patients. Arthritis Rheum. 1988;31:648–52.
383. Brandt KD. A pessimistic view of serologic markers for diagnosis and management of osteoarthritis. Biochemical, immunologic and clinicopathologic barriers. J Rheumatol Suppl. 1989;18:39–42.
384. Spector TD, Woodward L, Hall GM, Hammond A, Williams A, Butler MG, James IT, Hart DJ, Thompson PW, Scott DL. Keratan sulphate in rheumatoid arthritis, osteoarthritis, and inflammatory diseases. Ann Rheum Dis. 1992;51:1134–7.
385. Cohen NP, Foster RJ, Mow VC. Composition and dynamics of articular cartilage: structure, function, and maintaining healthy state. J Orthop Sports Phys Ther. 1998;28:203–15.
386. XL L, Mow VC, Guo XE. Proteoglycans and mechanical behavior of condylar cartilage. J Dent Res. 2009;88:244–8.
387. Bachrach NM, Mow VC, Guilak F. Incompressibility of the solid matrix of articular cartilage under high hydrostatic pressures. J Biomech. 1998;31:445–51.
388. Zheng W, Li X, Liu D, Li J, Yang S, et al. Mechanical loading mitigates osteoarthritis symptoms by regulating endoplasmic reticulum stress and autophagy. FASEB J. 2019;33(3):4077–88.
389. Kung LHW, Mullan L, Soul J, Wang P, Mori K, et al. Cartilage endoplasmic reticulum stress may influence the onset but not the progression of experimental osteoarthritis. Arthritis Res Ther. 2019;21(1):206.
390. Griffin TM, Guilak F. The role of mechanical loading in the onset and progression of osteoarthritis. Exerc Sport Sci Rev. 2005;33:195–200.
391. Sun HB. Mechanical loading, cartilage degradation, and arthritis. Ann N Y Acad Sci. 2010;1211:37–50.
392. Yokota H, Leong DJ, Sun HB. Mechanical loading: bone remodeling and cartilage maintenance. Curr Osteoporos Rep. 2011;9:237–42.
393. Mow VC, Holmes MH, Lai WM. Fluid transport and mechanical properties of articular cartilage: a review. J Biomech. 1984;17:377–94.
394. Mow VC, Wang CC, Hung CT. The extracellular matrix, interstitial fluid and ions as a mechanical signal transducer in articular cartilage. Osteoarthritis Cartilage. 1999;7:41–58.
395. Torzilli PA, Grigiene R, Huang C, Friedman SM, Doty SB, Boskey AL, Lust G. Characterization of cartilage metabolic response to static and dynamic stress using a mechanical explant test system. J Biomech. 1997;30:1–9.
396. Arokoski JP, Jurvelin JS, Vaatainen U, Helminen HJ. Normal and pathological adaptations of articular cartilage to joint loading. Scand J Med Sci Sports. 2000;10:186–98.
397. Bachrach NM, Valhmu WB, Stazzone E, Ratcliffe A, Lai WM, Mow VC. Changes in proteoglycan synthesis of chondrocytes in articular cartilage are associated with the time-dependent changes in their mechanical environment. J Biomech. 1995;28:1561–9.
398. Buschmann MD, Hunziker EB, Kim YJ, Grodzinsky AJ. Altered aggrecan synthesis correlates with cell and nucleus structure in statically compressed cartilage. J Cell Sci. 1996;109(Pt 2):499–508.
399. Steinmeyer J, Knue S. The proteoglycan metabolism of mature bovine articular cartilage explants superimposed to continuously applied cyclic mechanical loading. Biochem Biophys Res Commun. 1997;240:216–21.
400. Steinmeyer J, Knue S, Raiss RX, Pelzer I. Effects of intermittently applied cyclic loading on proteoglycan metabolism and swelling behaviour of articular cartilage explants. Osteoarthritis Cartilage. 1999;7:155–64.
401. Buschmann MD, Kim YJ, Wong M, Frank E, Hunziker EB, Grodzinsky AJ. Stimulation of aggrecan synthesis in cartilage explants by cyclic loading is localized to regions of high interstitial fluid flow. Arch Biochem Biophys. 1999;366:1–7.
402. Giannoni P, Siegrist M, Hunziker EB, Wong M. The mechanosensitivity of cartilage oligomeric matrix protein (COMP). Biorheology. 2003; 40:101–9.
403. Herger S, Vach W, Liphardt AM, Egloff C, Nüesch C, et al. Dose-response relationship between ambulatory load magnitude and load-induced changes in COMP in young healthy adults. Osteoarthritis Cartilage. 2019;27(1):106–13.
404. Hyldahl RD, Evans A, Kwon S, Ridge ST, Robinson E, Hopkins JT, Seeley MK. Running decreases knee intra-articular cytokine and cartilage oligomeric matrix concentrations: a pilot study. Eur J Appl Physiol. 2016;116:2305–14.

405. Monfort J, Garcia-Giralt N, Lopez-Armada MJ, Monllau JC, Bonilla A, Benito P, Blanco FJ. Decreased metalloproteinase production as a response to mechanical pressure in human cartilage: a mechanism for homeostatic regulation. Arthritis Res Ther. 2006;8:R149.
406. Kelly PA, O'Connor JJ. Transmission of rapidly applied loads through articular cartilage. Part 2: cracked cartilage. Proc Inst Mech Eng H J Eng Med. 1996;210:39–49.
407. Kelly PA, O'Connor JJ. Transmission of rapidly applied loads through articular cartilage. Part 1: uncracked cartilage. Proc Inst Mech Eng H J Eng Med. 1996;210:27–37.
408. Hatcher CC, Collins AT, Kim SY, Michel LC, Mostertz WC 3rd, Ziemian SN, Spritzer CE, Guilak F, DeFrate LE, McNulty AL. Relationship between T1rho magnetic resonance imaging, synovial fluid biomarkers, and the biochemical and biomechanical properties of cartilage. J Biomech. 2017;55:18–26.
409. Collins AT, Hatcher CC, Kim SY, Ziemian SN, Spritzer CE, et al. Selective enzymatic digestion of proteoglycans and collagens alters cartilage T1rho and T2 relaxation times. Ann Biomed Eng. 2019;47(1):190–201.
410. Lin PM, Chen CT, Torzilli PA. Increased stromelysin-1 (MMP-3), proteoglycan degradation (3B3- and 7D4) and collagen damage in cyclically load-injured articular cartilage. Osteoarthritis Cartilage. 2004;12:485–96.
411. Denning WM, Becker Pardo M, Winward JG, Hunter I, Ridge S, Hopkins JT, Reese CS, Parcell AC, Seeley MK. Ambulation speed and corresponding mechanics are associated with changes in serum cartilage oligomeric matrix protein. Gait Posture. 2016;44:131–6.
412. Denning WM, Winward JG, Pardo MB, Hopkins JT, Seeley MK. Body weight independently affects articular cartilage catabolism. J Sports Sci Med. 2015;14:290–6.
413. Luria A, Chu CR. Articular cartilage changes in maturing athletes: new targets for joint rejuvenation. Sports Health. 2014;6:18–30.
414. Mateer JL, Hoch JM, Mattacola CG, Butterfield TA, Lattermann C. Serum cartilage oligomeric matrix protein levels in collegiate soccer athletes over the duration of an athletic season: a pilot study. Cartilage. 2015;6:6–11.
415. Vuolteenaho K, Leppanen T, Kekkonen R, Korpela R, Moilanen E. Running a marathon induces changes in adipokine levels and in markers of cartilage degradation--novel role for resistin. PLoS One. 2014;9:e110481.
416. O'Kane JW, Hutchinson E, Atley LM, Eyre DR. Sport-related differences in biomarkers of bone resorption and cartilage degradation in endurance athletes. Osteoarthritis Cartilage. 2006;14:71–6.
417. Bartz RL, Laudicina L. Osteoarthritis after sports knee injuries. Clin Sports Med. 2005;24:39–45.

Part III

Knee Articular Cartilage Injury: Evaluation and Assessment

Acute and Chronic Traumatic Cartilage Injuries of the Knee

5

Henry B. Ellis Jr

5.1 Introduction

Of injuries treated by an orthopedic surgeon, trauma to the articular cartilage of any joint requires special attention. Articular cartilage is a sacred structure, which is highly respected by sports medicine health professionals. From the early works of Dr. Salter [1] to chondrocyte implantation, the drive to repair, restore, or regenerate articular cartilage remains ongoing.

Traumatic chondral injuries have four distinct and different patterns. An osteochondral (OC) fracture or an acute OC separation is due to a single traumatic event of both cartilage and subchondral bone from a shear force associated with an early effusion or hemarthrosis. Secondly, a defect in the articular cartilage, or a chondral defect, is a broad term used to define any lesion on the articular surface and the underlying hyaline cartilage. A chondral defect may or may not be symptomatic. Another chondral lesion is a bone contusion, sometimes referred to as a bone bruise. This is an impaction injury to the articular cartilage that is demonstrated by subchondral edema on advanced imaging. A bone contusion can also have an associated chondral defect. Lastly, repetitive supraphysiologic loading of the knee creates a chronic type of traumatic injury to the articular cartilage that is associated and frequently confused with primary idiopathic osteoarthritis (OA).

No matter what the cause of injury or the description of the lesion, a common goal exists to prevent progressive degeneration of the articular cartilage. Many injuries are common threads to articular damage, and frequently the treatment of articular cartilage is overshadowed by a more obvious and easily treated injury.

This chapter will focus on the natural history, classification, and incidence of knee injuries associated with acute and chronic traumatic articular cartilage injuries. We will also review patterns of cartilage damage seen in various sports. Treatment of these injuries is beyond the scope this chapter and will be discussed in Chaps. 11 and 12.

5.2 Natural History

The natural history of an isolated full-thickness chondral defect is not completely understood. Predictors of degenerative progression remain a mystery, as some chondral lesions continue to progress, while others have a natural ability to

H.B. Ellis Jr, MD (✉)
Department of Orthopaedic Surgery, University of Texas Southwestern Medical Center, Dallas, TX, USA

Department of Orthopaedic Surgery, Children's Health Dallas and Texas Scottish Rite Hospital for Children, Dallas, TX, USA
e-mail: henry.ellis@tsrh.org

H. K. Gahunia et al. (eds.), *Articular Cartilage of the Knee*,
https://doi.org/10.1007/978-1-4939-7587-7_5

heal and *fill* the defect [2–4]. A majority of full-thickness articular cartilage defects in adults do not spontaneously repair due to poor vascularity and subsequent lack of recruitment of progenitor repair cells [4, 5]. The size of the lesion (> 1 cm^2) may be a risk factor for progression of the lesion and thus, leading to OA [4, 6, 7]. Lesions to the cartilage deep zone tend to have more functional loss and have a higher prevalence of progression to degenerative arthritis [8]. Also, lateral condyle chondral injuries tend to subjectively do worse at long term than medial defects [9].

Biomechanical data have suggested that areas surrounding focal defects, whether considered articulating or non-articulating, see an increase in contact pressure [10]. Knee articular cartilage focal defects (due to injury, aging or disease) along with location-dependent cartilage mechanics alter the joint kinematics and deformation in the affected and opposing cartilages. Compared to healthy cartilage, the maximum compressive strains of small and average-sized focal defects are reported to increase by approximately 50% and 100%, respectively. Femoral defects affect the spatial distributions of deformation across the articular surfaces and also affect the opposing healthy tibial cartilage deformation [11]. There is also a tenfold increase in the shear strain on the opposing tissue around a focal defect [12]. Animal studies have demonstrated that focal chondral defects cause histologic cartilage changes not only in the affected compartment but also globally throughout the joint [13].

Despite these findings, clinical data have failed to show an inclusive progression to OA after focal chondral defects. Untreated lesions followed for 15 years demonstrated radiographic evidence of OA in only 39% of patients [14]. Patients with patellofemoral chondral defects were more likely to progress to OA. Regardless of the treatment, 5–8-year outcomes show improved knee function with no signs of degenerative arthritis [15].

Long-term data suggest that any significant knee injury increases one's risk of future development of OA [16]. The association of anterior cruciate ligament (ACL) injury and OA is well accepted; however, reports are conflicting on their relationship at long-term [17–19]. In a natural history study, Shelbourne reported on the untreated chondral defects identified during arthroscopy for an ACL reconstruction [9]. In this study, subjective scores at 6 years were worse in those with chondral defects than those without. At a 15-year follow-up of 36 patients after ACL reconstruction, Widuchowski reported no difference in the International Knee Documentation Committee (IKDC) subjective score, Tegner activity scale (TAS), or Lysholm score between patients with and without full-thickness chondral defects [20]. In both studies, there was no difference in radiographic appearance of OA between groups [9, 20]. Using a regression analysis, others have found medial compartment chondral defects to be a strong predictor of OA following an ACL injury [21].

The natural history of bone contusion is controversial and remains a topic of interest in the literature. Histologic samples obtained from articular cartilage overlying the subchondral edema represent degeneration or necrosis of the chondrocytes and loss of proteoglycan [22]. Most bone contusions resolve within 6 months; however, in some cases contusions can still be seen years after initial incident [23, 24]. The delay in resolution of a bone contusion is attributed either from continued subchondral stress, from lack of regression of the underlying edema, or from the trauma incurred during an ACL reconstruction [24]. Some early evidence suggests that there may be a future chondral thinning or cartilage degeneration occurring in areas with previous bone contusions, especially if there is damage on the chondral surface [22 , 25, 26].

A repetitive load on the articular surface of the knee may prevent adequate repair of surrounding chondrocytes when stressed. Prolonged activity beyond a certain threshold may lead to articular cartilage thinning and a reduction in the glycosaminoglycan concentration [27]. Repetitive supraphysiologic loading on the articular surface eventually causes a release of degradative enzymes and apoptosis of chondrocytes [28]. If the articular cartilage is unable to recover, a chondropenic response is initiated, and further deterioration to OA develops [5].

Overall, the natural history of untreated chondral lesions remains clinically unclear. Biomechanical and basic science data suggests the need to address these lesions to prevent further deterioration of the surrounding articular cartilage. In the coming years, long-term data with new management techniques and algorithms will further expand our understanding of the natural history of the chondral lesions and the need for treatment.

5.3 Classification Systems

In order to accurately assess, document, and communicate articular cartilage lesions, a surgeon needs to consider the size, depth, and anatomic location of the lesion as well as the patient age and activity level. As with any classification, the description must provide prognostic information or assist with treatment decisions. Even with many proposed classification systems, experienced arthroscopists agree that a classification for articular cartilage needs improvement [29]. Refer to Appendix A for arthroscopic classification systems for chondral injuries.

Historically, the name Outerbridge is synonymous with the classification of chondral defects. In 1961, Outerbridge described macroscopic changes seen on the undersurface of the patella while performing open meniscus surgery [30]. This original description of chondromalacia of the patella has later been adapted and popularized to chondromalacia and chondral injury at any location within the knee joint. The Outerbridge classification has also been adapted for assessing articular cartilage lesions in other large joints including the hip, ankle, shoulder, and elbow. A Grade 0 indicates intact and normal cartilage. Grade 1 describes softening, swelling, or blistering of the cartilage. In Grade 2, there is fragmentation and fissuring in an area half an inch or less in diameter. Grade 3 also has fragmentation and fissuring; however, the area is greater than half an inch in diameter. In Grade 4, there is erosion down to the bone with visible subchondral bone. In a survey reported in 2009, greater than 80% of experienced arthroscopic surgeons continue to use the Outerbridge classification [29]. A subsequent modification of this classification uses depth of fissuring as a distinction between Grades 2 and 3 rather than the size of the chondral defect (Table 5.1) [31].

The Outerbridge classification has moderate accuracy among surgeons in both intra- and interobserver testing [32, 33]. Interobserver reliability is substantial, with Cohen's kappa index ranging from 0.663 to 0.800 [33]. Patellar lesions are the most accurate between surgeons at an accuracy of 94%. As expected, surgeons with more experience tended to be more accurate [33]. Lower-grade lesions were less accurate than higher-grade lesions. However, there was still 81% and 94% agreement between Grades 2 and 3 lesions, respectively [32]. As reported by Marx, the tibial plateau lesions had decreased inter-observer reliability [32].

Critics of the original Outerbridge classification are concerned with the overlap in articular cartilage depth between Grades 2 and 3, as there may be treatment implications with differing depths of chondral lesions. Proposed additional classification systems [34-39] have failed to popularize partly due to their similarity or the complexity compared to the original Outerbridge classification and also due to the lack of available reliability. Further, these classifications have not proven to provide outcome or treatment data to date.

Both Insall [38] and Casscells [40] used classifications that are very similar to the modified version of the Outerbridge classification, making them difficult to differentiate. Ficat and Hungerford [39] presented a classification based on axial plain radiographs; however, classifying cartilage defects on plain radiographs is difficult and inaccurate. Bentley [37] felt that the size of the fissuring cartilage should guide treatment for

Table 5.1 Modified Outerbridge classification for articular cartilage defects

Grade 0: Normal intact articular cartilage
Grade 1: Chondral softening or blistering with an intact articular cartilage
Grade 2: Shallow superficial ulceration, fibrillation, or fissuring involving less than 50% of the depth of the articular cartilage
Grade 3: Deep ulceration, fibrillation, fissuring, or a chondral flap involving 50% or more of the depth of the articular cartilage without exposure of the subchondral bone
Grade 4: Full-thickness chondral wear with exposure of the underlying subchondral bone

Modified from Potter et al. [31]

symptomatic chondromalacia of the patella and further classified the fissuring cartilage by size. However, there is no grade for normal or intact lesions, as well as no grade for full-thickness lesions. The French Society of Arthroscopy (Société Francaise d' Arthroscopie, SFA) proposed a classification system to address the size, depth, and location of articular cartilage defect [36]. This system uses a visual analog scale (VAS) to quantify the depth of the defect to the subchondral bone. There is a substantial improvement in the inter-observer reliability in this classification after appropriate training [41].

The Noyes classification focuses on four pertinent variables [35]. These include the appearance of the articular surface, the depth of involvement, the size of the lesion diameter, and the location of the lesion. After scoring the chondral defects, this system assigns a percentage as a compartment score that can further be averaged to obtain a global knee joint score (100% indicating a normal joint or compartment). A limitation of this classification system is the weighted emphasis on the size of the lesion, as a 15-mm-sized lesion is twice the value of a 10 mm lesion. This ratio is also applicable to a 10 mm lesion, compared to a 24 mm lesion.

The International Cartilage Repair Society (ICRS) has further expanded the classification for articular cartilage defects and is included in the ICRS Cartilage Injury Evaluation Package, along with portions of the IKDC evaluation (Fig. 5.1) [42]. Grades 0–4 are similar to the modified Outerbridge classification previously mentioned. The ICRS classification includes additional subset that sets within Grades 1, 3, and 4. Grade 1a indicates only soft indentation, while Grade 1b has superficial fissures and cracks. ICRS Grade 3 has four additional subgroups. In Grade 3a, the depth of fissuring only includes greater than 50% of the cartilage depth, while Grade 3b fissuring goes down to the calcified cartilage layer. Fissuring to, but not through, the subchondral bone is a Grade 3c. Deep fissuring with surrounding blistering is a Grade 3d. Grades 4a and 4b are determined by the size and depth of defect through the subchondral bone (referred to an OC defect). The ICRS Cartilage Injury Evaluation Package also includes a detailed description of the size and location of the chondral defect and is extremely useful as a research tool. There is 80.9% agreement when comparing open versus arthroscopic grading using the ICRS classification [43]. However, interobserver reliability during an arthroscopy was poor with a Cohen's kappa index ranging from 0.052 to 0.308, depending on the compartment [44]. In one study, there was only 20% agreement between experienced surgeons using the ICRS classification intraoperatively [44].

In a comparison of arthroscopic classification with open assessment of chondral lesions, the mean size of the defects was overestimated arthroscopically, compared to the open measurements (5.69 cm^2 versus 4.54 cm^2, respectively) [43]. However, in general arthroscopy the smaller lesions tend to be overestimated while larger lesions tend to be underestimated.

Arthroscopy has become the gold standard for classifying articular cartilage defects. Potter demonstrated that magnetic resonance imaging (MRI) can also accurately assess and appropriately classify chondral lesions according to the modified Outerbridge classification, when compared to arthroscopy [31]. MRI had a sensitivity of 87%, a specificity of 94%, an accuracy of 92%, a positive predictive value of 85%, and a negative predictive value of 95% for detection of chondral lesions [31]. The use of MRI can also help a surgeon distinguish between an acute chondral lesion and a degenerative lesion arthroscopically [45].

There has been limited development of bone contusions classification system utilizing MRI. Costa-Paz and his associates developed a descriptive classification based on the MRI appearance of the bone contusion [46]. A type 1 bone contusion is a diffuse MR signal with a change of the medullary component. Often, this is reticular and distant from the subjacent articular surface. Type 2 is defined as a localized MR signal with contiguity to the subjacent articular surface. A disruption or depression of the normal cartilage surface is a type 3. More research is needed in this area to help quantify bone contusions and begin to predict the need for treatment if necessary, when a bone contusion is present.

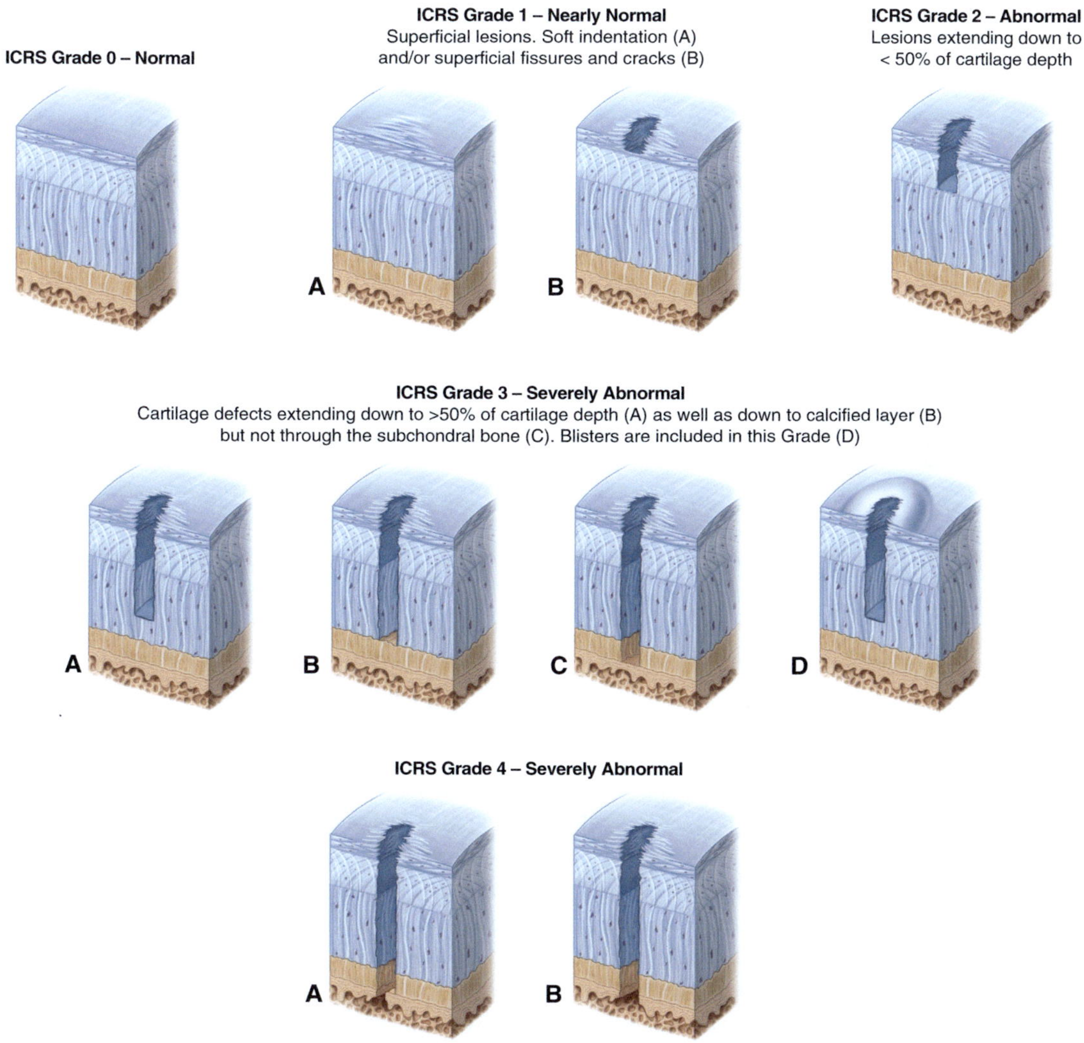

Fig. 5.1 The International Cartilage Repair Society classification with permission from the International Cartilage Repair Society

5.4 Incidence

The overall incidence of traumatic chondral injuries to the knee is probably unknown, since many of them may be clinically silent and never detected. There is also an overall difference between isolated chondral fractures and chondral lesions found during arthroscopy. Repetitive or chronic injuries are frequently confused with primary idiopathic OA, which also makes them difficult to quantify. A brief summary of the prevalence of these injuries is listed on Table 5.2.

Isolated chondral fractures occur in approximately one to four percent of all knee injuries requiring arthroscopic treatment [47, 48]. Forty-four to 85% of these isolated chondral fractures are from the medial femoral condyle [48, 49]. Interestingly, the tibial plateau is spared with less than 5% of the defects in the tibial plateau in either compartment [49]. These injuries are not clinically silent and require urgent attention from an orthopedic surgeon.

Five large studies report on the prevalence of chondral lesions among consecutive knee arthroscopies for an overall prevalence between 60%

Table 5.2 Prevalence summary of acute and chronic traumatic articular cartilage injuries (anterior cruciate ligament, ACL)

- 1–4% of knee injuries are osteochondral fractures
- 60–66% of all knee arthroscopies have chondral lesions
- Most chondral lesions and osteochondral fractures occur in the medial compartment
- 11% of chondral lesions identified during arthroscopy may be amendable to fixation
- Up to 60% of ACL tears have acute chondral damage
- Chronic ACL deficiency, male sex, and older patients have higher incidence of chondral damage with an ACL tear
- 80–100% of ACL injuries have bone contusions seen on MRI
- 57–71% of patella dislocations may have a chondral injury
- Half of chondral injuries may be missed on initial exam and plain radiographs

and 66% (Fig. 5.2) [48, 50–53]. Although the overall location of lesions is variable among different studies, the medial femoral condyle tends to have the most chondral defects by a factor of three. Patellar lesions are the second most common location for chondral defects. These valuable studies provide a cross-sectional analysis, or a snapshot, of articular cartilage lesions in the knee. A firm understanding of the prevalence of chondral lesions prior to undergoing a knee arthroscopy can help the surgeon's expectation. Eleven percent of lesions found during arthroscopy may be amenable to fixation [50]. Since many postoperative protocols for articular cartilage repair techniques are vastly different than that for a typical knee arthroscopy, the possibility of repairing a chondral defect may vary in time frame, depending on the surgeon's preoperative counseling with the patient.

Aroen et al. reported on 993 consecutive knee arthroscopies performed during a 6-month period at three collaborating hospitals, with a mean patient age of 35 years old [50]. Overall, 66% of all knee arthroscopies demonstrated some sort of chondral lesions. Of these, 44% were localized partial-thickness lesions, and 47% were localized full-thickness lesions. Twenty percent of the defects did not have evidence of surrounding degenerative changes. Not only were the most lesions in the medial femoral condyle, but they also tended to be the most serious lesions. Fifty-nine percent of the chondral lesions were thought to be from traumatic etiology, with sports participation (especially soccer) being the most common mechanism. A majority of the localized lesions were in the age group of less than 30 years, with only 27% localized lesions seen in patients over 45 years old.

In another comprehensive study with older population (mean age = 45 years), Curl noted 63% chondral lesions from 31,156 consecutive knee arthroscopies [48]. Patients with chondral lesions had an average of 2.7 lesions per knee. In this study, the male-to-female ratio was approximately 2:1. Using a modified Outerbridge classification, 10% of the lesions were Grade 1 lesions. Grades 2 and 3 lesions were seen in 28% and 41%, respectively. Subchondral bone (Grade 4) was seen in less than 20% of knees. The most common location for Grade 3 lesions was in the patella or medial femoral condyle. Seventy-two percent of Grade 4 lesions were noted in patients who were over 40 years old, whereas only 5% of all arthroscopies were accounted for by patients under 40 years old with Grade 4 chondral lesions. One-third of Grade 4 chondral lesions were seen with no associated meniscus or ligamentous pathology. Further, more than 80% of patients had no full-thickness lesions.

In a study of 1000 consecutive arthroscopies, Hjelle et al. reported chondral or osteochondral defects in 61% of patients, of which 19% were focal defects [52]. Sixty-one percent of these injuries, with a mean size of 2.1 cm^2, were related to a traumatic injury. As reported in the study by Curl et al. [48], Hjelle also found Grade 4 lesions to be rare in patients less than 40 years old.

Widuchowski et al. retrospectively reviewed 25,124 knee arthroscopies performed over a span of 15 years [51]. Sixty percent of the knees had evidence of a chondral lesion, with a male-to-female ratio of 2:1. Focal OC or chondral lesions were seen 67% of the time, with only 30% isolated lesions. Most of the lesions were from traumatic origin and were associated with a sporting activity. Football and skiing were the most common sport activities reported with these acute injuries. This study also quantified the size of the lesions, as 39% were less than 0.5 cm^2. Lesions

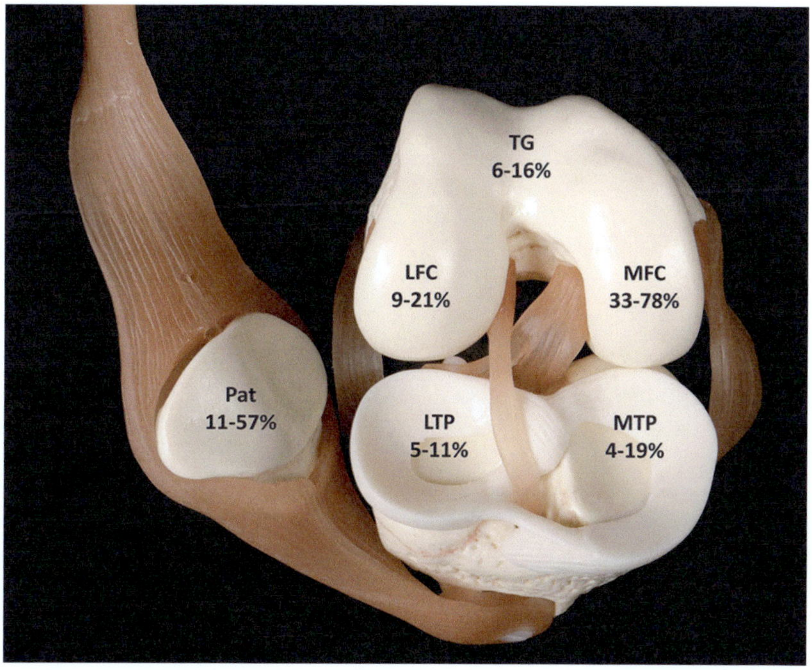

Fig. 5.2 Combined prevalence and location of chondral defects seen during (A) consecutive knee arthroscopic procedures [48, 50, 51–53]. MFC medial femoral condyle, LFC lateral femoral condyle, TG trochlear groove, MTP medial tibial plateau, LTP lateral tibial plateau, Pat patella *(Image courtesy of Texas Scottish Rite Hospital)*

between 0.5–1 cm^2 and 1–2 cm^2 were found in 25% and 29%, respectively. Only 7% of lesions were greater than 2 cm^2. According to the Outerbridge classification, one-fourth of the chondral injuries were Grade 3, while 12% were Grade 4 lesions.

A prospective review of 200 consecutive knee arthroscopies from 192 patients was performed by Zamber et al. [53]. The overall prevalence of a chondral defect was similar to previous studies at 61%. Medial compartment defects were more common. Unstable meniscus tears were associated with cartilage defects within the same compartment. Further, 75% of the knees with chronic ACL deficiency had chondral damage.

5.5 Clinical Presentation

Depending on the location of the chondral injury, articular cartilage defects, osteochondral fractures, or bone contusions can present with a variety of mechanisms of injuries. Sanders described five mechanisms of injuries and their associated bone marrow contusions [54]. These five patterns are useful in identifying specific injuries when static imaging only shows bone edema (i.e., a bone contusion on the medial patellar facet is suspicious for a patellar dislocation). In fact, these injuries are not just associated with bone marrow contusion but also with full-thickness chondral lesions.

The first mechanism is the *pivot shift injury* that occurs with a flexed knee and a valgus load with internal rotation of the femur on an externally rotated tibia causing an impaction of the posterior aspects of the lateral tibial plateau and the lateral femoral condyle. The pivot shift injury is associated with an ACL tear. The bone contusion pattern for a pivot shift injury is pathognomonic for an ACL tear (Fig. 5.3). The *dashboard injury* occurs during a front impact while driving on a flexed knee causing a tear of the posterior cruciate ligament (PCL) and a bone contusion on the anterior tibia. The *hyperextension injury* occurs when kicking a ball or landing on a hyperextended knee causing impaction of the anterior aspect of the femur on the tibia. This mechanism is associated with a posterolateral corner injury (Fig. 5.4). The *clip injury* is a lateral impact causing a valgus load on a knee that is associated with a medial

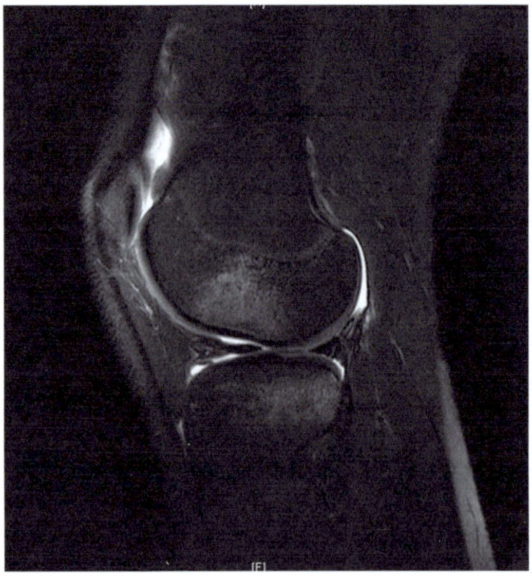

Fig. 5.3 Classic bone contusions seen with a tear of the ACL. During the pivoting mechanism, an impaction injury occurs with the lateral femoral condyle and the posterior aspect of the lateral tibial plateau. Even though a majority of the bone contusions occur in the lateral compartment, most chondral defects identified during an ACL reconstruction are in the medial compartment (*Image courtesy of Philip Wilson, MD)*

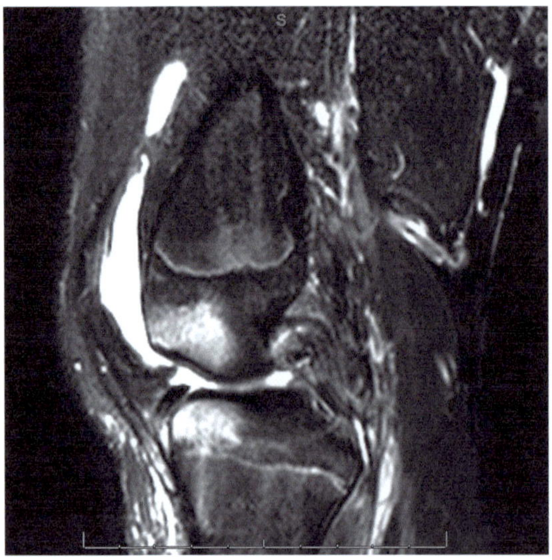

Fig. 5.4 Anterior bone contusions seen during a hyperextension injury associated with a concomitant injury to the posterolateral corner (*Image courtesy of Philip Wilson, MD)*

collateral ligament tear and sometimes an ACL tear. Impaction of the femur on the tibia occurs in the lateral compartment. The *lateral patellar dislocation* occurs during a variety of mechanisms, however, almost always a noncontact force on a flexed knee. Impaction occurs on the lateral aspect of the lateral femoral condyle and on the medial patellar facet (Fig. 5.5). All of the described patterns, except for the dashboard injury, have an effect on the articular cartilage. During the history and physical exam, one must perform a complete exam of the knee, as many traumatic chondral injuries are associated with additional injuries to the knee.

Patients may not recall a specific event that caused their traumatic chondral injury, and thus, presenting symptoms may be variable [49, 55]. Up to 60% of patients will complain of reduced function in the injured knee as compared to the contralateral knee [50]. The size of the lesion may have an effect on the symptoms, as smaller lesions tend to be more asymptomatic [56]. Many patients with isolated OC fractures recall a twisting injury to their knee, followed by an immediate effusion. These injuries are traditionally shearing injuries of the OC complex. A majority (70–95%) of athletes with a chondral injury will primarily complain of pain or recurrent swelling or effusion [49, 55]. Patients will have complaints similar to meniscus symptoms, except that only 18% will complain of locking of the knee [55]. Joint line tenderness is typically seen in about a third of patients [49].

The location of the chondral defect will also dictate the symptoms. Most patellar or trochlear lesions will present with anterior knee pain [57]. Patients may also complain of pain during jumping, deceleration, or the extension phase of kicking. Cartilage lesions on the anterior aspects of the condyle may present with pain during terminal extension or the extension phase of kicking, while lesions on the central portion of the condyle may produce pain with lateral movements of pivoting motion. Posterior condyle lesions will

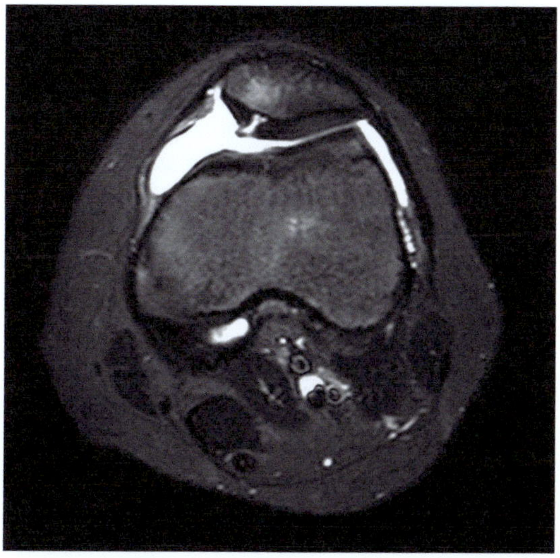

Fig. 5.5 Magnetic resonance imaging (MRI) following a patella dislocation The bone contusion (arrow) seen on the medial facet of the patella is a common location, along with the lateral femoral condyle. Note the full-thickness chondral flap caused by this mechanism

present with symptoms during deep knee bends or at positions of hyperflexion [49].

Outerbridge, when originally describing his articular cartilage classification, believed that chondromalacia of the patella was asymptomatic [30]. However in the later years, anterior knee pain has historically become a common complaint with a high rate of patellar articular cartilage lesion [38, 57–59]. Joensen further confirmed that athletes with anterior knee pain had patellofemoral chondral damages (17 out of 24 cases), compared to controls without anterior knee pain [57].

Osteochondral fractures have a higher prevalence in those under the age of 30 years [55]. A similar mechanism in a 40-year-old knee likely produces a chondral flap or a chondral separation, as opposed to a disruption in the subchondral bone. The reason for this is unclear; however, a weakness in the subchondral bone of adolescents and young adults has been proposed. A younger patient may, more likely, produce a higher shear force and thus, an OC fracture during twisting of the knee [60–62]. This may be due to their underlying ligament laxity. Flachsmann has proposed an explanation for this in a bovine model in which the structural changes occur in the anchoring region of the osteochondral junction during maturation [63]. Another theory is subclinical osteochondritis dissecans that weakens the underlying subchondral bone until a shearing force dislodges the fragment into an OC fracture.

A traumatic hemarthrosis is highly suspicious for an OC injury, especially in a child [64]. Up to three-fourths of acute traumatic hemarthrosis may have evidence of a chondral injury in a child [65–67]. In an adult, up to 40% of chondral injuries will present as a hemarthrosis [51]. A clinician should have a low threshold for pursuing an MRI in the face of an acute traumatic hemarthrosis. Timely diagnosis and treatment of these chondral fractures may have implications for healing. Many isolated chondral fractures should be addressed within 7–10 days of the injury.

Chronic traumatic lesions may not be symptomatic. There is no correlation between these chronic lesions or bone marrow edema on plain radiographs, MRI, and clinical symptoms [68]. Symptoms associated with chronic traumatic articular damage may not be present until later in life and will mimic primary OA with pain, stiffness, and swelling.

5.6 Associated Knee Tissue Injuries

5.6.1 Anterior Cruciate Ligament

Although several mechanisms have been proposed for an injury to the ACL, the common pivot shift mechanism is frequently associated with a lateral femoral condyle and posterolateral tibial plateau bone contusions [54]. The injury occurs when the knee is under a valgus moment with an internally rotated femur. When a pop and tear occur in the ACL, the posterior aspect of the tibial plateau impacts the lateral femoral condyle (Fig. 5.3). The location of the injury on the lateral femoral condyle is dependent on the knee flexion. The more flexion, the more posterior the chondral injury will be located. A depression of the lateral femoral condyle, referred to as a lateral femoral notch sign, is frequently seen on plain radiographs (Fig. 5.6) [69]. The femoral notch sign can also represent an OC fracture and should not be confused with the sulcus terminalis [70]. The posterolateral tibial plateau can be associated with an OC fracture during the same pivoting mechanism seen with an ACL injury [71, 72].

The presence of bone contusions, acute- or chronic-chondral lesions, is well-established associations with an ACL injury. The timing of ACL injury to treatment is an important distinction. Some have suggested that the greater the time between injury and treatment of the ACL increases the overall incidence of a chondral injury [73–75]. Other factors that affect the incidence and location of a chondral lesion associated with an ACL injury are gender, age, activity level, and mechanism of injury or sport. The overall incidence of significant articular cartilage damage in association with ACL injuries is between 16% and 60% [73, 74, 76–80]. Twenty-six to thirty six percent of chondral injuries seen on consecutive arthroscopies are associated with ACL tear [51, 52].

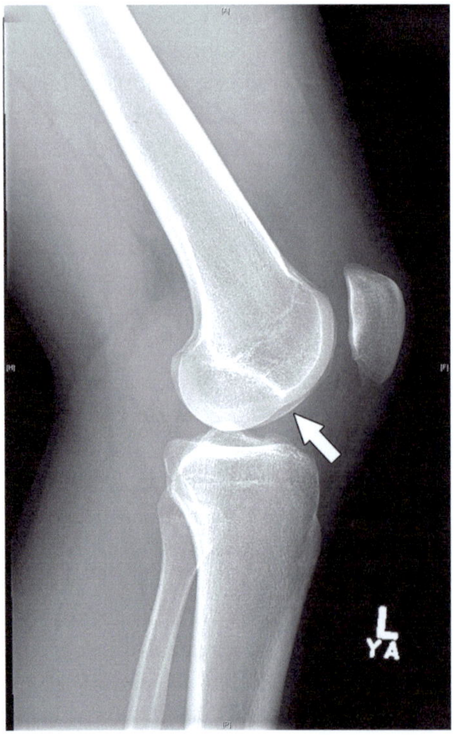

Fig. 5.6 A "femoral notch sign" on a lateral radiograph. This is seen with an impaction injury to the lateral femoral condyle after a pivoting injury. The lateral femoral notch sign (arrow) is seen with an acute tear to the ACL

In 1985, Indelicato and Bittar stated that articular cartilage disease increases from 23% to 54% in chronically lax ACL knees [81]. Not only is the overall prevalence higher the greater time between injury and treatment of chondral injuries, but more full-thickness defects are seen in those who wait longer until undergoing treatment for their deficient ACL [73]. The odds of a full-thickness cartilage lesion are 2.5 times greater than they would be at 1 year post-injury and 4.7 times greater when patients are more than 5 years after injury until seeking treatment [74]. Joseph reported that both athletes and nonathletes have a greater than 50% incidence of a chondral injury if more than 3 years from injury, as opposed to less than 20% if treatment is sooner than 3 months [79].

Recent data in the pediatric and adolescent age group also suggests an increased incidence of chondral injuries if ACL reconstruction is delayed [82–85]. Using logistic regression analysis, Lawrence found that a 12-week delay of ACL reconstruction in patient 14 years of age or younger was associated with medial and lateral compartment chondral injuries [82]. These chondral lesions were also found to be higher-grade cartilage injuries. When looking at the rate of chondral lesions alone, there is a strong evidence to consider an early ACL reconstruction without consideration of symptoms of instability. In a retrospective study including 130 pediatric patients (< 17 years; median age 14 years) who had 135 ACL reconstructions between the years of 2000 and 2012, Anderson corroborated the above findings that delayed ACL reconstruction increased the risks of secondary chondral injuries in pediatric patients [84]. Using ICRS criteria to document the location and grade of chondral injuries, arthroscopic assessment showed that 17 patients had 23 chondral injuries. The risk factors for chondral injury included increased time to surgery and any instability episode. Further, with increased grade of chondral injury, the risk factors were time to surgery (*P* </= 0.001) and any instability episode (*P* = 0.003). In another study, patients (*n* = 121; knees = 122; 93 males and 28 females; age range from 15 to 62 years; median age at surgery = 31 years) with posterior cruciate ligament (PCL) based multiligament knee injury or a minimum of three disrupted ligaments have also been reported with frequent occurrence of meniscal tears (67 knees; 55%) and chondral lesions (52 knees; 48%) [85]. Higher rates of articular cartilage lesions, especially in multiple compartments, were associated with longer interval from injury to surgical reconstruction.

In general, females are four times more likely to sustain a noncontact ACL injury compared to males [86]. Associated chondral injuries with an ACL injury occur twice as frequently in males than females [20]. Male basketball players with noncontact ACL injuries are three times more likely to have a chondral defect on the medial femoral condyle compared to females [87]. Males are also more likely to have lateral compartment articular cartilage injuries than females in the face of a concomitant ACL injury. Further, older patients tend to have more full-thickness injuries than younger patients [74].

As well, more chondral lesions are seen in competitive high school soccer players with an ACL injury than a recreational amateur soccer player [87]. When comparing incidence of chondral injury in athletes versus nonathletes, the overall incidence is not different; however, nonathletes tended to have more chondral defects if addressed less than 1 year from injury. The reason for this is unclear [79].

As expected because of the load on the lateral compartment, skiers have a greater tendency for lateral femoral condyle lesions compared to the medial compartment. The overall incidence of a chondral injury in an amateur skier is less than that for basketball and soccer.

The clinical significance of bone contusion in the face of an ACL injury is yet to be established. The incidence of bone bruises in association with an ACL tear is 80–98%, with a majority of lesions in the lateral compartment [78, 88]. The Multicenter Orthopaedic Outcomes Network (MOON) ACL reconstruction (ACLR) cohort study found that bone contusions typically occur in the younger patients and typically are seen in mechanisms that do not involve jumping and landing [89]. Seventy-five percent of chondromalacia seen during arthroscopy in the lateral compartment were associated with a bone bruise. The majority of bone edema associated with bone contusions resolved in the first 6 months; however, some may still be present after 1 year, especially if they have undergone an ACLR [90].

In the context of ACL tear, injuries to the meniscus and medial collateral ligament tended to increase the progression of the bone contusion [91]. The presence and location of a bone bruise do not correlate with a meniscal tear in a study by Frobell [88]. However, Nishimori found that 91% of bone bruises in the lateral compartment correlated with a tear of the lateral meniscus [92]. In contrast, only 25% of lateral meniscus tears were seen in patients without a bone contusion.

At this point, it is unclear whether there is a long-term effect with concomitant ACL injuries and chondral lesions. Data to date are based on gross appearance during arthroscopy and are conflicting [9, 20, 21, 93, 94]. In the earlier studies, missed subchondral injuries or bone contusions not seen during arthroscopy are likely the rationale for conflicting reports. Bone contusions in ACL injuries that are not visualized during arthroscopy may be at risk of future chondral thinning, particularly on the lateral femoral condyle [25]. With our expanding knowledge of bone contusions and improved MRI techniques [23, 95], future studies should evaluate the effect of chondral injuries with ACL tears on MRI and their long-term relationship in the progression of OA.

5.6.2 Patella Dislocation

Over one-fourth of patellar dislocations will have OC fractures fractures that are amenable to repair [96]. Articular cartilage injuries, of any kind, can be seen in 57–71% of patellar dislocations in those who underwent an arthroscopy [50, 97]. As discussed previously, the importance of determining the chondral injury in this population is often difficult and necessary prior to initiating conservative treatment for the patellar instability. Stanitski and Paletta assessed articular cartilage injury in 48 patients (24 boys and 24 girls; mean age 14 years), with acute, initial noncontact patellar dislocations. They found that only 23% of patients had a suspicion of a chondral injury on initial radiographic diagnosis; however, 71% had evidence of an articular injury on arthroscopy [98]. Approximately half of all chondral injuries, OC fractures, or loose bodies will be missed on conventional radiographs [98, 99].

A clinician should have a low threshold for an MRI following a first-time dislocation, and some clinicians may opt to perform an MRI on all first-time patellar dislocations. Sixty to hundred percent of patients will have a bone contusion on the patella or lateral femoral condyle after a patellar dislocation [97, 99]. Any evidence of mechanical symptoms (such as locked knee), patellofemoral crepitation or a hemarthrosis immediately after the injury, should warrant a MRI investigation [100]. MRI is reliable in assessing knee joint damage associated with patellar dislocation and in identifying risk factors for chronic patellar instability, which can thus provide valuable information for individually tailored treatment [99].

A majority of the articular cartilage defects occur on the patella, and up to 26% can present with OC fracture [96]. The incidence of injury to the patella and lateral femoral condyle is variable [96, 98]. However, in general, most injuries occur on the medial facet of the patella and the lateral femoral condyle (Fig. 5.5). OC fractures can occur on both surfaces [101] with a similar mechanism without a true patellar dislocation [102].

Isolated lesions to the patella or loose bodies should be surgically addressed within 7–10 days; however, these lesions may still be amendable to repair up to 3 months after the injury [99, 103, 104]. These injuries, in particular, compared to others, are typically in younger patients (mean age 13–23 years old) and respond very well to fixation [97, 103]. Focal defects of the patella will continue to progress, if not addressed [105].

5.6.3 Meniscus Tears

Approximately 36–40% of all acute chondral defects are associated with meniscus injuries [51, 52]. With a concomitant ACL injury, three-fourths of all chondral injuries are also seen with meniscus tears [73]. A bucket-handle meniscus tear is highly associated with advanced chondral changes in the medial compartment.

A chronic meniscus tear or a meniscectomy (partial or complete) is highly associated with future chondral damage [106–108]. This form of articular damage is more consistent with a chronic repetitive stress on the articular surface causing a gradual wear and tear on the joint. Since Fairbank's [109] original article, the changes to the joint surface and articular cartilage damage following a meniscectomy are well established. Radiographic changes seen after meniscectomy, or Fairbank's changes, include ridge formation, narrowing of the joint space, and flattening of the femoral condyle [109]. Minimizing meniscus debridement and resection is now common practice [110]. Following a meniscectomy, there is evidence of further arthritic degeneration, even compared to those with chondral damage without meniscus pathology [111].

5.6.4 Other Associated Injuries

Bone contusions are also seen with injuries to the PCL and posterolateral corner of the knee. Geeslin reviewed the MRI of consecutive patients with posterolateral corner injuries and found that 81% had bone contusions [112]. A majority (67%) of these injuries were located in the anteromedial femoral condyle (see Fig. 5.5). When a posterolateral corner injury was combined with an ACL injury, anteromedial bone contusions were seen more frequently than contusions seen on the lateral femoral condyle.

Miller et al. found that 45% of patients with medial collateral ligament injuries have evidence of trabecular microfracture or a bone contusion [113]. Almost all of these lesions occurred in the lateral compartment and had complete resolution at 4 months.

5.7 Repetitive Trauma

In 1996, Dye introduced the theory of the envelope of function for the knee [114]. The theory is based on the principle that the knee, as a source of biologic transmission of force, is limited by the applied load and frequency of this load. When a supraphysiologic load is applied to the knee and at a specific frequency, there can be subsequent failure of the biology or structure of the knee, in particular the extracellular matrix of the articular cartilage and subchondral bone. As an example, a basketball player landing from a lay-up is likely within the structural capacity of the knee; however, landing from a lay-up 100 times within an hour may be outside of the knee's capability to transmit the load without some form of structural damage. Although presented as a theory, recent data are now supporting this theory.

Preventable risk factors for chronic traumatic injuries to the knee articular cartilage include complete or partial meniscectomy, abnormal infrapatellar plica, and malalignment. As previously discussed, minimizing meniscus resection during arthroscopy is now common practice [110]. Osteonecrosis following a knee arthroscopy in an older patient may be due to a subtle subchondral fracture [115]. This may be due to a supraphysiologic load on weakened subchondral bone. In this situation, weight-bearing restrictions following a knee arthroscopy may be warranted. An abnormal and thickened infrapatellar plica increases the risk of chondral damage to the patellofemoral joint [116]. Resection of this may relieve underlying anterior knee pain and further chondral damage [117].

Running produces physiologic loads through a healthy knee joint without causing structural damage. However, when the same load is applied repetitively at a high frequency, as in running a marathon, this may cause chronic structural injury to the underlying cartilage. MRI before and after running marathons demonstrate signs of stress, and an effusion may be seen [118–120]. Long-distance running has demonstrated bone edema and early biochemical changes, specifically in the medial and patellofemoral compartments [118, 121, 122]. However, the long-term effects of this repetitive trauma remain controversial. The prevalence of OA in long-distance runners has been reported to be 14% higher than the average population [123]. However, Krampla demonstrated that seven long-distance runners followed for 10 years did not have an increased risk of OA due to repetitive loads on articular cartilage [119].

Recent 3-Tesla (3T) MRI technology has allowed us to visualize biochemical composition of articular cartilage. These techniques have been developed in order to quantify changes to the articular cartilage that are not visible with conventional MRI techniques. T1ρ is one such technique that detects damage to the cartilage collagen-proteoglycan matrix, which typically precedes loss of cartilage. T1ρ has been shown to be elevated even 3 months after running a marathon, indicating damage to the extracellular matrix of articular cartilage and thus, a supra physiologic load to the articular cartilage of the knee [121]. Having a better understanding of the biological changes seen with repetitive trauma will provide useful information in hope of treating, and perhaps preventing, the sequelae of repetitive trauma to the knee.

5.8 The Athlete and Articular Cartilage

An athlete, whether recreational or professional, exposes himself or herself to a sport-related injury each time he or she competes or even practices. An overall increase in competitive sports activity has led to an increase in knee injuries, including articular cartilage injuries [86, 124–129]. Not only is there current focus on identifying and treating these knee injuries, there has also been a recent push for injury prevention in athletics [130]. Although the incidence of acute chondral injuries is more frequently seen, the overall chronic repetitive load which athletes put through their knee joint has also caused an unacceptably high rate of OA in the athlete [123, 131, 132]. Athletes with isolated chondral defects have a good knee function at long term [132]. However, most competitive athletes, due to the nature of their profession, are at high risk of developing early OA of the knee [16, 123, 133–135]. The prevalence of OA in athletes is higher as they age [16]; as well, a high body mass index (BMI) may also be a risk factor [123]. Athletes involved in high-demand pivoting sports have a four- to five-fold increase in the development of OA [5].

Half of all soccer players retire due to injury, most of which are knee injuries [133]. The overall incidence of chondral injuries in soccer is unknown. This is likely because most injuries reported in soccer are either ligament injuries or meniscus tears, while the chondral injuries are typically secondary findings. Levy reported on 23 isolated chondral lesions in 15 soccer players, of which only a third were identified on MRI [19]. All lesions were reportedly full thickness and were treated with arthroscopic debridement. After return to play at an average of 10.8 weeks, one-fourth of players had recurrent chondral injuries that required repeated surgical intervention. In the long-term, soccer players have a higher than average rate of OA compared to the average population [123, 133, 134].

Acute or symptomatic chondral defect(s) in basketball players is relatively uncommon. However, 44–48% of asymptomatic professional and collegiate basketball players had articular cartilage lesions or bone marrow edema on MRI [136, 137]. A predilection of Outerbridge Grade 3 changes was seen on the patella and trochlea on both the jumping and non-jumping knees [136].

Knee injuries are extremely common in football [138]. Among many knee injuries seen in football, one-fifth of all players at the National Football League screening combine have asymptomatic full-thickness chondral injuries [139]. Linebackers and players with a higher BMI are more likely to have a knee chondral injury [139].

Marathon runners may be particularly susceptible to repetitive or chronic injury to the articular cartilage of the knee, at least in the short term. In 2006, MRI evaluation of long-distance runners before and after running a marathon did not reveal significant acute articular damage or bone marrow edema [140, 142]. However, recent 3T MRI techniques have been able to demonstrate cartilage biochemical composition changes that have not been previously available. The long-term effects are still being studied.

Additional activities associated with chondral lesions include racquet sports [142, 143], triathletes [144], dancing, and even video gaming [62]. Among athletes playing tennis, squash, badminton, or racquetball, a majority sought medical treatment for a twisting injury. More than 20% of these patients had symptomatic chondromalacia of the patella or another chondral lesion [143].

Regardless of articular cartilage repair technique, most high-level athletes are able to return to a pre-injury level of performance [145, 146]. Risk factors affecting return to sports include older age, longer duration of symptoms, large lesion size, higher number of previous surgeries, lower skill level, and those undergoing concomitant procedures [145].

With continued advances in the identification and treatment of articular cartilage defects, the overall long-term sequelae of such an injury will hopefully decrease the rate of OA, especially in the athlete. As with many medical situations, the most effective treatment is prevention. Not only is prevention important for the competitive athlete, but encouraging young adolescents to be active will, among other advantages, increase the thickness of their cartilage as they develop [147, 148].

5.9 Conclusions

Traumatic articular cartilage injuries occur in every compartment of the knee and most commonly in the medial compartment. Specific injuries and mechanisms are associated with common cartilage injury patterns. Repetitive impact activities, competitive sports for example, are associated with cartilage injuries.

References

1. Salter RB, Simmonds DF, Malcolm BW, Rumble EJ, MacMichael D, Clements ND. The biological effect of continuous passive motion on the healing of full-thickness defects in articular cartilage. An experimental investigation in the rabbit. J Bone Joint Surg Am. 1980;62(8):1232–51.

2. Heir S, Nerhus TK, Rotterud JH, et al. Focal cartilage defects in the knee impair quality of life as much as severe osteoarthritis: a comparison of knee injury and osteoarthritis outcome score in 4 patient categories scheduled for knee surgery. Am J Sports Med. 2010;38(2):231–7.
3. Alford JW, Cole BJ. Cartilage restoration, part 1: basic science, historical perspective, patient evaluation, and treatment options. Am J Sports Med. 2005;33(2):295–306.
4. Jackson DW, Lalor PA, Aberman HM, Simon TM. Spontaneous repair of full-thickness defects of articular cartilage in a goat model. A preliminary study. J Bone Joint Surg Am. 2001;83-A(1):53–64.
5. Mithoefer K, McAdams TR, Scopp JM, Mandelbaum BR. Emerging options for treatment of articular cartilage injury in the athlete. Clin Sports Med. 2009;28(1):25–40.
6. Guettler JH, Demetropoulos CK, Yang KH, Jurist KA. Osteochondral defects in the human knee: influence of defect size on cartilage rim stress and load redistribution to surrounding cartilage. Am J Sports Med. 2004;32(6):1451–8.
7. Papaioannou G, Demetropoulos CK, King YH. Predicting the effects of knee focal articular surface injury with a patient-specific finite element model. Knee. 2010;17(1):61–8.
8. Osti L, Papalia R, Del Buono A, Amato C, Denaro V, Maffulli N. Good results five years after surgical management of anterior cruciate ligament tears, and meniscal and cartilage injuries. Knee Surg Sports Traumatol Arthrosc. 2010;18(10):1385–90.
9. Shelbourne KD, Jari S, Gray T. Outcome of untreated traumatic articular cartilage defects of the knee: a natural history study. J Bone Joint Surg Am. 2003;85(A Suppl 2):8–16.
10. Simonian PT, Sussmann PS, Wickiewicz TL, Paletta GA, Warren RF. Contact pressures at osteochondral donor sites in the knee. Am J Sports Med. 1998;26(4):491–4.
11. Marchi BC, Arruda EM, Coleman R. The effect of articular cartilage focal defect size and location in whole knee biomechanics models. J Biomech Eng. 2019 doi: 10.1115/1.4044032. [Epub ahead of print].
12. Gratz KR, Wong BL, Bae WC, Sah RL. The effects of focal articular defects on intra-tissue strains in the surrounding and opposing cartilage. Biorheology. 2008;45(3–4):193–207.
13. Vaseenon T, Tochigi Y, Heiner AD, et al. Organ-level histological and biomechanical responses from localized osteoarticular injury in the rabbit knee. J Orthop Res. 2011;29(3):340–6.
14. Widuchowski W, Widuchowski J, Faltus R, et al. Long-term clinical and radiological assessment of untreated severe cartilage damage in the knee: a natural history study. Scand J Med Sci Sports. 2011;21(1):106–10.
15. Loken S, Heir S, Holme I, Engebretsen L, Aroen A. 6-year follow-up of 84 patients with cartilage defects in the knee. Knee scores improved but recovery was incomplete. Acta Orthop. 2010;81(5):611–8.
16. Bachmann GF, Basad E, Rauber K, Damian MS, Rau WS. Degenerative joint disease on MRI and physical activity: a clinical study of the knee joint in 320 patients. Eur Radiol. 1999;9(1):145–52.
17. Kessler MA, Behrend H, Henz S, Stutz G, Rukavina A, Kuster MS. Function, osteoarthritis and activity after ACL-rupture: 11 years follow-up results of conservative versus reconstructive treatment. Knee Surg Sports Traumatol Arthrosc. 2008;16(5):442–8.
18. Meuffels DE, Favejee MM, Vissers MM, Heijboer MP, Reijman M, Verhaar JA. Ten year follow-up study comparing conservative versus operative treatment of anterior cruciate ligament ruptures. A matched-pair analysis of high level athletes. Br J Sports Med. 2009;43(5):347–51.
19. Simon D, Mascarenhas R, Saltzman BM, Rollins M, Bach BR Jr, MacDonald P. The relationship between anterior cruciate ligament injury and osteoarthritis of the knee. Adv Orthop. 2015;2015:928301.
20. Widuchowski W, Widuchowski J, Koczy B, Szyluk K. Untreated asymptomatic deep cartilage lesions associated with anterior cruciate ligament injury: results at 10- and 15-year follow-up. Am J Sports Med. 2009;37(4):688–92.
21. Li RT, Lorenz S, Xu Y, Harner CD, FH F, Irrgang JJ. Predictors of radiographic knee osteoarthritis after anterior cruciate ligament reconstruction. Am J Sports Med. 2011;39(12):2595–603.
22. Nakamae A, Engebretsen L, Bahr R, Krosshaug T, Ochi M. Natural history of bone bruises after acute knee injury: clinical outcome and histopathological findings. Knee Surg Sports Traumatol Arthrosc. 2006;14(12):1252–8.
23. Theologis AA, Kuo D, Cheng J, et al. Evaluation of bone bruises and associated cartilage in anterior cruciate ligament-injured and -reconstructed knees using quantitative t(1rho) magnetic resonance imaging: 1-year cohort study. Arthroscopy. 2011;27(1):65–76.
24. Frobell RB. Change in cartilage thickness, posttraumatic bone marrow lesions, and joint fluid volumes after acute ACL disruption: a two-year prospective MRI study of sixty-one subjects. J Bone Joint Surg Am. 2011;93(12):1096–103.
25. Faber KJ, Dill JR, Amendola A, Thain L, Spouge A, Fowler PJ. Occult osteochondral lesions after anterior cruciate ligament rupture. Six-year magnetic resonance imaging follow-up study. Am J Sports Med. 1999;27(4):489–94.
26. Boks SS, Vroegindeweij D, Koes BW, Hunink MG, Bierma-Zeinstra SM. Follow-up of occult bone lesions detected at MR imaging: systematic review. Radiology. 2006;238(3):853–62.
27. Kiviranta I, Tammi M, Jurvelin J, Arokoski J, Saamanen AM, Helminen HJ. Articular cartilage thickness and glycosaminoglycan distribution in the

canine knee joint after strenuous running exercise. Clin Orthop Relat Res. 1992;283:302–8.
28. Vrahas MS, Mithoefer K, Joseph D. The long-term effects of articular impaction. Clin Orthop Relat Res. 2004;423:40–3.
29. Spahn G, Klinger HM, Hofmann GO. How valid is the arthroscopic diagnosis of cartilage lesions? Results of an opinion survey among highly experienced arthroscopic surgeons. Arch Orthop Trauma Surg. 2009;129(8):1117–21.
30. Outerbridge RE. The etiology of chondromalacia patellae. J Bone Joint Surg Br. 1961;43:752–7.
31. Potter HG, Linklater JM, Allen AA, Hannafin JA, Haas SB. Magnetic resonance imaging of articular cartilage in the knee. An evaluation with use of fast-spin-echo imaging. J Bone Joint Surg Am. 1998;80(9):1276–84.
32. Marx RG, Connor J, Lyman S, et al. Multirater agreement of arthroscopic grading of knee articular cartilage. Am J Sports Med. 2005;33(11):1654–7.
33. Cameron ML, Briggs KK, Steadman JR. Reproducibility and reliability of the outerbridge classification for grading chondral lesions of the knee arthroscopically. Am J Sports Med. 2003;31(1):83–6.
34. Bauer M, Jackson R, Ogilvie-Harris D, Morbidi M. Classificazione artroscopica delle lesioni condrali del ginocchio. Am J Sports Med. 1987;40:41–4.
35. Noyes FR, Stabler CL. A system for grading articular cartilage lesions at arthroscopy. Am J Sports Med. 1989;17(4):505–13.
36. Dougados M, Ayral X, Listrat V, et al. The SFA system for assessing articular cartilage lesions at arthroscopy of the knee. Arthroscopy. 1994;10(1):69–77.
37. Bentley G, Dowd G. Current concepts of etiology and treatment of chondromalacia patellae. Clin Orthop Relat Res. 1984;189:209–28.
38. Insall J, Falvo KA, Wise DW. Chondromalacia Patellae A prospective study. J Bone Joint Surg Am. 1976;58(1):1–8.
39. Ficat RP, Philippe J, Hungerford DS. Chondromalacia patellae: a system of classification. Clin Orthop Relat Res. 1979;144:55–62.
40. Casscells SW. Gross pathological changes in the knee joint of the aged individual: a study of 300 cases. Clin Orthop Relat Res. 1978;132:225–32.
41. Ayral X, Gueguen A, Ike RW, et al. Inter-observer reliability of the arthroscopic quantification of chondropathy of the knee. Osteoarthritis Cartilage. 1998;6(3):160–6.
42. The Cartilage Standard Evalution Form/Knee. In: ICRS Newsletter. ICRS 2000 Standards Workshop at Schloss Münchenwiler, Switzerland, January 27-30, 2000.
43. Niemeyer P, Pestka JM, Erggelet C, Steinwachs M, Salzmann GM, Sudkamp NP. Comparison of arthroscopic and open assessment of size and grade of cartilage defects of the knee. Arthroscopy. 2011;27(1):46–51.
44. Spahn G, Klinger HM, Baums M, Pinkepank U, Hofmann GO. Reliability in arthroscopic grading of cartilage lesions: results of a prospective blinded study for evaluation of interobserver reliability. Arch Orthop Trauma Surg. 2011;131(3):377–81.
45. Hempfling H, Bohndorf K, Roemer F. Acute, traumatic versus chronic cartilage lesions as terms of a medical expert's opinion. Zeitschrift fur Orthopadie und Unfallchirurgie. 2008;146(3): 381–91.
46. Costa-Paz M, Muscolo DL, Ayerza M, Makino A, Aponte-Tinao L. Magnetic resonance imaging follow-up study of bone bruises associated with anterior cruciate ligament ruptures. Arthroscopy. 2001;17(5):445–9.
47. Terry GC, Flandry F, Van Manen JW, Norwood LA. Isolated chondral fractures of the knee. Clin Orthop Relat Res. 1988;234:170–7.
48. Curl WW, Krome J, Gordon ES, Rushing J, Smith BP, Poehling GG. Cartilage injuries: a review of 31,516 knee arthroscopies. Arthroscopy. 1997;13(4):456–60.
49. Levy AS, Lohnes J, Sculley S, LeCroy M, Garrett W. Chondral delamination of the knee in soccer players. Am J Sports Med. 1996;24(5):634–9.
50. Aroen A, Loken S, Heir S, et al. Articular cartilage lesions in 993 consecutive knee arthroscopies. Am J Sports Med. 2004;32(1):211–5.
51. Widuchowski W, Widuchowski J, Trzaska T. Articular cartilage defects: study of 25,124 knee arthroscopies. Knee. 2007;14(3):177–82.
52. Hjelle K, Solheim E, Strand T, Muri R, Brittberg M. Articular cartilage defects in 1,000 knee arthroscopies. Arthroscopy. 2002;18(7):730–4.
53. Zamber RW, Teitz CC, McGuire DA, Frost JD, Hermanson BK. Articular cartilage lesions of the knee. Arthroscopy. 1989;5(4):258–68.
54. Sanders TG, Medynski MA, Feller JF, Lawhorn KW. Bone contusion patterns of the knee at MR imaging: footprint of the mechanism of injury. Radiographics. 2000;20:S135–51.
55. Johnson-Nurse C, Dandy DJ. Fracture-separation of articular cartilage in the adult knee. J Bone Joint Surg. 1985;67(1):42–3.
56. Mandelbaum BR, Browne JE, Fu F, et al. Articular cartilage lesions of the knee. Am J Sports Med. 1998;26(6):853–61.
57. Joensen AM, Hahn T, Gelineck J, Overvad K, Ingemann-Hansen T. Articular cartilage lesions and anterior knee pain. Scand J Med Sci Sports. 2001;11(2):115–9.
58. Kannus P, Natri A, Paakkala T, Jarvinen M. An outcome study of chronic patellofemoral pain syndrome. Seven-year follow-up of patients in a randomized, controlled trial. J Bone Joint Surg Am. 1999;81(3):355–63.
59. Outerbridge RE, Dunlop JA. The problem of chondromalacia patellae. Clin Orthop Relat Res. 1975;110:177–96.

60. Walsh SJ, Boyle MJ, Morganti V. Large osteochondral fractures of the lateral femoral condyle in the adolescent: outcome of bioabsorbable pin fixation. J Bone Joint Surg Am. 2008;90(7):1473–8.
61. Jehan S, Loeffler MD, Pervez H. Osteochondral fracture of the lateral femoral condyle involving the entire weight bearing articular surface fixed with biodegradable screws. J Pak Med Assoc. 2010;60(5):400–1.
62. Robinson RJ, Barron DA, Grainger AJ, Venkatesh R. Wii knee. Emerg Radiol. 2008;15(4):255–7.
63. Flachsmann R, Broom ND, Hardy AE, Moltschaniwskyj G. Why is the adolescent joint particularly susceptible to osteochondral shear fracture? Clin Orthop Relat Res. 2000;381:212–21.
64. Noyes FR, Bassett RW, Grood ES, Butler DL. Arthroscopy in acute traumatic hemarthrosis of the knee. Incidence of anterior cruciate tears and other injuries. J Bone Joint Surg Am. 1980;62(5):687–95.
65. Vellet AD, Marks PH, Fowler PJ, Munro TG. Occult posttraumatic osteochondral lesions of the knee: prevalence, classification, and short-term sequelae evaluated with MR imaging. Radiology. 1991;178(1):271–6.
66. Wessel LM, Scholz S, Rusch M, et al. Hemarthrosis after trauma to the pediatric knee joint: what is the value of magnetic resonance imaging in the diagnostic algorithm? J Pediatr Orthop. 2001;21(3):338–42.
67. Matelic TM, Aronsson DD, Boyd DW Jr, LaMont RL. Acute hemarthrosis of the knee in children. Am J Sports Med. 1995;23(6):668–71.
68. Link TM, Steinbach LS, Ghosh S, et al. Osteoarthritis: MR imaging findings in different stages of disease and correlation with clinical findings. Radiology. 2003;226(2):373–81.
69. Pao DG. The lateral femoral notch sign. Radiology. 2001;219(3):800–1.
70. Sharma G, Naik VA, Pankaj A. Displaced osteochondral fracture of the lateral femoral condyle associated with an acute anterior cruciate ligament avulsion fracture: a corollary of the lateral femoral notch sign. Knee Surg Sports Traumatol Arthrosc. 2011;20(8):1599–602.
71. Tei K, Kubo S, Matsumoto T, et al. Combined osteochondral fracture of the posterolateral tibial plateau and segond fracture with anterior cruciate ligament injury in a skeletally immature patient. Knee Surg Sports Traumatol Arthrosc. 2011;20(2):252–5.
72. Yoo JH, Yang BK, Ryu HK. A case of fracture of posterior margin of lateral tibial plateau by pivot shift mechanism in chronic ACL insufficiency. Arch Orthop Trauma Surg. 2009;129(3):363–7.
73. Maffulli N, Binfield PM, King JB. Articular cartilage lesions in the symptomatic anterior cruciate ligament-deficient knee. Arthroscopy. 2003;19(7):685–90.
74. Tandogan RN, Taser O, Kayaalp A, et al. Analysis of meniscal and chondral lesions accompanying anterior cruciate ligament tears: relationship with age, time from injury, and level of sport. Knee Surg Sports Traumatol Arthrosc. 2004;12(4):262–70.
75. Gregory T, Landreau P. Meniscus and cartilaginous lesions. Influence of the delay between ACL injury and ligament reconstruction in 40-year-old patients. Revue de chirurgie orthopedique et reparatrice de l'appareil moteur. 2008;94(6):566–72.
76. Drongowski RA, Coran AG, Wojtys EM. Predictive value of meniscal and chondral injuries in conservatively treated anterior cruciate ligament injuries. Arthroscopy. 1994;10(1):97–102.
77. Engebretsen L, Arendt E, Fritts HM. Osteochondral lesions and cruciate ligament injuries. MRI in 18 knees. Acta Orthop Scand. 1993;64(4):434–6.
78. Spindler KP, Schils JP, Bergfeld JA, et al. Prospective study of osseous, articular, and meniscal lesions in recent anterior cruciate ligament tears by magnetic resonance imaging and arthroscopy. Am J Sports Med. 1993;21(4):551–7.
79. Joseph C, Pathak SS, Aravinda M, Rajan D. Is ACL reconstruction only for athletes? A study of the incidence of meniscal and cartilage injuries in an ACL-deficient athlete and non-athlete population: an Indian experience. Int Orthop. 2008;32(1):57–61.
80. Brophy RH, Zeltser D, Wright RW, Flanigan D. Anterior cruciate ligament reconstruction and concomitant articular cartilage injury: incidence and treatment. Arthroscopy. 2010;26(1):112–20.
81. Indelicato PA, Bittar ES. A perspective of lesions associated with ACL insufficiency of the knee. A review of 100 cases. Clin Orthop Relat Res. 1985;198:77–80.
82. Lawrence JT, Argawal N, Ganley TJ. Degeneration of the knee joint in skeletally immature patients with a diagnosis of an anterior cruciate ligament tear: is there harm in delay of treatment? Am J Sports Med. 2011;39(12):2582–7.
83. Dumont GD, Hogue GD, Padalecki JR, Okoro N, Wilson PL. Meniscal and chondral injury in association with pediatric anterior cruciate ligament tears: relationship of treatment time and patient specific factors. Am J Sports Med. 2012;40(9):2128–33.
84. Anderson AF, Anderson CN. Correlation of meniscal and articular cartilage injuries in children and adolescents with timing of anterior cruciate ligament reconstruction. Am J Sports Med. 2015;43(2):275–81.
85. Krych AJ, Sousa PL, King AH, Engasser WM, Stuart MJ, Levy BA. Meniscal tears and articular cartilage damage in the dislocated knee. Knee Surg Sports Traumatol Arthrosc. 2015;23(10):3019–25.
86. Arendt E, Dick R. Knee injury patterns among men and women in collegiate basketball and soccer.

NCAA data and review of literature. Am J Sports Med. 1995;23(6):694–701.
87. Piasecki DP, Spindler KP, Warren TA, Andrish JT, Parker RD. Intraarticular injuries associated with anterior cruciate ligament tear: findings at ligament reconstruction in high school and recreational athletes. An analysis of sex-based differences. Am J Sports Med. 2003;31(4):601–5.
88. Frobell RB, Roos HP, Roos EM, et al. The acutely ACL injured knee assessed by MRI: are large volume traumatic bone marrow lesions a sign of severe compression injury? Osteoarthritis Cartilage. 2008;16(7):829–36.
89. Dunn WR, Spindler KP, Amendola A, et al. Which preoperative factors, including bone bruise, are associated with knee pain/symptoms at index anterior cruciate ligament reconstruction (ACLR)? A Multicenter Orthopaedic Outcomes Network (MOON) ACLR Cohort Study. Am J Sports Med. 2010;38(9):1778–87.
90. Frobell RB, Le Graverand MP, Buck R, et al. The acutely ACL injured knee assessed by MRI: changes in joint fluid, bone marrow lesions, and cartilage during the first year. Osteoarthritis Cartilage. Feb 2009;17(2):161–7.
91. Yoon KH, Yoo JH, Kim KI. Bone contusion and associated meniscal and medial collateral ligament injury in patients with anterior cruciate ligament rupture. J Bone Joint Surg Am. 2011;93(16):1510–8.
92. Nishimori M, Deie M, Adachi N, et al. Articular cartilage injury of the posterior lateral tibial plateau associated with acute anterior cruciate ligament injury. Knee Surg Sports Traumatol Arthrosc. 2008;16(3):270–4.
93. Neuman P, Englund M, Kostogiannis I, Friden T, Roos H, Dahlberg LE. Prevalence of tibiofemoral osteoarthritis 15 years after nonoperative treatment of anterior cruciate ligament injury: a prospective cohort study. Am J Sports Med. 2008;36(9):1717–25.
94. Swirtun LR, Renstrom P. Factors affecting outcome after anterior cruciate ligament injury: a prospective study with a six-year follow-up. Scand J Med Sci Sports. 2008;18(3):318–24.
95. Fleming BC, Oksendahl HL, Mehan WA, et al. Delayed gadolinium-enhanced MR imaging of cartilage (dGEMRIC) following ACL injury. Osteoarthritis Cartilage. 2010;18(5):662–7.
96. Sillanpaa PJ, Maenpaa HM, Mattila VM, Visuri T, Pihlajamaki H. Arthroscopic surgery for primary traumatic patellar dislocation: a prospective, nonrandomized study comparing patients treated with and without acute arthroscopic stabilization with a median 7-year follow-up. Am J Sports Med. 2008;36(12):2301–9.
97. Guerrero P, Li X, Patel K, Brown M, Busconi B. Medial patellofemoral ligament injury patterns and associated pathology in lateral patella dislocation: an MRI study. Sports Med Arthrosc Rehabil Ther Technol. 2009;1(1):17.
98. Stanitski CL, Paletta GA Jr. Articular cartilage injury with acute patellar dislocation in adolescents. Arthroscopic and radiographic correlation. Am J Sports Med. 1998;26(1):52–5.
99. Diederichs G, Issever AS, Scheffler S. MR imaging of patellar instability: injury patterns and assessment of risk factors. Radiographics. 2010;30(4):961–81.
100. Goh SK, Koh JS, Tan MH. Knee locking secondary to osteochondral fracture of the patella: an unusual presentation. Singapore Med J. 2008;49(6):505–6.
101. Callewier A, Monsaert A, Lamraski G. Lateral femoral condyle osteochondral fracture combined to patellar dislocation: a case report. Orthop Traumatol Surg Res. 2009;95(1):85–8.
102. Bhatt J, Montalban AS, Wang KH, Lee HD, Nha KW. Isolated osteochondral fracture of the patella without patellar dislocation. Orthopedics. 2011;34(1):54.
103. Chotel F, Knorr G, Simian E, Dubrana F, Versier G. Knee osteochondral fractures in skeletally immature patients: French multicenter study. Orthop Traumatol Surg Res. 2011;97(8 Suppl):S154–9.
104. Hoshino CM, Thomas BM. Late repair of an osteochondral fracture of the patella. Orthopedics. 2010;16:270–3.
105. Wong BL, Sah RL. Effect of a focal articular defect on cartilage deformation during patello-femoral articulation. J Orthop Res. 2010;28(12):1554–61.
106. Messner K, Fahlgren A, Persliden J, Andersson BM. Radiographic joint space narrowing and histologic changes in a rabbit meniscectomy model of early knee osteoarthrosis. Am J Sports Med. 2001;29(2):151–60.
107. Cicuttini FM, Forbes A, Yuanyuan W, Rush G, Stuckey SL. Rate of knee cartilage loss after partial meniscectomy. J Rheumatol. 2002;29(9):1954–6.
108. Allen PR, Denham RA, Swan AV. Late degenerative changes after meniscectomy. Factors affecting the knee after operation. J Bone Joint. 1984;66(5):666–71.
109. Fairbank TJ. Knee joint changes after meniscectomy. J Bone Joint Surg. 1948;30B(4):664–70.
110. Beaufils P, Hulet C, Dhenain M, Nizard R, Nourissat G, Pujol N. Clinical practice guidelines for the management of meniscal lesions and isolated lesions of the anterior cruciate ligament of the knee in adults. Orthop Traumatol Surg Res. 2009;95(6):437–42.
111. Maletius W, Messner K. The effect of partial meniscectomy on the long-term prognosis of knees with localized, severe chondral damage. A twelve- to fifteen-year followup. Am J Sports Med. 1996;24(3):258–62.
112. Geeslin AG, LaPrade RF. Location of bone bruises and other osseous injuries associated with acute grade III isolated and combined posterolateral knee injuries. Am J Sports Med. 2010;38(12):2502–8.

113. Miller MD, Osborne JR, Gordon WT, Hinkin DT, Brinker MR. The natural history of bone bruises. A prospective study of magnetic resonance imaging-detected trabecular microfractures in patients with isolated medial collateral ligament injuries. Am J Sports Med. 1998;26(1):15–9.
114. Dye SF. The knee as a biologic transmission with an envelope of function: a theory. Clin Orthop Relat Res. 1996;325:10–8.
115. MacDessi SJ, Brophy RH, Bullough PG, Windsor RE, Sculco TP. Subchondral fracture following arthroscopic knee surgery. A series of eight cases. J Bone Joint Surg Am. 2008;90(5):1007–12.
116. Ozcan M, Copuroglu C, Ciftdemir M, Turan FN, Calpur OU. Does an abnormal infrapatellar plica increase the risk of chondral damage in the knee. Knee Surg Sports Traumatol Arthrosc. 2011;19(2):218–21.
117. Boyd CR, Eakin C, Matheson GO. Infrapatellar plica as a cause of anterior knee pain. Clin J Sport Med. 2005;15(2):98–103.
118. Krampla W, Mayrhofer R, Malcher J, Kristen KH, Urban M, Hruby W. MR imaging of the knee in marathon runners before and after competition. Skeletal Radiol. 2001;30(2):72–6.
119. Krampla WW, Newrkla SP, Kroener AH, Hruby WF. Changes on magnetic resonance tomography in the knee joints of marathon runners: a 10-year longitudinal study. Skeletal Radiol. 2008;37(7):619–26.
120. Qiu L, Perez J, Emerson C, Barrera CM, Zhong J, et al. Biochemical changes in knee articular cartilage of novice half-marathon runners. J Int Med Res. 2019:300060519874140. doi: 10.1177/0300060519874140. [Epub ahead of print]
121. Luke AC, Stehling C, Stahl R, et al. High-field magnetic resonance imaging assessment of articular cartilage before and after marathon running: does long-distance running lead to cartilage damage? Am J Sports Med. 2010;38(11):2273–80.
122. Stahl R, Luke A, Ma CB, et al. Prevalence of pathologic findings in asymptomatic knees of marathon runners before and after a competition in comparison with physically active subjects-a 3.0 T magnetic resonance imaging study. Skeletal Radiol. 2008;37(7):627–38.
123. Kujala UM, Kettunen J, Paananen H, et al. Knee osteoarthritis in former runners, soccer players, weight lifters, and shooters. Arthritis Rheum. 1995;38(4):539–46.
124. Jones SJ, Lyons RA, Sibert J, Evans R, Palmer SR. Changes in sports injuries to children between 1983 and 1998: comparison of case series. J Public Health Med. 2001;23(4):268–71.
125. Murray IR, Benke MT, Mandelbaum BR. Management of knee articular cartilage injuries in athletes: chondroprotection, chondrofacilitation, and resurfacing. Knee Surg Sports Traumatol Arthrosc. 2016;24(5):1617–26.
126. Steadman JR, Hanson CM, Briggs KK, Matheny LM, James EW, Guillet A. Outcomes after knee microfracture of chondral defects in alpine ski racers. J Knee Surg. 2014;27(5):407–10.
127. Mithoefer K, Peterson L, Zenobi-Wong M, Mandelbaum BR. Cartilage issues in football-today's problems and tomorrow's solutions. Br J Sports Med. 2015;49(9):590–6.
128. Scillia AJ, Aune KT, Andrachuk JS, Cain EL, Dugas JR, Fleisig GS, et al. Return to play after chondroplasty of the knee in National Football League athletes. Am J Sports Med. 2015;43(3):663–8.
129. Field AE, Tepolt FA, Yang DS, Kocher MS. Injury Risk Associated With Sports Specialization and Activity Volume in Youth. Orthop J Sports Med. 2019;7(9):2325967119870124.
130. Bahr R, Engebretsen L, editors. Handbook of Sports Medicine and Science: Sports Injury Prevention. 1st ed. Wiley-Blackwell Publishing, Chichester, West Sussex, UK. 2009.
131. Felson DT, Lawrence RC, Dieppe PA, et al. Osteoarthritis: new insights. Part 1: the disease and its risk factors. Ann Intern Med. 2000;133(8):635–46.
132. Messner K, Maletius W. The long-term prognosis for severe damage to weight-bearing cartilage in the knee: a 14-year clinical and radiographic follow-up in 28 young athletes. Acta Orthop Scand. 1996;67(2):165–8.
133. Drawer S, Fuller CW. Propensity for osteoarthritis and lower limb joint pain in retired professional soccer players. Br J Sports Med. 2001;35(6):402–8.
134. Roos H. Are there long-term sequelae from soccer? Clin Sports Med. 1998;17(4):819–31. viii
135. Lohmander LS, Ostenberg A, Englund M, Roos H. High prevalence of knee osteoarthritis, pain, and functional limitations in female soccer players twelve years after anterior cruciate ligament injury. Arthritis Rheum. 2004;50(10):3145–52.
136. Kaplan LD, Schurhoff MR, Selesnick H, Thorpe M, Uribe JW. Magnetic resonance imaging of the knee in asymptomatic professional basketball players. Arthroscopy. 2005;21(5):557–61.
137. Major NM, Helms CA. MR imaging of the knee: findings in asymptomatic collegiate basketball players. AJR Am J Roentgenol. 2002;179(3):641–4.
138. Bradley J, Honkamp NJ, Jost P, West R, Norwig J, Kaplan LD. Incidence and variance of knee injuries in elite college football players. Am J Orthop (Belle Mead, NJ). 2008;37(6):310–4.
139. Hirshorn KC, Cates T, Gillogly S. Magnetic resonance imaging-documented chondral injuries about the knee in college football players: 3-year National Football League Combine data. Arthroscopy. 2010;26(9):1237–40.

140. Schueller-Weidekamm C, Schueller G, Uffmann M, Bader TR. Does marathon running cause acute lesions of the knee? Evaluation with magnetic resonance imaging. Eur Radiol. 2006;16(10):2179–85.
141. Schueller-Weidekamm C, Schueller G, Uffmann M, Bader T. Incidence of chronic knee lesions in long-distance runners based on training level: findings at MRI. Eur J Radiol. 2006;58(2):286–93.
142. Marans HJ, Kennedy DK, Kavanagh TG, Wright TA. A review of intra-articular knee injuries in racquet sports diagnosed by arthroscopy. Can J Surg. 1988;31(3):199–201.
143. Powell JM, Kavanagh TG, Kennedy DK, Marans HJ, Wright TA. Intra-articular knee injuries in racquet sports. A review of 128 arthroscopies. Surg Endosc. 1988;2(1):39–43.
144. Shellock FG, Hiller WD, Ainge GR, Brown DW, Dierenfield L. Knees of Ironman triathletes: magnetic resonance imaging assessment of older (>35 years old) competitors. J Magn Reson Imaging. 2003;17(1):122–30.
145. Mithoefer K, Hambly K, Della Villa S, Silvers H, Mandelbaum BR. Return to sports participation after articular cartilage repair in the knee: scientific evidence. Am J Sports Med. 2009;37(Suppl 1):167S–76S.
146. Harris JD, Brophy RH, Siston RA, Flanigan DC. Treatment of chondral defects in the athlete's knee. Arthroscopy. 2010;26(6):841–52.
147. Jones G, Bennell K, Cicuttini FM. Effect of physical activity on cartilage development in healthy kids. Br J Sports Med. 2003;37(5):382–3.
148. Gahunia HK, Pritzker KP. Effect of exercise on articular cartilage. Orthop Clin N Am. 2012;43(2):187–99.

6 Diagnostic Imaging of Knee Cartilage Injury: Evaluation and Assessment

Gaurav K. Thawait, Gustav Andreisek, and Avneesh B. Chhabra

6.1 Introduction

Articular cartilage abnormalities in the knee are a common source of pain and are difficult to diagnose on clinical examination or using plain radiographs. Articular cartilage lesions may be related to acute or chronic trauma, inflammatory (inflammatory arthritis, IA), or degenerative (osteoarthritis, OA) arthropathies. Because the adult articular cartilage is avascular and has no intrinsic regenerative capability, its injury can lead to progressive knee OA, which is a major cause of morbidity [1, 2]. This poses a serious clinical problem for the referring physicians and prompts a need for reliable means of cartilage injury evaluation before onset of any irreversible morphologic damage ensues. In recent years, magnetic resonance imaging (MRI) has become the mainstay of cartilage imaging and evaluation as it allows direct visualization of the cartilage morphology. With the increasing use of high-field MR scanners (1.5 T, 3 T, and 7 T), higher spatial and contrast resolution images are frequently acquired [3–7]. These allow a thorough morphologic assessment of articular cartilage and to develop a standardized MRI evaluation system for native, injured, and repaired cartilage.

Functionally, the knee comprises of two articulations: tibiofemoral and patellofemoral. The femoral condyles articulate with the corresponding tibial plateaus and the patella articulates with the trochlear groove of femur by the medial and lateral facets on the posterior surface of patella. The stability of the knee joint is dependent upon static (knee capsule, ligaments, and bone), and dynamic (muscles – muscular forces and joint stress) factors. The soft connective tissue structures include synovium, cartilage, menisci, and ligaments (cruciate, medial, and collateral) (Fig. 6.1). The knee has two types of cartilage:

G. K. Thawait, MBBS, MD (✉)
Russell H. Morgan Department of Radiology and Radiological Science, Johns Hopkins University, Baltimore, MD, USA

Department of Biomedical Engineering, Johns Hopkins University, Baltimore, MD, USA
e-mail: gthawai1@jhmi.edu

G. Andreisek, MD, MBA
Department of Radiology, University Hospital Zurich, University of Zurich, Zurich, Switzerland

Swiss Center for Musculoskeletal Imaging, Balgrist Campus AG, Zurich, Switzerland

Department of Radiology, St Claraspital, Basel, Switzerland

Department of Radiology, Spital Thurgau AG, Cantonal Hospital, Munsterlingen, Switzerland

A. B. Chhabra, MBBS, MD (✉)
Department of Radiology and Orthopedic Surgery, University of Texas Southwestern Medical Center, Dallas, TX, USA

Department of Musculoskeletal Radiology, Parkland Health and Hospital System, Dallas, TX, USA
e-mail: avneesh.chhabra@utsouthwestern.edu

H. K. Gahunia et al. (eds.), *Articular Cartilage of the Knee*,
https://doi.org/10.1007/978-1-4939-7587-7_6

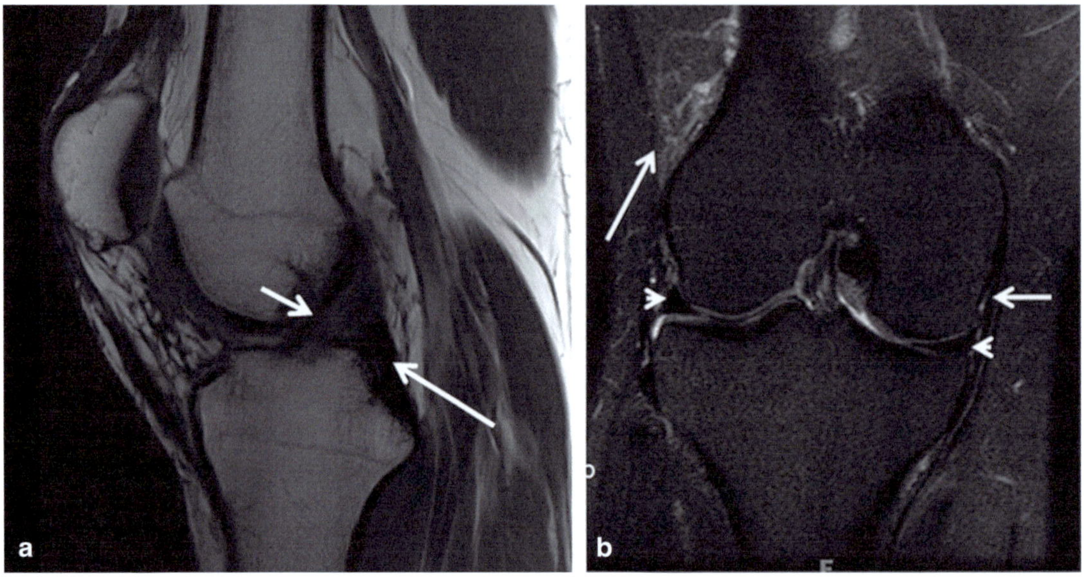

Fig. 6.1 Sagittal proton density-weighted (PDW) (**a**) and coronal fat suppressed (fs) PDW (**b**) MR images in a 16-year-old boy showing normal knee structures. (**a**) Shows the medial and lateral menisci (arrowheads), medial collateral ligament (small arrow), and iliotibial band (large arrow in **b**)

hyaline articular cartilage that covers the bone ends and menisci consisting of fibrocartilage between the bone ends. The patellar articular cartilage is the thickest in the body measuring around 4–6 mm in young healthy adults and is known to decrease with age [8, 9].

Understanding the MR imaging appearance of the normal and injured articular cartilage requires an understanding of its histologic and biochemical makeup. The hyaline cartilage is very hypocellular and is composed of about 4% chondrocytes by wet weight. Other major components include 70% water, 20% collagen, and 5–10% proteoglycans. The adult cartilage receives half of the oxygen and glucose by multiple small vascular branches near the tidemark zone and the other half through direct diffusion from the synovial fluid.

Histologically, hyaline cartilage reveals laminar (zonal) variation in cellular morphology, proteoglycan concentration, and collagen fiber size and orientation. The architecture and biochemical composition of the articular cartilage varies from superficial zone (SZ, toward the synovial fluid) to deeper zone (toward the subchondral bone). Also, regional differences in the cartilage exist, such as the weight-bearing portions of femorotibial articulation show a thicker radial deep zone (DZ) and a thinner transitional middle zone (MZ) due to more prevalent compression stresses. On the other hand, in the peripheral portions of the joint, the transitional zone occupies more space due to more prevalent shear stresses in that area. The tidemark anchors the cartilage to the underlying bone (Fig. 6.2). Refer to Chap. 1 for the in-depth knowledge of the knee articular cartilage structure and function.

With the technological advancements of hardware and software on high-field scanners, both morphologic and biochemical assessment of the articular cartilage can be reliably accomplished. A wide array of MR techniques have been employed for the assessment of the articular cartilage. This chapter reviews the advantages and disadvantages of various cartilage morphologic and biochemical MR imaging techniques. A thorough MR characterization of the various articular cartilage lesions is presented.

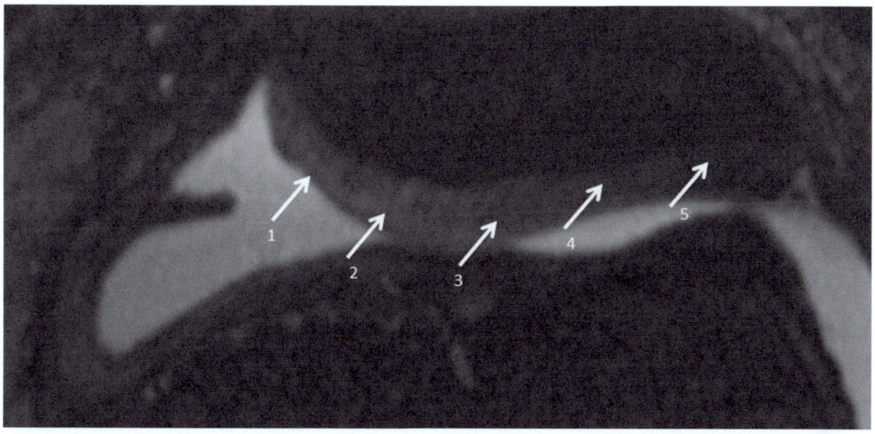

Fig. 6.2 Axial 3D dual excitation steady-state (DESS) sequence of patellofemoral cartilage showing five anatomic layers as shown with arrows 1–5 corresponding to the lamina splendens, superficial lamina, intermediate lamina, deep lamina, and tidemark, respectively

6.2 Articular Cartilage Specific MR Imaging

Ideally, an MR pulse sequence should display various cartilage zones referred to as "laminae" with optimal contrast and spatial resolution as well as changes to the subchondral bone plate, bone marrow edema, cysts, and granulation tissue. Using the appropriate high-resolution MR imaging technique, an analogous laminar anatomy of articular cartilage is often visible. On proton MR imaging, the characteristic gothic arch-like architecture of collagen fibers is responsible for the laminar MR appearance due to change in T2 signal intensity across the thickness of the cartilage [10]. The minimum T2 relaxation time in articular cartilage is approximately 10 ms, which implies that the tissue contrast depends on the T2 value even on T1-weighted and proton density-weighted images. In vitro and in vivo pulse sequences shows three distinct laminae: a hypointense superficial lamina, a hyperintense intermediate lamina, and a heterogeneous deep lamina that consists of alternating hyperintense and hypointense bands perpendicular to the subchondral bone [11, 12]. However, the various laminae may not be consistently identified due to the different angles and orientations of cartilage macromolecules that affect the internal water mobility and the dipole-dipole interactions of the collagen fibrils resulting in poorly demarcated layers. MR imaging pitfalls when imaging the knee articular cartilage and other joint tissues include regional anatomic variation, truncation artifact, partial volume effect, chemical shift, magic angle effects, and magnetic susceptibility effects. Although detection of early cartilage injury or disease remains elusive, MR imaging can demonstrate intermediate and advanced lesions.

6.2.1 Morphological Articular Cartilage MR Imaging (Qualitative)

Accurate evaluation of the articular cartilage in patients with acute or chronic injuries or joint disease is clinically significant. Identifying cartilage lesions or loss (focal or diffuse) can explain the cause of joint pain in symptomatic patients. Early diagnosis and appropriate treatment of cartilage lesions can reduce the associated pain and disability. The sensitivity and specificity of cartilage lesions detected on MR imaging, as correlated with reference standard of direct inspection on arthroscopy, vary from 60% to 95% depending upon the imaging technique used, patient population, and the reader's experience. Generally, best results are obtained from fast spin echo (FSE) and dual excitation steady-state (DESS) techniques, and the diagnostic perfor-

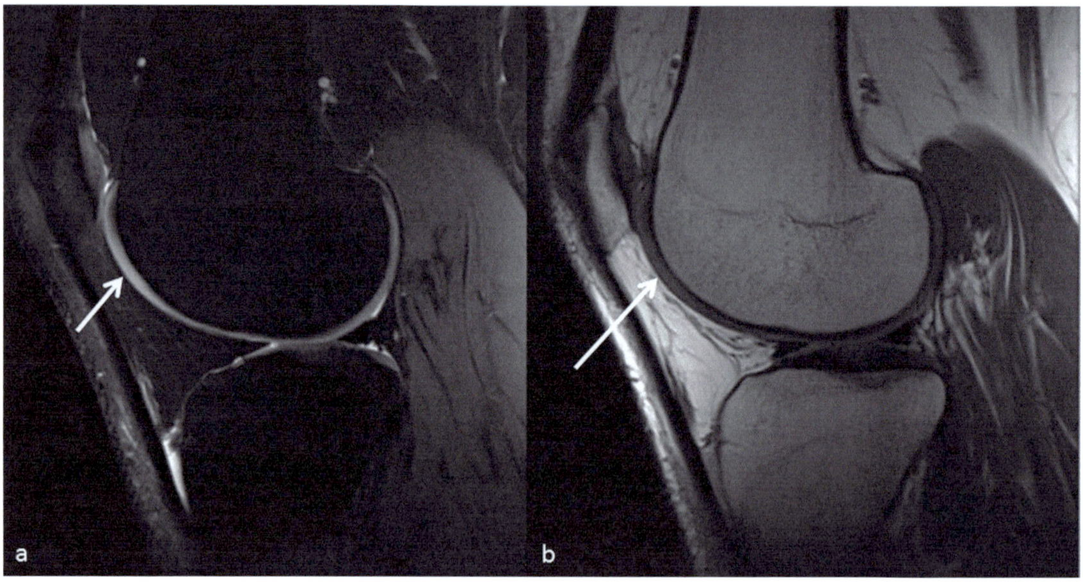

Fig. 6.3 Sagittal fs PDW (**a**) and sagittal PDW (**b**) MR images of the knee. The cartilage appears hyperintense (small arrow, **a**) but slightly less intense than joint fluid on fs PDW image, and shows intermediate signal intensity on PDW image (large arrow, **b**)

mance is highest on the thicker articular surfaces and larger/more deeper lesions, which is expected due to thin adult and aging knee cartilage and its complex geometry.

Evaluation of the cartilage macromolecular structure helps in providing an overview of the gross functional integrity of the tissue [13]. The various available morphologic MR techniques described below are easily applied and interpreted on regular picture archiving and communication system (PACS). On a routine protocol for joint imaging using fat-suppressed (fs) proton density-weighted (PDW) image, articular cartilage appears slightly hypointense to joint fluid, whereas on non-fs PDW images and three-dimensional (3D) DESS images, cartilage is seen as intermediate signal intensity (Fig. 6.3). An ideal combination for morphologic cum anatomic imaging is a combination of same plane fs and non-fs sequences (Fig. 6.3). Fat suppression techniques are used to increase dynamic range of contrast, especially at the subchondral bone-cartilage interface, and reduce chemical shift artifacts, usually at the expense of minimal loss of signal to noise ratio (SNR). Currently, MR arthrography is a commonly used method that can highlight early stage breach in articular cartilage surface integrity and continuity. MR arthrography provides a good contrast between the different joint structures with the excellent capability to show early signs of cartilage surface fibrillations as well as the integration site of repaired tissue with native cartilage [14, 15].

The most commonly used techniques for fat suppression include:

1. Chemically selective fat suppression pulses
2. Spatial-spectral pulses (water excitation)
3. Short inversion time (TI) inversion recovery (STIR) imaging
4. Iterative decomposition of water and fat with echo asymmetry and least-squares estimation (IDEAL) [16]

STIR imaging provides the most uniform fat suppression, however, at the expense of poorer SNR. Therefore, unless there is a large subject or presence of metal in the regional area, other methods do better than STIR imaging.

6.2.1.1 Two-Dimensional MR Imaging

Two-dimensional (2D) FSE, PDW and T2-weighted sequences are used for articular cartilage imaging. PDW sequence provides higher

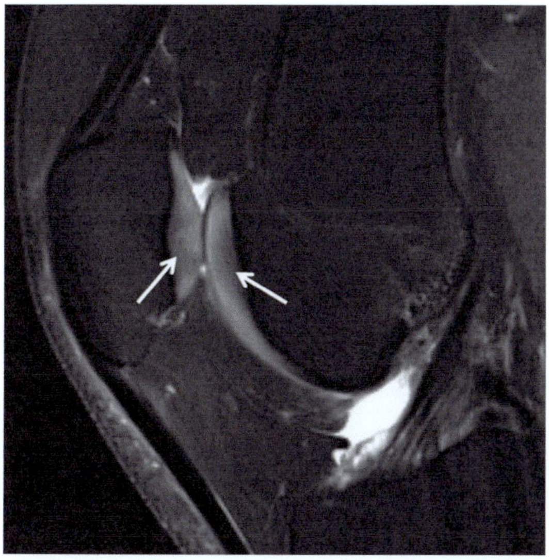

Fig. 6.4 Sagittal fs PDW image in a 40-year-old man shows normal trilaminar appearance of the articular cartilage of the patellofemoral joint. The trilaminar morphology corresponds to higher signal intensity of superficial and deep laminae with lower signal intensity of middle lamina

SNR but is more prone to magic angle artifacts as compared to T2-weighted images with longer echo times [17]. PDW images also frequently produce inadequate contrast with the surrounding synovial fluid. Although fs PDW images produce adequate contrast, this sequence may be prone to more blurring and lower SNR. As such, keeping echo times between 35 and 50 ms provides acceptable SNR and good quality images (Fig. 6.4). Also, the 2D imaging may lead to misdiagnosis of small cartilage lesions due to partial volume artifacts and imaging performed in only fixed planes.

6.2.1.2 Three-Dimensional MR Imaging

The common 3D FSE sequences include fast spin-echo CUBE (FSE- CUBE, General Electric Healthcare), sampling perfection with application optimized contrasts using different flip angle evolutions (SPACE, Siemens Medical Systems) (Fig. 6.5), and volumetric isotropic T2-weighted acquisition (VISTA, Philips Healthcare).These sequences use variable flip angle modulations to constrain T2 decay for an extended echo train producing intermediate-weighted images with bright synovial fluid [18]. The major advantage is that these images are acquired isotropically and can be reconstructed in any desired plane, reducing partial voluming artifacts. These images may also be simultaneously employed for the assessment of internal derangement findings. Additionally, due to avoidance of magnetization transfer effect-related cross-talk among adjacent slices, thinner slices with high resolution are possible than otherwise for 2D imaging on a 3 T scanner. However, there are some limitations to this technology. The cartilage to synovial fluid contrast is lower than using 2D FSE imaging; poor fat suppression may occur near the patellar surfaces and extremity curvatures; bone marrow edema is less conspicuous than using 2D fs FSE; and, imaging time is almost 2–3 times than using the 2D FSE sequence. In addition, if patient moves or imaging fails for some reason, the whole sequence needs to be repeated again. Finally, the reader's experience is required in order to appreciate the subtle findings of early cartilage abnormalities on these images.

The 3D gradient echo (3D GE) image datasets consist of volumetric acquisition of knee with isotropic voxels. The 3D GE imaging was the first to be used as 3D imaging of the cartilage. These sequences produce high spatial resolution images with multiplanar depiction, which shows bright synovial fluid and good cartilage-fluid differentiation. The 3D GE sequences include T2*-weighted gradient-recalled echo acquired in steady state (GRASS, General Electric Healthcare), gradient-recalled echo (GRE, Siemens Medical Systems), and T2-fast field echo (T2-FFE, Philips Healthcare). These images can be acquired faster than the 3D FSE images; however, they can be easily degraded by susceptibility artifacts from regional metal/air and provide suboptimal evaluation of adjacent subchondral bone, which is critical in cases of traumatic and degenerative cartilaginous lesions [17, 19, 20].

The 3D DESS sequence comprises of two or more gradients separated by a refocusing pulse. The data from these echoes result in higher T2* (gradient echo) weighting resulting in high signal intensity in cartilage and synovial fluid. An increase in flip angle has shown to increase the conspicuity between cartilage and synovial fluid [21]. The 3D DESS sequence is routinely used in clinical imaging as well as in OA initiative trial as it demonstrates the cartilage morphology with

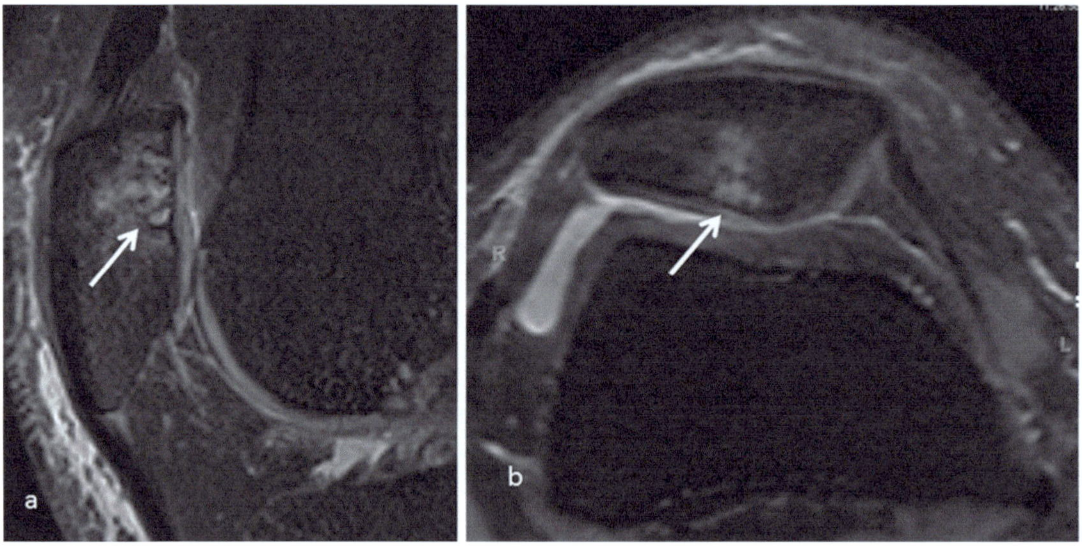

Fig. 6.5 Sagittal (**a**) and axial (**b**) isotropic reconstructions from a 3D SPACE imaging show high-grade cartilage defects of the lateral facet of patella with subchondral edema and cystic changes (arrows)

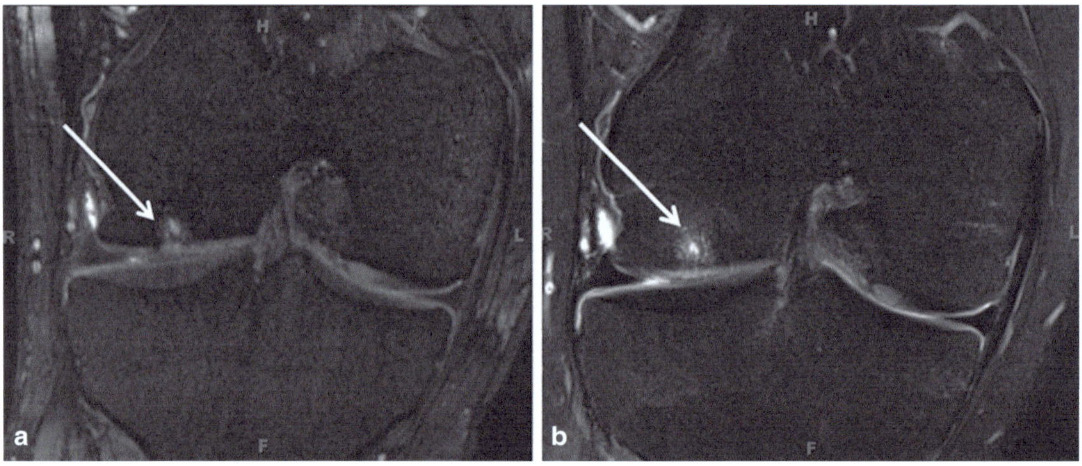

Fig. 6.6 Coronal 3D DESS (**a**) and corresponding fs PDW (**b**) MR images of the lateral femoral condyle of the knee in a 16-year-old boy shows subchondral cyst and marrow edema (arrows) related to overlying cartilage abnormality. The marrow edema and sharp meniscal definition is more apparent on the fs PDW image

higher SNR (cartilage appears thicker than FSE sequence), better tissue contrast, shorter acquisition time, and reduced motion artifacts. However, internal changes in cartilage signal intensity may be difficult to appreciate, bone marrow edema is less apparent, and it provides inferior SNR than the FSE sequence for internal derangement findings (Fig. 6.6) [22].

The 3D steady-state free precession (SSFP) sequences use symmetrical (balanced) gradient probing from different directions to produce images with high signal intensity (bright) fat, fluid, and hemorrhage); thus, good fat saturation is required for an ideal contrast of cartilage and synovial fluid. These sequences include fast imaging using steady-state acquisition (FIESTA, General Electric Healthcare), true fast imaging with steady-state precession (true FISP, Siemens Medical Systems) (Fig. 6.7), balanced FFE imaging (balanced FFE, Philips

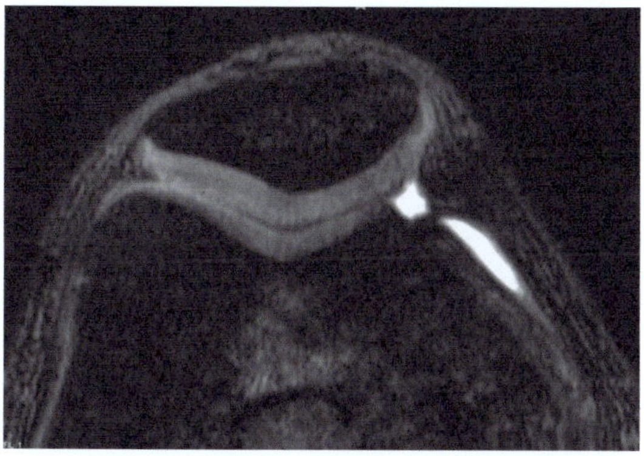

Fig. 6.7 Axial reconstruction from a fs TruFISP sequence demonstrating normal articular cartilage of the patellofemoral joint. The synovial fluid is uniformly bright providing a good cartilage to fluid contrast. Note the trilaminar morphology of articular cartilage

Healthcare), and their variants, such as fluctuating equilibrium MR (FEMR) and vastly undersampled isotropic projection steady-state free precession (VIPR-SSFP) [23, 24]. These sequences are promising; however, banding artifacts may frequently occur, and cartilage to synovial fluid contrast as well as fat suppression around the extremity curvatures is often limited. Additionally, similar to GRE techniques, the internal derangement findings are not optimally assessed.

6.2.2 Biochemical Articular Cartilage MR Imaging (Quantitative)

The biochemical properties of articular cartilage are influenced by the collagen and proteoglycan content and structure within the extracellular matrix. Quantitative MRI techniques have been developed to characterize the structure and composition of cartilage macromolecules. In normal articular cartilage, the fixed charge density of glycosaminoglycans chains of the proteoglycan increases with depth from the cartilage surface [25]. Further, proteoglycan depletion has been documented as the earliest findings in injured and diseased cartilage [26, 27]. The MR techniques sensitive to cartilage proteoglycan content/ depletion include:

1. Non contrast-enhanced techniques (such as sodium MR imaging or T1 rho mapping) [28–31]
2. Contrast-enhanced techniques (such as delayed gadolinium-enhanced MR imaging, dGEMRIC, and Gd-DTPA(2)-enhanced T1 imaging) [32–35]
3. MR techniques to determine glycosaminoglycan concentration (such as chemical exchange-dependent saturation transfer, gagCEST, imaging) [31, 36]

MR techniques indicative of the collagen content, integrity, and orientation along with water content and mobility can also be gauged by:

1. T2 relaxation time mapping [4, 37, 38]
2. Ultrashort echo time (UTE) imaging [39, 40]
3. Diffusion-weighted imaging (DWI) such as diffusion tensor imaging (DTI) [41, 42]
4. Magnetization transfer contrast (MTC) [12]

6.3 Magnetic Resonance Imaging of Articular Cartilage Injury

Injury to the articular cartilage in knee is a frequently encountered clinical problem, which may be confounded with meniscal or ligament injuries. Cartilage injury may include intraarticular or osteochondral lesions. Osteochondral lesions refer to combined injury to the cartilage and the underlying subchondral bone. It can be caused by trauma, osteochondritis dissecans (OCD), or insufficiency fractures (Fig. 6.8). While osteochondral lesions may be identified on plain radiographs, intraarticular lesions are best assessed on MRI.

Hyaline cartilage functions to resist the compression and shears forces as well as dissipate and/or distribute loading forces to a larger area in weight-bearing regions [43]. When a loading force is applied slowly, proteoglycan-bound water is squeezed into the uncompressed regions of the matrix distributing the forces. After removal of the load, osmotic pressure and dissolved electrolytes pull the water molecules back in the cartilage and restore equilibrium. In the

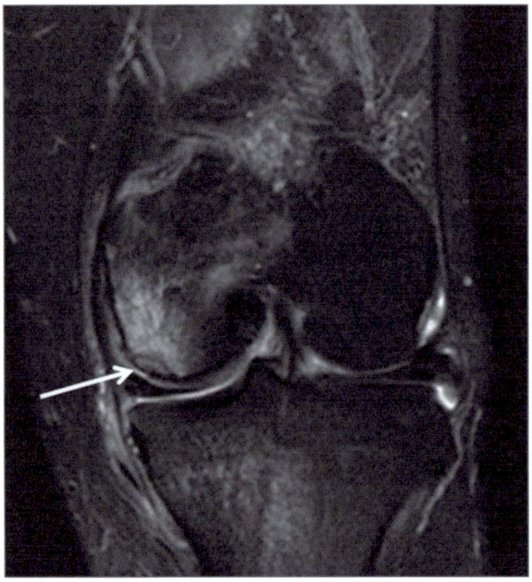

Fig. 6.8 Coronal fs PDW image in a 44-year-old man with acute medial knee pain. There is osteochondral fracture (arrow) of the medial femoral condyle with extensive bone marrow edema

event of significant trauma, the loading forces are too high or applied too rapidly, which results in unequal redistribution of the water molecules leading to disruption of the framework of articular cartilage. Similarly, in repetitive minor trauma, there is damage to the deeper layers of cartilage and subchondral bone which may occur without any apparent change in surface of the cartilage. Other predisposing factors of articular cartilage injury and/or loss include knee malalignment/maltracking, meniscal injury/extrusion, cruciate or collateral ligament injuries (Fig. 6.9), instability, inflammatory arthropathy, and finally osteochondral bodies, which may parasitize blood flow and growth – causing frictional cartilage loss.

6.3.1 Classification of Articular Cartilage Lesions

Over the years, several methods of classifying articular cartilage lesions have been proposed [44]. The arthroscopic staging criteria, Outerbridge, and its modified versions are outlined in Chap. 7, whereas the histopathological scoring system of cartilage lesion and OA is discussed in Chap. 15. The MR classification criteria for cartilage lesions and cartilage repair are presented in depth in Chaps. 13 and 14. Some of the commonly used MR scoring system for cartilage lesions includes whole-organ Magnetic Resonance Imaging Score (WORMS) [45], Boston-Leeds Osteoarthritis Knee Scoring System (BLOKS) [46], and Knee Osteoarthritis Scoring System (KOSS) [47]. For a reproducible assessment of the cartilage lesions, WORMS has been widely used [45]. The knee articular cartilage is subdivided by anatomic landmarks into 15 regions: medial and lateral facet of patella, medial and lateral femoral condyle (anterior/central/posterior), medial and lateral tibial plateau (anterior/central/posterior), and subspinous tibia.

It is a daunting task for the radiologists and referring physicians to remember and incorporate these ever-changing scoring systems in their practice. Additionally, with widespread MR imaging, it has become clear that not one scoring system fits all cartilage lesions. A variety of cartilage lesion morphologies are commonly observed. Further, the same compartment of the joint may have different lesions. Therefore, it is best to describe the lesion morphology, size, and extent in a structured radiology report rather than trying to fit the lesions in a particular scoring system. The following discussion will address and simplify the articular cartilage injury terms in common use and their respective meanings with relevant imaging examples.

6.3.2 Intraarticular Cartilage Lesions

Cartilage lesions of the knee can be grouped into three broad categories: acute chondral or osteochondral lesions, chronic lesions due to repetitive impaction, and lesions due to joint disorder such as OCD, OA, and IA. There are some dis-

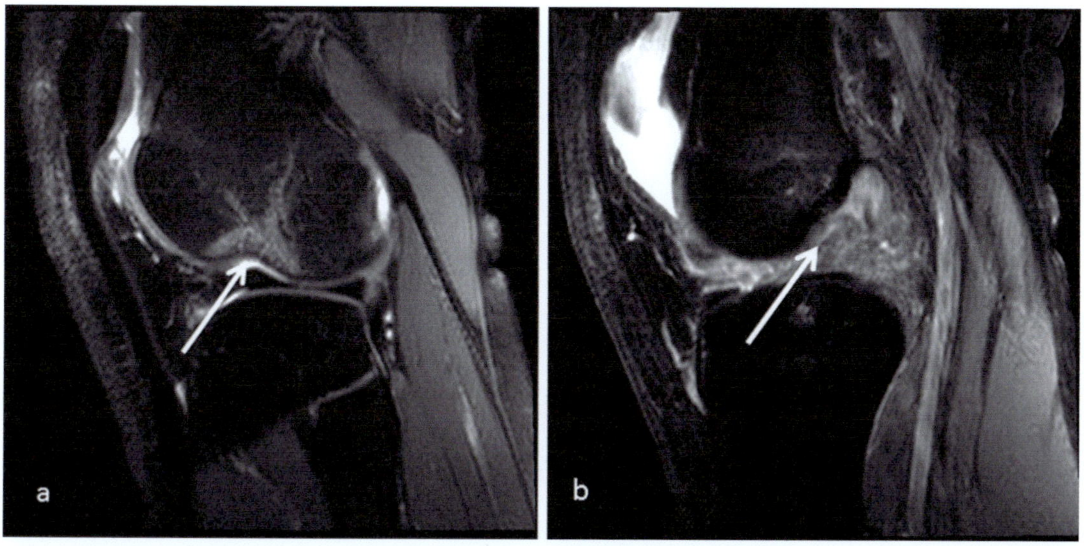

Fig. 6.9 Sagittal fs PDW images (**a**, **b**) of the knee in a 25-year-old woman with recent clipping injury. Note the osteochondral impaction fracture of the sulcus terminalis (**a**, arrow) from recent translational event and complete disruption of the anterior cruciate ligament (**b**, arrow)

tinguishing characteristics of each category. An acute lesion frequently occurs on weight-bearing area of the knee. It is characterized by sharp margins oriented perpendicular to the bone surface and exhibits subchondral bone marrow edema. At times lesions include fractured cartilage or cartilage and bone (osteochondral) that may break off as a "loose" fragment. In general, cartilage lesions have limited capacity to heal, and they often get worse with time. Visualizing and characterizing these lesions on MRI, particularly at an early stage prior to irreversible damage, are imperative because of the implications for surgery.

6.3.2.1 Chondromalacia

Chondromalacia is the earliest stage of cartilage injury that occurs without cartilage surface defect. It usually involves softening or blistering of the deeper cartilage lamina due to fluid imbibition, which is relatively soft "malacic" on arthroscopic probing. However, chondromalacia is a nonspecific finding and may be seen in asymptomatic subjects. MR imaging shows cartilage blister or softening as focal areas of increased T2 signal intensity in the deep cartilage lamina or loss of laminar differentiation with diffuse intraarticular increased signal intensity. This may be associated with focal or diffuse swelling of the articular cartilage (Fig. 6.10). T2 maps are useful for early identification of the above findings as it may not be apparent on anatomic imaging (Fig. 6.11).

6.3.2.2 Cartilage Repair Response

Degeneration, fibrocartilage, and chondrocalcinosis are the spectrum of a repair response to injury or microabrasion to the articular cartilage. Although spontaneous cartilage repair occurs, it often leads to the formation of biologically inefficient cartilage-like fibrotic tissue. MR imaging shows focal or diffuse areas of low signal intensity (signal heterogeneity) within the articular cartilage, especially the superficial and intermediate cartilage lamina. It is often difficult to differentiate the three entities; however, chondrocalcinosis may be well characterized on the GE imaging (Fig. 6.12).

6.3.2.3 Cartilage Fibrillation or Erosions

Fibrillations are vertical clefts between groups of chondrocyte resulting in "fingerlike" projections into the joint space. Fibrillation is an early

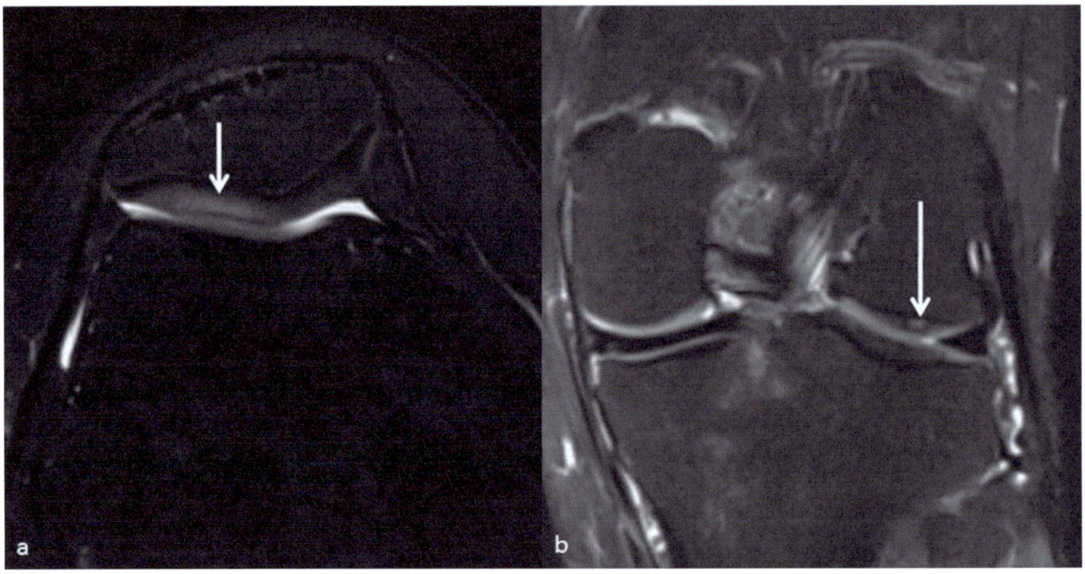

Fig. 6.10 Chondromalacia. Axial (**a**) and coronal (**b**) fs PDW MR images shows intraarticular focal areas of increased T2 signal intensity with loss of layered differentiation (**a**, small arrow). At times blister/focal softening with thickening of involved cartilage (**b**, large arrow) is seen

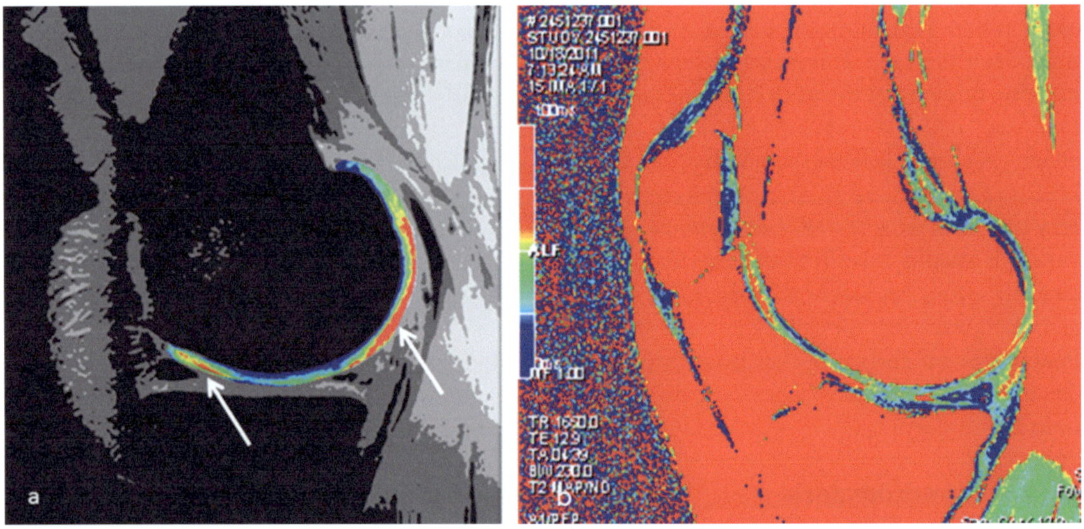

Fig. 6.11 Sagittal T2 map of the knee articular cartilage. Notice areas of chondromalacia (**a**, arrows) as compared to normal cartilage in **b**

stage of loss of cartilage surface integrity that may follow chondromalacia or may be a solitary finding, appropriately referred to as mild chondrosis. On MR imaging, the articular cartilage appears to be of near-normal thickness but shows uneven/irregular articular surface (lamina splendens) continuity (Fig. 6.13). It is commonly seen in frictional areas, such as the superior aspect of the lateral facets of the patellofemoral compartment and load-bearing area of femorotibial compartment.

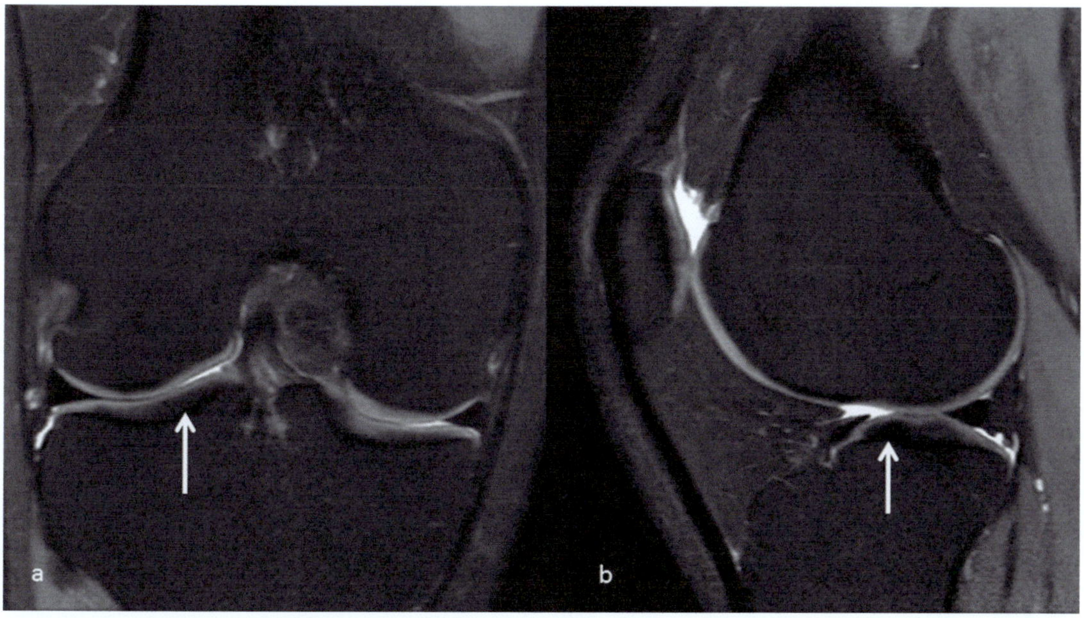

Fig. 6.12 Cartilage degeneration/fibrocartilage/chondrocalcinosis. Coronal (**a**) and sagittal (**b**) fs PDW MR images show focal areas of low signal intensity areas within the articular cartilage (arrows)

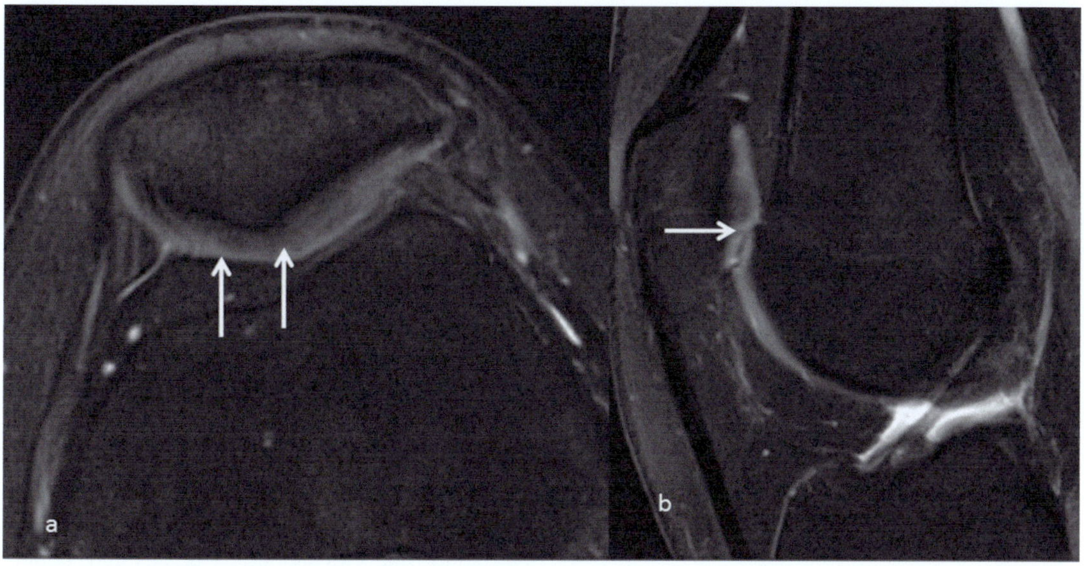

Fig. 6.13 Cartilage surface fibrillation/erosions. Axial (**a**) and sagittal (**b**) fs PDW MR images show the cartilage of normal thickness but with uneven articular surface (arrows)

6.3.2.4 Cartilage Fissure or Flap

Fissure or flaps are frequently caused by repetitive and prolonged overloading or traumatic injury to the articular cartilage. They can be low (< 50% of cartilage thickness) or high grade (> 50% of cartilage thickness) and can be solitary or multifocal. On MR imaging, a fissure is seen as linear T2 hyperintense signal, less than 2 mm transverse, which assumes vertical to minimally oblique orientation to the articular surface of the bone. A flap is formed by an obliquely oriented fissure, which causes elevation of the superficial

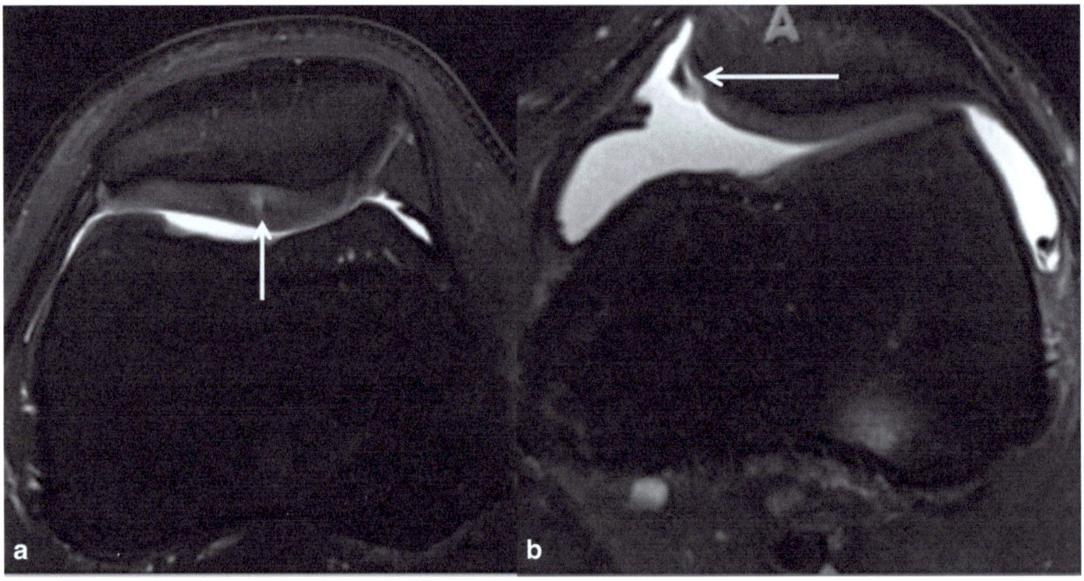

Fig. 6.14 Cartilage fissure/flap. Axial fs PDW MR images. (**a**) Shows a fissure which is a linear (< 2 mm) T2 hyperintense signal intensity and assumes a vertical/slightly oblique orientation and disrupts the articular surface (small arrow). (**b**) Shows a flap which is formed by an obliquely oriented fissure with elevation of the superficial semi-separated component (large arrow)

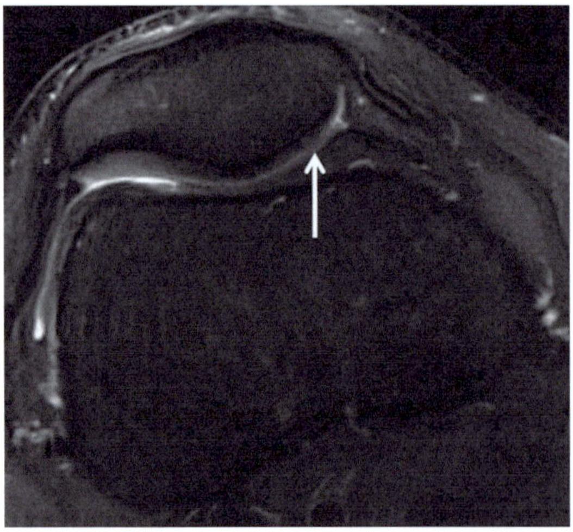

Fig. 6.15 Cartilage thinning. Axial fs PDW MR image shows diffuse thinning of the articular cartilage (arrow) of the medial facet of the patella

(< 50%) or deep (> 50%) semi-separated component of the articular cartilage (Fig. 6.14).

6.3.3 Articular Cartilage Thickness

Cartilage thinning or hypotrophy is frequently associated with chronic or recurrent cartilage injury (Figs. 6.15 and 6.16). This should also be classified as low or high grade using above-mentioned criteria. On MR imaging, the articular cartilage shows diffuse thinning with or without focal defects (Fig. 6.17). Comparison to the cartilage from normal appearing compartment of the knee is frequently used to make this diagnosis.

Increased relative thickness or hypertrophy of the cartilage at the lesion site may be apparent in few circumstances such as chondromalacia due to fluid imbibition, OCD due to osteochondrosis and abnormality of secondary physis and, hypertrophy observed as a complication of autologous chondrocyte implantation. The increased thickness of articular cartilage may lead to locking of knee with decreased joint motion with further cartilage damage. MR imaging shows increased thickness of the articular cartilage with respective findings of the underlying lesions as described above or surgical change from the cartilage replacement procedure.

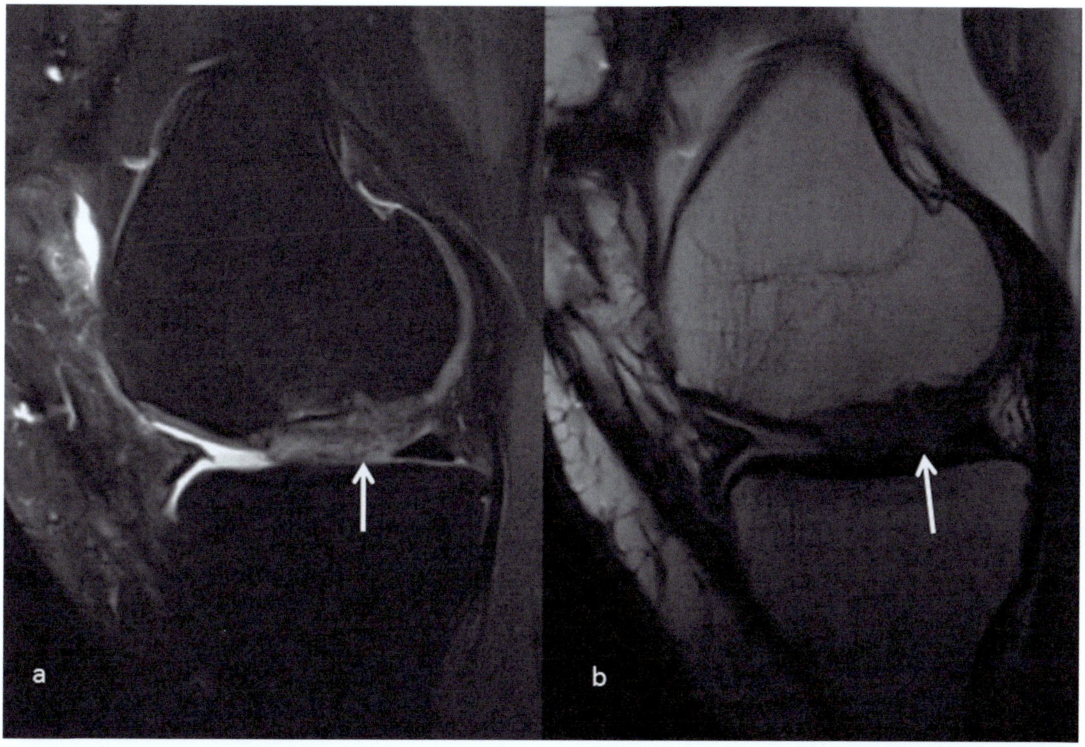

Fig. 6.16 Cartilage hypertrophy. Sagittal fs PDW (**a**) and PDW (**b**) MR images show increased thickness of articular cartilage (arrows) at the site of prior autologous cartilage implantation

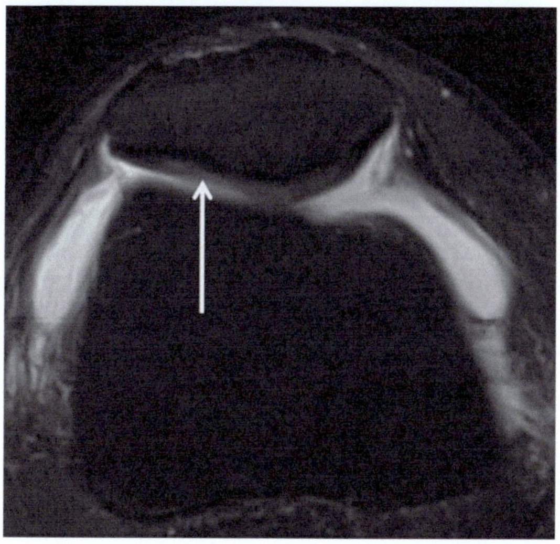

Fig. 6.17 Cartilage defect. Axial fs PDW MR image shows a fluid-filled hyperintense lesion (> 2 mm) of more than 50% of cartilage thickness, in keeping with a high-grade defect (arrow)

6.3.4 Articular Cartilage Defects

Cartilage defects are frank defects within the cartilage with transverse size more than 2 mm. These defects can vary in size and shape involving partial or complete loss of articular cartilage. They can be classified as low and high grade similar to fissures and flaps, based on the involved thickness. The defects may be single or multifocal. MR imaging shows a fluid-filled hyperintense lesion of more than 2 mm. In lesions related to arthritis, these defects appear as irregular lesions with obtuse margins while, in cases of trauma, a well-shouldered defect may be seen, which is high grade or associated with bone marrow changes. The latter may be best treated by surgery to prevent future progression.

Full-thickness cartilage defects results from the complete loss of articular cartilage leading to exposure of the subchondral bone. On MR imaging, full-thickness defect is often associated with a variable combination of bone marrow edema, cysts,

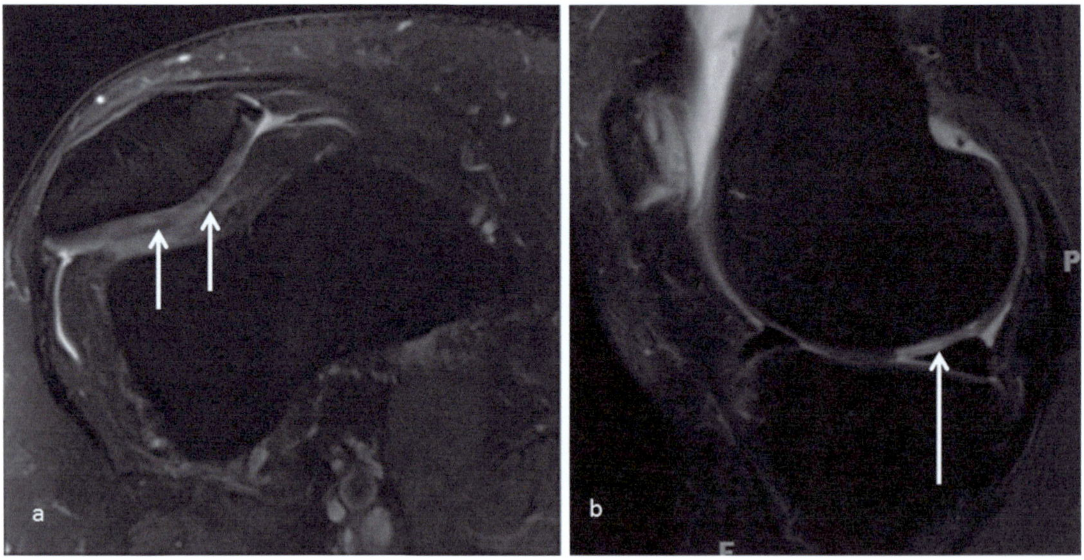

Fig. 6.18 Cartilage defects. Axial (**a**) and sagittal (**b**) fs PDW MR images show multifocal cartilage defects in the setting of arthritis as irregular obtuse margins (**a**, small arrows) and from trauma as a well-shouldered defect (**b**, large arrow)

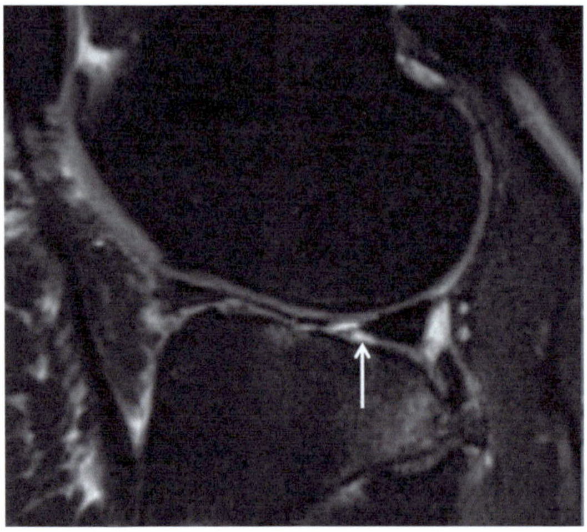

Fig. 6.19 Full-thickness cartilage defect. Sagittal fs PDW MR image shows exposed subchondral bone (arrow) in the posterolateral tibial plateau, which may be associated with reactive bone marrow change

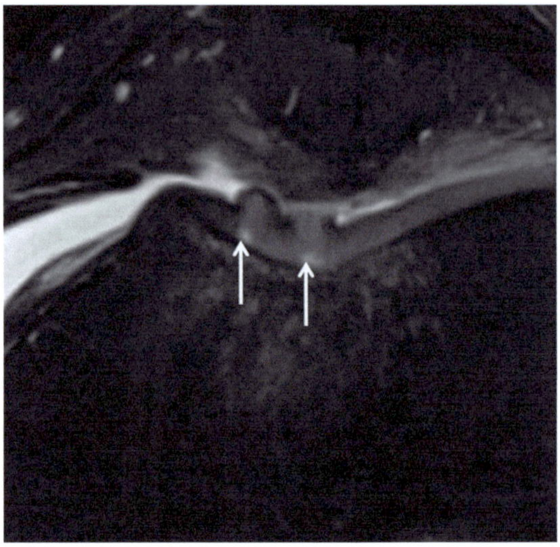

Fig. 6.20 Cartilage delamination. Axial fs PDW MR image shows high signal intensity fluid between the cartilage and subchondral bone (arrows) with buckling of the overlying debonded cartilage

and sclerosis; and, with further progression, underlying articular surface irregularity, depression, or osteophyte formation may be seen (Figs. 6.18 and 6.19).

6.3.4.1 Cartilage Delamination

Cartilage delamination refers to the separation (debonding) of the articular cartilage from the subchondral bone at the tidemark zone and is one of the worst cartilage lesions. MR imaging shows a high (fluid) signal intensity dissecting between the cartilage and bone with or without buckling of the delaminated cartilage (Fig. 6.20).

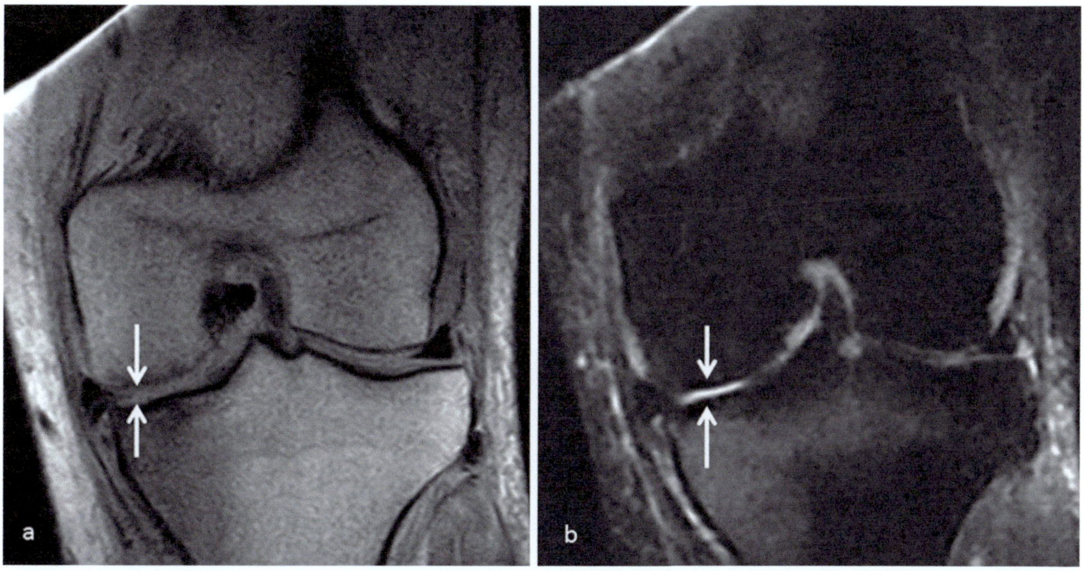

Fig. 6.21 Cartilage denudation. Coronal PDW (**a**) and T2-weighted (**b**) MR images shows complete absence of articular cartilage surface (**a**, arrows) in the medial compartment with complete denudation and reactive bone marrow change (**b**, arrows)

6.3.4.2 Cartilage Denudation

Cartilage denudation results from chronic progressive complete loss of cartilage from large areas of the bone. This lesion, if present in both opposing articular surfaces, as seen with severe arthritis, presents as painful bone on bone apposition due to reactive bone marrow changes. MRI shows complete absence of cartilage in the articular surface. Puddle sign on axial images can be seen when bone is exposed to synovial fluid. Reactive bone marrow edema, sclerosis, cysts, deformity, and/or osteophyte formation is nearly always present (Fig. 6.21).

6.3.5 Osteochondral Lesions

This is a traumatic lesion which causes the erosion/contusion of the articular cartilage at the impaction site with or without subchondral bone fracture. On MR imaging, overlying cartilage lesions (thinning, fissure, fibrillation, defect), underlying reactive bone marrow edema, or subchondral fracture (dark line in a cloud of edema) can be seen in acute stages (Fig. 6.22). In subacute and chronic stages, the edema evolves into subchondral cysts and sclerosis, with or without articular surface depression/loose body formation.

6.4 Articular Cartilage Lesions in Joint Disorder

The common joint disorders that affect the knee cartilage are OCD and arthritis (IA and OA). Using the appropriate pulse sequences, MR has shown much promise in identifying early signs of cartilage and bone lesions associated with these disorders.

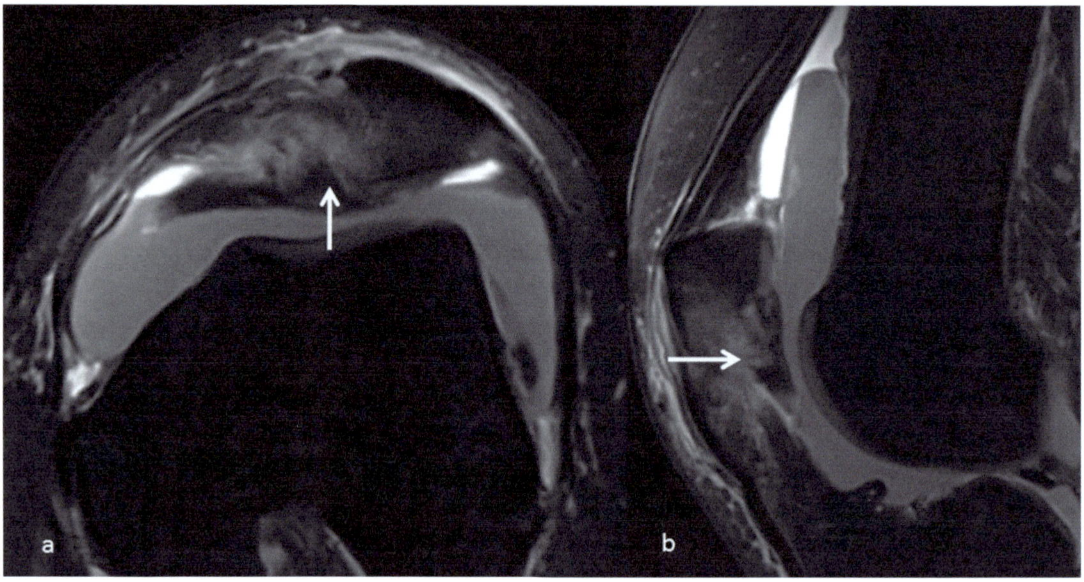

Fig. 6.22 (**a**, **b**) Osteochondral fracture. Axial (**a**) and sagittal (**b**) fs PDW MR images shows the eroded articular cartilage at the impaction injury with subchondral bone fracture (arrows)

6.4.1 Osteochondritis Dissecans

Osteochondritis dissecans is a joint disorder in which cracks form in the articular cartilage and the underlying subchondral bone. Eventually, fragmentation of both cartilage and bone occurs, called osteochondral fragment, releasing it within the joint space. Although rare (15–30 people out of 100, 000 in the general population affected each year), it is an important cause of joint pain in physically active adolescents [48, 49]. OCD reflects a disorder of secondary physis (beneath the articular cartilage) and in almost 50% of all cases, there is an underlying history of trauma. On MR imaging, it can be seen as half-moon-shaped lesion, usually in non-weight-bearing surface of the bone and may produce secondary bony changes as described above for the trauma-related osteochondral lesions (Fig. 6.22). Some locations are characteristic for this lesion, such as medial aspect of the lateral femoral condyle of the knee, talar dome, and capitellum. The overlying articular cartilage may be flush with the remaining cartilage, proud or, many times, deficient, depending upon the extent of the lesion. MRI plays an important role in determining the stability of the OCD defect. Stable lesions noted in MRI usually have good clinical outcome, whereas unstable lesions as detected by MRI are predicted to have poor clinical outcome. Signs of instability include full-thickness cartilage tearing, cystic change penetrating to deep lamina, osteochondral defect with fluid-filled cavity, and/or osteochondral fragment with high (fluid) signal intensity (Fig. 6.23). For in-depth discussion of OCD, refer to Chap. 10.

6.4.2 Inflammatory Arthritis

Inflammatory arthritis is a group of diseases characterized by inflammation of the joints and often other tissues, many of which are a result of autoimmunity. MRI is efficacious in initial disease detection and prognostication in patients with inflammatory arthritis as well as in monitoring of both disease progression and response to therapy. Subchondral bone marrow edema is the key imaging findings of inflammatory arthritis detectable by MRI and may be a forerunner of

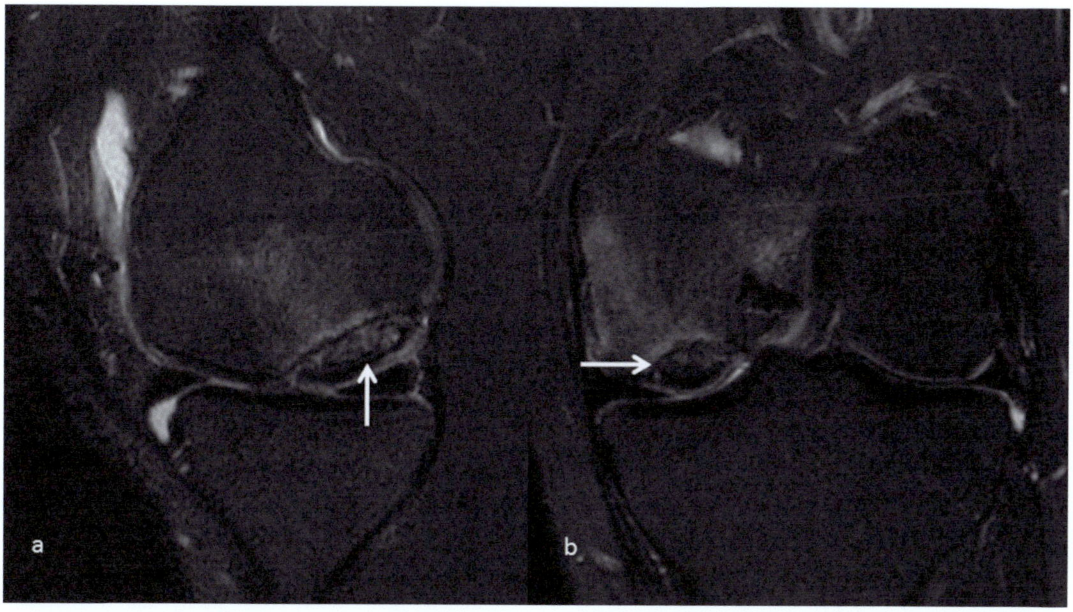

Fig. 6.23 Osteochondritis dissecans. Sagittal (**a**) and coronal (**b**) fs PDW MR images show half-moon-shaped lesion (arrows) in the lateral aspect of the medial femoral condyle, mildly proud as compared to the native cartilage. Notice bone marrow edema within the lesion and subjacent femoral condyle with early cyst formation

cartilage erosion, which is more diffuse and uniform. Other MR findings which include synovial thickening, synovitis, joint effusion, and chondrocalcinosis may also be seen, but focal lesions are not common.

6.4.3 Osteoarthritis

Osteoarthritis is a degenerative joint disease that results from aberrations of articular cartilage and the underlying subchondral bone. OA is believed to be caused by mechanical stress on the joint, and other causes include previous joint injury, abnormal join or limb development, and inherited factors; also, overweight individuals have a greater risk of developing knee OA. Changes in cartilage and subchondral bone composition are important to note in the progression of OA. In particular, bone marrow edema-like lesions, subchondral cyst, and subchondral bone aberrations are notable features indicating disease progression. Using the appropriate MR technique, the early stage of OA (proteoglycan loss and increased tissue fluid) corresponding to cartilage hypertrophy shows as increased MR signal intensity. MRI can also detect early signs of cartilage surface lesions (fissures), intraarticular lesions and focal or diffuse cartilage loss as well as joint space narrowing and changes in the subchondral bone surface, subchondral cysts, and early osteophytes as well as provide a baseline that can help predict the OA patient's individual risk for an incident total knee replacement 4–7 years later, and also the patient's risk of developing OA due to progressive knee articular cartilage degeneration secondary to other diseases such as diabetes [50, 51].

6.5 Conclusions

To conclude, articular cartilage architecture is complex and high resolution and high contrast MR imaging is essential to resolve the anatomy and its lesions. Reader skill and in-depth knowledge of cartilage anatomy and pathology is important for accurate diagnosis and follow-up of untreated and treated lesions.

References

1. Felson DT. Clinical practice. Osteoarthritis of the knee. N Engl J Med. 2006;354(8):841–8.
2. Helmick CG, Felson DT, Lawrence RC, Gabriel S, Hirsch R, Kwoh CK, et al. Estimates of the prevalence of arthritis and other rheumatic conditions in the United States Part I. Arthritis Rheum. 2008;58(1):15–25.
3. Cashman G, Attariwala R. Influence of MRI field strength on clinical decision making in knee cartilage injury – a case study. J Can Chiropr Assoc. 2014;58(4):395–400.
4. Andreisek G, Weiger M. T2* mapping of articular cartilage: current status of research and first clinical applications. Investig Radiol. 2014;49(1):57–62.
5. Chang G, Diamond M, Nevsky G, Regatte RR, Weiss DS. Early knee changes in dancers identified by ultra-high-field 7 T MRI. Scand J Med Sci Sports. 2014;24(4):678–82.
6. Jordan CD, Saranathan M, Bangerter NK, Hargreaves BA, Gold GE. Musculoskeletal MRI at 3.0 T and 7.0 T: a comparison of relaxation times and image contrast. Eur J Radiol. 2013;82(5):734–9.
7. Wyss M, Manoliu A, Marcon M, Spinner G, Luechinger R, et al. Clinical magnetic resonance imaging of the knee at 7 T: optimization of fat suppression. Invest Radiol. 2019;54(3):160–68.
8. Meachim G, Bentley G, Baker R. Effect of age on thickness of adult patellar articular cartilage. Ann Rheum Dis. 1977;36(6):563–8.
9. Faber SC, Eckstein F, Lukasz S, Muhlbauer R, Hohe J, Englmeier KH, et al. Gender differences in knee joint cartilage thickness, volume and articular surface areas: assessment with quantitative three-dimensional MR imaging. Skelet Radiol. 2001;30(3):144–50.
10. Xia Y, Farquhar T, Burton-Wurster N, Lust G. Origin of cartilage laminae in MRI. J Magn Reson Imaging. 1997;7(5):887–94.
11. Waldschmidt JG, Rilling RJ, Kajdacsy-Balla AA, Boynton MD, Erickson SJ. In vitro and in vivo MR imaging of hyaline cartilage: zonal anatomy, imaging pitfalls, and pathologic conditions. Radiographics. 1997;17(6):1387–402.
12. Rubenstein JD, Kim JK, Morova-Protzner I, Stanchev PL, Henkelman RM. Effects of collagen orientation on MR imaging characteristics of bovine articular cartilage. Radiology. 1993;188(1):219–26.
13. Gray ML, Burstein D. Molecular (and functional) imaging of articular cartilage. J Musculoskelet Neuronal Interact. 2004;4(4):365–8.
14. Ronga M, Angeretti G, Ferraro S, DEF G, Genovese EA, Cherubino P. Imaging of articular cartilage: current concepts. Joints. 2014;2(3):137–40.
15. Kalke RJ, Di Primio GA, Schweitzer ME. MR and CT arthrography of the knee. Semin Musculoskelet Radiol. 2012;16(1):57–68.
16. Bley TA, Wieben O, Francois CJ, Brittain JH, Reeder SB. Fat and water magnetic resonance imaging. J Magn Reson Imaging. 2010;31(1):4–18.
17. Link TM, Stahl R, Woertler K. Cartilage imaging: motivation, techniques, current and future significance. Eur Radiol. 2007;17(5):1135–46.
18. Notohamiprodjo M, Horng A, Pietschmann MF, Muller PE, Horger W, Park J, et al. MRI of the knee at 3T: first clinical results with an isotropic PDfs-weighted 3D-TSE-sequence. Investig Radiol. 2009;44(9):585–97.
19. Roemer FW, Hunter DJ, Guermazi A. MRI-based semiquantitative assessment of subchondral bone marrow lesions in osteoarthritis research. Osteoarthritis Cartilage. 2009;17(3):414–5. author reply 416-7
20. Disler DG, McCauley TR, Wirth CR, Fuchs MD. Detection of knee hyaline cartilage defects using fat-suppressed three-dimensional spoiled gradient-echo MR imaging: comparison with standard MR imaging and correlation with arthroscopy. AJR Am J Roentgenol. 1995;165(2):377–82.
21. Moriya S, Miki Y, Yokobayashi T, Ishikawa M. Three-dimensional double-echo steady-state (3D-DESS) magnetic resonance imaging of the knee: contrast optimization by adjusting flip angle. Acta Radiol. 2009;50(5):507–11.
22. Eckstein F, Hudelmaier M, Wirth W, Kiefer B, Jackson R, Yu J, et al. Double echo steady state magnetic resonance imaging of knee articular cartilage at 3 tesla: a pilot study for the osteoarthritis initiative. Ann Rheum Dis. 2006;65(4):433–41.
23. Gold GE, Hargreaves BA, Vasanawala SS, Webb JD, Shimakawa AS, Brittain JH, et al. Articular cartilage of the knee: evaluation with fluctuating equilibrium MR imaging--initial experience in healthy volunteers. Radiology. 2006;238(2):712–8.
24. Lu A, Barger AV, Grist TM, Block WF. Improved spectral selectivity and reduced susceptibility in SSFP using a near zero TE undersampled three-dimensional PR sequence. J Magn Reson Imaging. 2004;19(1):117–23.
25. Maroudas A, Muir H, Wingham J. The correlation of fixed negative charge with glycosaminoglycan content of human articular cartilage. Biochim Biophys Acta. 1969;177(3):492–500.
26. Burstein D, Gray M, Mosher T, Dardzinski B. Measures of molecular composition and structure in osteoarthritis. Radiol Clin N Am. 2009;47(4):675–86.
27. Dunn TC, Lu Y, Jin H, Ries MD, Majumdar S. T2 relaxation time of cartilage at MR imaging: comparison with severity of knee osteoarthritis. Radiology. 2004;232(2):592–8.
28. Duvvuri U, Charagundla SR, Kudchodkar SB, Kaufman JH, Kneeland JB, Rizi R, et al. Human knee: in vivo T1(rho)-weighted MR imaging at 1.5 T--preliminary experience. Radiology. 2001;220(3):822–6.
29. Stahl R, Luke A, Li X, Carballido-Gamio J, Ma CB, Majumdar S, et al. T1rho, T2 and focal knee cartilage abnormalities in physically active and sedentary

healthy subjects versus early OA patients--a 3.0-tesla MRI study. Eur Radiol. 2009;19(1):132–43.
30. Wang L, Regatte RR. T(1)rho MRI of human musculoskeletal system. J Magn Reso Imaging. 2015;41(3):586–600.
31. Schmitt B, Zbyn S, Stelzeneder D, Jellus V, Paul D, Lauer L, et al. Cartilage quality assessment by using glycosaminoglycan chemical exchange saturation transfer and (23)Na MR imaging at 7 T. Radiology. 2011;260(1):257–64.
32. Williams A, Sharma L, McKenzie CA, Prasad PV, Burstein D. Delayed gadolinium-enhanced magnetic resonance imaging of cartilage in knee osteoarthritis: findings at different radiographic stages of disease and relationship to malalignment. Arthritis Rheum. 2005;52(11):3528–35.
33. Wang L, Regatte RR. Quantitative mapping of human cartilage at 3.0T: parallel changes in T(2), T(1)rho, and dGEMRIC. Acad Radiol. 2014;21(4):463–71.
34. Bengtsson Mostrom E, Lammentausta E, Finnbogason T, Weidenhielm L, Janarv PM, Tiderius CJ. Pre- and postcontrast T1 and T2 mapping of patellar cartilage in young adults with recurrent patellar dislocation. Magn Reson Med. 2015;74(5):1363–9.
35. Bekkers JE, Bartels LW, Benink RJ, Tsuchida AI, Vincken KL, Dhert WJ, et al. Delayed gadolinium enhanced MRI of cartilage (dGEMRIC) can be effectively applied for longitudinal cohort evaluation of articular cartilage regeneration. Osteoarthritis Cartilage. 2013;21(7):943–9.
36. Ling W, Regatte RR, Navon G, Jerschow A. Assessment of glycosaminoglycan concentration in vivo by chemical exchange-dependent saturation transfer (gagCEST). Proc Natl Acad Sci U S A. 2008;105(7):2266–70.
37. Kijowski R, Blankenbaker DG, Munoz Del Rio A, Baer GS, Graf BK. Evaluation of the articular cartilage of the knee joint: value of adding a T2 mapping sequence to a routine MR imaging protocol. Radiology. 2013;267(2):503–13.
38. Koller U, Apprich S, Domayer S, Windhager R, Trattnig S. Magnetic resonance mapping of the rim of articular cartilage defects of the patella. Int Orthop. 2014;38(1):67–72.
39. Bae WC, Dwek JR, Znamirowski R, Statum SM, Hermida JC, D'Lima DD, et al. Ultrashort echo time MR imaging of osteochondral junction of the knee at 3 T: identification of anatomic structures contributing to signal intensity. Radiology. 2010;254(3):837–45.
40. Robson MD, Gatehouse PD, Bydder M, Bydder GM. Magnetic resonance: an introduction to ultrashort TE (UTE) imaging. J Comput Assist Tomogr. 2003;27(6):825–46.
41. Mamisch TC, Menzel MI, Welsch GH, Bittersohl B, Salomonowitz E, Szomolanyi P, et al. Steady-state diffusion imaging for MR in-vivo evaluation of reparative cartilage after matrix-associated autologous chondrocyte transplantation at 3 tesla--preliminary results. Eur J Radiol. 2008;65(1):72–9.
42. Raya JG. Techniques and applications of in vivo diffusion imaging of articular cartilage. J Magn Reson Imaging. 2015;41(6):1487–504.
43. Imhof H, Sulzbacher I, Grampp S, Czerny C, Youssefzadeh S, Kainberger F. Subchondral bone and cartilage disease: a rediscovered functional unit. Investig Radiol. 2000;35(10):581–8.
44. Pritzker KP, Gay S, Jimenez SA, Ostergaard K, Pelletier JP, Revell PA, et al. Osteoarthritis cartilage histopathology: grading and staging. Osteoarthritis Cartilage. 2006;14(1):13–29.
45. Peterfy CG, Guermazi A, Zaim S, Tirman PF, Miaux Y, White D, et al. Whole-organ magnetic resonance imaging score (WORMS) of the knee in osteoarthritis. Osteoarthritis Cartilage. 2004;12(3):177–90.
46. Hunter DJ, Lo GH, Gale D, Grainger AJ, Guermazi A, Conaghan PG. The reliability of a new scoring system for knee osteoarthritis MRI and the validity of bone marrow lesion assessment: BLOKS Boston Leeds osteoarthritis knee score. Ann Rheum Dis. 2008;67(2):206–11.
47. Kornaat PR, Ceulemans RY, Kroon HM, Riyazi N, Kloppenburg M, Carter WO, et al. MRI assessment of knee osteoarthritis: knee osteoarthritis scoring system (KOSS)--inter-observer and intra-observer reproducibility of a compartment-based scoring system. Skelet Radiol. 2005;34(2):95–102.
48. Obedian RS, Grelsamer RP. Osteochondritis dissecans of the distal femur and patella. Clin Sports Med. 1997;16(1):157–74.
49. Zanon G, Div G, Marullo M. Osteochondritis dissecans of the knee. Joints. 2014;2(1):29–36.
50. Heilmeier U, Wamba JM, Joseph GB, Darakananda K, Callan J, et al. Baseline knee joint effusion and medial femoral bone marrow edema, in addition to MRI-based T2 relaxation time and texture measurements of knee cartilage, can help predict incident total knee arthroplasty 4–7 years later: data from the Osteoarthritis Initiative. Skeletal Radiol. 2019;48(1):89–101.
51. Neumann J, Guimaraes JB, Heilmeier U, Joseph GB, Nevitt MC, et al. Diabetics show accelerated progression of knee cartilage and meniscal lesions: data from the osteoarthritis initiative. Skeletal Radiol. 2019;48(6):919–30.

7 Assessment of Knee Cartilage Injury: Arthroscopic Evaluation and Classification

Tim Dwyer and John S. Theodoropoulos

7.1 Introduction

In 1975, DeHaven and Collins described arthroscopy as the gold standard investigation of intra-articular pathology of the knee [1]. This statement remains true today, with evidence that many lesions remain undetected using today's magnetic resonance (MR) technology; nevertheless, as MR technology and magnetic field strength increases, the sensitivity of detecting and assessing cartilage lesions will undoubtedly improve [2, 3]. Although arthroscopy is invasive, it is still the most helpful diagnostic tool. Arthroscopy has the added advantage of allowing simultaneous diagnosis and treatment of chondral and associated lesions (i.e. meniscal tears, ligament tears) within the knee, as well as the ability to perform an examination under anaesthesia (EUA). The EUA is a critical component of arthroscopy, as coexisting knee disorders (anterior cruciate ligament – ACL injury, ligamentous laxity, biomechanical malalignment) can negatively impact any cartilage regeneration or repair surgery [4].

Up to 63% of patients undergoing knee arthroscopy have evidence of chondral pathology [5–9]. Many of these injuries are diffuse and not amenable to current repair techniques. The incidence of treatable focal and isolated lesions varies. In a prospective study of 1000 consecutive knee arthroscopies, Hjelle et al. identified focal chondral or osteochondral (OC) lesions in 19% of patients, whereas other investigators reported that between 4% and 10% of knee arthroscopy performed in patients under 40 years old have one or more well-defined International Cartilage Repair Society (ICRS, since 2018 renamed as International Cartilage Regeneration and Joint Preservation Society) scoring or Outerbridge grade 3 or 4 lesion [5–7] (see Appendix A – Arthroscopic Classification for Cartilage Injuries).

Accurate measurement of articular cartilage lesions using arthroscopy has been shown to be directly related to the arthroscopic experience of the surgeon [10]. The determination of a chondral defect's location, size, depth, morphology and degree of containment is extremely important, as it forms the basis of grading the lesion which guides treatment algorithms [11, 12]. In addition, the

T. Dwyer, MBBS, FRACS, FRCSC, PhD (✉)
Division of Orthopaedics, University of Toronto, Toronto, ON, Canada

University of Toronto Orthopaedic Sports Medicine, Women's College Hospital, Toronto, ON, Canada

Division of Orthopaedic Surgery, Women's College Hospital and Mount Sinai Hospital, Toronto, ON, Canada

J. S. Theodoropoulos, MD (✉)
Division of Orthopaedic Surgery, University of Toronto, Toronto, ON, Canada

University of Toronto Orthopaedic Sports Medicine Program, Women's College Hospital, Toronto, ON, Canada

Division of Orthopaedic Surgery, Women's College Hospital and Mount Sinai Hospital, Toronto, ON, Canada
e-mail: jtheodoropoulos@mtsinai.on.ca

H. K. Gahunia et al. (eds.), *Articular Cartilage of the Knee*,
https://doi.org/10.1007/978-1-4939-7587-7_7

measurement tool used by the surgeon may influence arthroscopic estimation of cartilage lesion size [13]. Also, chondral lesion factors, such as localisation and size (kissing vs. nonkissing lesions and multiple vs. single lesions), have been shown to influence symptoms and knee function [8]. It is recognised, however, that arthroscopy may not be the gold standard for the grading of articular cartilage defects, with some evidence that knee arthrotomy and direct measurement of a lesion's size and depth are more accurate [10]. Today, most surgeons use arthroscopy rather than arthrotomy for grading cartilage pathology.

The incidence, size and severity of chondral injury have been shown to increase with time from injury and increasing patient age [3, 14–16]. Amongst pediatric patients with ACL tears, those who underwent primary arthroscopic ACL reconstruction > 150 days after injury showed a higher rate of meniscal tears than those treated ≤ 150 days after injury [16]. The chondral injury significantly associated with the presence of meniscal tear in the same compartment of the knee.

Increased age and weight are independently associated with a higher rate of medial meniscal tear (MMT). Patients with ACL tears and MMT or lateral meniscal tear (LMT) are more likely to have a chondral injury in that particular compartment than those without meniscal tears. The effect of this is twofold. Firstly, these patients are more likely to require surgical intervention to address chondral lesions, which may have increased in both size and depth from the index event. Secondly, the number of patients who have disease affecting the opposing articular surface will increase, potentially precluding biological treatment options [17].

Careful and systematic examination of the knee joint is critically important in order to avoid missing significant joint tissue lesions. It is essential to evaluate the entire joint surface, as even minor areas of degeneration opposite a major cartilage defect can make achieving a satisfactory outcome challenging [17]. Commonly missed areas include the posterior femoral condyles and the trochlea. Furthermore, recognition that particular injuries may have chondral injury patterns (i.e. ACL rupture and patella dislocation) enables the surgeon to pay particular attention to those regions.

This chapter will focus on the classification of chondral lesions arthroscopically; detail the assessment of these lesions in regard to their location, size and depth; and discuss the articular cartilage injury patterns seen with common knee pathology and trauma.

7.2 Classification Systems for Chondral Lesions

Classification and scoring systems have been devised to quantify the severity of cartilage damage, allowing the creation of treatment algorithms and the assessment of clinical outcomes. Without accurate reporting of chondral lesions, research into proper treatment modalities is limited. Only two of the many classification systems will be discussed in this chapter, whereas other arthroscopic classification systems (Noyes Classification and Oswestry Arthroscopy Score) are outlined in Appendix A. The Outerbridge classification is mentioned for historical reasons, whereas the ICRS classification is mentioned because it has become adapted for use by most of the modern literature and researchers in the field of cartilage regeneration.

7.2.1 Outerbridge Classification

The Outerbridge classification was first described in 1961 and was based on the assessment of patella chondromalacia visualised whilst performing open medial meniscectomy [18]. Divided into four grades, its major limitation is that the differentiation between grade 2 and grade 3 lesions depends on the diameter rather than depth [19] (Table 7.1. Also refer to Appendix A for the modified version).

Table 7.1 Outerbridge classification

Grade	Description of the Lesion
I	Softening and swelling of the cartilage
II	Fragmentation and fissuring in an area half an inch or less in diameter
III	Same as grade 2 but an area more than half an inch in diameter is involved
IV	Erosion of cartilage down to the subchondral bone

Brismar et al. examined the reliability of the Outerbridge classification by using 19 videotaped knee arthroscopies in patients with mild to moderate knee osteoarthritis (OA) [20]. The data was analysed by four orthopedic surgeons. Reliability, as judged by intra-observer kappa value, was only fair to good, with an intra-observer reliability best for normal cartilage (grade 0) and advanced changes (grade 4). However, the inter-observer reliability/overall percentage agreement was only 61%, which was felt to be likely due to the fact that OA is a continuum of changes. Other studies reported moderate intra-observer and inter-observer reproducibility and accuracy using the arthroscopy Outerbridge classifications for chondral lesions [21–23]. Trisolino et al. assessed the reliability of the videotape scoring system in fifty-seven patients who underwent arthroscopic treatment of meniscal tears. Using the Outerbridge classification system, assessment of articular cartialge lesions at six sites showed substantial interobserver and intra-observer reliability, and moderate consistency with the intra-operative score provided by the surgeon [21].

7.2.2 The International Cartilage Repair Society Classification

The International Cartilage Repair Society classification was originally described in 1998 and modified in 2003 [19, 24]. This commonly used grading system is similar to Outerbridge but distinguishes between grade 2 and 3 lesions based on the depth of the cartilage defect. The ICRS grade 2 chondral lesions (abnormal) involve less than 50% of the cartilage depth, and the ICRS grade 3 lesions (severely abnormal) involve more than 50% of the cartilage depth (Fig. 7.1, Table 7.2 and Appendix A). Validation of ICRS for the arthroscopic assessment of cartilage repair has been found to be statistically reliable and repeatable with good intraobserver and interobserver reliability [25, 26]. Further, the arthroscopic ICRS grading of chondral lesions in cadavers correlated well with the histological grades of lesion depth [26].

Table 7.2 Arthroscopic grading of chondral injuries using the International Cartilage Repair Society (ICRS) classification

Grade	Description of the Lesion
0	Normal
1A	Superficial fibrillation or softening
1B	Superficial fissures and lacerations
2	Defect less than 50% of depth
3A	Defect more than 50% but not down to the calcified layer
3B	Defect more than 50% down to the calcified layer
3C	Defect down to but not through the subchondral bone plate
3D	Defect more than 50% with blisters
4A	Defect includes superficial subchondral bone plate
4B	Defect down to deep subchondral bone

7.3 Assessment of Articular Cartilage Defects

The main goal in the arthroscopic evaluation of a chondral injury is to appropriately classify the lesion(s), allowing the application of treatment algorithms. Each cartilage defect must be identified and carefully evaluated in regard to the lesion location, size, depth and containment.

7.3.1 Articular Cartilage Appearance

It is important to be able to distinguish between hyaline cartilage and fibrocartilage (Fig. 7.2). Normal hyaline cartilage has a glossy, bluish white and homogeneous appearance.

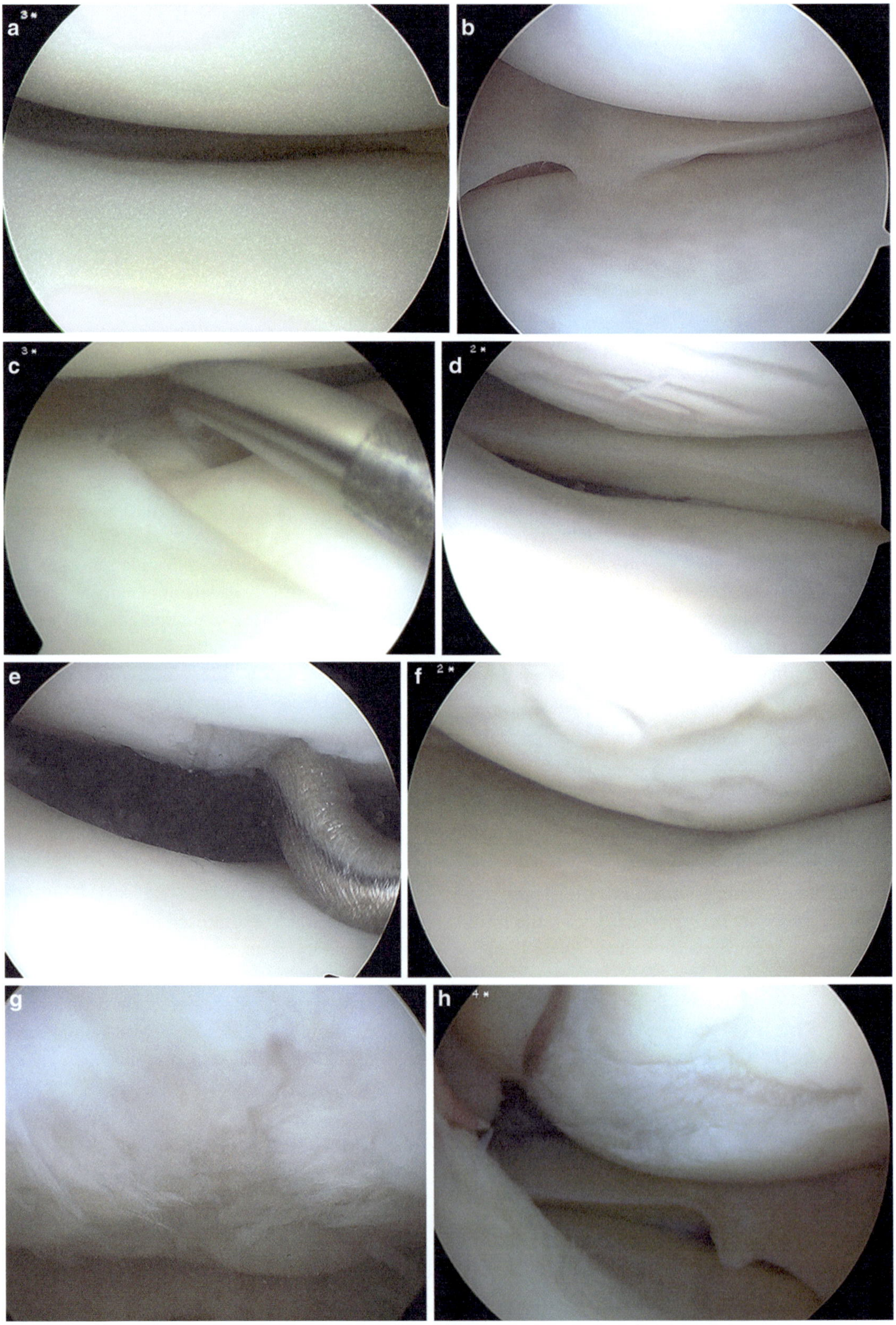

Fig. 7.1 (continued)

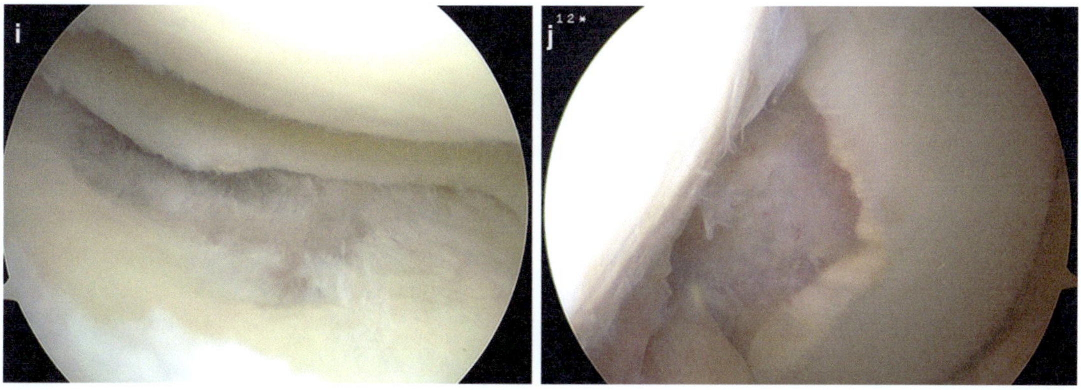

Fig. 7.1 Arthroscopic photographs of knee chondral lesions graded according to the International Cartilage Repair Society (ICRS) classification system. (**a**) Normal with grade 0; (**b**) Grade 1A with cartilage softening; (**c**) Grade 1B with superficial lacerations; (**d**) Grade 2 with lesions less than 50% of cartilage depth; (**e**) Grade 3A with lesions extending to more than 50% of uncalcified cartilage depth; (**f**) Grade 3B with lesions extending up to the calcified cartilage; (**g**) Grade 3C with lesions extending up to but not through the subchondral bone; (**h**) Grade 3D showing defect more than 50% with blisters; (**i**) Grade 4A with defect extending to the superficial subchondral bone plate; and (**j**) Grade 4B with defect extending deep into the subchondral bone

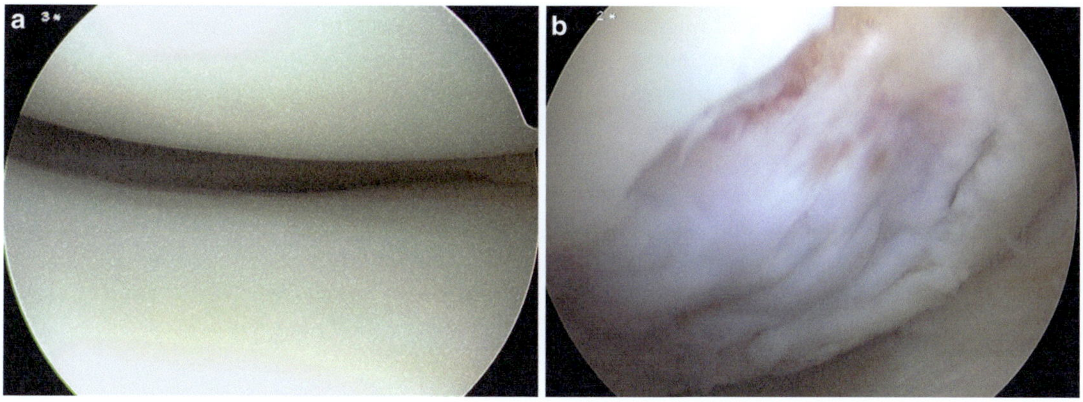

Fig. 7.2 Arthroscopic photographs showing: (**a**) Normal hyaline cartilage. (**b**) Fibrocartilaginous repair tissue

Fibrocartilage consists of cartilaginous and fibrous components in varying proportions, which is most likely be encountered after a repair procedure (i.e. a successful microfracture, MFX) or an ICRS - 4 chondral lesion that has had an element of fibrocartilage healing response (Fig. 7.2a). Fibrocartilage is not biomechanically adapted to serve as articular cartilage, with its higher proportion of type I rather than type II collagen; it is designed to resist loading in tension rather than compression [27].

7.3.2 Chondral Lesion Location

Specifying the location of chondral lesions is important as chondral lesions of different regions of the knee have varying treatment options and may have different prognosis. Further, an accurate description of the lesion is important for the interpretation of clinical outcomes. Certainly some areas of the knee, such as the medial femoral condyle (MFC) or knee with medial tibiofemoral offset, are more prone to chondral injury [14, 28].

Various systems for the reporting of chondral defect locations have been published. The most commonly used and simple method divides the knee into six regions: the patella (medial and lateral), trochlea, MFC, lateral femoral condyle (LFC), medial tibial plateau (MTP) and lateral tibial plateau (LTP). In 2001, Hunt et al. proposed a system for evaluating knee chondral lesions (N = 1,553 in 853 patients) at arthroscopy [29]. This complex chondral mapping tool was designed to increase accuracy and to provide a meaningful analysis of patterns of articular cartilage damage. This mapping tool divides the patella into six zones, the tibia into ten zones and the femur into ten zones. This system takes into account the location of tibial lesions in relation to the menisci, as well as whether femoral lesions are weight bearing in extension or flexion. A similar chondral lesion mapping system has been adapted as part of the ICRS Cartilage Injury Evaluation Package, using a grid system of the tibial and femur as shown in Fig. 7.3.

Studies reporting the location of chondral lesions at knee arthroscopy demonstrate that the MFC is consistently the most common site of focal chondral lesions, followed by the patella and the LFC, whilst the MTP is least commonly affected [3, 5, 7] (Table 7.3). In regard to the isolated grade 4 lesions identified in 1277 patients, Curl et al. corroborated the above findings by documenting that lesions on the MFC were the most common, followed by the LFC and the patella [6].

7.3.3 Chondral Lesion Size and Diameter

Measurement of the size of a focal lesion, an important factor in treatment algorithms, usually involves the use of a scaled, hooked, arthroscopic instrument or probe with marked 5 mm increments. Lesions are measured in length and width, which assumes that a defect is basically rectangular, hence generating a defect area in cm^2 [19] (Fig. 7.4).

An accurate measurement of the chondral defect size is difficult and is related to the arthroscopic experience of the surgeon. In a study of over 400 patients with chondral injuries, lesions were measured arthroscopically at the time of chondral biopsy and also 3–4 weeks later at arthrotomy for the subsequent autologous chondrocyte implantation (ACI) procedure [9]. The result showed a significant overestimation of the defect size at arthroscopy, with surgeons of all experience levels. The average arthroscopic estimation exceeded the real defect size by more than 1 cm^2; the greatest overestimation was with small defects < 4 cm^2. Accuracy was improved by surgeon's experience, both with surgeons who had performed > 100 knee arthroscopies and surgeons who had performed > 1000 knee arthroscopies. Interestingly, there was no statistically significant difference based on location of chondral lesions within the knee.

7.3.4 Chondral Lesion Depth

The depth of the chondral lesion is a critical component of the ICRS classification, with grade 3 and 4 lesions generally accepted as requiring treatment. The prognosis for ICRS - 2 lesions in patients treated with simple debridement has been shown to be good [30, 31]. There is some evidence that partial-thickness chondral injuries (grade 1 and 2), at least in rabbits, may undergo spontaneous repair due to stem cell migration from adjacent synovium [30].

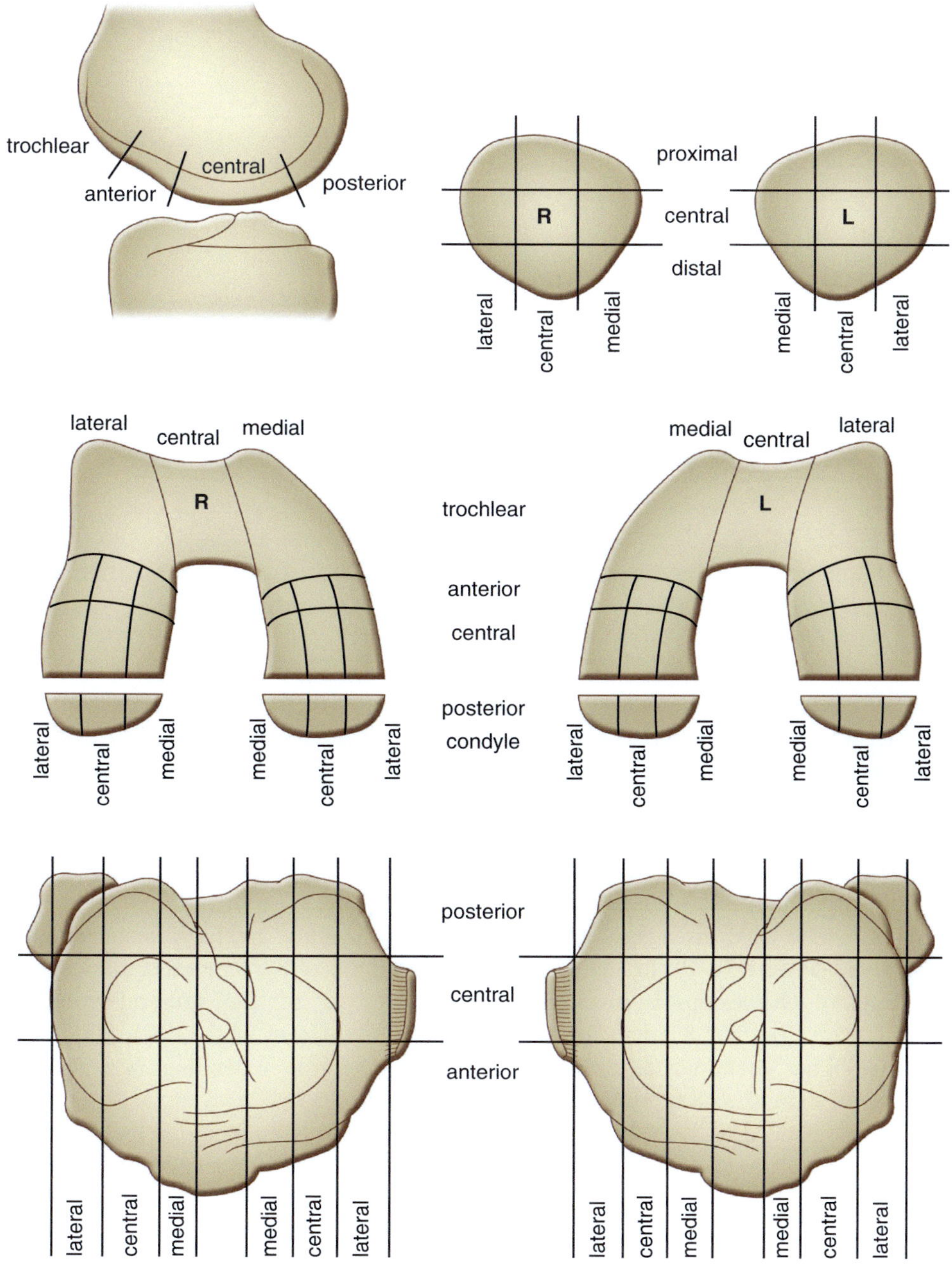

Fig. 7.3 The International Cartilage Repair Society (ICRS) knee cartilage lesion mapping system (Reprinted from the ICRS Cartilage Injury Evaluation Package [www.cartilage.org], with permission from the ICRS)

Table 7.3 Location of chondral lesions at knee arthroscopy

Reference	Patient # (*N*)	MFC	LFC	MTP	LTP	Patella	Trochlea
Widuchowski et al. (2006)	10,574	34%	9%	6%	7%	36%	8%
Figueroa et al. (2007)	82	32.2%	14.8%	2.6%	7.8%	33%	9.6%
Hjelle et al. (2002)	193	58%	9%	5%	11%	11%	6%

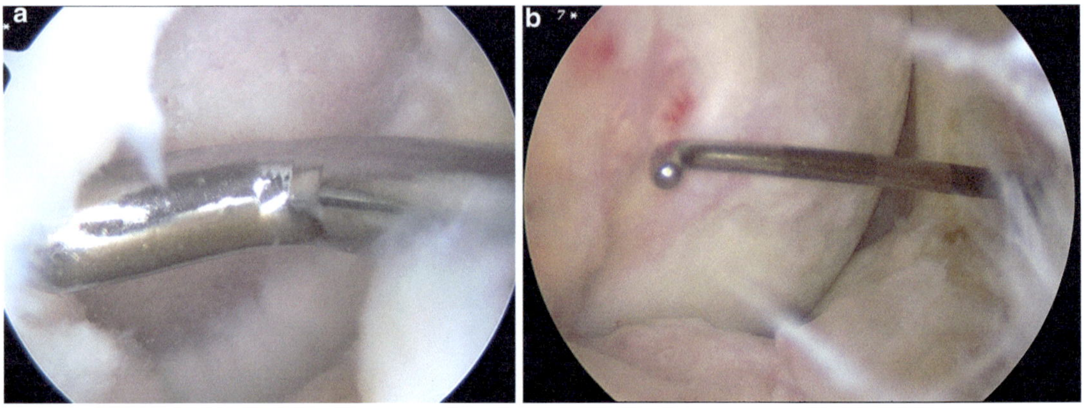

Fig. 7.4 Arthroscopic photographs showing measurement of the size of chondral lesions. (**a**) 7 mm wide lesion. (**b**) 15 mm wide lesion

Broadly speaking, the goal of the surgeon is to distinguish superficial partial-thickness injuries (< 50%), from deeper lesions (> 50%), using the graduated probe to estimate the depth of chondral lesions as per the ICRS classification (Fig. 7.5f). Important techniques involve probing the individual fissures, thus ensuring that crevices do not extend to bone, as well as the debridement of flaps of cartilage that may be hiding grade 3 or 4 articular cartilage injuries [19] (Figs. 7.5a, b). Surrounding cartilage must also be carefully evaluated, as it may have disengaged from the underlying bone (Figs. 7.5c, d). In addition, the absolute depth of OC lesions is important to ascertain, as lesions less than 8 mm in depth may heal with autologous chondrocyte implantation, whilst defects of more than 8 to 10 mm require bone grafting in association with ACI or osteochondral autograft transfer system (OATS) procedures [32] (Fig. 7.5e).

To investigate the accuracy of grading chondral lesions (450 focal lesions in 407 patients) using ICRS classification, Niemeyer et al. compared the ICRS grades obtained arthroscopically versus open techniques [9]. Using open surgery as the gold standard, they found that 80.9% of lesions were correctly graded using arthroscopy. Interestingly, there was no difference in grading accuracy between surgeons with different levels of experience.

7.3.5 Chondral Defect Contained/Uncontained

The containment of the lesion is one of the prognostic factors for clinical outcomes of arthroscopic bone marrow stimulation. A contained chondral lesion is surrounded with a stable, functional, native articular cartilage, whereas uncontained chondral lesions do not have a cartilage margin surrounding the entire defect (Fig. 7.6b). Uncontained chondral lesions are more likely to occur along the lateral margins of the femoral condyles, the posterior aspects of the femoral condyles, the posterior surfaces of the tibial plateau and any chondral lesion extending into intercondylar notch [4].

The issues stemming from the treatment of the uncontained defect relate to both MFX and to chondrocyte implantation techniques. In the MFX technique, a fibrin clot forms in the defect from the initial haematoma or blood clot, with mesenchymal stem cell migration occurring from the marrow cavity to populate this fibrin clot [33]. In the absence of a healthy cartilaginous rim, containment of the blood clot proves difficult; further, a steep wall also allows for the attachment of fibrous tissue [34]. In both ACI and matrix-induced autologous chondrocyte implantation (MACI) techniques, a cartilage margin is required

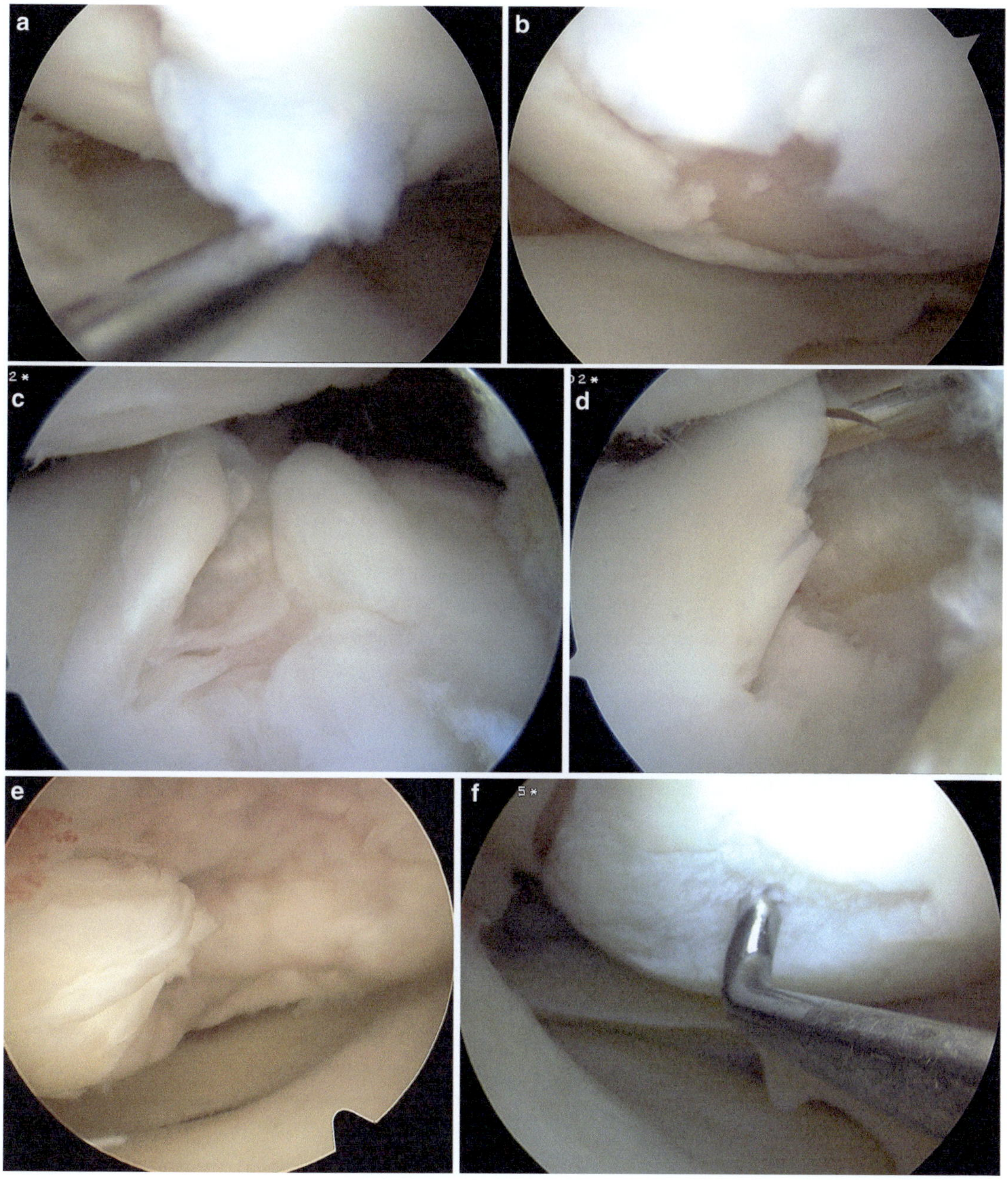

Fig. 7.5 Arthroscopic photographs showing: (**a**) Chondral flap. (**b**) ICRS - Grade 4 lesion revealed after debridement of flap seen in **a**. (**c**) Trochlea chondral flap. (**d**) Cartilage in the trochlea seen in Fig. 7.5c has disengaged from subchondral bone. (**e**) Osteochondral lesion. (**f**) Measurement of depth of ICRS - Grade 3 lesion

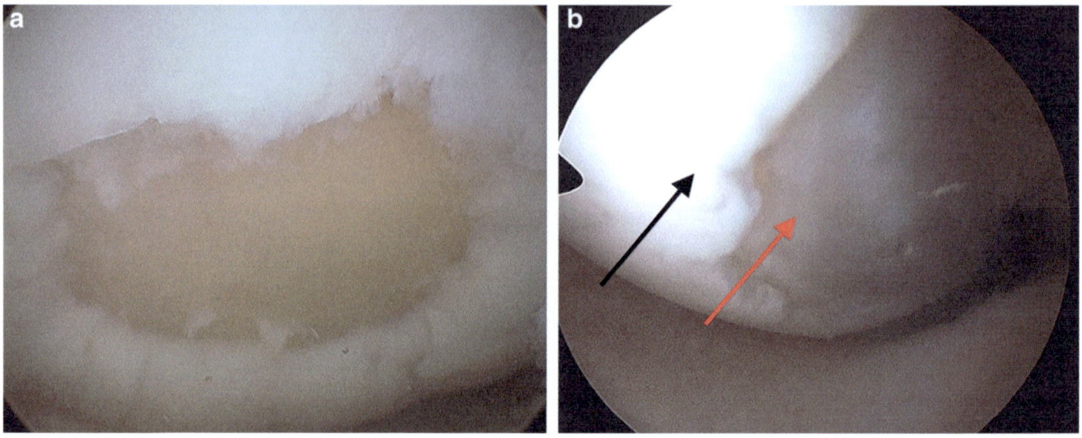

Fig. 7.6 Arthroscopic photographs showing: (**a**) Contained chondral defect where cartilage rim surrounds entire defect. (**b**) Uncontained chondral defect of the right MFC extending into the intercondylar notch with the black arrow showing normal cartilage and red arrow showing cartilage defect that has extended into the intercondylar notch.

to suture either periosteal grafts (ACI) or contain/suture the membrane (MACI) [4]. In the absence of a full cartilage margin, these techniques are either contraindicated or margins have to be created using techniques such as OATS or allograft.

7.4 Associated Knee Injuries

The recognition and treatment of associated knee injuries, such as loose bodies, meniscal tears and ACL ruptures, is an important aspect of knee arthroscopy. Rarely is articular cartilage damage sustained in isolation, and cartilage restoration algorithms require that lower limb malalignment, meniscal deficiency and cruciate ligament injuries be addressed in order to improve patient outcomes [4, 17, 24]. This section will address the most commonly associated pathologies, patterns of chondral injury and aspects of management.

7.4.1 Loose Bodies

Full-thickness chondral and OC defects may be associated with loose bodies, which are sometimes repairable in the acute setting. Otherwise, loose bodies must be removed to prevent mechanical symptoms such as locking and avoid potentially catastrophic chondral damage. Careful evaluation of preoperative imaging (X-ray, CT, MRI) aids the diagnosis and location of loose bodies prior to arthroscopy, along with complete and systematic arthroscopic examination of the entire knee. The surgeons' ability to examine the posterior compartments of the knee is an important skill in locating loose bodies. Accessory posteromedial and posterolateral portals may be required in order to remove chondral and OC fragments (Fig. 7.7).

7.4.2 Meniscal Tears

The presence of medial meniscal tears (MMT), especially bucket handle meniscal lesions, increases the incidence of chondral injuries on the MFC, especially in the weight-bearing aspect [35]. The meniscal loss was associated with a threefold increase in chondral injury or loss [36]. Also, the lateral meniscal tears (LMT) correlated with LFC and LTP damage. Posterior meniscal and lateral anterior meniscal tears have been commonly noted with advanced chondral lesions [37]. Posterior MMT with associated chondral lesions have been shown to predominate in females [38]. An investigation of 252 patients diagnosed with discoid LMT during arthroscopy 26.6% ($N = 67$) also had articular cartilage lesions, which was

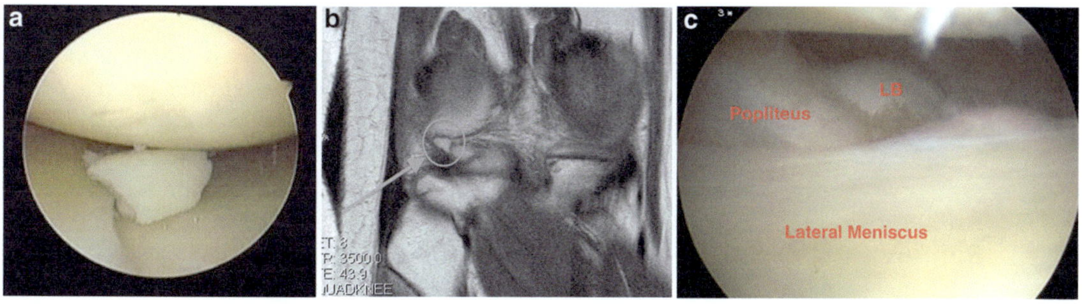

Fig. 7.7 Photographs showing: (**a**) Chondral loose body at arthroscopy. (**b**) Coronal MRI demonstrating a loose body in the posterolateral compartment (grey arrow). (**c**) Loose body (marked LB) in the posterolateral compartment of the knee at arthroscopy

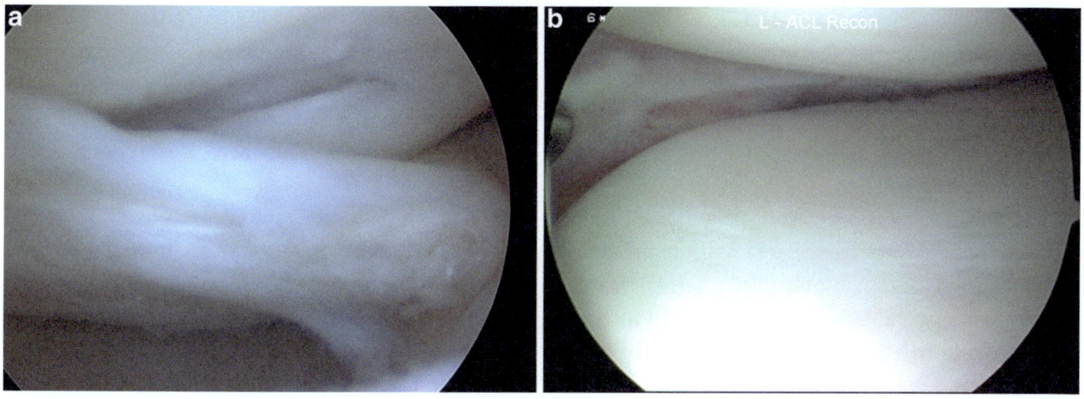

Fig. 7.8 Arthroscopic photographs showing: (**a**) Bucket handle meniscal tear causing a grade 4 medial femoral condyle (MFC) chondral lesion. (**b**) Subtotal medial meniscectomy

most commonly located on the LTP [38]. In another study of 378 patients (age range 16 to 50 years), with ACL tears undergoing knee arthroscopy, patients with a meniscal tear had a greater degree of articular cartilage damage than knees without a meniscal tear, whilst patients with a bucket handle tear of the medial meniscus had greater degeneration of the MFC than those patients with other types of meniscal tears [14] (Fig. 7.8a).

Patients who have undergone total or subtotal meniscectomy may warrant meniscal transplant, as it is established that cartilage degeneration and OA often follows meniscal resection [19, 39–42] (Fig. 7.8b). Following partial medial meniscectomy in 14 patients (9 male and 5 female; mean age 48 ± 12 years), Eichinger documented a significant increase in the severity of cartilage lesions in the medial tibial plateau [43]. Further, the size of the cartilage lesions significantly increased in both the femoral condyles and patella [43]. Traditional indications for meniscal allograft transplantation (MAT) have been suggested for symptomatic post-meniscectomy knees in patients with Outerbridge grade 2 articular cartilage damage or less. However, statistically significant improvements have been demonstrated in patients undergoing combined MAT and ACI/osteochondral allograft (OCA) in the medial and lateral compartments of the knee. These improvements were seen in all standardised outcomes scores at a minimum of 2-year follow-up [44, 45]. Such procedures often need to be combined with other surgery, including anterior cruciate reconstruction, high tibial osteotomy and tibial tubercle osteotomy [46].

7.4.3 Anterior Cruciate Ligament Rupture

A systematic review of acute ACL tears (< 3 months from injury) found that the incidence of articular cartilage injury was between 16% and 46% [47, 48]. In a retrospective study with a subset of 487 patients (350 non-athlete and 137 athlete) requiring acute ACL reconstruction (ACLR), the incidence of chondral lesions at time of presentation < 3 months of injury showed that 16% had a grade 3 or 4 lesion [49]. Another study consisted of a group of 15 patients, during arthroscopy with ACL tear and concominant grade – 3 or – 4 (Outerbridge classification) articular cartilage injuries (up to 2 cm in diameter) without meniscal and any other ligamentous injuries [50]. These patients underwent ACLR with chondroplasty via the drilling or MFX technique. The Lysholm knee score for each patient at 6 and 12 months showed good results with patient satisfaction and improvement in their quality of life (QoL).

The pattern of chondral injury with ACL tears may vary depending on whether knee arthroscopy is performed in the acute or chronic setting [14, 51, 52] (Table 7.4). In a prospective study of patients undergoing ACLR within 3 months of injury, lesions were most commonly seen on the LFC [51]. Some lesions were LFC impaction fractures, corresponding to the area of bone bruise which was commonly seen in the acute ACL injured knee on MRI (Fig. 7.9c).

In a study series looking at both acute and chronic ACL tears, the most common location for chondral injury was noted on the MFC, especially in the weight-bearing area [14]. In 2001, Hunt et al. investigated 145 patients with ACL ruptures and chondral injuries and reported that the lesions were commonly found in the lateral compartment of the knee. However, the authors did not discriminate between acute and chronic injuries and did not provide specifics on lesion location [29]. Further study is required to determine if chondral injury patterns differ in the acute and chronic setting of ACL rupture.

As the length of time between the ACL injury and knee arthroscopy increases, so does the incidence of severe chondral lesions [14, 15]. In a study of 764 patients with ACL tears seen at arthroscopy, there was a 6.1% incidence of ICRS - 3 and ICRS - 4 at 1 year post injury, 14.8% incidence at 2 - 5 years post injury and 44.8% incidence at greater than 5 years post injury [15].

Shelbourne and Gray reported that articular cartilage damage was the most important predictor of poor outcome after ACL reconstruction [53]. Combined treatment of chondral pathology and ACL tears was first described in 1993 [54]. It is now generally accepted that chondral restoration procedures such as ACI or autologous osteochondral transplantation should be combined with ACL reconstruction [54–56]. Good patient outcomes have been reported with this procedure. However, to date, there is lack of studies focussing specifically on the outcome of combined MFX and ACL reconstruction [47].

Table 7.4 Location of chondral lesions in ACL-deficient knees at arthroscopy

Reference	Study Type	N	MFC	LFC	MTP	LTP
Spindler et al. (1993)	Acute ACLR < 3 m	25	11	15	3	7
Drongowski et al. (1994)	Acute tear	32	4	19	2	7
Maffulli et al. (2003)	Acute + chronic	163	77	16	8	21

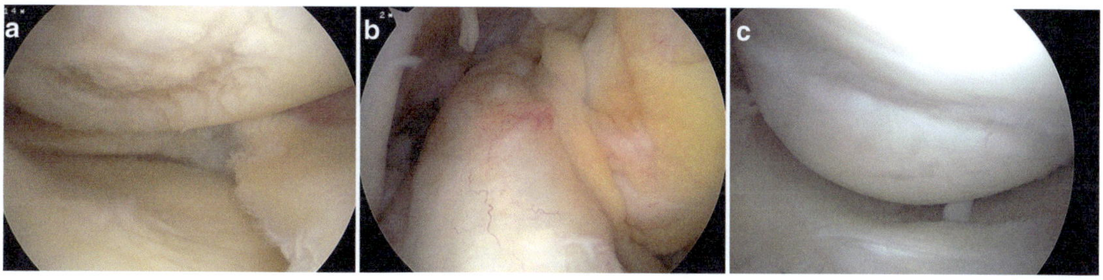

Fig. 7.9 Arthroscopic photographs showing: (**a**) medial femoral condyle (MFC) lesion in association with anterior cruciate ligament (ACL) rupture. (**b**) ACL rupture. (**c**) lateral femoral condyle (LFC) post ACL rupture

7.4.4 Posterior Cruciate Ligament Rupture

Geissler et al. reviewed the arthroscopic findings of 88 patients with proven, isolated, posterior cruciate ligament (PCL) tears in symptomatic patients [57]. Of patients with acute injuries (< 3 weeks post injury), chondral defects were seen in 12% of patients, affecting both the LFC and the patella. In patients with chronic injuries (> 1 month post injury), chondral defects were seen in 49% of patients, most commonly in the MFC and the patellofemoral joint (PFJ). Overall, 49% of patients with PCL injury had articular defects; nearly half of the defects arose from the PFJ articulation.

In a study involving patients with chronic PCL instability, 48% had moderate to severe MFC cartilage injury with only 31% showing radiographic evidence of the cartilage damage [58]. Similar to ACL rupture, the incidence of cartilage damage increases with time between injury and PCL reconstruction.

7.4.5 Lateral Patella Dislocation

Chondral injuries are extremely common following acute patella dislocation, requiring a high degree of clinical suspicion, especially in the patient with hemarthrosis [59]. In an arthroscopic study of 39 consecutive knees less than 3 weeks after lateral patella dislocation, 95% had articular cartilage injury. Of these lesions, 72% were OC fractures. The majority of damage was sustained to the medial facet of the patella, with a quarter of patients sustaining articular cartilage damage to the LFC [60] (Fig. 7.10a).

Stanitski and Paletta reviewed patella dislocations in 48 adolescents in 24 boys and 24 girls (mean age, 14 years) [61]. They documented that 34/48 (71%) patients had arthroscopic evidence of cartilage damage, mostly (94%) were OC lesions with relatively equal rates of injury to the patella and the LFC. Of concern was the fact that only one-third of these patients had evidence of OC fracture on x-ray. This finding has prompted some authors to suggest that arthroscopy may be warranted in children with patella dislocation and knee hemarthrosis [59]. Certainly, further imaging such as CT or MRI is mandatory in such cases. Recent advances in MR technology has provided an overall high arthroscopy-validated diagnostic accuracy of 91% and good-to-very good interreader reliability for the diagnosis of internal knee derangements in children with painful knee conditions [62, 63]

7.4.6 Medial Plica

The medial patella plica is an embryological remnant of the synovial cavity that arises from the medial aspect of the knee joint and inserts onto the infrapatellar fat pad. Medial patella plica is present in between 19% and 70% of knees [64]. Whilst usually an incidental finding in asymptomatic patients, medial plica can become pathological, causing catching symptoms, pain and chondral damage [65]. Pathological plica are characterised by thickened, fibrotic synovial tissue that may be

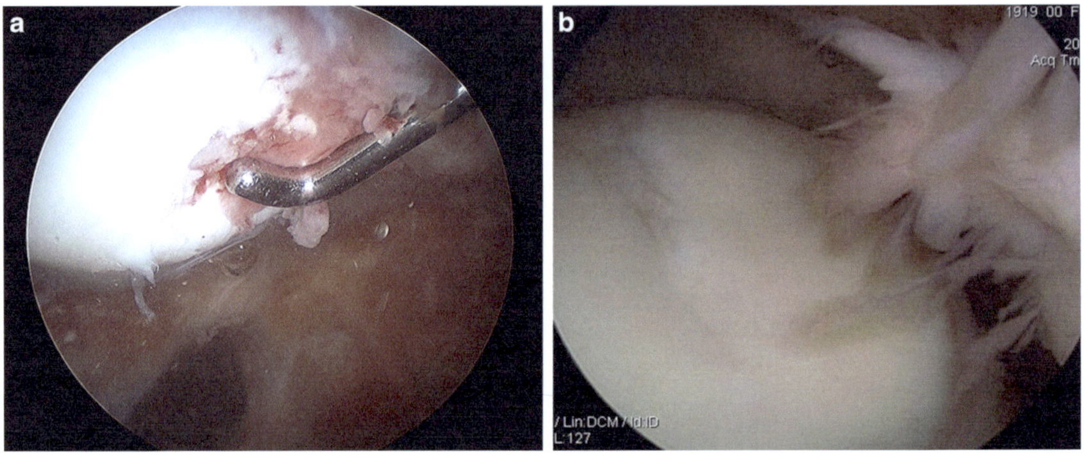

Fig. 7.10 Arthroscopic photographs showing: (**a**) Medial patella chondral lesion after patella dislocation. (**b**) Medial femoral condyle (MFC) chondral lesion associated with pathological medial plica

inflamed; typically they are associated with chondral lesions on the anterior half of the weight-bearing surface of the MFC [29, 66] (Fig. 7.10b).

7.5 Treatment Review

It is important to have a management algorithm at the forefront of the surgeon's mind when performing knee arthroscopy, which is briefly discussed in this section but more in-depth in Chap. 11. Not all treatment modalities are available at all centres or within each surgeon's skill set; however, such knowledge enables appropriate initial treatment and referral if necessary.

There are two main types of lesions: chondral defects of various uncalcified articular cartilage thickness and OC defects, where the injury has extended into the subchondral bone. As previously mentioned, ICRS - 2 lesions, when treated with the debridement of any potentially unstable cartilage fragments to a stable base, have a good prognosis [31]. Grade 3 and 4 lesions are generally accepted as requiring further treatment, especially when symptomatic [19].

Broadly speaking, treatments for full-thickness chondral defects fall into two main categories. The first category encompasses articular cartilage regeneration techniques, with marrow stimulation secondary to abrasion, drilling or MFX; arthroscopy is ideally suited to these bone marrow stimulation techniques. The second category involves articular cartilage reconstruction, utilising ACI, mosaicplasty or OC allografts [67].

Niemeyer et al. proposed a basic guideline to the management of full-thickness chondral defects (ICRS - 3 and ICRS - 4) [10]. Lesions < 4 cm^2 are treated with MFX, whilst lesions > 4 cm^2, or any failed MFX lesions > 2 cm^2, are treated with ACI. In their algorithm, OC defects are treated with autologous OC graft or by supplementing ACI with a bone grafting procedure.

In a review article published in 2009, Cole et al. uses a treatment algorithm for focal chondral lesions that varies depending on patient activity level and on the location of the lesion (PFJ versus femoral condyle) [17]. Lesions of the femoral condyle < 2 – 3 cm^2 in size are treated with MFX or OATS, whilst lesions > 2 – 3 cm^2 are treated with OCA or ACI. In regard to lesions within the PFJ, these are treated with MFX in low-demand patients, or ACI/OATS/OCA in high-demand patients, and are usually combined with an anteromedialisation (AMZ) procedure [17, 68] (Fig. 7.11).

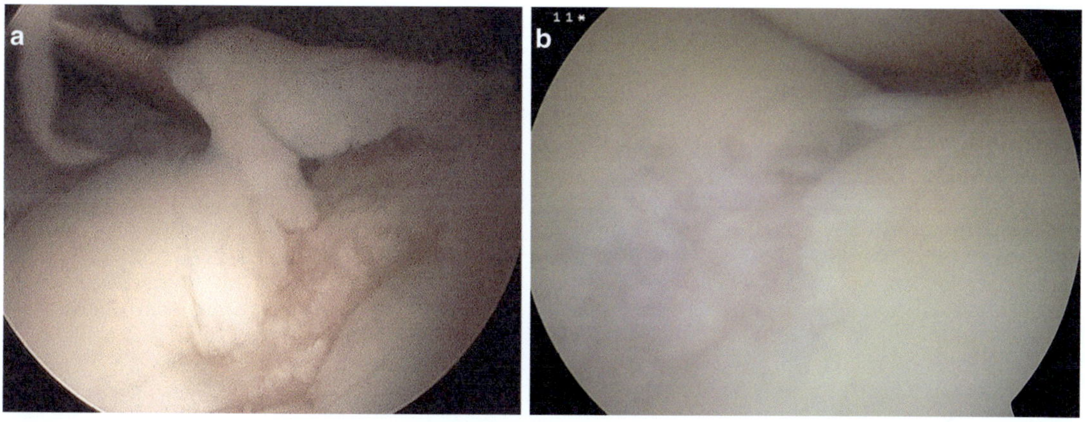

Fig. 7.11 Arthroscopic photographs showing chondral lesion of trochlea. (**a**) ICRS grade 4. (**b**) ICRS grade 3

7.6 Conclusions

Arthroscopy is a crucial tool in the diagnosis, evaluation and management of chondral injuries. Knowledge, skill and experience are required in order to recognise and correctly classify articular cartilage lesions, the first step to optimal management.

7.7 Acknowledgement

Arthroscopic images used with permission of www.boneschool.com.

References

1. DeHaven KE, Collins HR. Diagnosis of internal derangements of the knee. The role of arthroscopy. J Bone Joint Surg Am. 1975;57(6):802–10.
2. Eckstein F, et al. Accuracy and precision of quantitative assessment of cartilage morphology by magnetic resonance imaging at 3.0T. Arthritis Rheum. 2005;52(10):3132–6.
3. Figueroa D, et al. Knee chondral lesions: incidence and correlation between arthroscopic and magnetic resonance findings. Arthroscopy. 2007;23(3):312–5.
4. Brittberg M, et al. Articular cartilage engineering with autologous chondrocyte transplantation. A review of recent developments. J Bone Joint Surg Am. 2003;85-A(Suppl 3):109–15.
5. Hjelle K, et al. Articular cartilage defects in 1,000 knee arthroscopies. Arthroscopy. 2002;18(7):730–4.
6. Curl WW, et al. Cartilage injuries: a review of 31,516 knee arthroscopies. Arthroscopy. 1997;13(4):456–60.
7. Widuchowski W, Widuchowski J, Trzaska T. Articular cartilage defects: study of 25,124 knee arthroscopies. Knee. 2007;14(3):177–82.
8. Solheim E, Krokeide AM, Melteig P, Larsen A, Strand T, Brittberg M. Symptoms and function in patients with articular cartilage lesions in 1,000 knee arthroscopies. Knee Surg Sports Traumatol Arthrosc. 2016;24(5):1610–6.
9. Hiranaka T, Furumatsu T, Kamatsuki Y, Sugiu K, Okazaki Y, et al. Posttraumatic cartilage degradation progresses following anterior cruciate ligament reconstruction: a second-look arthroscopic evaluation. J Orthop Sci. 2019;24(6):1058–63. https://doi.org/10.1016/j.jos.2019.08.001.
10. Niemeyer P, et al. Comparison of arthroscopic and open assessment of size and grade of cartilage defects of the knee. Arthroscopy. 2011;27(1):46–51.
11. Jones KJ, Sheppard WL, Arshi A, Hinckel BB, Sherman SL. Articular cartilage lesion characteristic reporting is highly variable in clinical outcomes studies of the knee. Cartilage. 2018;1:1947603518756464. https://doi.org/10.1177/1947603518756464. Epub ahead of print.
12. Lewandrowski KU, Ekkernkamp A, Dávid A, Muhr G, Schollmeier G. Classification of articular cartilage lesions of the knee at arthroscopy. Am J Knee Surg. 1996;9(3):121–8.
13. Flanigan DC, Carey JL, Brophy RH, Graham WC, DiBartola AC, Hamilton D, Nagaraja HN, Lattermann C. Interrater and intrarater reliability of arthroscopic measurements of articular cartilage defects in the knee. J Bone Joint Surg Am. 2017;99(12):979–88.
14. Maffulli N, Binfield PM, King JB. Articular cartilage lesions in the symptomatic anterior cruciate ligament-deficient knee. Arthroscopy. 2003;19(7):685–90.
15. Tandogan RN, et al. Analysis of meniscal and chondral lesions accompanying anterior cruciate ligament

tears: relationship with age, time from injury, and level of sport. Knee Surg Sports Traumatol Arthrosc. 2004;12(4):262–70.
16. Dumont GD, Hogue GD, Padalecki JR, Okoro N, Wilson PL. Meniscal and chondral injuries associated with pediatric anterior cruciate ligament tears: relationship of treatment time and patient-specific factors. Am J Sports Med. 2012;40(9):2128–33.
17. Cole BJ, Pascual-Garrido C, Grumet RC. Surgical management of articular cartilage defects in the knee. J Bone Joint Surg Am. 2009;91(7):1778–90.
18. Outerbridge RE. The etiology of chondromalacia patellae. J Bone Joint Surg Br. 1961;43-B:752–7.
19. Brittberg M, Winalski CS. Evaluation of cartilage injuries and repair. J Bone Joint Surg Am. 2003;85-A(Suppl 2):58–69.
20. Brismar BH, et al. Observer reliability in the arthroscopic classification of osteoarthritis of the knee. J Bone Joint Surg Br. 2002;84(1):42–7.
21. Trisolino G, Favero M, Lazzaro A, Martucci E, Strazzari A, Belluzzi E, Goldring SR, Goldring MB, Punzi L, Grigolo B, Olivotto E. Is arthroscopic videotape a reliable tool for describing early joint tissue pathology of the knee? Knee. 2017;24(6):1374–82.
22. Lasmar NP, Lasmar RC, Vieira RB, de Oliveira JR, Scarpa AC. Assessment of the reproducibility of the Outerbridge and FSA classifications for chondral lesions of the knee. Rev Bras Ortop. 2015;46(3):266–9.
23. Cameron ML, Briggs KK, Steadman JR. Reproducibility and reliability of the outerbridge classification for grading chondral lesions of the knee arthroscopically. Am J Sports Med. 2003;31(1):83–6.
24. Brittberg M, Peterson L. Introduction to an articular cartilage classification. ICRS Newsletter. 1998;1:8–8.
25. Smith GD, et al. Arthroscopic assessment of cartilage repair: a validation study of 2 scoring systems. Arthroscopy. 2005;21(12):1462–7.
26. Dwyer T, Martin CR, Kendra R, Sermer C, Chahal J, Ogilvie-Harris D, Whelan D, Murnaghan L, Nauth A, Theodoropoulos J. Reliability and validity of the arthroscopic international cartilage repair society classification system: correlation with histological assessment of depth. Arthroscopy. 2017;33(6):1219–24.
27. Freemont AJ, Hoyland J. Lineage plasticity and cell biology of fibrocartilage and hyaline cartilage: its significance in cartilage repair and replacement. Eur J Radiol. 2006;57(1):32–6.
28. Siriwanarangsun P, Chen KC, Finkenstaedt T, Bae WC, Statum S, et al. Patterns of cartilage degeneration in knees with medial tibiofemoral offset. Skeletal Radiol. 2019;48(6):931–37.
29. Hunt N, et al. Chondral lesions of the knee: a new localization method and correlation with associated pathology. Arthroscopy. 2001;17(5):481–90.
30. Hunziker EB, Rosenberg LC. Repair of partial-thickness defects in articular cartilage: cell recruitment from the synovial membrane. J Bone Joint Surg Am. 1996;78(5):721–33.
31. Messner K, Maletius W. The long-term prognosis for severe damage to weight-bearing cartilage in the knee: a 14-year clinical and radiographic follow-up in 28 young athletes. Acta Orthop Scand. 1996;67(2):165–8.
32. Peterson L, et al. Autologous chondrocyte transplantation. Biomechanics and long-term durability. Am J Sports Med. 2002;30(1):2–12.
33. Williams RJ 3rd, Harnly HW. Microfracture: indications, technique, and results. Instr Course Lect. 2007;56:419–28.
34. Asik M, et al. The microfracture technique for the treatment of full-thickness articular cartilage lesions of the knee: midterm results. Arthroscopy. 2008;24(11):1214–20.
35. Jones S, Caplan N, St Clair Gibson A, Kader N, Kader D. Interactions between severity a nd location of chondral lesions and meniscal tears found at arthroscopy. Knee Surg Sports Traumatol Arthrosc. 2011;19(10):1699–703.
36. Murrell GA, et al. The effects of time course after anterior cruciate ligament injury in correlation with meniscal and cartilage loss. Am J Sports Med. 2001;29(1):9–14.
37. Unay K, Akcal MA, Gokcen B, Akan K, Esenkaya I, Poyanlı O. The relationship between intra-articular meniscal, chondral, and ACL lesions: finding from 1,774 knee arthroscopy patients and evaluation by gender. Eur J Orthop Surg Traumatol. 2014;24(7):1255–62.
38. Fu D, Guo L, Yang L, Chen G, Duan X. Discoid lateral meniscus tears and concomitant articular cartilage lesions in the knee. Arthroscopy. 2014;30(3):311–8.
39. Nakamae A, Adachi N, Deie M, Ishikawa M, Nakasa T, Ikuta Y, Ochi M. Risk factors for progression of articular ca rtilage damage after anatomical anterior cruciate ligament reconstruction. Bone Joint J. 2018;100-B(3):285–93.
40. Lee CR, Bin SI, Kim JM, Lee BS, Kim NK. Arthroscopic partial meniscectomy in young patients with symptomatic discoid lateral meniscus: an average 10-year follow-up study. Arch Orthop Trauma Surg. 2018;138(3):369–76.
41. Eijgenraam SM, Reijman M, Bierma-Zeinstra SMA, van Yperen DT, Meuffels DE. Can we pred ict the clinical outcome of arthroscopic partial meniscectomy? A systematic review. Br J Sports Med. 2018;52(8):514–21.
42. Chahla J, Cinque ME, Godin JA, Sanchez G, Lebus GF, Whalen JM, Price MD, Kennedy NI, Moatshe G, LaPrade RF, Provencher MT. Meniscectomy and resultant articular cartilage lesions of the knee among prospective national football league players: an imaging and performance analysis. Am J Sports Med. 2018;46(1):200–7.

43. Eichinger M, Schocke M, Hoser C, Fink C, Mayr R, Rosenberger RE. Changes in articular cartilage following arthroscopic partial medial meniscectomy. Knee Surg Sports Traumatol Arthrosc. 2016;24(5):1440–7.
44. Rue JP, et al. Prospective evaluation of concurrent meniscus transplantation and articular cartilage repair: minimum 2-year follow-up. Am J Sports Med. 2008;36(9):1770–8.
45. Noyes FR, Barber-Westin SD, Rankin M. Meniscal transplantation in symptomatic patients less than fifty years old. J Bone Joint Surg Am. 2004;86-A(7):1392–404.
46. Farr J, Rawal A, Marberry KM. Concomitant meniscal allograft transplantation and autologous chondrocyte implantation: minimum 2-year follow-up. Am J Sports Med. 2007;35(9):1459–66.
47. Brophy RH, et al. Anterior cruciate ligament reconstruction and concomitant articular cartilage injury: incidence and treatment. Arthroscopy. 2010;26(1):112–20.
48. Salem HS, Shi WJ, Tucker BS, Dodson CC, Ciccotti MG, Freedman KB, Cohen SB. Contact versus noncontact anterior cruciate ligament injuries: is mechanism of injury predictive of concomitant knee pathology? Arthroscopy. 2018;34(1):200–4.
49. Joseph C, et al. Is ACL reconstruction only for athletes? A study of the incidence of meniscal and cartilage injuries in an ACL-deficient athlete and non-athlete population: an Indian experience. Int Orthop. 2008;32(1):57–61.
50. Tahami SM, Rad SM. Outcome of ACL reconstruction and concomitant articular injury treatment. Arch Bone Jt Surg. 2015;3(4):260–3.
51. Spindler KP, et al. Prospective study of osseous, articular, and meniscal lesions in recent anterior cruciate ligament tears by magnetic resonance imaging and arthroscopy. Am J Sports Med. 1993;21(4):551–7.
52. Drongowski RA, Coran AG, Wojtys EM. Predictive value of meniscal and chondral injuries in conservatively treated anterior cruciate ligament injuries. Arthroscopy. 1994;10(1):97–102.
53. Shelbourne KD, Gray T. Results of anterior cruciate ligament reconstruction based on meniscus and articular cartilage status at the time of surgery. Five- to fifteen-year evaluations. Am J Sports Med. 2000;28(4):446–52.
54. Matsusue Y, Yamamuro T, Hama H. Arthroscopic multiple osteochondral transplantation to the chondral defect in the knee associated with anterior cruciate ligament disruption. Arthroscopy. 1993;9(3):31 8–21.
55. Klinger HM, et al. Anterior cruciate reconstruction combined with autologous osteochondral transplantation. Knee Surg Sports Traumatol Arthrosc. 2003;11(6):366–71.
56. Peterson L, et al. Two- to 9-year outcome after autologous chondrocyte transplantation of the knee. Clin Orthop Relat Res. 2000;374:212–34.
57. Geissler WB, Whipple TL. Intraarticular abnormalities in association with posterior cruciate ligament injuries. Am J Sports Med. 1993;21(6):846–9.
58. Clancy WG Jr, et al. Treatment of knee joint instability secondary to rupture of the posterior cruciate ligament. Report of a new procedure. J Bone Joint Surg Am. 1983;65(3):310–22.
59. Vahasarja V, Kinnuen P, Serlo W. Arthroscopy of the acute traumatic knee in children. Prospective study of 138 cases. Acta Orthop Scand. 1993;64(5):580–2.
60. Nomura E, Inoue M, Kurimura M. Chondral and osteochondral injuries associated with acute patellar dislocation. Arthroscopy. 2003;19(7):717–21.
61. Stanitski CL, Paletta GA Jr. Articular cartilage injury with acute patellar dislocation in adolescents. Arthroscopic and radiographic correlation. Am J Sports Med. 1998;26(1):52–5.
62. Fritz J, Ahlawat S, Fritz B, Thawait GK, Stern SE, Raithel E, Klyce W, Lee RJ. 10-min 3D turbo spin echo MRI of the knee in children: arthroscopy-validated accuracy for the diagnosis of internal derangement. J Magn Reson Imaging. 2019;49(7):e139–51.
63. Fritz J, Fritz B, Zhang J, Thawait GK, Joshi DH, et al. Simultaneous multislice accelerated turbo spin echo magnetic resonance imaging: comparison and combination with in-plane parallel imaging acceleration for high-resolution magnetic resonance imaging of the knee. Invest Radiol. 2017;52(9):529–37.
64. Dupont JY. Synovial plicae of the knee. Controversies and review. Clin Sports Med. 1997;16(1):87–122.
65. Flanagan JP, et al. Arthroscopic excision of symptomatic medial plica. A study of 118 knees with 1-4 year follow-up. Acta Orthop Scand. 1994;65(4):408–11.
66. Lyu SR, Hsu CC. Medial plicae and degeneration of the medial femoral condyle. Arthroscopy. 2006;22(1):17–26.
67. Onoi Y, Hiranaka T, Nishida R, Takase K, Fujita M, et al. Second-look arthroscopic findings of cartilage and meniscus repair after injection of adipose-derived regenerative cells in knee osteoarthrits: report of two cases. Regen Ther. 2019;11:212–6.
68. Farr J. Autologous chondrocyte implantation improves patellofemoral cartilage treatment outcomes. Clin Orthop Relat Res. 2007;463:187–94.

Part IV

Repair of Knee Articular Cartilage Injury: Non-surgical Approaches

Physical and Rehabilitative Therapy for Knee Articular Cartilage Injury and Disease

8

Joseph B. Houpt, Harpal K. Gahunia, and Kenneth P. H. Pritzker

8.1 Introduction

The knee is composed of specialized connective tissues which act synergistically to deal with the mechanical loads encountered over a lifetime [1, 2, 3]. The integrity of articular cartilage and its shock absorbing property are essential for normal joint nutrition. The knee articular cartilage volume, joint space, and pathogenesis of knee osteoarthritis (OA) are associated with the genetic makeup of the individual [4–12]. Also, playing a role in the differences in cartilage structure between individuals is the functional adaptation of cartilage to biomechanical stresses [13].

Articular cartilage adapts to mechanical stimuli by altering its morphology, architecture (specifically its thickness), and composition (proteoglycan – PG, collagen, and interstitial water content). Each of the components of the cartilage matrix contributes to the strength, longevity and resilience of this tissue. When performing various tasks such as standing, walking, and running, the knee frequently encounters forces of several magnitudes relative to body weight (BW) [14–16]. In adults, increased loading due to sports does not appear to be associated with increased cartilage thickness, whereas in children and adolescents, such loading has been shown to increase cartilage thickness [17]. Once skeletal maturity is attained at adolescence, i.e., closure of articular epiphyseal plate and maturation of the articular-epiphyseal cartilage complex (AECC), the mature articular cartilage has limited capacity to increase its mass as a result of mechanical stimulation. Knee cartilage appears to display atrophic (thinning) changes during reduced loading conditions or unloading which may be accompanied with extracellular matrix (ECM) compositional changes [18–22]. With aging, knee articular cartilage thinning and degradation are related to the pressure of loading over the years which contributes to less hydration and less capacity by chondrocytes to synthesize PGs [23].

During childhood, running, jumping, and other high impact activities benefit bone health by increasing the size and strength of the growing skeleton. The benefits in bone size and strength induced by exercise during growth persist lifelong. However in both elite and amateur athletes, due to the significant acute and chronic joint

J. B. Houpt, MD, FRCPC (✉)
Faculty of Medicine, University of Toronto, Toronto, ON, Canada
e-mail: jbhoupt@sympatico.ca

H. K. Gahunia, MSc, PhD
Orthopaedic Science Consulting Services, Oakville, ON, Canada

K. P. H. Pritzker, MD, FRCPC
Department of Laboratory Medicine and Pathobiology, Department of Surgery, and Institute of Biomaterials and Biomedical Engineering, University of Toronto, Toronto, ON, Canada

Department of Pathology and Laboratory Medicine, Mount Sinai Hospital, Toronto, ON, Canada

H. K. Gahunia et al. (eds.), *Articular Cartilage of the Knee*,
https://doi.org/10.1007/978-1-4939-7587-7_8

stress associated with excessive impact forces, articular cartilage injury of the knee is frequently observed [24–36]. Among elite football players, significant increase in the magnetic resonance imaging (MRI) $T2^*$ relaxation times, predominantly in the superficial zone (SZ) of articular cartilage, was noted compared to amateur athletes [37]. This increase in $T2^*$ relaxation times is indicative of increased fluid content and degradative changes in the cartilage collagen structure and architecture.

Articular cartilage is subjected to deformation under physiologic loading conditions and the magnitude to which these mechanical signals are transmitted to the cartilage matrix and chondrocytes vary during activities of daily living. The extent of cartilage deformation varies at the different compartments of the knee, and the way the load is distributed through the knee determines which tissues are subjected to mechanical stress. Patellar articular cartilage deformation is greater at regions of more intense loading, whereas, in the tibiofemoral cartilage, relatively little deformation occurs except during high impact activities [38]. Knee pain may arise when runners increase the duration and frequency of the loading through the lower limb. In the adolescent athlete, anterior knee pain is a common presenting symptom in sports medicine clinics due to patellofemoral instability. This may result from sports-related subluxation events leading to patellofemoral cartilage injuries. Later in life, superimposed on previous injury, this cartilage is subject to continuing degeneration due to wear. The articular cartilage injury may eventually lead to chronic joint changes and functional disability. Due to the high mechanical demands of athletic activity, the treatment of articular cartilage lesions in the athletes presents a therapeutic challenge, and skeletal maturity often dictates what procedures can be safely attempted [39–43].

Static and dynamic lower limb mechanics, footwear, and floor surface may influence the knee symptomatology of the joint and periarticular soft tissues. During normal activities, adult human cartilage deforms very little and recovers from deformation within 90 min after loading [44]. Although physical training exercise does not seem to affect cartilage deformational behavior, with increasing age cartilage deformation seems to decrease. Likely this is because of accumulation of the collagen and non-collagen proteins as well as decreased PGs and cartilage hydration during aging. Differences in cartilage deformability perhaps explain the high frequency of patellofemoral OA and that OA is more likely to start in the patellofemoral joint in individuals with symptoms of early knee OA [45, 46].

Although the therapeutic value of exercise to cartilage is now known, injuries to the knee and adjacent soft tissues may occur acutely as a result of sports or trauma injury (direct blow) or progressively over time from lesser but persistent impacts, e.g., jogging on concrete [47]. This is characterized by progressive loss of cartilage structure and function. The process begins with cartilage softening due to edema, acute injury, or repeated acute injury, which then progresses to fragmentation. As the articular cartilage is lost, the underlying subchondral bone (having less protection against the normal forces) initially shows signs of stress and microfractures which then leads to OA. The biomechanical factors that can contribute to this process include twisting injuries, meniscal fragmentation, and collateral ligamentous changes contributing to joint instability. The symptoms of OA-related cartilage injuries may include knee joint pain and swelling, locking, catching, or instability.

Non-surgical, non-pharmacological management of cartilage lesions due to injury or disease includes weight loss, targeted physical activities, and rehabilitation treatment modalities to overcome trauma-associated pain. To review the structural and functional changes of articular cartilage with aging, refer to Chap. 3. The pharmacological approach to reduce knee pain and repair damaged cartilage is described in Chap. 9.

8.2 Lifestyle Modifications

The average human life expectancy is currently 83 years compared to 69 years in 1979 [48]. Lifestyle modifications to manage joint pain and inflammation may enable patients to manage injured or aging knees while maintaining a relatively active lifestyle. These modifications such as dietary weight loss, physical activity, and routine exercise can be overall health-enhancing activities which may play a role in maintaining the health of the knee articular cartilage. Further, when knee cartilage is damaged due to injury, disease, or old age, the lifestyle changes along with therapeutic exercise, physiotherapy, and rehabilitation serve as early treatment strategies that may prevent further cartilage damage.

8.2.1 Weight Loss

Being overweight places increased load and stress on lower extremity joints which further accelerates knee cartilage degradation. Losing weight and maintaining weight loss can reduce knee problems [49, 50]. Weight loss has been shown to decrease knee pain and inflammation, increase mobility, and improve the quality of life (QoL) [49–54]. Weight loss should be attempted through diet with reduced caloric intake and by increasing the level of regular activities such as walking, cycling (including stationary bicycle), swimming, and regular exercise.

Weight loss may also help slow the progression of knee OA. It has been noted that the adverse effects of increasing weight are stronger in the offspring of people who have had knee replacement for knee OA. A genetics-environment interaction with regard to overweight with a body mass index (BMI) of 25 to < 30 and obesity with a BMI higher than 30 has been observed in the pathogenesis of knee OA [55]. An 18-month study reviewed a weight loss program in 142 sedentary, overweight, and obese adults [52]. By the end of the study, participants had lost an average of 2% of their BW and lowered their BMI by 3%. It was determined that for every pound of weight lost, there was a 4-pound reduction in the load placed on the knee for each step. The accumulated reduction in knee load for a 1-pound loss in weight would be more than 4800 pounds per mile walked [52]. For people losing 10 pounds, each knee would be subjected to 48,000 pounds less in compressive load per mile walked. The limitation of this study was the lack of correlation of their findings (decreased BW/BMI and load placed on the knee) with the patient's knee symptoms. Although there are no longitudinal studies indicating that weight loss in humans slows the progression of knee OA, weight reduction is often clinically relevant [54, 56]. Further research is required to investigate the potential of weight loss to slow or even prevent the progression of knee OA.

In another 18-month single-blind, randomized controlled trial, the effects of dietary weight loss and exercise on the health-related QoL were investigated in a total of 316 overweight and obese older adults (age > 60 years) with symptomatic knee OA [56, 57]. The adult cohort (BMI $\geq$ 28 kg/m^2) was randomly assigned to one of four groups: dietary weight loss, exercise, dietary weight loss and exercise, or healthy lifestyle control. Participants completed measures of stair climb time and 6-min walk distance, self-efficacy for completing each mobility task, and self-reported pain at baseline, 6 months and 18 months during the trial period. The results demonstrated that compared with the healthy lifestyle control group, the dietary weight loss intervention along with exercise produced greater improvements in mobility-related self-efficacy, stair climb and 6-min walk performance, and pain reduction [57]. Also, results showed that the combined diet and exercise intervention had a consistently positive effect on the health-related QoL as measured using 36-Item Short-Form (SF-36) Health Survey (refer to Appendix B for details) and satisfaction with body function and appearance [56]. The results of these and other studies confirm the significant treatment effects of dietary weight loss combined with regular exercise [49, 58]. In another 4-year study, adult participants with or at risk of knee OA were categorized based on obesity (normal or high BMI) and waist circumference (small/medium and large) [59]. Participants with obesity and a large waist circumference had 2.4 times the risk of developing the inability to walk 400 m compared with those with a healthy BMI and small/medium waist circumference. This study suggests that waist circumference may be an indicator for developing knee symptomatology with fast walking or running in adults with or at risk of knee OA.

8.2.2 Physical Activity and Exercise

The term "physical activity" encompasses all forms of activity that involves expenditure of calories with an increased heart rate. Physical activities include everyday activity (daily walking within and out of the house, housework, gardening, cycling, pleasure- or work-related activity), active recreation (recreational walking, cycling, dancing), sport (informal or structured competitive), and exercise. Physical activity in childhood has been shown to be positively associated with cartilage growth and development in randomly selected healthy children without knee pain or injury [60]. Among young adults (31–41 years old), physical activity has been shown to be associated with an increased tibial cartilage volume and reduced cartilage defects [61]. Among adults (51–81 years old) participating in more frequent occupational physical activities, individuals with high baseline cartilage volume modified their risk for knee OA; however, individuals with low baseline cartilage volume had greater medial cartilage volume loss compared to those who were relatively more inactive [62].

Aging of joint and periarticular tissues may be accelerated by joint injury. With joint pain, maintaining an active life and participating in sports can be challenging. Joint inactivity or microgravity has been associated with tissue atrophy, whereas physical exercise has been shown to increase blood circulation to the joint tissues which helps to reduce inflammation [63–65]. The latter was corroborated in a study that showed running decreased knee intra-articular pro-inflammatory cytokine concentration [66].

High impact exercises (such as running and jumping) and weight-bearing exercises (such as strength training, jogging, tennis, running, and weightlifting) which involves work force against gravity can put "stress" on the bones [67]. For instance, the jolting motions involved in running can cause an impact of 2.5 times the runner's body weight with each step. In response to this "stress," the osteoblasts build new dense bone and maintain bone mass [68]. On the other hand, low impact exercises like yoga, biking or swimming place less stress on the bones. Moderate physical activity, including regular walking, was associated with a lower incidence of bone marrow lesions. Research on the effect of exercise on cartilage show its tendency to weaken without regular loading, similar to muscle, bone, ligament, and tendon [69–71]. There are differences in cartilage thickness between individuals, but what remains unclear is whether physical activity or certain exercises are significant contributors to this finding.

In healthy individuals, regular activity facilitates cycles of ECM turnover within cartilage and chondrocytes maintain the cartilage homeostasis. Daily regular activities and mobility are sufficient to maintain adequate knee cartilage lubrication and diffusion of nutrients through the cartilage. Besides strengthening joint tissues (muscle, bone, articular cartilage, ligaments, and tendons), moderate activities also enhance articular cartilage lubrication. The production of synovial fluid that maintains joint lubrication increases with exercise. Excessive synovial fluid produced by the synovial membrane is a short-term or acute response to aggressive exercise [72]. However, too little exercise or immobilization eventually compromises the lubricant properties of cartilage. With long periods of immobility, the joints may become stiff and lose some of their movement range. Knee mobility exercises such as knee bending may encourage a steady supply of normal synovial fluid. This suggests that joints require a basal amount of exercise to stay lubricated, nourished, and healthy.

Some studies implicate physical activity in provoking knee OA, while others suggest that physical activity may actually protect the knee from the disease [62]. Conflicting reports of the effect of physical activity on knee cartilage may be due to the heterogeneity of populations examined and, in particular, the underlying health of the knee in the study populations. The influence of recreational and occupational physical activity on cartilage volume loss was investigated [62]. In this study, individuals with less baseline cartilage volume were more at risk of structural knee damage with either heavy occupational or recreational workloads or both, whereas individuals with high baseline cartilage volume who participated in more frequent occupational physical activities advantageously modified their risk for knee OA [62]. In another study, the effect of physical activity performed in various degrees of intensity, frequency, and duration on the knee was investigated [73]. The study cohort comprised of a total of 257 healthy adults (age range, 50–79 years), with no history of knee injury or OA. MRI was used to assess tibiofemoral cartilage defects and bone marrow lesions, as well as measure cartilage volume, an indicator of cartilage health and strength. Participants answered specific questions regarding their exercise and walking habits, as well as routine activity at home and at work, to determine their level of physical activity in both the 6 months and 7 days prior to the study. To create a baseline for each subject, past information on weight, height, BMI, and physical activity from questionnaires completed for a previous 4-year period was obtained. Results showed that weight-bearing vigorous activity increased the tibial cartilage volume and was inversely associated with cartilage defects. Also, regular walking was associated with reduced risk of bone marrow lesions.

Though both the intensity and duration of physical activity have a significant positive impact on cartilage, the ideal amount of physical activity for joint health remains unclear. A recent study shows that middle-aged men and women who engage in high levels of physical activity at home, work, or gym may cause damage to the knee increasing their risk for OA [74]. This study involved 136 women and 100 men, ages 45–55 years, within a healthy weight range (BMI of 19 to 27), and without knee pain or other symptoms. The participants were separated into low-, middle-, and high-activity groups based on their level of physical activities. A person whose activity level was classified as high typically might engage in several hours of walking, sports, or other types of exercise per week. MRI scans showed that knee damage, including cartilage and ligament lesions and bone marrow edema, was more common and more severe among those individuals who engaged in the highest levels of physical activity involving high impact, weight-bearing activities such as running and jumping which may carry a greater risk of injury over time. Conversely, low impact activities, such as swimming and cycling, may protect diseased cartilage and prevent healthy cartilage from developing disease. For example, 93% of people in the high-activity groups suffered cartilage damage compared to 60% in the low-activity group. Cartilage damage was three times more severe in the high-activity group. The participants' age or sex did not affect the risk of knee injury [74].

Individuals of all ages benefit from mild to moderate exercise which contributes to cartilage healing and reduces the risk for injury. However, excessive exercise may be associated with cartilage injury eventually leading to degenerative changes. Among elite athletes, the strenuous physical activity may place continuous stress on the knee that can result in articular cartilage microtrauma and degeneration. The risk for OA increases in athletes excessively participating in high impact sports resulting in their knees being exposed to long duration, high-intensity and high-frequency physical training, acute repetitive impact, and torsional loading [29, 3, 75]. These results corroborated the study of the rabbit knee model whereby exercise of physiologic magnitude but excessive intensity (chronic loading) led to cartilage degeneration and chondrocyte necrosis [76].

MRI exams revealed that light exercisers had the healthiest knee cartilage among all exercise levels and patients with minimal strength training had healthier cartilage than patients with either no strength training or frequent strength training [77]. The results of moderate to strenuous exercise in women who did any amount of strength training were associated with higher fluid content and more degenerated collagen architecture in the knee. This result indicates that moderate to strenuous exercise may accelerate cartilage degeneration, hence subjecting these women to greater risk of developing OA. Further, frequent knee-bending activities, such as climbing up at least ten flights of stairs a day, lifting objects weighing more than 25 pounds, squatting, kneeling, or deep knee bending for at least 30 min per day, were associated with higher fluid content and cartilage abnormalities [77]. This study indicates that light exercise, particularly frequent walking, is a safe choice in maintaining healthy cartilage [77].

8.3 Post-injury Knee Rehabilition

Rest, physical therapy, and exercise are often the first-line treatments for patients with knee pain and joint tissue injury. Physiotherapy can help restore joint function and heal injured cartilage. An individualized exercise program should be designed for each patient's specific condition, with the inclusion of strength and flexibility training. Rebuilding the quadriceps, hamstrings, and calf muscles that support and stabilize the knee is essential after knee injury. An early start to the guided exercises is extremely beneficial for the joint healing process and return to normal daily function. These exercises are performed with slow and steady movements using both legs to maintain the balance and proprioception. However, with supervised physiotherapy, the use of special equipment may be required for some patients.

Various experimental and clinical investigations have shown that continuous passive motion (CPM) enhances the metabolic activity of the joint tissues, healing, and regeneration of articular cartilage by stimulating pluripotential cells to differentiate into chondroblasts and chondrocytes and has significant stimulatory effects on articular cartilage and periarticular tissues [78–86]. CPM machines have been used to alleviate joint stiffness, swelling, and pain as well as to enhance functional ability by continuously bending and straightening the joint [87, 88]. Several studies have also shown the benefit of CPM to increase range of motion and scar tissue formation during the first few days and weeks of post-injury and surgery. However, recent clinical data indicated the lack of the long-term benefit of CPM (6 to 8 weeks post knee or anterior cruciate ligament surgery) and its limited effectiveness in returning knee range of motion [89–92]. Obesity may have a negative impact on the beneficial effect of CPM [93].

8.3.1 Elevation, Ice Application, and Heat Therapy

Post knee injury, elevation of the leg, and early icing may help relieve pain by controlling the bleeding, swelling, and discomfort. Icing is effective when applied consecutively for a few days for about 45 min, several times a day. Subsequent heat applications to the injured knee may improve circulation, promote muscle relaxation, relieve joint pain and stiffness, and allow early range of joint movement exercises. Various forms of heat therapy may be used with attention to skin protection. These include dry or moist heat, diathermy, and ultrasound. For dry heat, a therapeutic infrared heat lamp, hot water bottles, or electric heating pads also may be used. Wet heat can be applied by hot tub baths or by means of a warm towel applied to the injured knee. Whirlpool baths are also effective.

8.3.2 Crutches and Canes

In some cases of moderate knee cartilage injury, the use of crutches at the early stage could enhance the healing phase by keeping the body weight (totally or partially) off the knee. At times patients are allowed to weight bear by using crutches to walk as tolerated, on tiptoe or on the heel. The use of crutches provides a tool to apply the concept of CPM to improve the circulation and expedite the cartilage healing process [80, 85]. Even if still on crutches and not fully weight-bearing, the patient is encouraged to walk cautiously as soon as possible.

A cane held in the contralateral hand while walking may be useful [94]. In practice, as the symptomatic leg is put forward, so is the cane held in the opposite hand. This results in one half of the total body weight supported by the cane and only the other half of body weight supported by the symptomatic knee. Contralateral cane use has been shown to significantly reduce medial knee load [95].

8.3.3 Splinting or Bracing

Splinting (or bracing) is another tool to improve knee function and assist in healing cartilage injury. Joint malalignment is a marker of disease severity and/or its progression [96]. Bracing should improve knee alignment, thereby reducing pain. Bracing will also provide some additional stability to the knee and prevent the knee from giving out during activity. Several types of knee braces are available that may provide support while standing or exercising. For mildly unstable symptomatic knee, a simple "tensor" sleeve with lateral and medial stays may provide stability. The use of both the knee "tensor" and cane held in the opposite hand may be very useful.

8.3.4 Walking

Post knee injury, walking assists in regaining the range of movement in the knee. Walking, using a slow-speed treadmill, or working out on static exercise bike can help build strength in all areas of the knees. While walking downhill is usually tolerated well by healthy people, however, excessive overuse or other deformity may cause cartilage damage under the patella. The heel slide exercises enhance the range of motion and reduce knee pain. Walking in a swimming pool can provide relief to the injured knee cartilage. The pool water provides resistance to the knee and helps to regain the range of motion. Walking on ground or water must be comfortable and not induce significant pain. The shoes should provide a good arch support and with a semisoft thick sole.

8.3.5 Therapeutic Exercises

An individual approach is important to determine which treatment plan is most appropriate for the patient for the management of knee pain and articular cartilage healing post-injury and in the symptomatic OA knee. The use of non-pharmacological, nonsurgical, treatment with physiotherapy is most effective when utilized in combination with other post knee injury management strategies.

Therapeutic knee exercises are performed for a variety of reasons: building strength and stability, treating an injury, and alleviating arthritis symptoms. Physical therapists carefully tailor and implement the exercises to help improve knee motion and muscle function inhibited by pain and to assist patients ensuring that a safe amount of weight is placed on the injured leg. Initial emphasis is placed on light exercises of the knee to enhance circulation, reduce inflammation, and strengthen periarticular soft tissue. As the program progresses, more emphasis is on knee strength and function through more challenging exercises.

During the course of knee rehabilitation after knee injury, the intensity of the exercises will usually depend on the area the rehabilitation is focused on. It is important to start controlled strengthening exercises to build up strength as soon as possible. Exercises focused on building strength should be performed with a resistance that is light enough for several repetitions, whereas stretching exercise done as part of knee rehabilitation typically focuses on the quadriceps and hamstring muscles. Stretches of the hamstrings and quadriceps are important to ensure more flexibility to the muscles around the knee. Stretching the legs and knees before and after exercise is beneficial to prevent patellar subluxation. When strengthening and stretching the muscles around the knee, it is important to work on range-of-motion exercises to promote knee strength. Beneficial knee exercises are those that work both the front and back of the joint equally, enabling a person to balance their knee strength.

In addition to therapeutic exercise, physical therapists also use cardio training, ice massage, deep heat, and nerve stimulation to assist patients with their pain, range of motion, and strength. Pain may signal inflammation or overactivity. Rest and leg elevation along with pain medication can help relieve the discomfort. The post-injury recovery time varies markedly from patient to patient and depends on the extent of joint injury, patient's ability to heal, and type of rehabilitation.

The overall health of the knee dictates the health of cartilage structure and function. Moderate exercise may be beneficial to improve the joint symptom and function and also to enhance the articular cartilage glycosaminoglycan (GAG) content in patients at high risk of developing knee OA [47]. In a study comprised of patients who had undergone meniscus repair within the past 3–5 years, subjects (29 men and 16 women; age range, 35–50 year) were randomly assigned to a control or an exercise group

[47]. The exercise group was enrolled in a supervised program of aerobic and weight-bearing moves for 1 h, three times weekly for 4 months. At the study's onset and follow-up, subjects from both groups underwent MRI scans to evaluate knee cartilage GAG content. Further, they also responded to a series of questions pertaining to their knee pain and stiffness, as well as their general activity level. Of the original 45 subjects, only 30 ($n = 16$ in the exercise group and $n = 14$ in the control group) completed the trial and all post-trial assessments. In the exercise group, many subjects reported gains in physical activity and functional performance tests compared with subjects in the control group. MRI measures of the GAG content showed a strong correlation with the increased physical training of the subjects who had regularly participated in moderate, supervised exercise. However, the long-term effect of exercise on adult articular cartilage in subjects at risk for OA remains unclear.

8.3.6 Swimming or Water Aerobics

Swimming and water aerobics are non-weight-bearing exercises that are performed without the impact of working out on land. There is strong evidence that suggest aquatic exercise can alleviate joint pain and improve self-addressed and measured joint function [97–105]. Exercise in water can involve aerobics, walking, jogging, or swimming. With swimming, the knees are supported by the water resulting in decreased load on the knee cartilage. Investigation of the efficacy of aquatic resistance training on the macromolecular composition of tibiofemoral cartilage in postmenopausal women with mild OA showed an improvement in the integrity of the cartilage collagen-interstitial water ambiance as reflected by low T2 values [106]. This response may be attributed to the low shear and compressive forces the knee cartilage is subjected to during aquatic resistance training. Results from an animal study on the effect of swimming on cartilage formation suggested that this activity could induce systemic hormonal and/or metabolic changes that promote cartilage formation [107].

8.3.7 Cycling

Cycling is a low impact exercise modality that may be considered for knee rehabilitation after joint injury as well as management of knee OA [108]. Cycling is an excellent knee rehabilitation tool that involves a non-weight-bearing, controlled cyclic movement with variable resistance that helps to increase or restore the knee range of movement, improve knee mobility and stability, decrease or eliminate pain, and prevent reoccurrence of the knee injury [109]. Importantly, cycling stimulates the cartilage repair within the knee by nourishing the joint cartilage.

8.3.8 Laser Treatment

Laser-assisted treatments which are currently experimental have been tested in several cartilage injury and OA animal models [110–114]. These studies reported the genesis of hyaline-like repair tissue at the site of chondral lesions. Further, low-power helium-neon laser for experimental OA treatment has shown zonal variation in the capability of chondrocytes from different cartilage zones to produce GAGs [115]. Low-energy laser therapy has also been shown to be effective in reducing joint inflammation, inhibit activation of proteases such as gelatinase, and stimulate collagen production in the experimental model of acute arthritis [111, 112, 114]. Also, an in vitro study demonstrated that low-pulse laser is capable of stimulating articular chondrocyte proliferation and matrix secretion [114]. Only a small number of studies have been conducted to investigate the pro-repair and anti-inflammatory effects of laser treatment on human knee cartilage [116–118]. Short-term studies showed improved range of motion or functionality demonstrating the anti-inflammatory and swelling reduction effects of light laser treatment. Long-term studies showing significant pain relief and improved functionality could be attributed to cartilage regeneration. However, the utility and effectiveness of laser therapy for repair of knee cartilage requires further investigation in randomized controlled trials in humans with knee injury and OA patients. The use of low-pulse laser treatment may be promising in the treatment of mild or early moderate cartilage lesions in young patients [116].

Beside its use to assist in articular cartilage repair, laser abrasion technique is utilized to excise loose cartilage post knee injury. It uses heat to induce alterations in the ECM, which results in cartilage morphological change. Improving this therapy to make it more spatially selective may avoid excessive tissue damage such as air bubble formation, tissue necrosis, reactive synovitis, chondrolysis, and subsequent acceleration of articular cartilage degeneration.

8.3.9 Pulsed Electromagnetic Field Therapy

Over the last four decades, pulsed electromagnetic field (PEMF) therapy protocol for joint pain has come into use, without any known side effects. This therapy involves the use of PEMF delivered through a mat placed on the joint surface. Recent animal studies on the application of PEMF post joint injury have suggested the capacity to heal cartilage and delay OA [119]. In a Hartley guinea pig study, PEMF preserved the morphology of articular cartilage and slowed the development of OA lesions in the experimental group compared with a control group [120]. The study concluded that PEMF was disease modifying in this animal model. Recent in vitro study of human chondrocytes showed an increased cell proliferation with exposure to PEMF [121]. The study noted that electric and electromagnetic fields increased gene expression and synthesis of growth factors, which may amplify field effects through autocrine and paracrine signaling. A study involving biophysical stimulation of osteonecrosis of the human femoral head with PEMF treatment indicated the benefit of this treatment in the early stage through reduction or relief of pain [122]. In bovine articular cartilage explants, PEMF exposure on articular cartilage in vitro demonstrated a chondroprotective effect by promoting anabolic activities and PG synthesis [123–125]. Although not clearly understood, it is thought that the short-term effect of PEMF stimulation could protect the articular cartilage from the catabolic effect of inflammation and subchondral bone marrow edema, whereas the long-term effect of PEMF stimulation could promote osteogenic activity at the osteonecrotic area and prevent trabecular fracture and subchondral bone collapse.

8.4 Conservative Treatment of Cartilage Injuries in Knee Joint Diseases

The appropriate treatment for the asymptomatic knee with the incidental finding of chondral injury is problematic. However, if left untreated, asymptomatic lesions may deteriorate to permanent knee damage. The conservative treatment of chondral lesions on symptomatic knee depends on factors such as patient age, daily and sport activities, etiology, quality of the lesion, and disease stage. Conservative treatments are usually the first choice for the management of knee degeneration with the goal of reducing symptoms, especially in the early phase of disease.

8.4.1 Treatment of Osteochondritis Dissecans

Osteochondritis dissecans (OCD) is a joint disorder most often noted in children, adolescents, and young adults. The most common joint affected by OCD is the knee, ankle, and elbow although it can also occur in other joints. Typically, this condition affects one joint; however, some children can develop OCD in several joints. The etiology of OCD is most likely due to injury to an area of the joint with fairly tenuous blood supply where the OC fragment separates from a normal vascular bony bed. As a consequence of blood deprivation and loss of blood flow in the subchondral bone, a small segment of bone begins to separate from its surrounding region forming fissures and fragmentation in the articular cartilage that may extend to the underlying subchondral bone. The most common initial symptoms of OCD are pain and inflammation of the affected joint that develops gradually and is often more pronounced during sports, physical activity, or exercise. Advanced cases of OCD may cause joint catching, locking, popping noises, and/or buckling during movement that could restrict the range of movement. Refer to Chap. 10 for an in-depth description, pathophysiology and current treatment strategies for OCD.

In many cases of OCD, children with skeletally immature bone and articular cartilage, with a relatively small, intact lesion and the absence of loose bodies, the cartilage and bone heal on their own. Non-surgical and non-pharmacological management often include activity modification, restricted weight-bearing (partial or non-weight-bearing) for 6–8 weeks, and joint immobilization to promote cartilage healing and to prevent potential subchondral bone fracture and collapse. Resting, activity modification, and avoiding vigorous sports until symptoms resolve often relieve pain and swelling. Due to the capability of immature cartilage to repair to some degree, more than 90% of the OCD lesions of the knee often heal within 3–6 months [126]. If symptoms do not subside after a reasonable amount of time, then the use of crutches, splinting, or casting of the affected joint for a short period of time often helps in the cartilage and bone healing process. In general, most children start to feel better over a 2- to 4-month course of rest and non-surgical treatment. They usually return to all activities as symptoms improve. Most OCD patients do well without long-term sequelae.

In a recent systematic review comprising 27 studies for a total of 908 knees, among different nonsurgical, conservative treatment options for knee OCD lesions, restriction of sport and strenuous activities appeared as a favorable approach, possibly in combination with physiokinesitherapy [127]. Patients with large OCD lesion size, severe stage, older age and skeletal maturity, and clinical presentation with swelling or locking showed negative prognostic factors.

However, once skeletal maturity is attained in grown children and young adults, OCD can have more severe effects with higher incidence of the OCD lesions separating from the surrounding bone and cartilage to detach and float inside the joint space. Surgical intervention is recommended in failed conservative treatment and in patients close to skeletal maturity or older. Candidates for surgery include those with severe OCD lesion(s) separated or detached from the surrounding bone and cartilage and those with very large lesions greater than 1 centimeter in diameter.

8.4.2 Treatment of Osteoarthritis

Osteoarthritis is the leading cause of disability among adults. OA pain has been shown to be associated with synovial hypertrophy, synovial effusions, signs of joint instability, and pain on various ranges of movement. In patients with knee OA and meniscal tear, the presence of extensive effusion-synovitis is associated with subsequent progression of articular cartilage damage over 18 months [128]. Subchondral bone marrow edema and microfracture of the articular plate may be seen with cartilage-specific imaging studies [129]. Arthritis education and structured land-based exercise programs (with or without dietary weight management) constitutes the non-surgical, core treatments for knee OA. Based on objective review of high-quality meta-analytic data, Bannuru et al. expanded upon prior OARSI guidelines by developing a comprehensive and patient-centered treatment algorithm to facilitate individualized non-surgical treatment decisions for the management of knee OA [130]. Applications of heat or cold may be used in the management of OA for symptom relief [131]. Therapeutic exercise aimed to diminish pain is of major importance in the physical therapy program for the OA patient [132]. The use of a patellar brace in patients with patellofemoral OA for symptom relief has been shown to alter the patellar weight-bearing region and to increase the contact area between the patella and femoral trochlea [133].

The effect of strength training and other training modalities has been investigated in OA patients. It is possible to increase stability by strengthening the muscles around the hip and knee. Strength training as well as low impact exercises such as cycling, tai chi, and swimming also can reduce pain in the knee caused by OA [134–137]. A Cochrane report concluded that there is at least a short-term benefit from exercise in terms of reduced knee pain and improved physical function for individuals with knee OA. The magnitude of the treatment effect was small, and the study duration was short-term, but the claimed effect was comparable to the effect of nonsteroidal anti-inflammatory drugs [138]. There is good evidence that joint cartilage will undergo atrophy under reduced loading, such as postoperative immobilization and paraplegia [139, 140]. On the other hand, adult cartilage will not become thicker after increased load such as intensive running and similar exercises [44]. To what degree, if any, the morphology of injured cartilage can be influenced by training and exercise is unknown [85].

People at risk for OA may be able to delay the onset of the disease or even prevent it with simple changes to their physical activity [77]. Frequent movement of the knee, including mild to moderate weight-bearing exercise such as walking or running, can relieve the symptoms of OA. Moderate exercise has been shown to reduce pain and improve function in patients with OA of the knee and hip [47]. The impact of moderate exercise was investigated on the knee cartilage of 45 subjects (mean age, 46 years; BMI, 26.6) who underwent partial medial meniscus resection 3–5 years prior and were at high risk for developing OA [47]. This study suggested that compositional changes occur in adult knee cartilage as a result of increased exercise. The changes imply that human cartilage responds to physiologic loading in a way similar to that exhibited by muscle and bone and that positive symptomatic effect of exercise in patients with OA may occur by improving the quality of knee cartilage.

Moderate exercise as an effective way to reduce pain and improve function in patients with knee OA was studied by the National Institutes of Health (NIH) OA Initiative. Enrolled were 128 asymptomatic participants at risk for knee OA as well as 33 age and BMI-matched controls [77]. The study participants with BMI of 18 to 27 kg/m^2 (99 women and 66 men; age range, 45–55 years) were grouped into three exercise and strength-training levels, based on their responses to the Physical Activity Scale for the Elderly (PASE) questionnaire. The exercise levels included sedentary individuals, light exercisers, and those who were moderate to strenuous exercisers. The strength-training groups included none, minimal, and frequent knee strengthening. Self-reported knee-bending activities were also analyzed. Using Whole-organ Magnetic Resonance Imaging Score (WORMS), the articular cartilage of the right knee was graded, and compartment-specific T2 values were determined for each of the cartilage segments. Among subjects with risk factors for knee OA, the light exercisers showed lower T2 values when compared with sedentary and moderate/strenuous exercisers. Females who were moderate/strenuous exercisers had higher T2 values (more tissue fluid) compared with sedentary individuals and light exercisers. The T2 values did not show significant differences based on exercise level in subjects without risk factors for knee OA. However, frequent knee-bending activities were associated with higher T2 values in both participants with and those without OA risk factors with more severe cartilage lesions in the group with risk factors. As such, engaging in light exercise and refraining from frequent knee-bending activities may protect against the onset of the disease. However, high impact activity, such as running, more than 1 h per day at least three times a week appears to be associated with more degenerated cartilage and potentially a higher risk for development of OA.

In early postmenopausal women with mild knee OA, progressive implementation of high impact and intensive exercise for a period of 1 year has been shown to exert a favorable effect on patellar cartilage [141]. Asymptomatic middle-aged individuals from an OA initiative incidence cohort study have been shown to have a high prevalence of cartilage lesions with high level of physical activity [74]. Over a short period, high impact exercises may have a beneficial effect on cartilage; however, further investigation is required to determine if long-term (several years) effect of high impact exercises can harm knee articular cartilage.

8.5 Conclusions

The ultimate goal of a rehabilitation program is to restore function of the patient's knee for the long term. As described in this chapter, there are many modalities to assist rehabilitation following injury or disease to the knee. However, the principal indicators of clinical progress remain crude: pain, capacity for extension, and endurance of movement. None of these parameters are specific for which rehabilitation modalities might be applied to best expedite healing and restoration of function.

References

1. Arokoski JP, Jurvelin JS, Väätäinen U, Helminen HJ. Normal and pathological adaptations of articular cartilage to joint loading. Scand J Med Sci Sports. 2000;10(4):186–98.
2. Cohen NP, Foster RJ, Mow VC. Composition and dynamics of articular cartilage: structure, function, and maintaining healthy state. J Orthop Sports Phys Ther. 1998;28(4):203–15.
3. Gahunia HK, Pritzker KP. Effect of exercise on articular cartilage. Orthop Clin North Am. 2012;43(2):187–99.
4. Ding C, Cicuttini F, Scott F, Stankovich J, Cooley H, Jones G. The genetic contribution and relevance of knee cartilage defects: case-control and sib-pair studies. J Rheumatol. 2005;32(10):1937–42.
5. Duren DL, Sherwood RJ, Czerwinski SA, Chumlea WC, Lee M, Demerath EW, Sun SS, Siervogel RM, Towne B. Genetic architecture of knee radiographic joint space in healthy young adults. Hum Biol. 2008;80(1):1–9.
6. Hunter DJ, Snieder H, March L, Sambrook PN. Genetic contribution to cartilage volume in women: a classical twin study. Rheumatology (Oxford). 2003;42(12):1495–500.
7. Khan HI, Aitken D, Chou L, McBride A, Ding C, Blizzard L, Pelletier JP, Pelletier JM, Cicuttini F, Jones G. A family history of knee joint replacement increases the progression of knee radiographic osteoarthritis and medial tibial cartilage volume loss over 10 years. Osteoarthritis Cartilage. 2015;23(2):203–9.
8. Kraus VB, Jordan JM, Doherty M, Wilson AG, Moskowitz R, Hochberg M, Loeser R, Hooper M, Renner JB, Crane MM, Hastie P, Sundseth S, Atif U. The Genetics of Generalized Osteoarthritis (GOGO) study: study design and evaluation of osteoarthritis phenotypes. Osteoarthritis Cartilage. 2007;15(2):120–7.
9. Moazedi-Fuerst FC, Hofner M, Gruber G, Weinhaeusel A, Stradner MH, Angerer H, Peischler D, Lohberger B, Glehr M, Leithner A, Sonntagbauer M, Graninger WB. Epigenetic differences in human cartilage between mild and severe OA. J Orthop Res. 2014;32(12):1636–45.
10. Pan F, Khan H, Ding C, Winzenberg T, Martel-Pelletier J, Pelletier JP, Cicuttini F, Jones G. Familial effects on structural changes relevant to knee osteoarthritis: a prospective cohort study. Osteoarthritis Cartilage. 2015;23(4):559–64.
11. Zhai G, Ding C, Stankovich J, Cicuttini F, Jones G. The genetic contribution to longitudinal changes in knee structure and muscle strength: a sibpair study. Arthritis Rheum. 2005;52(9):2830–4.
12. Zhai G, Stankovich J, Ding C, Scott F, Cicuttini F, Jones G. The genetic contribution to muscle strength, knee pain, cartilage volume, bone size, and radiographic osteoarthritis: a sibpair study. Arthritis Rheum. 2004;50(3):805–10.
13. Leong DJ, Hardin JA, Cobelli NJ, Sun HB. Mechanotransduction and cartilage integrity. Ann N Y Acad Sci. 2011;1240:32–7.
14. Liemohn W. Exercise and arthritis. Exercise and the back. Rheum Dis Clin N Am. 1990;16(4):945–70.
15. Ounpuu S. The biomechanics of running: a kinematic and kinetic analysis. Instr Course Lect. 1990;39:305–18.
16. Wu G, Ladin Z. Limitations of quasi-static estimation of human joint loading during locomotion. Med Biol Eng Comput. 1996;34(6):472–6.
17. Zhang BT, Liu L, Zheng J, Dai YM, SN Y, Liu GF, Liu L. Effect of snow sports on knee cartilage maturation in children and adolescent with MRI quantitative analysis Zhang. Zhonghua Yi Xue Za Zhi. 2016;96(43):3499–503.
18. Carter DR, Wong M, Orr TE. Musculoskeletal ontogeny, phylogeny, and functional adaptation. J Biomech. 1991;24(Suppl 1):3–16.
19. Huiskes R, Ruimerman R, van Lenthe GH, Janssen JD. Effects of mechanical forces on maintenance and adaptation of form in trabecular bone. Nature. 2000;405(6787):704–6.
20. King KB, Opel CF, Rempel DM. Cyclical articular joint loading leads to cartilage thinning and osteopontin production in a novel in vivo rabbit model of repetitive finger flexion. Osteoarthritis Cartilage. 2005;13(11):971–8.
21. Nomura M, Sakitani N, Iwasawa H, Kohara Y, Takano S, Wakimoto Y, Kuroki H, Moriyama H. Thinning of articular cartilage after joint unloading or immobilization. An experimental investigation of the pathogenesis in mice. Osteoarthritis Cartilage. 2017;25(5):727–36.

22. Pauwels F. Biomechanics of the locomotion apparatus. Berlin: Springer; 1980.
23. Novelli C, Costa JBV, Souza RR. Effects of aging and physical activity on articular cartilage: a literature review. J Morphol Sci. 2012;29(1):1–7.
24. Hirshorn KC, Cates T, Gillogly S. Magnetic resonance imaging-documented chondral injuries about the knee in college football players: 3-year National Football League Combine data. Arthroscopy. 2010;26(9):1237–40.
25. Lattermann C, Jacobs CA, Proffitt Bunnell M, Huston LJ, Gammon LG, Johnson DL, Reinke EK, Huebner JL, Kraus VB, Spindler KP. A Multicenter Study of early anti-inflammatory treatment in patients with acute anterior cruciate ligament tear. Am J Sports Med. 2017;45(2):325–33.
26. Mithoefer K, Hambly K, Logerstedt D, Ricci M, Silvers H, Della Villa S. Current concepts for rehabilitation and return to sport after knee articular cartilage repair in the athlete. J Orthop Sports Phys Ther. 2012;42(3):254–73.
27. Mithoefer K, Steadman RJ. Microfracture in football (soccer) players: a case series of professional athletes and systematic review. Cartilage. 2012;3(Suppl 1):18S–24S.
28. Pappas GP, Vogelsong MA, Staroswiecki E, Gold GE, Safran MR. Magnetic resonance imaging of asymptomatic knees in collegiate basketball players: the effect of one season of play. Clin J Sport Med. 2016;26(6):483–9.
29. Saxon L, Finch C, Bass S. Sports participation, sports injuries and osteoarthritis: implications for prevention. Sports Med. 1999;28(2):123–35.
30. Smith MV, Nepple JJ, Wright RW, Matava MJ, Brophy RH. Knee Osteoarthritis is associated with previous meniscus and anterior cruciate ligament surgery among elite college American football athletes. Sports Health. 2017;9(3):247–51.
31. Sonnery-Cottet B, Archbold P, Thaunat M, Carnesecchi O, Tostes M, Chambat P. Rapid chondrolysis of the knee after partial lateral meniscectomy in professional athletes. Knee. 2014;21(2):504–8.
32. Steadman JR, Hanson CM, Briggs KK, Matheny LM, James EW, Guillet A. Outcomes after knee microfracture of chondral defects in alpine ski racers. J Knee Surg. 2014;27(5):407–10.
33. Wissman RD, England E, Mehta K, d'Heurle A, Langenderfer E, Mangine R, Kenter K. The trochlear cleft: initial experience in elite athletes. J Comput Assist Tomogr. 2014;38(4):499–502.
34. Mithoefer K, McAdams TR, Scopp JM, Mandelbaum BR. Emerging options for treatment of articular cartilage injury in the athlete. Clin Sports Med. 2009;28(1):25–40.
35. DePhillipo NN, Cinque ME, Kennedy NI, Chahla J, Moatshe G, LaPrade RF. Patellofemoral chondral defect in a preadolescent skier: A case report in early sport specialiazation. Int J Sports Phys Ther. 2018;13(1):131–6.
36. Culvenor AG, Wirth W, Maschek S, Boeth H, Diederichs G, Duda G, Eckstein F. Longitudinal change in patellofemoral cartilage thickness, cartilage T2 relaxation times, and subchondral bone plate area in adolescent vs mature athletes. Eur J Radiol. 2017;92:24–9.
37. Behzadi C, Welsch GH, Laqmani A, Henes FO, Kaul MG, Schoen G, Adam G, Regier M. Comparison of T2* relaxation times of articular cartilage of the knee in elite professional football players and age- and BMI-matched amateur athletes. Eur J Radiol. 2017;86:105–11.
38. Eckstein F, Lemberger B, Gratzke C, Hudelmaier M, Glaser C, Englmeier KH, Reiser M. In vivo cartilage deformation after different types of activity and its dependence on physical training status. Ann Rheum Dis. 2005;64(2):291–5.
39. Bessette M, Saluan P. Patellofemoral pain and instability in adolescent athletes. Sports Med Arthrosc Rev. 2016;24(4):144–9.
40. Fabricant PD, Yen YM, Kramer DE, Kocher MS, Micheli LJ, Lawrence JTR, Ganley TJ, Heyworth BE. Fixation of Traumatic Chondral-Only Fragments of the Knee in Pediatric and Adolescent Athletes: A Retrospective Multicenter Report. Orthop J Sports Med. 2018;6(2):1–7. https://doi.org/10.1177/2325967117753140.
41. Browne GJ, Barnett P. Common sports-related musculoskeletal injuries presenting to the emergency department. J Paediatr Child Health. 2016;52(2):231–6.
42. Fabricant PD, Yen YM, Kramer DE, Kocher MS, Micheli LJ, Heyworth BE. Fixation of chondral-only shear fractures of the knee in pediatric and adolescent athletes. J Pediatr Orthop. 2017;37(2):156.
43. Hancock KJ, Westermann RR, Shamrock AG, Duchman KR, Wolf BR, et al. Trends in knee articular cartilage treatments: an American board of orthopaedic surgery database study. J Knee Surg. 2019;32(1):85–90.
44. Eckstein F, Hudelmaier M, Putz R. The effects of exercise on human articular cartilage. J Anat. 2006;208(4):491–512.
45. Lankhorst NE, Damen J, Oei EH, Verhaar JA, Kloppenburg M, Bierma-Zeinstra SM, van Middelkoop M. Incidence, prevalence, natural course and prognosis of patellofemoral osteoarthritis: the cohort hip and cohort knee study. Osteoarthritis Cartilage. 2017;25(5):647–53.
46. Stefanik JJ, Guermazi A, Roemer FW, Peat G, Niu J, Segal NA, Lewis CE, Nevitt M, Felson DT. Changes in patellofemoral and tibiofemoral joint cartilage damage and bone marrow lesions over 7 years:

the multicenter osteoarthritis study. Osteoarthritis Cartilage. 2016;24(7):1160–6.
47. Roos EM, Dahlberg L. Positive effects of moderate exercise on glycosaminoglycan content in knee cartilage: a four-month, randomized, controlled trial in patients at risk of osteoarthritis. Arthritis Rheum. 2005;52(11):3507–14.
48. World Health Statistics. Monitoring the health goal-indicators of overall progress. Edited by World Health Organization. 2016, p. 7–13 and p. 43.
49. Christensen R, Henriksen M, Leeds AR, Gudbergsen H, Christensen P, Sorensen TJ, Bartels EM, Riecke BF, Aaboe J, Frederiksen R, Boesen M, Lohmander LS, Astrup A, Bliddal H. Effect of weight maintenance on symptoms of knee osteoarthritis in obese patients: a twelve-month randomized controlled trial. Arthritis Care Res. 2015;67(5):640–50.
50. Burn E, Murray DW, Hawker GA, Pinedo-Villanueva R, Prieto-Alhambra D. Lifetime risk of knee and hip replacement following a GP diagnosis of osteoarthritis: a real-world cohort study. Osteoarthritis Cartilage. 2019;27(11):1627–35.
51. Messier SP. Diet and exercise for obese adults with knee osteoarthritis. Clin Geriatr Med. 2010;26(3):461–77.
52. Messier SP, Gutekunst DJ, Davis C, DeVita P. Weight loss reduces knee-joint loads in overweight and obese older adults with knee osteoarthritis. Arthritis Rheum. 2005;52(7):2026–32.
53. Nicklas BJ, Ambrosius W, Messier SP, Miller GD, Penninx BW, Loeser RF, Palla S, Bleecker E, Pahor M. Diet-induced weight loss, exercise, and chronic inflammation in older, obese adults: a randomized controlled clinical trial. Am J Clin Nutr. 2004;79(4):544–51.
54. Miller GD, Nicklas BJ, Davis C, Loeser RF, Lenchik L, Messier SP. Intensive weight loss program improves physical function in older obese adults with knee osteoarthritis. Obesity (Silver Spring). 2006;14(7):1219–30.
55. Pan F, Blizzard L, Tian J, Cicuttini F, Winzenberg T, Ding C, Jones G. The interaction between weight and family history of total knee replacement with knee cartilage: a 10-year prospective study. Osteoarthritis Cartilage. 2017;25(2):227–33.
56. Rejeski WJ, Focht BC, Messier SP, Morgan T, Pahor M, Penninx B. Obese, older adults with knee osteoarthritis: weight loss, exercise, and quality of life. Health Psychol. 2002;21(5):419–26.
57. Focht BC, Rejeski WJ, Ambrosius WT, Katula JA, Messier SP. Exercise, self-efficacy, and mobility performance in overweight and obese older adults with knee osteoarthritis. Arthritis Rheum. 2005;53(5):659–65.
58. Fransen M. Dietary weight loss and exercise for obese adults with knee osteoarthritis: modest weight loss targets, mild exercise, modest effects. Arthritis Rheum. 2004;50(5):1366–9.
59. Gill SV, Hicks GE, Zhang Y, Niu J, Apovian CM, White DK. The association of waist circumference with walking difficulty among adults with or at risk of knee osteoarthritis: the osteoarthritis initiative. Osteoarthritis Cartilage. 2017;25(1):60–6.
60. Jones G, Glisson M, Hynes K, Cicuttini F. Sex and site differences in cartilage development: a possible explanation for variations in knee osteoarthritis in later life. Arthritis Rheum. 2000;43(11):2543–9.
61. Antony B, Venn A, Cicuttini F, March L, Blizzard L, Dwyer T, Cross M, Jones G, Ding C. Association of physical activity and physical performance with tibial cartilage volume and bone area in young adults. Arthritis Res Ther. 2015;17:298.
62. Teichtahl AJ, Wang Y, Heritier S, Wluka AE, Strauss BJ, Proietto J, Dixon JB, Jones G, Cicuttini FM. The interaction between physical activity and amount of baseline knee cartilage. Rheumatology (Oxford). 2016;55(7):1277–84.
63. Booth FW. Terrestrial applications of bone and muscle research in microgravity. Adv Space Res. 1994;14(8):373–6.
64. Keller TS, Strauss AM, Szpalski M. Prevention of bone loss and muscle atrophy during manned space flight. Microgravity Q. 1992;2(2):89–102.
65. Anghelina M, Sjostrom D, Perera P, Nam J, Knobloch T, Agarwal S. Regulation of biomechanical signals by NF-kappaB transcription factors in chondrocytes. Biorheology. 2008;45(3-4):245–56.
66. Hyldahl RD, Evans A, Kwon S, Ridge ST, Robinson E, Hopkins JT, Seeley MK. Running decreases knee intra-articular cytokine and cartilage oligomeric matrix concentrations: a pilot study. Eur J Appl Physiol. 2016;116:2305–14.
67. Maimoun L, Mariano-Goulart D, Couret I, Manetta J, Peruchon E, Micallef JP, Verdier R, Rossi M, Leroux JL. Effects of physical activities that induce moderate external loading on bone metabolism in male athletes. J Sports Sci. 2004;22:875–83.
68. Multanen J, Nieminen MT, Hakkinen A, Kujala UM, Jamsa T, Kautiainen H, Lammentausta E, Ahola R, Selanne H, Ojala R, Kiviranta I, Heinonen A. Effects of high-impact training on bone and articular cartilage: 12-month randomized controlled quantitative MRI study. J Bone Miner Res. 2014;29(1):192–201.
69. Foley S, Ding C, Cicuttini F, Jones G. Physical activity and knee structural change: a longitudinal study using MRI. Med Sci Sports Exerc. 2007;39(3):426–34.
70. Hohmann E, Wortler K, Imhoff A. Osteoarthritis from long-distance running? Sportverletzung Sportschaden. 2005;19(2):89–93.
71. Wren TA, Beaupre GS, Carter DR. A model for loading-dependent growth, development, and adaptation of tendons and ligaments. J Biomech. 1998;31(2):107–14.
72. Renstrom P. Sports traumatology today. A review of common current sports injury problems. Ann Chir Gynaecol. 1991;80(2):81–93.

73. Racunica TL, Teichtahl AJ, Wang Y, Wluka AE, English DR, Giles GG, O'Sullivan R, Cicuttini FM. Effect of physical activity on articular knee joint structures in community-based adults. Arthritis Rheum. 2007;57(7):1261–8.
74. Stehling C, Lane NE, Nevitt MC, Lynch J, McCulloch CE, Link TM. Subjects with higher physical activity levels have more severe focal knee lesions diagnosed with 3T MRI: analysis of a non-symptomatic cohort of the osteoarthritis initiative. Osteoarthritis Cartilage. 2010;18(6):776–86.
75. Ozkan C, Sarpel Y, Bicer OS. The effects of exercise on articular cartilage. Acta Orthop Traumatol Turc. 2007;41(Suppl 2):13–8.
76. Horisberger M, Fortuna R, Valderrabano V, Herzog W. Long-term repetitive mechanical loading of the knee joint by in vivo muscle stimulation accelerates cartilage degeneration and increases chondrocyte death in a rabbit model. Clin Biomech (Bristol, Avon). 2013;28(5):536–43.
77. Hovis KK, Stehling C, Souza RB, Haughom BD, Baum T, Nevitt M, McCulloch C, Lynch JA, Link TM. Physical activity is associated with magnetic resonance imaging-based knee cartilage T2 measurements in asymptomatic subjects with and those without osteoarthritis risk factors. Arthritis Rheum. 2011;63(8):2248–56.
78. Moran ME, Kim HK, Salter RB. Biological resurfacing of full-thickness defects in patellar articular cartilage of the rabbit Investigation of autogenous periosteal grafts subjected to continuous passive motion. J Bone Joint Surgery Br. 1992;74(5):659–67.
79. O'Driscoll SW, Salter RB. The repair of major osteochondral defects in joint surfaces by neochondrogenesis with autogenous osteoperiosteal grafts stimulated by continuous passive motion. An experimental investigation in the rabbit. Clin Orthop Relat Res. 1986;208:131–40.
80. Salter RB. The biologic concept of continuous passive motion of synovial joints. The first 18 years of basic research and its clinical application. Clin Orthop Relat Res. 1989;242:12–25.
81. Salter RB. The physiologic basis of continuous passive motion for articular cartilage healing and regeneration. Hand Clin. 1994;10(2):211–9.
82. Salter RB. History of rest and motion and the scientific basis for early continuous passive motion. Hand Clin. 1996;12(1):1–11.
83. Salter RB, Bell RS, Keeley FW. The protective effect of continuous passive motion in living articular cartilage in acute septic arthritis: an experimental investigation in the rabbit. Clin Orthop Relat Res. 1981;159:223–47.
84. Salter RB, Hamilton HW, Wedge JH, Tile M, Torode IP, O'Driscoll SW, Murnaghan JJ, Saringer JH. Clinical application of basic research on continuous passive motion for disorders and injuries of synovial joints: a preliminary report of a feasibility study. J Orthop Res. 1984;1(3):325–42.
85. Salter RB, Simmonds DF, Malcolm BW, Rumble EJ, MacMichael D, Clements ND. The biological effect of continuous passive motion on the healing of full-thickness defects in articular cartilage. An experimental investigation in the rabbit. J Bone Joint Surg Am. 1980;62(8):1232–51.
86. Ferretti M, Srinivasan A, Deschner J, Gassner R, Baliko F, Piesco N, Salter R, Agarwal S. Anti-inflammatory effects of continuous passive motion on meniscal fibrocartilage. J Orthop Res. 2005;23(5):1165–71.
87. Trzeciak T, Richter M, Ruszkowski K. Effectiveness of continuous passive motion after total knee replacement. Chir Narzadow Ruchu Ortop Pol. 2011;76:345–9.
88. O'Driscoll SW, Giori NJ. Continuous passive motion (CPM): theory and principles of clinical application. J Rehabil Res Dev. 2000;37(2):179–88.
89. Bakirhan S, Unver B, Karatosun V. Effects of two different continuous passive motion protocols on the functional activities of total knee arthroplasty inpatients. Acta Orthop Traumatol Turc. 2015;49(5):497–502.
90. Gatewood CT, Tran AA, Dragoo JL. The efficacy of post-operative devices following knee arthroscopic surgery: a systematic review. Knee Surg Sports Traumatol Arthrosc. 2017;25(2):501–16.
91. Lenssen TA, van Steyn MJ, Crijns YH, Waltje EM, Roox GM, Geesink RJ, van den Brandt PA, De Bie RA. Effectiveness of prolonged use of continuous passive motion (CPM), as an adjunct to physiotherapy, after total knee arthroplasty. BMC Musculoskelet Disord. 2008;9:60.
92. Denis M, Moffet H, Caron F, Ouellet D, Paquet J, Nolet L. Effectiveness of continuous passive motion and conventional physical therapy after total knee arthroplasty: a randomized clinical trial. Phys Ther. 2006;86(2):174–85.
93. Liao CD, Huang YC, Chiu YS, Liou TH. Effect of body mass index on knee function outcomes following continuous passive motion in patients with osteoarthritis after total knee replacement: a retrospective study. Physiotherapy. 2017;103(3):266–75.
94. McAlindon TE, Bannuru RR, Sullivan MC, Arden NK, Berenbaum F, Bierma-Zeinstra SM, Hawker GA, Henrotin Y, Hunter DJ, Kawaguchi H, Kwoh K, Lohmander S, Rannou F, Roos EM, Underwood M. OARSI guidelines for the non-surgical management of knee osteoarthritis. Osteoarthritis Cartilage. 2014;22(3):363–88.
95. Simic M, Bennell KL, Hunt MA, Wrigley TV, Hinman RS. Contralateral cane use and knee joint load in people with medial knee osteoarthritis: the effect of varying body weight support. Osteoarthritis Cartilage. 2011;19(11):1330–7.
96. Gross KD, Hillstrom H. Knee osteoarthritis: primary care using noninvasive devices and biomechanical principles. Med Clin North Am. 2009;93(1):179–200. xii.

97. Bartels EM, Juhl CB, Christensen R, Hagen KB, Danneskiold-Samsoe B, Dagfinrud H, Lund H. Aquatic exercise for the treatment of knee and hip osteoarthritis. Cochrane Database Syst Rev. 2016;3:CD005523.
98. Bartels EM, Lund H, Hagen KB, Dagfinrud H, Christensen R, Danneskiold-Samsoe B. Aquatic exercise for the treatment of knee and hip osteoarthritis. Cochrane Database Syst Rev. 2007;4:CD005523.
99. Batterham SI, Heywood S, Keating JL. Systematic review and meta-analysis comparing land and aquatic exercise for people with hip or knee arthritis on function, mobility and other health outcomes. BMC Musculoskelet Disord. 2011;12:123.
100. Foley A, Halbert J, Hewitt T, Crotty M. Does hydrotherapy improve strength and physical function in patients with osteoarthritis--a randomised controlled trial comparing a gym based and a hydrotherapy based strengthening programme. Ann Rheum Dis. 2003;62(12):1162–7.
101. Gill SD, McBurney H, Schulz DL. Land-based versus pool-based exercise for people awaiting joint replacement surgery of the hip or knee: results of a randomized controlled trial. Arch Phys Med Rehabil. 2009;90(3):388–94.
102. Lim JY, Tchai E, Jang SN. Effectiveness of aquatic exercise for obese patients with knee osteoarthritis: a randomized controlled trial. PM R. 2010;2(8):723–31. quiz 793.
103. Waller B, Munukka M, Multanen J, Rantalainen T, Poyhonen T, Nieminen MT, Kiviranta I, Kautiainen H, Selanne H, Dekker J, Sipila S, Kujala UM, Hakkinen A, Heinonen A. Effects of a progressive aquatic resistance exercise program on the biochemical composition and morphology of cartilage in women with mild knee osteoarthritis: protocol for a randomised controlled trial. BMC Musculoskelet Disord. 2013;14:82.
104. Wang TJ, Belza B, Elaine Thompson F, Whitney JD, Bennett K. Effects of aquatic exercise on flexibility, strength and aerobic fitness in adults with osteoarthritis of the hip or knee. J Adv Nurs. 2007;57(2):141–52.
105. Wyatt FB, Milam S, Manske RC, Deere R. The effects of aquatic and traditional exercise programs on persons with knee osteoarthritis. J Strength Cond Res. 2001;15(3):337–40.
106. Munukka M, Waller B, Rantalainen T, Hakkinen A, Nieminen MT, Lammentausta E, Kujala UM, Paloneva J, Sipila S, Peuna A, Kautiainen H, Selanne H, Kiviranta I, Heinonen A. Efficacy of progressive aquatic resistance training for tibiofemoral cartilage in postmenopausal women with mild knee osteoarthritis: a randomised controlled trial. Osteoarthritis Cartilage. 2016;24(10):1708–17.
107. Yamada A, Maruoka Y, Asahi K, Iimura T, Oida S, Ezawa I, Goseki-Sone M. The effect of swimming on cartilage formation. J Nutr Sci Vitaminol (Tokyo). 2002;48(3):238–41.
108. Kutzner I, Heinlein B, Graichen F, Rohlmann A, Halder AM, Beier A, Bergmann G. Loading of the knee joint during ergometer cycling: telemetric in vivo data. J Orthop Sports Phys Ther. 2012;42(12):1032–8.
109. Asplund C, St Pierre P. Knee pain and bicycling: fitting concepts for clinicians. Phys Sportsmed. 2004;32(4):23–30.
110. Alves AC, Albertini R, Dos Santos SA, Leal-junior EC, Santana E, Serra AJ, Silva JA Jr, de Carvalho Pde T. Effect of low-level laser therapy on metalloproteinase MMP-2 and MMP-9 production and percentage of collagen types I and III in a papain cartilage injury model. Lasers Med Sci. 2014;29(3):911–9.
111. Carlos FP. de Paula Alves d, Silva M, de Lemos Vasconcelos Silva Melo E, Costa MS, Zamuner SR. Protective effect of low-level laser therapy (LLLT) on acute zymosan-induced arthritis. Lasers Med Sci. 2014;29(2):757–63.
112. IRV C, Santisteban Valenzuela JM, Gomez-Villamandos RJ, Redondo JI, Gomez-Villamandos RJ, Jurado IA. Histological and clinical responses of articular cartilage to low-level laser therapy: experimental study. Lasers Med Sci. 1997;12:117–21.
113. Archakova LIG VN, Yemelyanova AA, Serdyuchenko NS, Soroka NF. Effects of laser and magnetolaser treatment on the growth and maturation of repairing hyaline cartilage cells in the knee joint of rabbits in different postoperative periods. Minsk, Republic of Belarus: Edited by The Belaruskaya Navuka Publishing House; 2002. p. 42–53.
114. Jia YL, Guo ZY. Effect of low-power he-ne laser irradiation on rabbit articular chondrocytes in vitro. Lasers Surg Med. 2004;34(4):323–8.
115. Lin YS, Huang MH, Chai CY. Effects of helium-neon laser on the mucopolysaccharide induction in experimental osteoarthritic cartilage. Osteoarthritis Cartilage. 2006;14(4):377–83.
116. Zati A, Desando G, Cavallo C, Buda R, Giannini S, Fortuna D, Facchini A, Grigolo B. Treatment of human cartilage defects by means of Nd:YAG Laser Therapy. J Biol Regul Homeost Agents. 2012;26(4):701–11.
117. Shibata Y, Ogura N, Yamashiro K, Takashiba S, Kondoh T, Miyazawa K, Matsui M, Abiko Y. Anti-inflammatory effect of linear polarized infrared irradiation on interleukin-1beta-induced chemokine production in MH7A rheumatoid synovial cells. Lasers Med Sci. 2005;20(3-4):109–13.
118. Gur A, Cosut A, Sarac AJ, Cevik R, Nas K, Uyar A. Efficacy of different therapy regimes of low-power laser in painful osteoarthritis of the knee: a double-blind and randomized-controlled trial. Lasers Surg Med. 2003;33(5):330–8.
119. Ongaro A, Pellati A, Masieri FF, Caruso A, Setti S, Cadossi R, Biscione R, Massari L, Fini M, De Mattei M. Chondroprotective effects of pulsed electromagnetic fields on human cartilage explants. Bioelectromagnetics. 2011;32(7):543–51.

120. Ciombor DM, Aaron RK, Wang S, Simon B. Modification of osteoarthritis by pulsed electromagnetic field--a morphological study. Osteoarthritis Cartilage. 2003;11(6):455–62.
121. Anbarasan S, Baraneedharan U, Paul SF, Kaur H, Rangaswami S, Bhaskar E. Low dose short duration pulsed electromagnetic field effects on cultured human chondrocytes: an experimental study. Indian J Orthop. 2016;50(1):87–93.
122. Massari L, Fini M, Cadossi R, Setti S, Traina GC. Biophysical stimulation with pulsed electromagnetic fields in osteonecrosis of the femoral head. J Bone Joint Surg Am. 2006;88(Suppl 3):56–60.
123. Massari L, Benazzo F, De Mattei M, Setti S, Fini M, Group CS. Effects of electrical physical stimuli on articular cartilage. J Bone Joint Surg Am. 2007;89(Suppl 3):152–61.
124. De Mattei M, Pasello M, Pellati A, Stabellini G, Massari L, Gemmati D, Caruso A. Effects of electromagnetic fields on proteoglycan metabolism of bovine articular cartilage explants. Connect Tissue Res. 2003;44(3-4):154–9.
125. De Mattei M, Pellati A, Pasello M, Ongaro A, Setti S, Massari L, Gemmati D, Caruso A. Effects of physical stimulation with electromagnetic field and insulin growth factor-I treatment on proteoglycan synthesis of bovine articular cartilage. Osteoarthritis Cartilage. 2004;12(10):793–800.
126. Williams JS Jr, Bush-Joseph CA, Bach BR Jr. Osteochondritis dissecans of the knee. Am J Knee Surg. 1998;11(4):221–32.
127. Andriolo L, Candrian C, Papio T, Cavicchioli A, Perdisa F, Filardo G. Osteochondritis dissecans of the knee–Conservative treatment strategies: a systematic review. Cartilage. 2018. Feb 1:1947603518758435. https://doi.org/10.1177/1947603518758435. (Epub ahead of print).
128. MacFarlane LA, Yang H, Collins JE, Jarraya M, Guermazi A, et al. Association of changes in effusion-synovitis with progression of cartilage damage over eighteen months in patients with osteoarthritis and meniscal tear. Arthritis Rheumatol. 2019;71(1):73–81.
129. Conaghan PG, Felson DT. Structural associations of osteoarthritis pain: lessons from magnetic resonance imaging. Novartis Found Symp. 2004;260:191–201. discussion 201–205, 277–9.
130. Bannuru RR, Osani MC, Vaysbrot EE, Arden NK, Bennell K, et al. OARSI guidelines for the non-surgical management of knee, hip, and polyarticular osteoarthritis. Osteoarthritis Cartilage. 2019;27(11):1578–89.
131. Zhang W, Moskowitz RW, Nuki G, Abramson S, Altman RD, Arden N, Bierma-Zeinstra S, Brandt KD, Croft P, Doherty M, Dougados M, Hochberg M, Hunter DJ, Kwoh K, Lohmander LS, Tugwell P. OARSI recommendations for the management of hip and knee osteoarthritis, part I: critical appraisal of existing treatment guidelines and systematic review of current research evidence. Osteoarthritis Cartilage. 2007;15(9):981–1000.
132. Ikuta F, Takahashi K, Hashimoto S, Mochizuki Y, Yuzawa Y, et al. Effect of physical therapy on early knee osteoarthritis with medial meniscal posterior tear assessed by MRI T2 mapping and 3D-to-2D registration technique: a prospective intervention study. Mod Rheumatol. 2019;6:1–10.
133. Callaghan MJ, Guney H, Reeves ND, Bailey D, Doslikova K, Maganaris CN, Hodgson R, Felson DT. A knee brace alters patella position in patellofemoral osteoarthritis: a study using weight bearing magnetic resonance imaging. Osteoarthritis Cartilage. 2016;24(12):2055–60.
134. Chang WD, Chen S, Lee CL, Lin HY, Lai PT. The effects of tai chi Chuan on improving mind-body health for knee osteoarthritis patients: a systematic review and meta-analysis. Evid Based Complement Alternat Med. 2016;2016:1813979.
135. Alkatan M, Baker JR, Machin DR, Park W, Akkari AS, Pasha EP, Tanaka H. Improved function and reduced pain after swimming and cycling training in patients with osteoarthritis. J Rheumatol. 2016;43(3):666–72.
136. Salacinski AJ, Krohn K, Lewis SF, Holland ML, Ireland K, Marchetti G. The effects of group cycling on gait and pain-related disability in individuals with mild-to-moderate knee osteoarthritis: a randomized controlled trial. J Orthop Sports Phys Ther. 2012;42(12):985–95.
137. Nejati P, Farzinmehr A, Moradi-Lakeh M. The effect of exercise therapy on knee osteoarthritis: a randomized clinical trial. Med J Islam Repub Iran. 2015;29:186.
138. Fransen M, McConnell S. Exercise for osteoarthritis of the knee. Cochrane Database Syst Rev. 2008;4:CD004376.
139. Vanwanseele B, Eckstein F, Knecht H, Stussi E, Spaepen A. Knee cartilage of spinal cord-injured patients displays progressive thinning in the absence of normal joint loading and movement. Arthritis Rheum. 2002;46(8):2073–8.
140. Vanwanseele B, Lucchinetti E, Stussi E. The effects of immobilization on the characteristics of articular cartilage: current concepts and future directions. Osteoarthritis Cartilage. 2002;10(5):408–19.
141. Koli J, Multanen J, Kujala UM, Hakkinen A, Nieminen MT, Kautiainen H, Lammentausta E, Jamsa T, Ahola R, Selanne H, Kiviranta I, Heinonen A. Effects of exercise on patellar cartilage in women with mild knee osteoarthritis. Med Sci Sports Exerc. 2015;47(9):1767–74.

9 Pharmacologic Agents for Knee Articular Cartilage Injury and Disease

Joseph B. Houpt, Kenneth P. H. Pritzker, and Harpal K. Gahunia

9.1 Introduction

There is an increased awareness of the impact that knee injuries have on patients' quality of life (QoL) and the heavy burden of joint diseases on the health-care system [1–3]. Articular cartilage can be injured by trauma related to accident, sports or diseases such as osteoarthritis (OA) and inflammatory arthritis (IA). Primary cartilage injury directly affects the articular cartilage, whereas secondary cartilage injury is a consequence of damage to other joint tissues such as ligaments, tendons, meniscus, or subchondral bone, which then result in cartilage structural damage. Joint malalignment, congenital disease, and obesity are factors that play a role in the damage to the knee cartilage. The social impact of knee joint disease results in high costs in terms of treatments and loss of income [1, 2, 4]. The trend of current cartilage research is directed toward the prevention, diagnosis, and treatment of chondral and osteochondral (OC) injuries. Several available options are directed toward the early stages of cartilage structural damage in an attempt to enhance cartilage regeneration, restore normal function, and reduce degenerative mechanisms by halting or delaying the progression of cartilage degeneration.

In children, adolescents and young adults, normal knee use, such as running, squatting, or jumping, is beneficial to the growth of articular cartilage [5]. However, in middle-aged and older adults the safety threshold for these activities is determined most likely on an individual basis and the nature of activities (frequency, intensity and duration) and by their genetic constitution [6–10]. Focal chondral and OC defects in adults have poor intrinsic healing capacity that may lead to symptomatic degeneration of the joint. The goal of non-surgical treatment of symptomatic cartilage injuries affecting the knee is to reduce pain, restore joint function, and prevent or delay the onset of degenerative arthritis. The choice of an appropriate treatment should be made on an individual basis, with consideration for the patient's age, activity level, and specific goals such as pain reduction and functional improvement. The extent of the lesion (size: length, width, and depth) and defect location in the joint (weight-bearing or non-weight-bearing

J. B. Houpt, MD, FRCPC (✉)
Faculty of Medicine, University of Toronto, Toronto, ON, Canada
e-mail: jbhoupt@sympatico.ca

K. P. H. Pritzker, MD, FRCPC
Department of Laboratory Medicine and Pathobiology, Department of Surgery, and Institute of Biomaterials and Biomedical Engineering, University of Toronto, Toronto, ON, Canada

Department of Pathology and Laboratory Medicine, Mount Sinai Hospital, Toronto, ON, Canada

H. K. Gahunia, MSc, PhD
Orthopaedic Science Consulting Services, Oakville, ON, Canada

H. K. Gahunia et al. (eds.), *Articular Cartilage of the Knee*,
https://doi.org/10.1007/978-1-4939-7587-7_9

area) may also determine the treatment recommendation.

A conservative approach should be the first choice for the management of knee cartilage injuries, in particular following trauma and in the early stage of OA. A wide spectrum of treatments is available including non-pharmacological strategies (refer to Chap. 8), dietary supplements, analgesic herbal medicines, pharmacologic therapies, as well as minimally invasive procedures involving intra-articular injections of various chondroprotective agents aiming to restore cartilage homeostasis and provide symptomatic relief [3, 11]. Numerous pharmacologic agents have been proposed, but the long-term effectiveness, optimal dose, and administration modalities still need to be clarified.

The term nutraceuticals (commonly used in marketing but without regulatory definition) was introduced to include food or extract of food components in the form of dietary supplements that have potential medical or health benefit [12]. Common food items such as olive oil, fish oil, ginger, avocado/soybean unsaponifiables, and saturated or omega-6 polyunsaturated fatty acids have been documented to have regulatory function on the homeostasis of cartilage metabolism [13–17]. However, due to the lack or limited scientific evidence as well as uncertainties pertaining to the quality, safety, efficacy, possible side effects, and interaction with other pharmacologic drugs, the use of nutraceuticals is not without risks. Clinical studies have documented the chondroprotective function and reduction of pain including joint stiffness with the use of dietary supplement of glucosamine, chondroitin sulfate (CS), collagen hydrolysate, and vitamins C and D as well as viscosupplementation with hyaluronic acid (HA) and platelet-rich plasma (PRP) [18–21].

A surgical approach to knee cartilage repair and knee replacement is only recommended after all conservative treatment options have failed to provide symptomatic relief. A biological approach to articular cartilage healing and repair has led to the development of medications and injections aimed to reduce pain and perhaps heal cartilage injury. The focus of this chapter is to review the non-surgical, pharmacologic approaches to the treatment of cartilage injuries and healing. The surgical approach to repair cartilage is described in depth in Chaps. 11 and 12, whereas the details of cell-seeded and non-cell-seeded matrix implants are found in Chaps. 16, 17, and 18.

9.2 Conservative Approach to Cartilage Injury in Children

The immature cartilage of children and adolescents has more metabolically active chondrocytes with better intrinsic potential to self-repair than the adult cartilage. This important aspect is associated with the phase of cartilage growth, varying degree of vascularization, and abundance of pluripotent stem cells in children. As described in Chap. 2, during endochondral ossification, besides the growth and elongation of long bones, the growth plate also provides the cell source for cartilage growth. Further, vascularization provides the nutrients to the growing, immature cartilage enhancing the regenerative capability within the defective articular cartilage. Therefore, chondral and OC lesions in children have greater potential for healing compared to the similar size lesions in adults.

The term *acute knee injury* is applied to knee injuries due to sudden trauma. Acute knee injuries occur frequently in children and skeletally immature adolescents [22, 23]. Among children, the most common cause of knee injury occurs during competitive or recreational sports and during accidental falls. The largest number of sports-related knee injury among children occurs during soccer, football, basketball, and hockey. Accidental falls from a bicycle ride, trampoline, and skating also pose risks for knee injury. Post-injury knee pain is considered acute or subacute if the pain resolves within 6 weeks. Pain resulting from acute knee injury often prevents the person from completing their activity. Sequelae such as intra-articular bleeding, soft tissue swelling, and/or joint effusion often accompany acute knee injuries. Acute pain may also be associated with overuse of the joint experienced after strenuous activity.

Chronic knee injury can arise from an acute injury that does not heal properly (e.g., anterior cruciate ligament tear that is not fully rehabilitated), due to insidious onset of pain without specific injury related to excessive activity or repetitive microtrauma of the subchondral bone (e.g., iliotibial band syndrome in a soccer player or runner), or pain associated with certain preexisting conditions (such as IA, hemophilia, osteomyelitis, or septic arthritis) [24–31]. Chronic knee pain persists longer than 6 weeks. While the 6-week threshold is arbitrary, it can be useful since many self-limited acute injuries (contusions) heal by the end of 6 weeks with appropriate rest.

The involvement of articular cartilage in knee injuries could be primary or secondary to other injury such as ligament tears, sprains or strains, meniscal injuries, fractures, and patellar dislocations [32–41]. Osteochondral fractures may result in OC fragments being released into the synovial space, resulting in mechanical symptoms such as catching, locking, or buckling. If untreated, these fractures may progress to OC defects and eventually cause OA. Typically, patients with OC injury complain of knee pain and swelling that may result in mechanical discomfort, tightness, and reduced activity. At rest, patients may report no pain, but when active, they experience pain with resulting restricted activity.

A conservative treatment approach is the first choice in children when the chondral or OC defect is very small ($\leq$1cm^2) and the OC unit is still intact such as in early-stage lesions in conditions like osteochondritis dissecans. At this stage, the child usually does not exhibit the symptoms at rest but may complain of pain or discomfort during and/or after activity. When cartilage injury is due to sports, it is essential that the child eliminate or reduce sporting activity for a period of 6–15 weeks and non-weight-bearing may be recommended for 2–3 months with gradual return to normal activity with physiotherapy and strengthening exercises, if needed.

With increased intensities of sports activities and repetitive impact on the knee with certain sports, especially those involved in competitive sports or dance, overuse knee injuries are commonly encountered in children [42, 43]. Knee pain during such activities is not normal and is an indicator of knee overuse. These warning signs of joint overuse may require modification, reduction, or, with severe continued pain, discontinuation of the activity. Among children and skeletally immature adolescents, conservative treatment can be very effective. Favorable results are usually obtained treating children conservatively; nevertheless, cases with more serious injury involving severe cartilage lesion(s) may warrant surgical intervention [41].

9.3 Pharmacologic Approach to Cartilage Injury in Adults

The natural history of a focal chondral lesion in the adult is poorly understood. In the symptomatic knee, management of malalignment, ligament insufficiency, and inflammation are helpful. A meniscal tear may present with acute pain and swelling mimicking an acute process due to OA and should be treated conservatively. Acute synovitis due to sepsis, gout (urate crystals), or pseudogout (calcium pyrophosphate crystals) may mimic an osteoarthritic process and may require appropriate joint aspiration, synovial fluid culture, and crystal identification.

When adult hyaline cartilage is injured as a result of accident or sports-related trauma, or due to gradual wear and tear which may be related to excessive activity, occupation, or aging, patients may experience symptoms of severe joint pain, and normal joint mobility may become limited. Treatment options include nonsteroidal anti-inflammatory drugs (NSAIDs), various non-opioid analgesics including acetaminophen, judicious use of corticosteroid injections, topical cream with NSAIDS, and/or use of oral or injectable chondroprotective agents.

9.3.1 Pain Management and Systemic Medications

Articular cartilage injury in adults can occur primarily as an isolated incident, secondary to other joint tissue injury (ligament, meniscus, tendon), or in conjunction with other knee injuries. Sports-related injuries to the articular cartilage may result from torsional stresses or from direct impact on the knee joint. Acute injury to articular cartilage often results in joint inflammation and pain. Conservative management of mild articular cartilage injury may involve rest for several weeks and partial or non-weight-bearing followed by rehabilitation with gentle strengthening exercises. To address the pain and swelling, oral NSAID medications may be prescribed. In conjunction, non-pharmacologic conservative approaches (described in Chap. 8) may also be implemented such as ice and elevation to help minimize the swelling. If the cartilage injury is not severe, then non-surgical, conservative treatment may result in healing of the cartilage injury.

Painful chronic cartilage conditions may be treated with long-term oral NSAIDs, potent analgesics, prudent corticosteroid injections, and, if indicated, with surgery. NSAIDS have been a remarkable addition to the treatment of articular diseases, but they have significant side effects. Acute gastrointestinal (GI) bleeding, chronic upper and lower GI symptomatology, hypertension and fluid retention, increased frequency of myocardial ischemia, and infarction are some of the more serious side effects that may be seen with these potent agents [44–46]. Strong opiate analgesics are discouraged due to the potential for addiction. Also, frequent intra-articular steroid injections are discouraged as they have been associated with avascular necrosis [47, 48]. In addition, repeated intra-articular corticosteroid injections are discouraged as they have been associated with generalized osteoporosis, compression vertebral fractures, or infection; and, in experimental animals with articular cartilage calcification [49–51]. Further, the long-term use of repeated corticosteroid injections in chronic painful tendinopathy has been shown to be ineffective [52]. Intra-articular steroid, once absorbed, has a similar effect on lowering the adrenal endogenous production of steroid as oral steroids and should be noted if the patient is in a "stressful" situation such as requiring an anaesthetic and supplemental oral steroids [53–55].

9.3.2 Topical Medications

Opinions differ on the effectiveness of over-the-counter topical pain medications. While there are claims that these products help relieve joint pain, scientific studies reveal only modest benefits. Some suggest that topical NSAID creams and gels work as well as oral NSAIDS. For those who cannot tolerate oral NSAIDs, topical NSAIDs may be useful.

9.4 Chondroprotective Agents

Chondroprotective agents are compounds that inhibit cartilage degradation and prevent fibrin formation in the subchondral and synovial vasculature. These agents function to regulate the extracellular matrix (ECM) metabolism and to stimulate chondrocyte synthesis of collagen and proteoglycans. Examples of compounds that exhibit some of these characteristics are endogenous molecules of articular cartilage such as HA, glucosamine and CS, as well as PRP.

9.4.1 Glucosamine

Glucosamine is a compound that is naturally synthesized in human articular cartilage. Studies have demonstrated that glucosamine, when given to athletes (bicycle racers and soccer players), stimulates the chondrocytes to synthesize collagen type II and also prevent collagen type II degradation [56–58]. Commercially available glucosamine products are obtained from the exoskeleton of crustaceans. The sulfate and hydrochloride salts vary substantially in molecular form, pharmaceutical and dose regime [59]. Although both forms have been shown to have mild anti-inflammatory activity and analgesic properties when used for prolonged periods of time, a recent study reported that the crystalline glucosamine sulfate form demonstrated improved treatment selection, increased treatment adherence, and optimized clinical benefit in OA, relative to other forms [59–61]. In short-term clinical trials, glucosamine has provided effective symptomatic relief of knee pain in some patients [62–64]. Although a number of clinical trials have been considered to have a negative outcome, a subgroup of patients with the most advanced clinical and radiologic OA seemed to have had a significant benefit [63, 65]. A placebo-controlled double-blind trial was unable to show any significant beneficial effect on radiologic joint space widening, although the authors suggested that the subset of those patients with Kellgren-Lawrence (K/L) grade 2 may have had some benefit compared to placebo. A selection of other reports of randomized double-blind, placebo-controlled trials of glucosamine for pain identified various influences that explain the heterogeneity and discordant results in various trials of glucosamine [64].

9.4.2 Chondroitin Sulfate

Chondroitin sulfate is the most abundant glycosaminoglycan (GAG) in articular cartilage. It plays an important structural role in articular cartilage, notable for its role in binding with collagen fibrils. As a chondroprotective agent, it has a metabolic effect as well: its action is to competitively inhibit many of the degradative enzymes that break down the cartilage matrix and synovial fluid in OA. However, a meta-analysis based on 20 trials (3846 patients) revealed a high degree of heterogeneity among the trials, and the symptomatic benefit of chondroitin by itself was minimal or nonexistent. The authors concluded that the routine use of chondroitin alone has no therapeutic effect [66].

9.4.3 Glucosamine and Chondroitin Combined

Glucosamine and CS are agents that occur naturally in the body, but can be supplemented in over-the-counter capsule form. Glucosamine stimulates the formation and repair of articular cartilage, while CS prevents other body enzymes from breaking down the building blocks of joint cartilage. Many believe that glucosamine and chondroitin have anti-inflammatory effects that help relieve the pain of OA, with fewer side effects than NSAIDs. Whether they actually slow the degenerative process or restore cartilage in arthritic joints has not been determined.

When used together, it seems that glucosamine and chondroitin sulfate combine effects to stimulate the metabolism of chondrocytes and synoviocytes, inhibit degradative enzymes, and reduce fibrin thrombi in peri-articular microvasculature. Numerous animal studies performed on horses at US veterinary schools have supported this combination and synergistic effect [67, 68]. However, illustrative of the dilemma regarding the efficacy of these compounds in humans are the results of a large double-blind National Institutes of Health (NIH) trial comparing glucosamine sulfate, with and without chondroitin sulfate, to the potent NSAID celecoxib. This trial was considered to have a negative effect. However there was a significant positive effect in the subgroup of their patients considered to have severe knee OA [64, 65].

9.5 Viscosupplementation Therapy

Viscosupplementation is a therapy that aims to be chondroprotective by restoring the fluid properties of the tissue matrix by means of intra-articular injections of highly purified "viscoelastic" solutions of sodium hyaluronate. Viscosupplementation can be considered when the patient has not found pain relief from other therapies.

HA is a physiologic component of the synovial fluid with viscoelastic properties that acts as a shock absorber and lubricant in the knee. Intra-articular injections of HA prepared commercially from chicken combs are widely used in the Asian and European orthopedic communities for controlling the pain and loss of joint function resulting from OA [69]. It is claimed that intra-articular injection of HA has a protective effect on articular cartilage and functions to restore the normal articular homoeostasis. Further, HA therapy is reported to provide anti-inflammatory relief through a number of different pathways, including the suppression of pro-inflammatory cytokines and chemokines [70]. Viscosupplementation can be considered when the patient has not found pain relief from other therapies. HA is well tolerated with no demonstrable toxicity and minimal side effects. Possible mechanisms by which HA may act therapeutically include providing additional lubrication of the synovial membrane, controlling permeability of the synovial membrane, thereby controlling effusions and directly blocking inflammation. However, the exact mechanisms of action, articular cartilage changes, and short- and long-term results remain unknown. Although some studies indicated the importance of molecular weight of the HA preparation in the clinical outcome, other studies suggested that there is no correlation between molecular weight and the HA treatment efficacy [71–72]. Because these viscosupplements are claimed to work by physical action (increasing elastoviscosity) and not by chemical action, they are classified by the Food and Drug Administration (FDA) as devices rather than as drugs.

9.6 Platelet-Rich Plasma Therapy

Growth factors play an important role in chondrogenesis and in prevention of joint degeneration. The biological potential of platelets in the cartilage healing process is attributed to its bioactive proteins and numerous growth factors, including platelet-derived growth factor, insulin-like growth factor (IGF), transforming growth factor (TGF), epidermal growth factor (EGF), fibroblast growth factor (FGF), and vascular endothelial growth factor (VEGF) [73, 74].

PRP was first introduced in 1987 by Ferrari et al. in open heart surgery [75]. PRP has been shown to have anti-inflammatory agents including hepatocyte growth factor (HGF) [76, 77]. These properties suggested the potential of PRP to enhance cartilage regeneration and reduce catabolic factors that lead to cartilage degradation [73, 78]. Subsequently, studies have been reported in an attempt to understand the biological effects of PRP and its potential in regenerative therapy for cartilage repair [18, 74, 76, 79–81]. Due to its versatility, biocompatibility, and low costs, the therapeutic use of PRP has gained popularity in clinical practice and has shown promising results for the treatment and management of some musculoskeletal problems including knee cartilage disorders [73, 82]. In vitro studies have shown that PRP stimulates mesenchymal cells adhesion, migration, and proliferation as well as enhances chondrocyte proliferation and chondrogenic differentiation [83, 84]. Also, PRP have shown to stimulate the superficial zone protein and enhance the cartilage lubrication [85]. Further, PRP maintains chondrocyte phenotype and increases GAG synthesis and col-II level [79, 84, 86]. The efficacy of autologous PRP has been linked to stimulating chondrocyte proliferation and collagen synthesis [87].

The PRP administration is through intra-articular injections as an outpatient procedure. As an autologous blood product, PRP is safe. In the knee, platelet concentrates have been used to reduce pain as well as improve knee function and QoL in younger patients with a lesser degree of articular cartilage degeneration [88]. Improvements in function and symptoms were achieved in younger (less than 50 years) and more active patients with a low degree of cartilage degeneration, whereas a worse outcome was noted in more degenerated joints and in older patients [88]. PRP has shown to provide symptomatic relief and improve knee function and QoL with short-term efficacy [80, 89–91]. However, after multiple PRP injections, an increased risk of local adverse reactions and inconsistent clinical outcome pertaining to its use has been noted [89, 92].

Studies have suggested that PRP injections are either as effective or more efficacious than HA, highlighting the potential of PRP injections as an option for knee cartilage treatment [74, 93–95].

Conflicting results have been published when HA injection results have been compared to PRP injections [93, 96–98]. In one study comprising end career professional soccer athletes, each patient received three intra-articular injections of either high molecular weight HA (24 patients) or PRP (23 patients). At 3- and 6-month follow-ups, patients who received HA injections showed a significant clinical improvement compared to the PRP group, but there was loss of this significant difference between the two groups at a 12-month follow-up [96].

9.7 Conservative Management of the Osteoarthritic Knee

Osteoarthritis is a multifactorial, degenerative disease that is considered as one of the most significant causes of disability. The genetic and anatomic factors contributing to the development of adult knee OA are poorly understood. Further, OA progresses at different rates in different individuals, and even within the same individual, it may progress at a different rate between different joint compartments. Often, pain relief, preservation of function, and delay in knee arthroplasty can be achieved by assiduous exercise such as that on a stationary bicycle [99]. This activity promotes muscle strengthening around the knee, flow of metabolites in that region, and perhaps partial repair of cartilage and bone within the articular plate.

Studies of cartilage biochemistry and pathogenesis of OA have focused research on slowing the progression of degeneration and promoting cartilage regeneration. It is unclear as to whether any pharmacologic intervention alters the natural history of progressive cartilage degeneration. The early preclinical lesions of non-traumatic OA may be asymptomatic. OA processes of the knee over time may gradually degrade the articular cartilage resulting in the development of subchondral bone sclerosis, osteophytes, cysts, and joint effusions. These further damage the articular cartilage, leading to varying degree of joint stiffness, swelling, pain, and loss of mobility.

Evaluation of treatment modalities in patients with OA has proven to be difficult due to the natural history of the processes, the variable effects of self-administered analgesics, the effects of weight loss, symptom effects of changes in barometric pressure, walking aids such as canes, and the crucial assessment of the role of testimonials in the "health food" industry [64]. Various assessment tools have been helpful in determining the effectiveness of treatment modalities of musculoskeletal disorders (see Appendix B).

The management of OA consists of conservative (non-pharmacologic and/or pharmacologic) and surgical approaches. The management is individualized based on the patient's OA severity, level of activity, function and expectation, sports, needs or other interests, occupation, and the presence of any other underlying or coexisting medical conditions. The goal of conventional pharmacologic therapy for OA is focused on symptomatic relief from pain and inflammation, to minimize disability and to improve the quality of life and return to normal function. For details on conservative, non-pharmacologic interventions, refer to Chap. 8. The pharmacological treatment of patients with symptomatic knee OA includes oral or intra-articular administration of pharmacologic agents, analgesics such as acetaminophen and NSAIDs, intra-articular injections of viscosupplements, or chondromodulators. Patients with severe OA should not routinely be prescribed narcotics for pain management. Topical NSAID preparations play a minor role in the management of pain due to OA of the knee.

In many OA knees, the synovial fluid is less viscous and less elastic than that found in healthy knees [100]. Several studies have shown the efficacy of HA for the treatment of mild to moderate knee OA, with positive effects on pain and articular function as assessed by the Western Ontario and McMaster Universities Arthritis Index (WOMAC), Lequesne Index (LI), Range of Motion (ROM), subjective global assessment, and reduction in NSAID consumption [69, 96, 101–104]. HA injections are indicated for the pain in the knee of OA patients who have failed to respond to other conservative measures. A preparation of HA is injected into the arthritic knee joint several times over several weeks. Usually, the benefit is evident within several weeks and may persist for 6–12 months. The therapy is well tolerated with only limited local transient discomfort. In one meta-analysis, the authors concluded that such viscosupplementation had a moderate to significant effect compared to placebo. Some investigators have claimed that the effect is comparable to NSAIDS and intra-articular corticosteroid [105, 106]. Some patients obtain pain relief through viscosupplementation that may last several months. Patients with mild to moderate OA also reported improvement. Whether viscosupplementation has any beneficial effect on focal cartilage defects in patients is unknown.

Clinical trials, involving intra-articular PRP injection into OA knees, have shown promise for achieving symptomatic relief of pain and improving function. Injection of autologous PRP was first reported by Mei-Dan et al. in a prospective randomized study in 30 patients (18–60 years) affected by talar OA lesions [107]. This study investigated the short-term efficacy and safety of PRP and HA [107]. Each patient received three intra-articular injections consecutively, one per week with up to 28 weeks of follow-up with evaluation of pain, stiffness, and function. Decreased pain and disability and increased function with minimal adverse effects were reported. Further, results suggested that PRP treatment was more efficacious than HA injection in reducing symptoms, as corroborated by other studies [93, 94]. In another study, 150 patients with symptomatic knee OA were treated weekly with three PRP intra-articular injections and at follow-up 2- and 6-month [94]. The PRP-treated patients showed more and longer efficacy compared with those who received either low or high molecular weight HA injections. A recent systematic review and meta-analysis of 14 randomized controlled trials (RCTs) comprising 1423 patients was aimed to investigate the efficacy of PRP for treating knee OA [108]. The pooled control cohort included those injected with saline placebo, HA, ozone, and corticosteroids. Using WOMAC pain subscores at 3-, 6-, and 12-month follow-up, PRP injections showed significant reduction in pain subscores and improved physical function subscores compared with controls. This study also suggested the superiority of intra-articular PRP injections compared with HA injections. However, other discordant studies have shown that HA injection in OA knee provided a superior clinical improvement in knee pain and function for up to 26 weeks compared to PRP injection [97, 98, 101]. Recently, a study reported slight reduction in the clinical signs of the knee OA (stage II/III) without adverse effects after intra-articular injection of a single dose of bone marrow-derived mononuclear cell [109]. Although the use of placental tissues (amnion, chorion, amniotic fluid, and the umbilical cord) for intra-articular therapies has shown promising results in modulating knee pain and inflammation in OA, future basic science and clinical research should be conducted to better understand the anti-inflammatory and chondroregenerative properties of amniotic tissue [110]. Intra-articular injection of a single dose of bone marrow-derived mesenchymal stromal cells for treatment of patients with severe knee OA resulted in mitigation of synovial inflammation and overall improvement in joint pain [111].

The use of nutraceuticals or dietary compounds has been promoted by the Health Food Industry for the management of OA [13, 18, 112, 113]. It has been suggested, without convincing success, that these dietary compounds play a regulatory function on homeostasis of cartilage metabolism [13].

9.8 Conclusions

Assessment of the various modalities of nonsurgical management of knee articular cartilage injury and OA has proven to be challenging. The various studies reported in this chapter have shown inconsistent results pertaining to the efficacy of the treatment modalities. This may be a reflection of the heterogeneity of study design, varying preparations of pharmaceutical agents, degree of knee injury or arthritis, and varying differences in response to treatment. Patient and investigator bias including industry sponsorship may also play a role in the inconsistency in the evaluation of treatment effects. With regard to OA, the multifactorial natural history including asymptomatic initial stage, degree of disability, and duration of treatment are contributing factors to the discrepancies of the therapeutic claims for the various treatment modalities. In the face of discrepant evidence for efficacy, for individual patients with chronic articular pain, pharmacologic agents including nutraceuticals should be offered with due attention to observing objective improvement.

References

1. Brown TD, Johnston RC, Saltzman CL, Marsh JL, Buckwalter JA. Posttraumatic osteoarthritis: a first estimate of incidence, prevalence, and burden of disease. J Orthop Trauma. 2006;20:739–44.
2. Nunez M, Nunez E, Segur JM, Macule F, Sanchez A, Hernandez MV, Vilalta C. Health-related quality of life and costs in patients with osteoarthritis on waiting list for total knee replacement. Osteoarthritis Cartilage. 2007;15:258–65.
3. Arnold W, Fullerton DS, Holder S, May CS. Viscosupplementation: managed care issues for osteoarthritis of the knee. J Manag Care Pharm. 2007;13:S3–19. quiz S20–12
4. Mather RC 3rd, Hug KT, Orlando LA, Watters TS, Koenig L, Nunley RM, Bolognesi MP. Economic evaluation of access to musculoskeletal care: the case of waiting for total knee arthroplasty. BMC Musculoskelet Disord. 2014;15:22.
5. Gahunia HK, Pritzker KP. Effect of exercise on articular cartilage. Orthop Clin North Am. 2012;43:187–99. v
6. Hyldahl RD, Evans A, Kwon S, Ridge ST, Robinson E, Hopkins JT, Seeley MK. Running decreases knee intra-articular cytokine and cartilage oligomeric matrix concentrations: a pilot study. Eur J Appl Physiol. 2016;116:2305–14.
7. Ding C, Cicuttini F, Scott F, Glisson M, Jones G. Sex differences in knee cartilage volume in adults: role of body and bone size, age and physical activity. Rheumatology (Oxford). 2003;42:1317–23.
8. Hinterwimmer S, Feucht MJ, Steinbrech C, Graichen H, Eisenhart-Rothe v. R: the effect of a six-month training program followed by a marathon run on knee joint cartilage volume and thickness in marathon beginners. Knee Surg Sports Traumatol Arthrosc. 2014;22:1353–9.
9. Racunica TL, Teichtahl AJ, Wang Y, Wluka AE, English DR, Giles GG, O'Sullivan R, Cicuttini FM. Effect of physical activity on articular knee joint structures in community-based adults. Arthritis Rheum. 2007;57:1261–8.
10. Teichtahl AJ, Wluka AE, Wang Y, Forbes A, Davies-Tuck ML, English DR, Giles GG, Cicuttini FM. Effect of long-term vigorous physical activity on healthy adult knee cartilage. Med Sci Sports Exerc. 2012;44:985–92.
11. Teymouri S, Rakhshandeh H, Baghdar HN, Yousefi M, Salari R. Analgesic herbal medicines in treatment of knee osteoarthritis: A systematic review. Curr Rheumatol Rev. 2019;15(4):290–303.
12. Kalra EK. Nutraceutical--definition and introduction. AAPS PharmSci. 2003;5:E25.
13. Castrogiovanni P, Trovato FM, Loreto C, Nsir H, Szychlinska MA, Musumeci G. Nutraceutical supplements in the management and prevention of osteoarthritis. Int J Mol Sci. 2016;17:2042.
14. Musumeci G, Trovato FM, Pichler K, Weinberg AM, Loreto C, Castrogiovanni P. Extra-virgin olive oil diet and mild physical activity prevent cartilage degeneration in an osteoarthritis model: an in vivo and in vitro study on lubricin expression. J Nutr Biochem. 2013;24:2064–75.
15. CL W, Jain D, McNeill JN, Little D, Anderson JA, Huebner JL, Kraus VB, Rodriguiz RM, Wetsel WC, Guilak F. Dietary fatty acid content regulates wound repair and the pathogenesis of osteoarthritis following joint injury. Ann Rheum Dis. 2015;74:2076–83.
16. Christiansen BA, Bhatti S, Goudarzi R, Emami S. Management of Osteoarthritis with avocado/soybean Unsaponifiables. Cartilage. 2015;6:30–44.
17. McAlindon TE. Nutraceuticals: do they work and when should we use them? Best Pract Res Clin Rheumatol. 2006;20:99–115.
18. Zaslav K, McAdams T, Scopp J, Theosadakis J, Mahajan V, Gobbi A. New Frontiers for cartilage repair and protection. Cartilage. 2012;3:77S–86S.
19. Clark KL, Sebastianelli W, Flechsenhar KR, Aukermann DF, Meza F, Millard RL, Deitch JR, Sherbondy PS, Albert A. 24-week study on the use of collagen hydrolysate as a dietary supplement in athletes with activity-related joint pain. Curr Med Res Opin. 2008;24:1485–96.
20. Bottegoni C, Muzzarelli RA, Giovannini F, Busilacchi A, Gigante A. Oral chondroprotection with nutraceuticals made of chondroitin sulphate plus glucosamine sulphate in osteoarthritis. Carbohydr Polym. 2014;109:126–38.
21. Mobasheri A, Vannucci SJ, Bondy CA, Carter SD, Innes JF, Arteaga MF, Trujillo E, Ferraz I, Shakibaei M, Martin-Vasallo P. Glucose transport and metabolism in chondrocytes: a key to understanding chondrogenesis, skeletal development and cartilage degradation in osteoarthritis. Histol Histopathol. 2002;17:1239–67.
22. Gage BE, McIlvain NM, Collins CL, Fields SK, Comstock RD. Epidemiology of 6.6 million knee injuries presenting to United States emergency departments from 1999 through 2008. Acad Emerg Med. 2012;19:378–85.
23. Ferry T, Bergstrom U, Hedstrom EM, Lorentzon R, Zeisig E. Epidemiology of acute knee injuries seen at the emergency Department at Umea University Hospital, Sweden, during 15 years. Knee Surg Sports Traumatol Arthrosc. 2014;22:1149–55.
24. Finlayson C. Knee injuries in the young athlete. Pediatr Ann. 2014;43(12):e282–90.

25. Taylor R 2nd. Sports medicine in children: knee pain. FP Essent. 2014;417:26–9.
26. Houghton KM1. Review for the generalist: evaluation of anterior knee pain. Pediatr Rheumatol Online J. 2007;5:8.
27. Strauss EJ1, Kim S, Calcei JG, Park D. Iliotibial band syndrome: evaluation and management. J Am Acad Orthop Surg. 2011;19(12):728–36.
28. Atanda A Jr, Ruiz D, Dodson CC, Frederick RW. Approach to the active patient with chronic anterior knee pain. Phys Sportsmed. 2012;40(1):41–50.
29. Yen YM1. Assessment and treatment of knee pain in the child and adolescent athlete. Pediatr Clin North Am. 2014;61(6):1155–73.
30. Blatnik TR1, Briskin S. Bilateral knee pain in a high-level gymnast. Clin J Sport Med. 2013;23(1):77–9.
31. EC1 R-M. Prevention of the musculoskeletal complications of hemophilia. Adv Prev Med. 2012;2012:201271.
32. Bessette M, Saluan P. Patellofemoral pain and instability in adolescent athletes. Sports Med Arthrosc Rev. 2016;24:144–9.
33. Kim HK, Shiraj S, Kang CH, Anton C, Kim DH, Horn PS. Patellofemoral instability in children: correlation between risk factors, injury patterns, and severity of cartilage damage. AJR Am J Roentgenol. 2016;206:1321–8.
34. Mitchell J, Graham W, Best TM, Collins C, Currie DW, Comstock RD, Flanigan DC. Epidemiology of meniscal injuries in US high school athletes between 2007 and 2013. Knee Surg Sports Traumatol Arthrosc. 2016;24:715–22.
35. Metzler AV, Lattermann C, Johnson DL. Cartilage lesions of the patella: management after acute patellar dislocation. Orthopedics. 2015;38:310–4.
36. Zheng L, Shi H, Feng Y, Sun BS, Ding HY, Zhang GY. Injury patterns of medial patellofemoral ligament and correlation analysis with articular cartilage lesions of the lateral femoral condyle after acute lateral patellar dislocation in children and adolescents: an MRI evaluation. Injury. 2015;46:1137–44.
37. Krych AJ, Sousa PL, King AH, Engasser WM, Stuart MJ, Levy BA. Meniscal tears and articular cartilage damage in the dislocated knee. Knee Surg Sports Traumatol Arthrosc. 2015;23:3019–25.
38. Seeley MA, Knesek M, Vanderhave KL. Osteochondral injury after acute patellar dislocation in children and adolescents. J Pediatr Orthop. 2013;33:511–8.
39. Seeley M, Bowman KF, Walsh C, Sabb BJ, Vanderhave KL. Magnetic resonance imaging of acute patellar dislocation in children: patterns of injury and risk factors for recurrence. J Pediatr Orthop. 2012;32:145–55.
40. Dumont GD, Hogue GD, Padalecki JR, Okoro N, Wilson PL. Meniscal and chondral injuries associated with pediatric anterior cruciate ligament tears: relationship of treatment time and patient-specific factors. Am J Sports Med. 2012;40:2128–33.
41. Panni AS, Vasso M, Cerciello S. Acute patellar dislocation. What to do? Knee Surg Sports Traumatol Arthrosc. 2013;21:275–8.
42. Launay F. Sports-related overuse injuries in children. Orthop Traumatol Surg Res. 2015;101:S139–47.
43. Cassas KJ, Cassettari-Wayhs A. Childhood and adolescent sports-related overuse injuries. Am Fam Physician. 2006;73:1014–22.
44. Hamilton K, Davis C, Falk J, Singer A, Bugden S. Assessing prescribing of NSAIDs, antiplatelets, and anticoagulants in Canadian family medicine using chart review. Int J Clin Pharm. 2016;38:1094–102.
45. Morrison A, Ramey DR, van Adelsberg J, Watson DJ. Systematic review of trials of the effect of continued use of oral non-selective NSAIDs on blood pressure and hypertension. Curr Med Res Opin. 2007;23:2395–404.
46. Shau WY, Chen HC, Chen ST, Chou HW, Chang CH, Kuo CW, Lai MS. Risk of new acute myocardial infarction hospitalization associated with use of oral and parenteral non-steroidal anti-inflammation drugs (NSAIDs): a case-crossover study of Taiwan's National Health Insurance claims database and review of current evidence. BMC Cardiovasc Disord. 2012;12:4.
47. Kontovazenitis PI, Starantzis KA, Soucacos PN. Major complication following minor outpatient procedure: osteonecrosis of the knee after intraarticular injection of cortisone for treatment of knee arthritis. J Surg Orthop Adv. 2009;18:42–4.
48. McCarty DJ, McCarthy G, Carrera G. Intraarticular corticosteroids possibly leading to local osteonecrosis and marrow fat induced synovitis. J Rheumatol. 1991;18:1091–4.
49. Doss A. Non surgical repair of tendon, Cartilage & Neurogenic Conditions - a paradigm shift in musculoskeletal medicine and pain management by percutaneous regenerative intervention (Orthopaedics mini review). EC Orthopaedics. 2015;2(5): 159–67.
50. Glade MJ, Krook L, Schryver HF, Hintz HF. Calcium metabolism in glucocorticoid-treated pony foals. J Nutr. 1982;112:77–86.
51. Glade MJ, Krook L, Schryver HF, Hintz HF. Morphologic and biochemical changes in cartilage of foals treated with dexamethasone. Cornell Vet. 1983;73:170–92.
52. Coombes BK, Bisset L, Vicenzino B. Efficacy and safety of corticosteroid injections and other injections for management of tendinopathy: a systematic review of randomised controlled trials. Lancet. 2010;376:1751–67.
53. MacMahon PJ, Eustace SJ, Kavanagh EC. Injectable corticosteroid and local anesthetic preparations: a review for radiologists. Radiology. 2009;252: 647–61.
54. Habib GS. Systemic effects of intra-articular corticosteroids. Clin Rheumatol. 2009;28:749–56.

55. Tehranzadeh J, Booya F, Root J. Cartilage metabolism in osteoarthritis and the influence of viscosupplementation and steroid: a review. Acta Radiol. 2005;46:288–96.
56. Igarashi M, Sakamoto K, Nagaoka I. Effect of glucosamine on expression of type II collagen, matrix metalloproteinase and sirtuin genes in a human chondrocyte cell line. Int J Mol Med. 2017;39:472–8.
57. Momomura R, Naito K, Igarashi M, Watari T, Terakado A, Oike S, Sakamoto K, Nagaoka I, Kaneko K. Evaluation of the effect of glucosamine administration on biomarkers of cartilage and bone metabolism in bicycle racers. Mol Med Rep. 2013;7:742–6.
58. Yoshimura M, Sakamoto K, Tsuruta A, Yamamoto T, Ishida K, Yamaguchi H, Nagaoka I. Evaluation of the effect of glucosamine administration on biomarkers for cartilage and bone metabolism in soccer players. Int J Mol Med. 2009;24:487–94.
59. Saengnipanthkul S, Waikakul S, Rojanasthien S, Totemchokchyakarn K, Srinkapaibulaya A, Cheh Chin T, Mai Hong N, Bruyere O, Cooper C, Reginster JY, Lwin M. Differentiation of patented crystalline glucosamine sulfate from other glucosamine preparations will optimize osteoarthritis treatment. Int J Rheum Dis. 2017. Epub: PMID: 28332780. https://doi.org/10.1111/1756-185X.13068
60. Reginster JY, Deroisy R, Rovati LC, Lee RL, Lejeune E, Bruyere O, Giacovelli G, Henrotin Y, Dacre JE, Gossett C. Long-term effects of glucosamine sulphate on osteoarthritis progression: a randomised, placebo-controlled clinical trial. Lancet. 2001;357:251–6.
61. Kahan A, Uebelhart D, De Vathaire F, Delmas PD, Reginster JY. Long-term effects of chondroitins 4 and 6 sulfate on knee osteoarthritis: the study on osteoarthritis progression prevention, a two-year, randomized, double-blind, placebo-controlled trial. Arthritis Rheum. 2009;60:524–33.
62. Matheson AJ, Perry CM. Glucosamine: a review of its use in the management of osteoarthritis. Drugs Aging. 2003;20:1041–60.
63. Houpt JB, McMillan R, Wein C, Paget-Dellio SD. Effect of glucosamine hydrochloride in the treatment of pain of osteoarthritis of the knee. J Rheumatol. 1999;26:2423–30.
64. Vlad SC, LaValley MP, McAlindon TE, Felson DT. Glucosamine for pain in osteoarthritis: why do trial results differ? Arthritis Rheum. 2007;56:2267–77.
65. Clegg DO, Reda DJ, Harris CL, Klein MA, O'Dell JR, Hooper MM, Bradley JD, Bingham CO 3rd, Weisman MH, Jackson CG, Lane NE, Cush JJ, Moreland LW, Schumacher HR Jr, Oddis CV, Wolfe F, Molitor JA, Yocum DE, Schnitzer TJ, Furst DE, Sawitzke AD, Shi H, Brandt KD, Moskowitz RW, Williams HJ. Glucosamine, chondroitin sulfate, and the two in combination for painful knee osteoarthritis. N Engl J Med. 2006;354:795–808.
66. Reichenbach S, Sterchi R, Scherer M, Trelle S, Burgi E, Burgi U, Dieppe PA, Juni P. Meta-analysis: chondroitin for osteoarthritis of the knee or hip. Ann Intern Med. 2007;146:580–90.
67. Forsyth RK, Brigden CV, Northrop AJ. Double blind investigation of the effects of oral supplementation of combined glucosamine hydrochloride (GHCL) and chondroitin sulphate (CS) on stride characteristics of veteran horses. Equine Vet J Suppl. 2006;38:622–5.
68. Frisbie DD, McIlwraith CW, Kawcak CE, Werpy NM. Evaluation of intra-articular hyaluronan, sodium chondroitin sulfate and N-acetyl-D-glucosamine combination versus saline (0.9% NaCl) for osteoarthritis using an equine model. Vet J. 2013;197:824–9.
69. Aviad AD, Houpt JB. The molecular weight of therapeutic hyaluronan (sodium hyaluronate): how significant is it? J Rheumatol. 1994;21:297–301.
70. Altman R, Bedi A, Manjoo A, Niazi F, Shaw P, et al. Anti-inflammatory effects of intra-articular hyaluronic acid: a systematic review. Cartilage. 2019;10(1):43–52.
71. Moreland LW. Intra-articular hyaluronan (hyaluronic acid) and hylans for the treatment of osteoarthritis: mechanisms of action. Arthritis Res Ther. 2003;5:54–67.
72. Asari A, Miyauchi S, Matsuzaka S, Ito T, Kominami E, Uchiyama Y. Molecular weight-dependent effects of hyaluronate on the arthritic synovium. Arch Histol Cytol. 1998;61:125–35.
73. Abrams GD, Frank RM, Fortier LA, Cole BJ. Platelet-rich plasma for articular cartilage repair. Sports Med Arthrosc Rev. 2013;21:213–9.
74. PI W, Diaz R, Borg-Stein J. Platelet-rich plasma. Phys Med Rehabil Clin N Am. 2016;27:825–53.
75. Ferrari M, Zia S, Valbonesi M, Henriquet F, Venere G, Spagnolo S, Grasso MA, Panzani I. A new technique for hemodilution, preparation of autologous platelet-rich plasma and intraoperative blood salvage in cardiac surgery. Int J Artif Organs. 1987;10(1):47–50.
76. Bendinelli P, Matteucci E, Dogliotti G, Corsi MM, Banfi G, Maroni P, Desiderio MA. Molecular basis of anti-inflammatory action of platelet-rich plasma on human chondrocytes: mechanisms of NF-kappaB inhibition via HGF. J Cell Physiol. 2010;225:757–66.
77. Sundman EA, Cole BJ, Karas V, Della Valle C, Tetreault MW, Mohammed HO, Fortier LA. The anti-inflammatory and matrix restorative mechanisms of platelet-rich plasma in osteoarthritis. Am J Sports Med. 2014;42:35–41.
78. Vannini F, Di Matteo B, Filardo G. Platelet-rich plasma to treat ankle cartilage pathology - from translational potential to clinical evidence: a systematic review. J Exp Orthop. 2015;2:2.
79. Akeda K, An HS, Okuma M, Attawia M, Miyamoto K, Thonar EJ, Lenz ME, Sah RL, Masuda K. Platelet-

rich plasma stimulates porcine articular chondrocyte proliferation and matrix biosynthesis. Osteoarthritis Cartilage. 2006;14:1272–80.
80. Filardo G, Kon E, Roffi A, Di Matteo B, Merli ML, Marcacci M. Platelet-rich plasma: why intra-articular? A systematic review of preclinical studies and clinical evidence on PRP for joint degeneration. Knee Surg Sports Traumatol Arthrosc. 2015;23:2459–74.
81. Mascarenhas R, Saltzman BM, Fortier LA, Cole BJ. Role of platelet-rich plasma in articular cartilage injury and disease. J Knee Surg. 2015;28:3–10.
82. Metcalf KB, Mandelbaum BR, McIlwraith CW. Application of platelet-rich plasma to disorders of the knee joint. Cartilage. 2013;4:295–312.
83. Mishra A, Tummala P, King A, Lee B, Kraus M, Tse V, Jacobs CR. Buffered platelet-rich plasma enhances mesenchymal stem cell proliferation and chondrogenic differentiation, tissue engineering part C. Methods. 2009;15:431–5.
84. Spreafico A, Chellini F, Frediani B, Bernardini G, Niccolini S, Serchi T, Collodel G, Paffetti A, Fossombroni V, Galeazzi M, Marcolongo R, Santucci A. Biochemical investigation of the effects of human platelet releasates on human articular chondrocytes. J Cell Biochem. 2009;108:1153–65.
85. Sakata R, McNary SM, Miyatake K, Lee CA, Van den Bogaerde JM, Marder RA, Reddi AH. Stimulation of the superficial zone protein and lubrication in the articular cartilage by human platelet-rich plasma. Am J Sports Med. 2015;43:1467–73.
86. Park SI, Lee HR, Kim S, Ahn MW, Do SH. Time-sequential modulation in expression of growth factors from platelet-rich plasma (PRP) on the chondrocyte cultures. Mol Cell Biochem. 2012;361:9–17.
87. Fallouh L, Nakagawa K, Sasho T, Arai M, Kitahara S, Wada Y, Moriya H, Takahashi K. Effects of autologous platelet-rich plasma on cell viability and collagen synthesis in injured human anterior cruciate ligament. J Bone Joint Surg Am. 2010;92:2909–16.
88. Kon E, Buda R, Filardo G, Di Martino A, Timoncini A, Cenacchi A, Fornasari PM, Giannini S, Marcacci M. Platelet-rich plasma: intra-articular knee injections produced favorable results on degenerative cartilage lesions. Knee Surg, Sports Traumatol, Arthrosc. 2010;18:472–9.
89. Campbell KA, Saltzman BM, Mascarenhas R, Khair MM, Verma NN, Bach BR Jr, Cole BJ. Does intra-articular platelet-rich plasma injection provide clinically superior outcomes compared with other therapies in the treatment of knee osteoarthritis? A systematic review of overlapping meta-analyses. Arthroscopy. 2015;31:2213–21.
90. Filardo G, Kon E, Buda R, Timoncini A, Di Martino A, Cenacchi A, Fornasari PM, Giannini S, Marcacci M. Platelet-rich plasma intra-articular knee injections for the treatment of degenerative cartilage lesions and osteoarthritis. Knee Surg Sports Traumatol Arthrosc. 2011;19:528–35.
91. Sucuoğlu H, Üstünsoy S. The short-term effect of PRP on chronic pain in knee osteoarthritis. Agri. 2019;31(2):63–9.
92. Jayabalan P, Hagerty S, Cortazzo MH. The use of platelet-rich plasma for the treatment of osteoarthritis. Phys Sportsmed. 2014;42:53–62.
93. Raeissadat SA, Rayegani SM, Hassanabadi H, Fathi M, Ghorbani E, Babaee M, Azma K. Knee osteoarthritis injection choices: platelet- rich plasma (PRP) versus hyaluronic acid (a one-year randomized clinical trial). Clin Med Insights Arthritis Musculoskelet Disord. 2015;8:1–8.
94. Kon E, Mandelbaum B, Buda R, Filardo G, Delcogliano M, Timoncini A, Fornasari PM, Giannini S, Marcacci M. Platelet-rich plasma intra-articular injection versus hyaluronic acid viscosupplementation as treatments for cartilage pathology: from early degeneration to osteoarthritis. Arthroscopy. 2011;27:1490–501.
95. Di Martino A, Di Matteo B, Papio T, Tentoni F, Selleri F, et al. Platelet-rich plasma versus hyaluronic acid injections for the treatment of knee osteoarthritis: results at 5 years of a double-blind, randomized controlled trial. Am J Sports Med. 2019;47(2):347–54.
96. Papalia R, Zampogna B, Russo F, Vasta S, Tirindelli MC, Nobile C, Di Martino AC, Vadala G, Denaro V. Comparing hybrid hyaluronic acid with PRP in end career athletes with degenerative cartilage lesions of the knee. J Biol Regul Homeost Agents. 2016;30:17–23.
97. Filardo G, Di Matteo B, Di Martino A, Merli ML, Cenacchi A, Fornasari P, Marcacci M, Kon E. Platelet-rich plasma intra-articular knee injections show no superiority versus Viscosupplementation: a randomized controlled trial. Am J Sports Med. 2015;43:1575–82.
98. Filardo G, Kon E, Di Martino A, Di Matteo B, Merli ML, Cenacchi A, Fornasari PM, Marcacci M. Platelet-rich plasma vs hyaluronic acid to treat knee degenerative pathology: study design and preliminary results of a randomized controlled trial. BMC Musculoskelet Disord. 2012;13:229.
99. Kon E, Filardo G, Drobnic M, Madry H, Jelic M, van Dijk N, Della Villa S. Non-surgical management of early knee osteoarthritis. Knee Surg Sports Traumatol Arthrosc. 2012;20:436–49.
100. LaPrade RF, Swiontkowski MF. New horizons in the treatment of osteoarthritis of the knee. JAMA. 1999;281:876–8.
101. Campbell KA, Erickson BJ, Saltzman BM, Mascarenhas R, Bach BR Jr, Cole BJ, Verma NN. Is local Viscosupplementation injection clinically superior to other therapies in the treatment of osteoarthritis of the knee: a systematic review of overlapping meta-analyses. Arthroscopy. 2015;31:2036–45. e2014

102. Askari A, Gholami T, NaghiZadeh MM, Farjam M, Kouhpayeh SA, Shahabfard Z. Hyaluronic acid compared with corticosteroid injections for the treatment of osteoarthritis of the knee: a randomized control trail. Springerplus. 2016;5:442.
103. Balazs EA. Analgesic effect of elastoviscous hyaluronan solutions and the treatment of arthritic pain. Cells Tissues Organs. 2003;174:49–62.
104. Barakat AS, Ibrahim NM, Elghobashy O, Sultan AM, Abdel-Kader KFM. Prevention of post-traumatic osteoarthritis after intra-articular knee fractures using hyaluronic acid: a randomized prospective pilot study. Int Orthop. 2019. https://doi.org/10.1007/s00264-019-04360-8. [Epub ahead of print]
105. Bellamy N, Campbell J, Robinson V, Gee T, Bourne R, Wells G. Viscosupplementation for the treatment of osteoarthritis of the knee. Cochrane Database Syst Rev. 2006; CD005321.
106. Bellamy N, Campbell J, Robinson V, Gee T, Bourne R, Wells G. Intraarticular corticosteroid for treatment of osteoarthritis of the knee. Cochrane Database Syst Rev. 2006; CD005328.
107. Mei-Dan O, Carmont MR, Laver L, Mann G, Maffulli N, Nyska M. Platelet-rich plasma or hyaluronate in the management of osteochondral lesions of the talus. Am J Sports Med. 2012;40:534–41.
108. Shen L, Yuan T, Chen S, Xie X, Zhang C. The temporal effect of platelet-rich plasma on pain and physical function in the treatment of knee osteoarthritis: systematic review and meta-analysis of randomized controlled trials. J Orthop Surg Res. 2017;12:16.
109. Goncars V, Kalnberzs K, Jakobsons E, Enĝele I, Briede I, et al. Treatment of knee osteoarthritis with bone marrow-derived mononuclear cell injection: 12-month follow-up. Cartilage. 2019;10(1):26–35.
110. Hannon CP, Yanke AB, Farr J. Amniotic tissue modulation of knee pain-a focus on osteoarthritis. J Knee Surg. 2019;32(1):26–36.
111. Chahal J, Gómez-Aristizábal A, Shestopaloff K, Bhatt S, Chaboureau A, et al. Bone marrow mesenchymal stromal cell treatment in patients with osteoarthritis results in overall improvement in pain and symptoms and reduces synovial inflammation. Stem Cells Transl Med. 2019;8(8):746–57.
112. Leslie M. Knee osteoarthritis management therapies. Pain Manag Nurs. 2000;1:51–7.
113. Henrotin Y, Lambert C, Couchourel D, Ripoll C, Chiotelli E. Nutraceuticals: do they represent a new era in the management of osteoarthritis? – a narrative review from the lessons taken with five products. Osteoarthritis Cartilage. 2011;19:1–21.

Part V

Repair of Knee Articular Cartilage: Surgical Approaches

10 Osteochondritis Dissecans of the Knee: Pathophysiology and Treatment

Charles A. Popkin

10.1 Introduction

Osteochondritis dissecans (OCD) is a poorly understood localized process involving injury to the subchondral bone, which can progress to destabilization of the overlying articular cartilage [1, 2]. This condition is currently seen with increased frequency, possibly because of the rapid rise in younger athletes participating in competitive sports and the increased use of magnetic resonance imaging (MRI) [3]. The incidence of OCD has been estimated to be between 0.02% and 0.03% by radiography and as high as 1.2% by arthroscopy [4, 5]. Prevalence of this condition ranges between 0.01% and 0.06% in European and North American populations [6]. The literature reveals that this condition affects males more commonly than females with ratios as high as 2:1 [7, 8]. A population-based study of 302 individuals diagnosed with knee OCD lesions showed the highest incidence for both males and females occurs between the ages 11 and 15 years [9]. Among 122 adult patients with a total of 124 lesions, knee OCD was 3.6 times higher for men than women [10]. Females with patellar lesions and unstable lesions are at risk for persistent knee pain [11]. OCD involves both knees in 15–30% of cases, making assessment of the contralateral knee an important part of the evaluation [7]. In Aichroth's classic paper, the most common location of an OCD lesion was in the posterolateral aspect of the medial femoral condyle (MFC) (69%) [12]. The lateral femoral condyle (LFC) was involved in 15% of the lesions and the patella in 5%. A subsequent large European study reported on location in 509 knees (318 juvenile, 191 adults) and found a slightly different breakdown of OCD lesion location [7]. The classic location on the lateral aspect of the MFC remained the most common; however, it was involved only 51% of the time, whereas the LFC was 16.5%, and the patella was 6.5%.

Osteochondritis dissecans resulting from osteonecrosis of subchondral bone was first described by Ambroise Pare in 1558 after finding loose bodies in a patient's knee. Paget named the process "quiet necrosis" when describing two patients with knee pain in 1870 [13, 14]. Osteochondritis means an inflammation of the osteochondral joint surface. The Latin word "dissecans" means to separate. From 1887 to 1888, Konig was given credit for his theory that the loose bodies resulted from a combination of trauma acting on the necrotic lesion underneath.

The author has nothing to disclose.

C.A. Popkin, MD (✉)
Orthopedic Surgery and Sports Medicine, Columbia University Medical Center, New York, NY, USA

Department of Orthopedic Surgery, Sports Medicine Center for the Developing Athlete, Presbyterian Morgan Stanley Children's Hospital, New York, NY, USA
e-mail: cp2654@cumc.columbia.edu

H. K. Gahunia et al. (eds.), *Articular Cartilage of the Knee*,
https://doi.org/10.1007/978-1-4939-7587-7_10

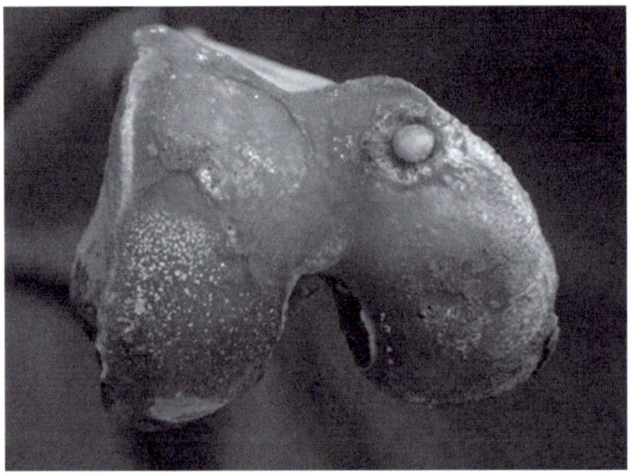

Fig. 10.1 Right femoral osteochondritis dissecans lesion in a 4000-year-old mummy (middle-aged female) from Northern Chile (Reprinted with permission from Kothari et al. [17])

The term "osteochondritis dissecans" was first coined in the late 1880s by König [15]. Subsequent study of OCD since König's paper has not confirmed inflammation to be a cause of this condition [16]. Nevertheless, the misnomer "osteochondritis dissecans" has persisted in the literature.

There is evidence of OCD involving both knees in a 4000-year-old female mummy found in Northern Chile [17] (Fig. 10.1). Despite afflicting knees for thousands of years and being a recognized disease entity in the medical literature for over 120 years, there remain considerable debate and no clear consensus as to the etiology of OCD. There are many theories, which can be broadly grouped into hereditary, vascular, and traumatic causes [18, 19]. None of these theories are universally accepted and none to date has completely explained all OCD lesions [20].

Numerous predispositions to OCD have been identified in the literature. A recent systematic review of the knee OCD literature performed on the PubMed and Cochrane databases (86 studies) suggested that the etiology of OCD could be of biological or mechanical origin [21]. The biological hypothesis (40 articles) included genetic causes, ossification center deficit, and endocrine disorders, whereas the mechanical hypothesis (52 articles) included injury/overuse, tibial spine impingement, discoid meniscus, and biomechanical alterations as the cause of the onset of OCD. These biological and mechanical factors were found to result in subchondral bone remodeling alterations, acting independently or more likely synergically in the onset and progression of knee OCD.

Associations with a subgroup of multiple epiphyseal dysplasia was first reported in 1955 [22]. Two additional studies have confirmed a familial pattern of OCD associated with short stature and early osteoarthritis (OA) [23, 24]. A retrospective study on a heterogeneous cohort of pediatric patients treated for OCD (N = 103) showed that the proportion of patients with a positive family history of OCD was 14% [25]. However, a study by Petrie of 34 patients with radiographic evidence of OCD of the knee showed only 1 case of an OCD identified by clinical and radiographic examinations of 86 first-degree relatives [26]. Despite the work by Petrie, subsequent studies have found an association of OCD with an assortment of conditions including short stature [27], Stickler syndrome [28, 29], Osgood-Schlatter disease [7], juvenile idiopathic arthritis [30], and tibia vara [2].

There is also some evidence that accessory femoral ossification centers may play a role in the etiology of OCD. Caffey et al. found that 66% of boys and 41% of girls had abnormalities in ossification of the distal femur [31]. They postulated that the cause of the abnormal ossification occurred during periods of rapid growth at the distal femur when the process of cartilage proliferation and provisional calcification is uncoupled. These lesions are usually not pathologic and resolve without any sequelae. However, other authors have advocated that these areas of abnormalities may be precursor lesions and break away from the epiphysis [22, 26].

A vascular etiology has also been postulated as a cause for OCD. Several prominent historical figures in orthopedics have advocated an ischemic cause for OCD lesions including Ficat and Paget [2, 21]. Enneking and Dunham attributed OCD formation to insufficiency of the end arterial blood supply to the subchondral bone, with weak contributing anastamoses from the surrounding vessels [32]. Proponents of the vascular theory reference a cadaveric study from Atlanta that identified a potential watershed area with diminished intraosseous and extraosseous blood supply to the medial femoral condyle [33]. In addition, several authors have tried to prove a vascular cause using histologic studies. Unfortunately, many of the studies using histology were hampered by some significant limitations. Small sample size [34], no reporting on the location of the specimen from within the OCD lesions [35], reporting on histology of only the loose fragment and not the underlying (basal) side [36], and the substantial variety in physeal status of the samples may help explain the wide array of histologic results. For example, one report demonstrated no histopathologic evidence for necrosis in completely detached lesions [37]. In contrast, Linden and Telhag performed a histologic study on 14 adult patients with OCD, and evidence of scattered ischemic necrosis was found in all specimens with more involvement on the detached side of the OCD than the base [38]. Uozomi et al., in their histologic study taken from 11 classically located OCD lesions harvested with an osteochondral autograft transplantation (OATS, Arthrex™, Naples, FL), found evidence of ischemic subchondral necrosis in only 2 of the specimens [34]. It is unclear from the current body of literature if ischemia is the cause of OCD or the result of the healing and remodeling process.

Recently, Kessler et al. investigated the association of childhood obesity with OCD of the knee in a population-based cohort of 269 children and adolescents [39]. Based on the body mass index (BMI) for age, each patient in the cohort was grouped under one of the five weight classes (underweight, normal weight, overweight, moderately obese, and extremely obese). Results showed that extreme obesity strongly associated with an increased risk of OCD overall (knee, elbow, and ankle) and moderately obese patients had a 1.8 times increased risk of knee OCD as compared to children with normal weight. Patients with OCD were found to have a significantly greater average BMI when compared with patients without OCD.

Traumatic injury has been reported in up to 40% of patients with a diagnosis of OCD [2]. It has been suggested by many authors that repetitive microtrauma may be responsible for shear forces and a stress reaction of the underlying bone seen with many OCD lesions [19]. Fairbank championed a model of repetitive microtrauma resulting from the tibial spine impinging on the lateral aspect of MFC with internal rotation [40]. This idea has been supported by a biomechanical study that showed the lateral aspect of the MFC receives a significant amount of shear forces when the knee is flexed, internally rotated and loaded [41]. While this may account for OCD lesions seen in the most common location (lateral aspect of the MFC), it does not account for OCD lesions seen elsewhere in the knee. However, another study highlighted a relationship between the mechanical axis and the location of OCD in the knee [6]. Medial lesions were seen with varus alignment and lateral lesions with valgus alignment. This suggests abnormal alignment may be a possible factor in the development of OCD lesions and may help explain those lesions in the atypical lateral location (valgus alignment).

Additional work since Fairbank's article has highlighted the relationship between athletic participation and the development of OCD lesions in the knee. Aichroth's study showed that more than 60% of OCD lesions developed in patients who participated in a high level of sports [12]. A multicenter study from Europe demonstrated that close to 55% of patients with an OCD lesion were active in sports or participated in strenuous athletic activity [7]. While there is no definite answer, there is a growing consensus that repetitive microtrauma plays a fundamental role in the pathophysiology of this condition.

10.2 Clinical Presentation

Initial presentation of the OCD lesion traditionally consists of nonspecific knee pain, often made worse with activity. If the OCD is unstable, mechanical symptoms, giving-way episodes, and recurrent effusions are commonly noted. The patients may ambulate with an externally rotated gait. On physical exam, there may be an effusion and point tenderness over the involved condyle. The classic physical examination maneuver is Wilson's test, which aims to impinge the tibial spine on the OCD lesion located in the classic position on the lateral aspect of the MFC [42]. This is performed with internal rotation of the involved knee while extending the knee from 90 degrees of flexion. The pain is relieved when the same motion is performed with the knee externally rotated. Though helpful when present, this physical sign lacks sufficient sensitivity and specificity to be of significant value in the diagnosis of OCD. However, some authors recommend using Wilson's test to monitor clinical response to treatment [43].

10.3 Classification and Diagnostic Imaging

Classification systems in orthopedics serve three essential purposes [44]. The first is to describe lesions or injuries so they can be divided into various groups. Once the various groups are established, a good classification system will use these different groups to guide clinical treatment choices. Finally, and most importantly, a good classification system will help the clinician predict clinical outcome. This can allow the orthopedist at the time the lesion is recognized to counsel patients regarding the expected outcome. Significant time and effort over the years have been spent attempting to classify OCD lesions. Outcomes in the orthopedic literature for OCD have identified two significant prognostic factors: patient's skeletal maturity and lesion stability. Also, lesion size has been identified as an important factor [45, 46]. Smillie described the first classification system; and, distinguished two main types, juvenile and adult [47]. Since this designation, other authors have added adolescent as a subtype [48, 49]. This has been added because the outcomes for adolescents with closing physes are not as promising as younger children but better than adults with closed physes. A more accurate assessment of the patient's physeal status can significantly alter the expected outcome.

Conventional radiographs allow for determination of location and the size of the lesion, as well as assessment of the skeletal maturity of the patient. Radiographic evaluation of patients with suspected OCD should include anteroposterior (AP), lateral, tunnel, and Merchant views. The tunnel view allows improved visualization of the posterior femoral condyle, as it is brought into view with increased knee flexion. The Merchant view provides visualization of the femoral trochlea, an uncommon but potentially problematic location for OCD lesions.

Smillie's classification for OCD was based upon plain radiographs and expanded by Cahill and Berg in 1983 [50]. In this classification system, OCD lesions are localized using 15 distinct zones based on an alphanumeric assignment (Fig. 10.2). On the AP radiograph, the zones are numbered 1 through 5 medial to lateral across the knee (Fig. 10.2a). On the lateral radiograph, Blumensaat's line and the posterior cortical line are used to divide the knee into three zones assigned letters A to C: A is anterior, B is central, and C is assigned to posteriorly located lesions (Fig. 10.2b). The classic lesion in the knee is a 2B. This classification is primarily used for research and has not found regular use in the clinical setting.

Perilesional sclerosis has been identified as a prognostic indicator in evaluating OCD lesions on radiographs [51]. In this study, OCD lesions were staged as follows: Stage 0, if there was no evidence of perilesional sclerosis on either AP or lateral radiograph; Stage 1, if there was a rim of sclerosis on either AP or lateral radiograph; and Stage II, if there was a perifocal ring of sclerosis visible on both radiographic views around the OCD. The authors grouped the patients by age (years): 12 years or younger (juvenile), 12 to 15 years (adolescent), and 15 years or older. They found that OCD lesions without perilesional sclerosis healed in all cases. Stage I and II lesions that received drilling healed more reliably than Stage I and II lesions treated conservatively. Finally, children younger than 12 years did better than those aged 15 years or older. Radiographs provide important

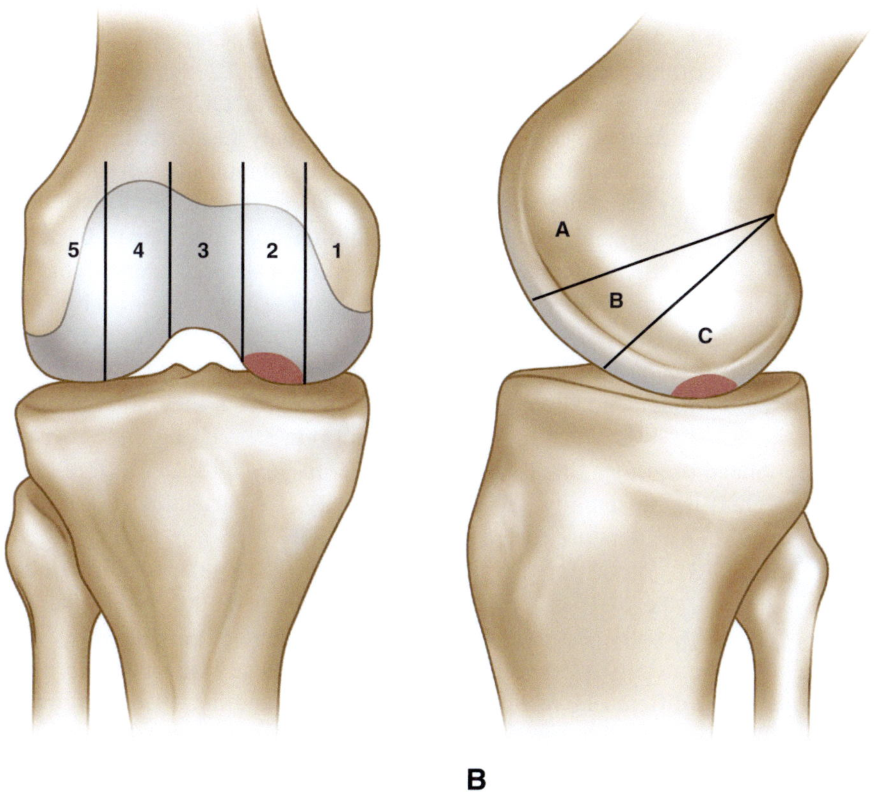

Fig. 10.2 Schematic diagram of Cahill and Berg's classification for anatomic location of the osteochondritis dissecans knee lesions seen on the (**a**) Anteroposterior and (**b**) Lateral view [50]

information about OCD lesion location, size, and the presence or absence of sclerosis. However, for treatment recommendations, additional advanced imaging is necessary to make more informed decisions about lesion prognosis [4]. Although recent advances in ultrasound technology qualifies it as an appropriate tool for the screening and monitoring of OCD's stages II to IV, ultrasonic examination has limitations in assessing the OCD stage 1; hence, is not suitable for evaluating the early stage of OCD [52].

Bone scintigraphy was initially utilized quite extensively in the diagnosis and determination of appropriate treatment of OCD lesions by many authors [50, 53]. However, bone scan provides no information about the overlying articular cartilage. In addition, the significant overlap of findings with stable and unstable lesions made routine bone scan unreliable in guiding clinical decisions.

Magnetic resonance imaging is now the advanced imaging modality of choice used to confirm the presence of an OCD lesion and to assess its stability. Patient demographics, clinical presentation, and the role of trauma are critical for differential diagnosis of osteochondral (OC) defect, which can develop from acute traumatic injury or as an end result of several chronic conditions. The MRI features of OC defect include the location and extent of bone marrow edema, the presence of a fracture line, deformity of the subchondral bone plate, and a hypointense area subjacent to the subchondral bone plate [18, 54]. The characteristic MRI features of OCD lesions with a subchondral region demarcated from the surrounding bone reveal a laminar or "double-line sign" at the demarcation, which is typical of avascular necrosis or findings of instability and often seen with cyst-like foci in the subchondral bone and bone marrow edema pattern on proton density- or T2-weighted images [54, 55]. As mentioned above, stability is an important prognostic factor for determining the likelihood of an OCD lesion to heal with nonoperative therapy [3, 46, 56]. There are four criteria on T2 - weighted images that have been described by De Smet and colleagues as correlating with instability found at arthroscopy [57, 58]. These MRI criteria include a high-signal-intensity rim surrounding an OCD lesion, a high-signal-intensity fracture line extending through the articular cartilage, and a defect in the articular cartilage and subchondral cysts.

Despite the continued use of De Smet's criteria in determining OCD lesion stability, there is no apparent consensus in the literature regarding the most appropriate MRI criteria for defining OCD instability. Further, the MRI criteria for OCD instability in the pediatric knee do not always correlate with the necessity for surgery [59–61]. The widespread differences of opinion in the literature regarding the most appropriate MRI criteria for OCD instability may relate to a lack of distinction in the De Smet study between adult, adolescent, and juvenile forms of OCD. In their initial study, the majority of the patients were adults.

Several authors have reported that the initial De Smet criteria may not be applicable to juvenile patients. O'Connor et al. reported that a high-signal T2 line (one of the four De Smet criteria) was a predictor of instability in the juvenile lesions only when it was accompanied by a break in the cartilage that could be detected on T1-weighted images [62]. Using this modification, the ability of the MRI to predict instability verified at arthroscopy jumped from 45 to 85%. Samora et al. also found that MRI frequently overcalled instability not confirmed arthroscopically in juvenile patients [63]. Similarly, Yoshida et al. found a very high rate of healing of OCD lesions treated conservatively despite the presence of a high-signal T2 line [64].

In an attempt to improve accuracy in predicting instability in juvenile OCD patients, revised criteria have been established. Kijowski et al., in a study of 32 skeletally immature patients (25 boys and 7 girls; mean age, 14 years) utilizing arthroscopy as the reference standard, found that the presence of T2 signal intensity rim or cysts surrounding an OCD lesion may be signs of instability only in adults [65]. In their study, a high T2 signal intensity rim surrounding an OCD lesion indicated instability only if it had the same signal intensity as adjacent joint fluid, was surrounded by a second outer rim of low T2 signal intensity, or was accompanied by multiple breaks in the subchondral bone plate. Cysts surrounding a juvenile OCD lesion were indicative of instability only if they were multiple or large (> 5 mm) in size. Using these revised secondary criteria in juvenile OCD, the sensitivity and specificity for detecting instability increased substantially.

Despite the popularity of the De Smet criteria and Kijowski's modifications, there is no apparent consensus in the literature regarding the most appropriate MR imaging criteria for defining OCD instability. The widespread difference of opinion may relate to a lack of distinction between the juvenile and adult forms of OCD and due to the potentially different imaging features of stability/instability seen between juvenile and adult forms of the disease. The use of a 3 Tesla (T) magnet can enhance resolution and potentially increase diagnostic accuracy. In addition, T2 mapping and the use of delayed gadolinium-enhanced magnetic resonance imaging of cartilage (dGEMRIC) hold promise in being able to assess OCD lesion instability as well as document healing of these lesions. At this time, the utility of either a 3T magnet or dGEMRIC imaging in evaluating OCD lesions is uncertain.

Arthroscopy remains the gold standard for confirming OCD lesion instability with direct visualization. The Guhl classification is useful for communicating not only lesion stability but also integrity of the overlying articular cartilage [66]. A similar arthroscopic classification system is also used in the literature, the Ewing and Voto [67]. Both classification systems are in four stages (Table 10.1). It should be noted that arthroscopic assessment should not be limited to either of these classification systems alone. The OCD lesion size

Table 10.1 Arthroscopic classification systems for osteochondritis dissecans lesions of the knee. (*A*) Guhl and (*B*) Ewing and Voto classification

Stage	Arthroscopic Finding of OCD Lesions
Guhl Arthroscopic Classification System [66]	
Type I	Softening without breach of the cartilage surface
Type II	Breached cartilage that is stable
Type III	A flap lesion
Type IV	Loose body
Ewing and Voto Arthroscopic Classification System [67]	
Stage I	Intact lesion
Stage II	Early cartilage separation
Stage III	Partially attached lesion
Stage IV	Crater lesion-loose body

and location, number of loose bodies, bone presence on the back side of the loose fragment, lesion repairability, donor site condition, and overall condition of the surrounding non-OCD cartilage should be documented.

10.4 Natural History of Osteochondritis Dissecans

At this time, very little is known about the natural history of OCD. In addition, there are no randomized control trials looking at nonsurgical versus surgical management of OCD involving the knee. The only randomized control trial to date involving any aspect of the treatment for OCD in the knee was done in Lithuania and reported in 2009 [68]. This study compared microfracture (MFX) with mosaic-type OAT for OCD lesions in the femoral condyles of patients under 18 years of age. Using International Cartilage Repair Society (ICRS) score, return to play (RTP), and MRI, the authors concluded that OATS had superior results. These authors had conducted a previous randomized control trial in 2005, but this included OC defects and OCD lesions together in patients younger than 40 years of age [69]. Unfortunately, surgical intervention to date for OCD lesions is heavily based on recommendations from many Level IV retrospective studies, case series, and reports. Complicating the interpretation is the fact that many studies do not differentiate juvenile from adult and present a wide range of indications for surgery. At this time in reviewing the best available literature, a few keys facts remain clear: young patients with wide open physes have the best prognosis. Those patients with closed physes, unstable lesions, or large lesions ($> \cong 2$–$3\ cm^2$) are all poor prognostic factors and likely to require surgical intervention [7, 45].

A large, multicentered review from the European Paediatric Orthopaedic Society (EPOS) reported findings on 509 knees and reached some noteworthy findings. Outcome is better if there is no evidence of instability at initial diagnosis. Pain and swelling are not good predictors of instability; results depend on the location of the lesion; and those lesions in the classic position on the lateral aspect of the MFC have the best outcome. Nonathletic patients have a better outcome than their athletic counterparts; and lesions larger than 2 cm have a worse prognosis [7].

The American Academy of Orthopedic Surgeons (AAOS) published guidelines on the treatment of OCD lesions in Journal of the American Academy of Orthopedic Surgeons (JAAOS) in 2011 [70]. Not surprisingly, this systematic review of the literature on diagnosis and treatment of OCD lesions was not able to generate one recommendation that received a strong grade. In fact, based on the available literature, the group was only able to reach consensus on 4 of 16 recommendations reviewed. They agreed on the following: symptomatic skeletally mature and immature patients with salvageable unstable and/or displaced lesions should be offered surgery; physical therapy should be recommended after surgery to treat OCD lesions; finally, they reached agreement that in the absence of reliable evidence, patients remaining symptomatic after treatment for OCD lesions undergo history, physical examination, radiographs, and/or MRI to assess healing.

10.5 Treatment of Osteochondritis Dissecans

Care must be taken to review the imaging for the OCD lesion's size, location, and stability [1]. In addition, the status of the growth plate is critical for making initial management decision for the patient with an OCD. Nonoperative treatment, with an emphasis on activity modification, is an appropriate initial treatment in a stable lesion in a juvenile or adolescent with an open physis [71]. Whether or not to include immobilization, and for how long, is open to considerable debate. There are two schools of thought concerning nonoperative management. Those that favor protecting the subchondral bone argue that the lesion should be treated like a fracture and immobilized. This can be in a long leg or cylinder cast [45]. However, after careful review of the literature, the duration and weight-bearing status for immobilization are not certain. The other school of thought embraces Salter's concepts of continuous motion to preserve articular cartilage and, thus, favors a treatment protocol geared toward maintaining motion and cartilage health. At this time, there is no consensus in the literature, and nonoperative protocols and recommendations vary from casting to a standard knee immobilizer to custom unloader knee braces or as little as restricting only sports participation [3]. This substantial variation in treatments makes the interpretation of the results in the literature difficult.

Although OCD has been a recognized condition for more than 100 years, there are no natural history studies at this time to verify a correct time period for conservative treatment in the juvenile patients [72]. There is a general consensus that up to 6 months is a reasonable trial period for juvenile patients with OCD lesions. Complete resolution of symptoms and radiographic evidence of healing can take several months in OCD lesions. As the patients near skeletal maturity, the clinician should be wary of prolonged immobilization. It should be noted that in adult patients with OCD lesions, nonoperative treatment has a limited role [73, 74]. Adults do not possess the same healing potential after the closure of the physes compared to children and adolescents with open physes. As such, adults will most likely require operative intervention to preserve joint integrity.

The success of nonoperative treatment for stable juvenile OCD lesions ranges from 50 to 66% [45, 75, 76]. Arthritis after nonoperative treatment of OCD lesions is a challenging problem. In a study of 86 patients (mean age, 21 years) with OCD lesions of the knee treated nonoperatively, an estimated 30% cumulative incidence of arthritis was reported at 35 years post OCD diagnosis [77]. In addition to failure of nonoperative management, other operative indications include lesions with physeal closure impending within 6 months, unstable/hinged lesions, detached lesions (loose bodies), and full-thickness loss of overlying articular cartilage identified by MRI. When planning operative intervention, the treating physician should focus on the three essential factors for the OCD. First, the physeal status of the patient; second, the lesion stability; and finally, the lesion size. Size of the lesion will help dictate treatment options available if the lesion is not salvageable. From these factors, the following treatment algorithm for approaching surgical OCD lesions was derived (Fig. 10.3).

While the search for the cause of OCD is ongoing, there has been a substantial evolution in the surgical treatment of OCD lesions since Paré first described the removal of loose bodies over 170 years ago [78]. Articular cartilage resurfacing with OATS and allograft OATS, MFX, and autologous chondrocyte implantation (ACI) are now available options [3, 19, 79, 80]. Results on biomimetic nanostructured OC scaffold and "one-step" bone marrow-derived cell transplantation techniques have also been published [81–84]. Despite these advancements, current treatments are not uniformly successful in addressing challenging OCD lesions, and new treatment options are in development. The goals of surgery are twofold. First and foremost, the emphasis is on preserving native articular cartilage whenever possible. When this is not possible and the articular cartilage is not salvageable, cartilage restoration procedures are utilized.

Arthroscopic drilling of a stable lesion that has failed nonoperative management is well supported in the literature [85]. There are two options when performing drilling of these lesions: transarticular and retroarticular. There are advantages and disadvantages of both techniques. The transarticular method is straightforward, well visualized, and accurate but

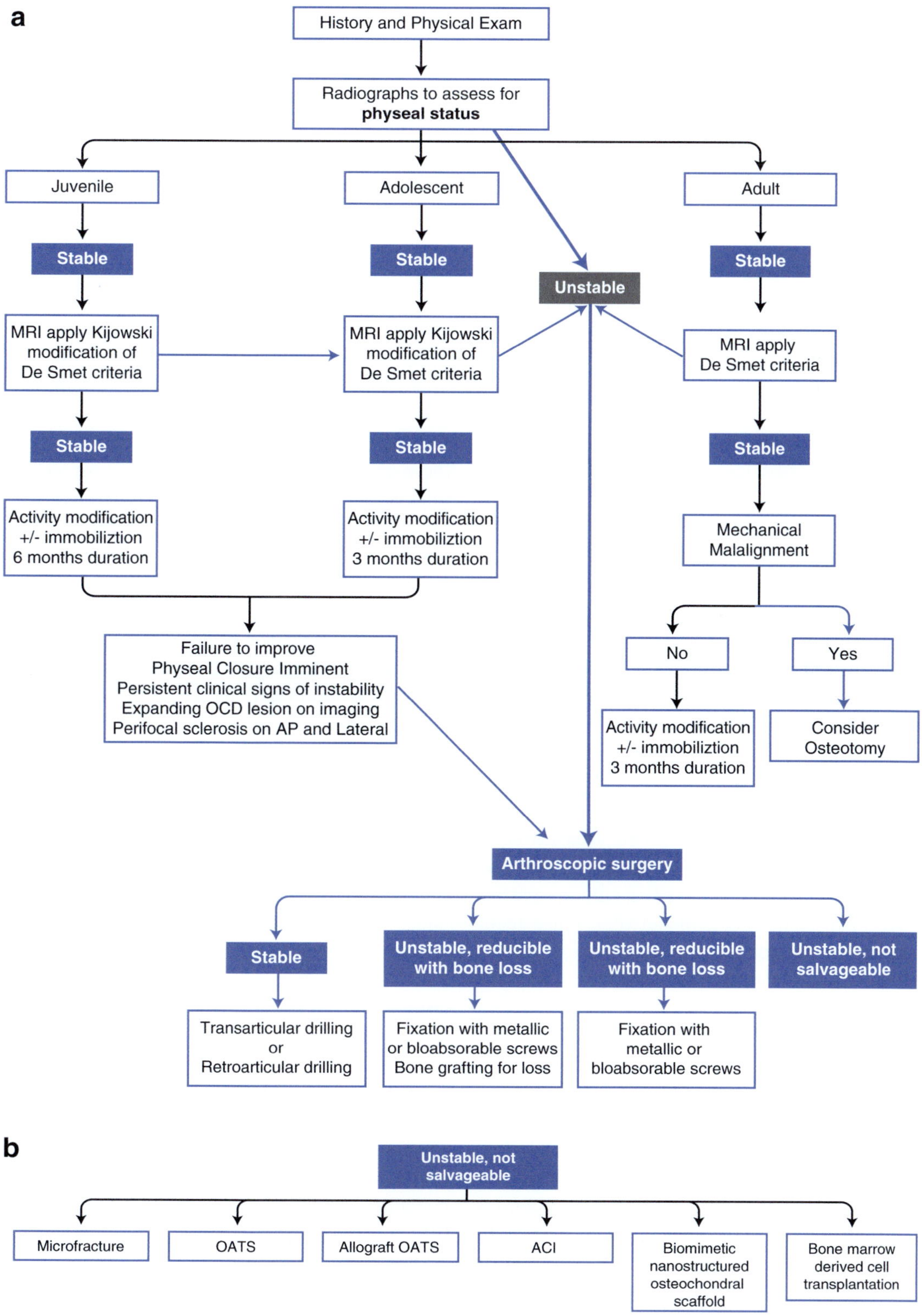

Fig. 10.3 Treatment algorithm for osteochondritis dissecans lesions of the knee

requires breaching of the articular surface. The retroarticular technique requires fluoroscopy, is technically more demanding, possesses a higher risk for inadequate drilling, but spares the overlying joint cartilage. The purpose of the drilling is to create vascular channels to stimulate revascularization and promote healing of the lesion [86]. Donaldson and Wotjys reported that 11 out of 12 patients had excellent results after retroarticular drilling [87]. Similar results were found in a study from Japan examining 20 skeletally immature knees with OCD (10 boys and 2 girls; mean age, 12 years; range, 9–15 years) after failure of 6 months of nonoperative treatment. Significant improvement in the Lysholm score (72.3–95.8) was found postoperatively, and only 1 of the 20 surgically treated lesions did not heal after the retrograde drilling [88].

Kocher et al. studied transarticular drilling in 30 knees in 23 skeletally immature patients (mean age, 12 years; range, 8–16 years) and found evidence of radiographic healing in all knees at a mean of 4.4 months [89]. Kawasaki et al. described a technique of drilling involving the intercondylar bare area, thus removing one of the major disadvantages of the transarticular technique, damage to the articular cartilage. They achieved healing in all 16 cases and saw an increase in the Lysholm knee score (70.4–97.8) [86]. Currently, the transarticular and retroarticular techniques are employed, and the decision should be based on surgeon preference [90]. A comparison between these techniques is an active area of interest in the Research in Osteochondritis Dissecans of the Knee (ROCK) Group.

For OCD lesions that are unstable, fibrous tissue located between the subchondral bone and cartilage should be debrided. If the lesions have bone loss, the lesions should be packed with autogenous bone graft before internal fixation. For Guhl Type II–IV lesions, the initial treatment involves internal fixation, curettage of any fibrous tissue, and bone grafting as necessary for those lesions with subchondral bone loss. This can be done arthroscopically or, if necessary, with use of an arthrotomy to gain necessary access to the lesion. Fixation of the lesion can be achieved with metallic or bioabsorbable implants. Internal fixation of both "classic" and cartilage-only OCD lesions has shown to have strong outcomes in managing challenging cases [91].

10.5.1 Fixation of Lesion with Metallic Screws

Metallic implants have a long track record in orthopedics for achieving compression and stability. There are two significant disadvantages to using metallic screws. First, they can abrade the opposing joint surface cartilage, and second, they may require a second surgical procedure for screw removal. Despite these disadvantages, there are good results from retrospective studies in the literature for OCD lesions treated with metallic screws. Johnson et al. reported their results using headed compression screws in 35 cases of OCD lesions [92]. At second-look arthroscopy to remove the screw, 94% of the lesions had evidence of healing confirmed by subsequent radiographs. Loosening of four fragments was observed, requiring additional surgery. This group reported 88% good to excellent results at a minimum of 2 years follow-up. Magnussen et al. reported their results using headed compression screws in 12 patients with Guhl Type IV lesions [93]. At second-look arthroscopic removal of the screw, 11 of the 12 had evidence for healing. Two of the 12 patients had evidence of scuffing of the adjacent tibial plateau cartilage. At 9-year follow-up, these patients did not have lower Knee Injury and Osteoarthritis Outcome Score (KOOS) for pain, lower activities of daily living (ADL), or less sports function than their age-matched controls. Gomoll et al. in a study using a variety of compression screws (8 headless, 4 AO 3.5 mm compression screws) obtained healing in all OCD lesions (N = 12) in adolescent and young adult patients (mean age 16 years; range, 12–19 years) [94].

The use of headless compression screws is also advocated as this can minimize damage to the opposing joint surface and, in some cases, may not necessitate planned second surgical

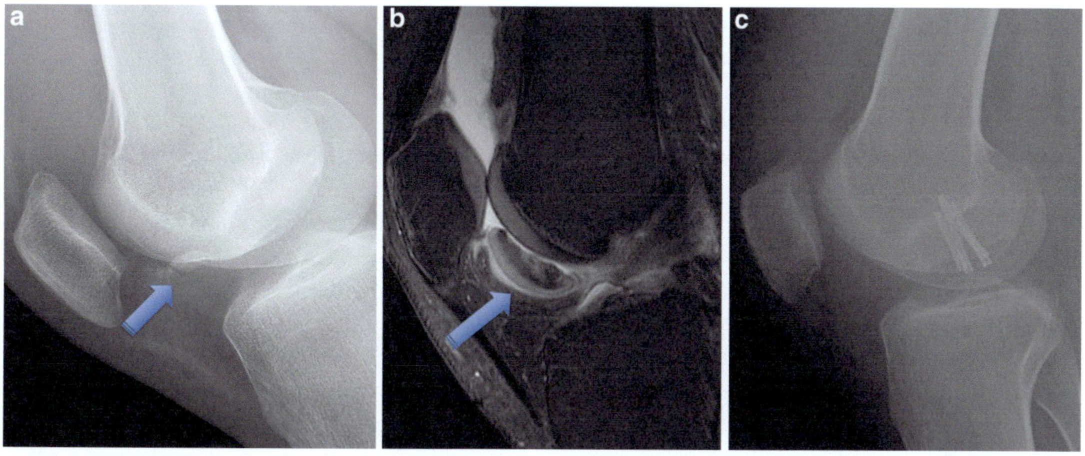

Fig. 10.4 Large partly non-ossified osteochondral fragment of the right knee. (**a**) Lateral radiograph and (**b**) sagittal fast spin-echo T2-weighted MR image demonstrate the significant discrepancy in the mostly non-ossified displaced osteochondral fragment situated anterior to the femoral trochlea (arrow). Large osteochondral defect at the lateral femoral condyle is also noted. (**c**) Postoperative lateral radiograph following rigid fixation of displaced osteochondral fragment with multiple fixation pins

removal (Fig. 10.4). Makino et al. studied OCD lesions fixed with titanium Herbert screws in 15 knees (age range 12–35 years) [95]. They verified healing at second-look arthroscopy to remove the screw and with follow-up MRI which showed healing in 14 of the 15 knees. At final follow-up, Lysholm scores increased from 79 to 97 in 13 of the 15 patients. Other studies using headless screws for fixation have documented similar results with successful outcomes and healing in a range from 82 to 90% [96, 97].

10.5.2 Fixation of Lesion with Bioabsorbable Screws

Bioabsorbable screws offer some attractive advantages compared to metallic fixation. The bioabsorbable screws are intended to absorb over time, do not interfere with subsequent knee imaging, and do not require planned surgical removal. Disadvantages of bioabsorbable implants are the risk of cyst formation, inciting synovitis in the joint, breakage, sterile abscesses, and loss of fixation [93].

In a study of 12 adolescent patients with stable OCD (mean age 15 years) who failed conservative treatment, the OCD lesions were treated with bioabsorbable smart nails for arthroscopic Guhl Type I and II lesions [94]. The authors used a mean of four nails per case. Postoperatively, patients were evaluated with several functional tests and scoring systems, including Lysholm, International Knee Documentation Committee (IKDC), and KOOS. At MRI follow-up with a mean of 32 months, all lesions healed. One patient developed synovitis that resolved with nonsteroidal anti-inflammatory drug (NSAID) treatment. However, it should be noted that these patients failed only 6 weeks of nonoperative treatment before arthroscopy, which is a considerably shorter period compared to other similar studies in the literature.

Tabaddor et al. reported their findings on 24 knees treated with similar bioabsorbable fixation 96 L/4D lactide copolymer nails [98]. The mean age in this study was 14 years with average almost 40 months of follow-up. Tabbador et al. were able to obtain MRIs in 17 patients at a mean of 22 months of which 16 patients showed evidence of healing. They reported good and excellent results in 22 of 24 knees. Kubota et al. reported good mid- and long-term outcomes (12 years) after OCD fixation using bioabsorbable pins [99]. Of note, one of the failures was in an Ewing and Voto Type IV lesion (completely detached loose body). In their concluding remarks, the authors have cautioned against bioabsorbable fixation in Type IV lesions.

In a larger retrospective study on the treatment of OCD, Kocher et al. studied unstable OCD lesions in 26 patients fixed with a wide array of metallic and bioabsorbable implants. Using Ewing and Voto classification system, 9 patients scored Stage II, 11 patients scored Stage III, and 6 patients scored Stage IV. They found an overall healing rate of 84% with no statistical difference between the groups by stage [100]. While there have been encouraging results in retrospective studies using internal fixation when the lesion is salvageable, this procedure is not without difficulty. Loosening, failure of hardware to maintain compression, broken hardware, abrasion to opposing cartilage surface, loose bodies, and hemarthroses are all reported complications of internal fixation, regardless if metallic or bioabsorbable screws were used.

10.5.3 Unsalvageable Lesions

It is not uncommon for the surgeon to encounter a detached or loose fragment that is not salvageable. This can occur with significant lesion fragmentation, prolonged period of detachment, and inadequate bony backing (< 2 mm) [3]. Under these conditions, excision may be required. This should be avoided if possible, as multiple studies have confirmed that excision of a large OCD can be associated with a poor outcome and the development of OA [101–104]. Options available to the surgeon in this situation include MFX, OATS (autograft/allograft), and ACI. Newer techniques with very little or long-term follow-up data have also been discussed recently and include biomimetic nanostructured OC scaffold and "one-step" bone marrow-derived cell transplantation technique as well as matrix-assisted autologous chondrocyte transplantation technique with autologous bone grafting [84 , 105, 106]. In combination to these surgical techniques, the administration of platelet-rich plasma or the use of orthobiologic scaffolds have shown promising long-term results [107–109].

Microfracture is thought to be a useful treatment option because it promotes filling of the defect with pluripotential cells that result in fibrocartilage formation [111]. This technique can be utilized for smaller, well-contained lesions. However, OCD lesions have some important differences from traumatic cartilage lesions. These bear mentioning with regard to the efficacy of the MFX treatment. First, traumatic cartilage lesions tend to have intact subchondral bone, whereas in OCD lesions, the subchondral bone is thought to be part of the primary pathophysiology and is more heavily involved. Second, after debridement, OCD lesions can lack a substantial amount of bone, leading to the question whether MFX can adequately restore support to the affected area [112].

In a randomized control trial, Gudas et al. compared the outcomes of the arthroscopic mosaic-type OAT and MFX procedures for the treatment of OCD lesions in 50 children mean age of 14 years; age range of 12 to 18 years) [68]. Their inclusion criteria included the following: ICRS score of 3 or 4, defect size between 2 and 4 cm^2, and the patient age of 18 years or younger. Despite randomization, the OATS group had 4 more (5 to 1) large lesions between 3 and 4 cm^2 compared to the MFX group. For the OATS technique, 5 and 6 mm diameter plugs were used and an average of 4 to 5 plugs per case. While both groups showed substantial initial improvement at 1-year follow-up; at 4.2 years follow-up, the OATS group had 83% of patients with good or excellent results compared with only 63% for the MFX group. None of the OATS patients had a clinical failure at final follow-up. The study indicates that for lesions smaller than 4 cm^2, OATS offers a more reliable clinical result than MFX. Other authors have shown OATS to be a viable and intriguing option for treatment of unsalvageable OCD lesions. OATS involves transferring cartilage from a non-weightbearing part of the joint to the symptomatic area. Classically, plugs are taken from the medial or lateral trochlea and the intercondylar notch. Several authors have reported good results in retrospective studies and case series [112, 113]. There is a range of recommended plug size. Concern has been expressed for plugs smaller than 3.5 mm diameter because of inadequate biomechanical strength. Similarly, plugs greater than 6.5 mm diameter may have problems filling in and can accelerate patella-femoral joint wear.

Several studies investigated the treatment outcomes of unstable OCD lesions using plug diameter ranging from 2.7 mm to 10 mm [113–115]. In a study of 20 patients (mean age 14 years) with unstable OCD lesions of the knee, Miniaci et al. arthroscopically assessed the OCD lesions and then fixed in situ by placing multiple 4.5 mm OC plugs (average 4 plugs per case) [114]. Using IKDC, the knee scores all normalized after surgery, and the authors reported no donor site complications related to the harvest. Fonseca et al. used smaller plugs with diameters between 2.7 mm and 3.5 mm in their study of 20 knees (mean age 27 years) with unstable ICRS III and IV OCD lesions [113]. Miura et al., in a study of mosaicplasty from Japan, used a range of plug diameters from 5 to 10 mm (mean 7 mm) in 12 patients (mean age 16 years) with knee OCD (1 patient scored ICRS II, 8 scored ICRS III and 3 scored ICRS IV) [115]. The authors obtained MRI evidence of healing in 3 months in all patients with Hughston scale scores of 8 (excellent), 3 (good), and 1 (fair). They also reported no donor site complications.

Secondary reconstruction of the cartilage with fresh allograft has been successfully performed and is on the algorithm for large, unsalvageable OCD lesions greater than 3 cm^2. There is no donor site morbidity with this procedure; however there are concerns about chondrocyte viability, graft availability, and disease transmission. The largest study in the literature looking specifically at fresh allograft in OCD patients to date consisted of 66 patients (mean age 28 years) with OCD lesions of the distal femur [116]. All patients had undergone a mean of 1.7 procedures prior to the allograft procedure. The mean size of allograft used in this study was 7.5 cm^2. The authors reported 70% good to excellent results after fresh allograft reconstruction. Fresh allograft can be a valuable salvage operation for larger lesions.

Autologous chondrocyte implantation technique was first started in Sweden in the late 1980s. Brittberg et al. published their initial trial in the New England Journal of Medicine in 1994 [117]. A two-stage procedure, this technique attempts to replace the damaged articular surface with viable chondrocytes. During the first stage at initial knee arthroscopy, chondrocytes are harvested from the intercondylar notch or the nonweightbearing surface of the medial trochlea. The sample is then sent for processing and expansion. The second stage involves implanting the expanded autologous chondrocytes from the original sample into the defect and covering it with a periosteal patch.

Currently, there is a role for ACI in the treatment of OCD lesions 2–10 cm^2 in size with success rates ranging between 80 and 91% depending on the study. Peterson's study of 58 patients with OCD and a mean lesion size of 5.7 cm^2 treated with ACI demonstrated greater than 90% good or excellent results [118]. They had two early failures causing graft delamination, which the authors attributed to the patients' early return to high-impact sports. In a study from Boston, Mithöfer et al. examined ACI in the treatment of full-thickness cartilage lesions (mean size 6.4 cm^2) in 23 adolescent athletes [119]. Fourteen of these were OCD lesions. Before ACI implantation, patients had a mean of 2.5 procedures performed. Of note, the authors reported results similar to Peterson's; 96% of these patients returned to high-impact sports. Krishnan et al. reported on their 2–7 year results on ACI for OCD of the knee in 37 patients (28 juvenile, 9 adult) with mean lesion size of 5.9 cm^2 [120]. They reported clinical results slightly lower than the two previous sets of authors at 82% with excellent and good results. However, at second-look arthroscopy 1 year later, visualization of the ACI demonstrated ICRS scores of 1 or 2 in 87.5% of patients. Furthermore, in 23 biopsies taken, 47.5% showed hyaline cartilage or a mix of hyaline and fibrocartilage. The above studies suggest there may be a role for ACI in cases of OCD that are refractory to other previously mentioned treatment options.

There are some newer techniques to treat unsalvageable OCD lesions, and there is initial research to support their use [121]. Biomimetic nanostructured OC scaffold and bone marrow-derived cell transplantation have compared favorably in small studies to ACI results for OCD but with the advantage of requiring only one operation [84, 105]. More study is required before definitive recommendations on these new techniques can be made.

10.6 Return to Play and Osteochondritis Dissecans

For many patients with OCD lesions, return to previous activity and sports is an important priority after surgery. Depending on the type of surgical intervention, there is a broad range of RTP in the literature after OCD surgery. Edmonds et al. reported on 59 patients who failed conservative treatment and were treated with retroarticular drilling [122]. The mean age in their study was 13 years, and the mean lesion size was 3.2 mm^2. On average, patients returned to full activities at 2.1 months (range 1.3–13 months). Using retroarticular drilling, Donaldson and Wotjys reported an average RTP at 8.5 months (range 5–14 months) for their patients (mean age 12 years) [87]. No additional information on lesion size was included. For transarticular drilling, Yonetani et al. reported all 19 patients treated returned to sports by 6 months [123].

Kramer et al. evaluated the functional outcomes of surgical management of OCD lesions of the patella and trochlea in a total of 26 pediatric patients (9 females and 17 males; mean age 14 years; range 9–18 years) and their ability to return to sports [124]. A total of 29 OC lesions were identified (3 with bilateral lesions) of which 21 knees with lesions (72%) had open physes and median follow-up of 3.8 years (range, 1–9 years). Twenty-two lesions (76%) underwent transarticular drilling (N = 14) or drilling with fixation (N = 8), while seven underwent excision and marrow stimulation. At the final follow-up, 48% (14 knees) were pain-free, and 48% had mild residual pain, and 85% (22 patients) returned to sports. Transarticular drilling and surgical excision with marrow stimulation treatment of patellofemoral OCD in children and adolescents produced a high rate of satisfaction and return to sports.

Din et al. reported that all 12 of their patients with stable OCD lesions treated with bioabsorbable implants had returned to sports by 8 months after surgery [101]. In a study from Boston, utilizing metallic and bioabsorbable fixation for unstable OCD lesions, Kocher et al. found their patients returned to sports at a mean of 8.3 months after the procedure [100].

For unsalvageable lesions, the return to play tends to be more delayed. In the only randomized controlled trial to date on OCD lesions, Gudas et al. reported the average RTP for their MFX and ACI patients [68]. The patients treated with MFX had only 7 out of 22 patients returned to sports. Their return averaged 14.1 months (range 10–16 months). At 4-year follow-up, only 3 of the 22 initial MFX patients were playing sports. For the OATS patients, 21 of the 25 patients returned to sports at an average of 11.7 months (range 9–14 months). Seventeen of the 21 OATS patients were continuing athletics at the 4-year follow-up. A higher return to sport and activity with OATS compared with MFX has been confirmed in a large review [125].

For RTP after ACI, in the Mithöfer study (a mix of traumatic cartilage lesions and OCD), 96% of athletes returned to high-impact sports and 60% to a level equal or higher than before the injury [119]. They allowed RTP at 12 months after surgery. Of note the authors found that patients with symptoms before surgery of less than 12 months all returned to play compared to only 33% in those patients with more than a year of symptoms. For ACI in higher level athletes, the RTP has not been as encouraging. In a study from Greece, only 6 of 19 athletes were able to resume their previous level of activity. While not all of these lesions were OCD (traumatic cartilage lesions were included as well), this suggests returning younger high-impact patients to their previous activity may not be as likely as other studies have suggested. Higher level athletes should be cautioned that their RTP may not be as high as previous studies have indicated.

Mithöfer et al. published a review of RTP after articular cartilage procedures in 2009 [125]. This review encompassed all types of cartilage lesions, not exclusively OCD lesions. The main results of this study are worth repeating. Younger age was a positive prognostic factor for return to sport, regardless of surgical technique. If symptoms were present for less than 12 months before surgery, results on RTP with MFX was 66% and for ACI 67%. Rates dropped to 14% and 15%, respectively, if symptoms were present for more than 1 year. RTP was statistically much quicker in competitive athletes than recreational (14 vs 22 months) who underwent ACI procedures. Overall RTP rates after articular cartilage surgery were 73%, with the highest RTP with OATS (91% OATS, 67% ACI, and 66% MFX).

10.7 Conclusions

Osteochondritis dissecans has remained a challenging and evasive clinical problem since König first described it back in 1888. It is not a benign condition of the knee, even in the skeletally immature. The potential for an OCD to evolve into arthritis and degeneration is a significant concern. After this review, it should become apparent there remains a substantial amount of work to be done to elucidate OCD's cause as well as to optimize its treatment. Most of the current research to date consists of case series, expert opinion, and retrospective review. Despite these limitations, several points should be remembered when treating patients with OCD lesions. Factors associated with a good outcome include open growth plates, stable lesions, and smaller lesions. Closed physes, unstable lesions, and larger lesions are all more likely to necessitate surgery. While treatment of OCD lesions has evolved from simple excision, the current available treatments available continue to lack uniform success. Future research aims should look to identify clearly the natural history of these lesions, standardize nonoperative treatment protocols and compare outcomes in different surgical treatment approaches to maintain joint congruity for unsalvageable OCD lesions.

Critical Points

Osteochondritis dissecans is a disease of the subchondral bone that can develop into secondary problems with the involvement of the overlying articular cartilage. It should not be confused with an OC defect.

The etiology of OCD is unknown at this time and likely multifactorial in nature. The growing consensus is that microtrauma plays a fundamental role in pathophysiology of OCD.

The natural history of OCD lesions is not clearly defined at this time.

On MRI, a high-signal T2 rim alone is not indicative of instability in juvenile patients unless it is accompanied by a break in the articular cartilage as seen on T1-weighted images, multiple fractures are seen in the subchondral plate, and/or a low-signal T2 rim is seen in the host bone.

Although the treatment of OCD is dictated by many factors, the physeal status, lesion stability, and size are the most important.

Conservative treatment with an emphasis on activity modification is an appropriate treatment in stable OCD lesion in young patients with an open physis; however, conservative treatment plays a minimal role for adults with OCD lesions.

OATS provides a more durable result than MFX for OCD lesions between 2 and 4 cm^2 in diameter. For larger defects > 4 cm^2, ACI and allograft OATS should be considered.

References

1. Heywood CS, Benke MT, Brindle K, Fine KM. Correlation of magnetic resonance imaging to arthroscopic findings of stability in juvenile osteochondritis dissecans. Arthroscopy. 2011;27(2):194–9.
2. Crawford DC, Safran MR. Osteochondritis dissecans of the knee. J Am Acad Orthop Surg. 2006;14(2):90–100.
3. Kocher MS, Tucker R, Ganley TJ, Flynn JM. Management of osteochondritis dissecans of the knee: current concepts review. Am J Sports Med. 2006;34(7):1181–91.
4. Bradley J, Dandy DJ. Osteochondritis dissecans and other lesions of the femoral condyles. J Bone Joint Surg Br. 1989;71(3):518–22.

5. Linden B. The incidence of osteochondritis dissecans in the condyles of the femur. Acta Orthop Scand. 1976;47(6):664–7.
6. Jacobi M, Wahl P, Bouaicha S, Jakob RP, Gautier E. Association between mechanical axis of the leg and osteochondritis dissecans of the knee: radiographic study on 103 knees. Am J Sports Med. 2010;38(7):1425–8.
7. Hefti F, Beguiristain J, Krauspe R, et al. Osteochondritis dissecans: a multicenter study of the European Pediatric Orthopedic Society. J Pediatr Orthop B. 1999;8(4):231–45.
8. Hughston JC, Hergenroeder PT, Courtenay BG. Osteochondritis dissecans of the femoral condyles. J Bone Joint Surg Am. 1984;66(9):1340–8.
9. Pareek A, Sanders TL, Wu IT, Larson DR, Saris DBF, Krych AJ. Incidence of symptomatic osteochondritis dissecans lesions of the knee: a population-based study in Olmsted County. Osteoarthritis Cartilage. 2017;25(10):1663–71.
10. Weiss JM, Shea KG, Jacobs JC Jr, Cannamela PC, Becker I, Portman M, Kessler JI. Incidence of osteochondritis dissecans in adults. Am J Sports Med. 2018;46(7):1592–5.
11. Hevesi M, Sanders TL, Pareek A, Milbrandt TA, Levy BA, Stuart MJ, Saris DBF, Krych AJ. Osteochondritis dissecans in the knee of skeletally immature patients: rates of persistent pain, osteoarthritis, and arthroplasty at mean 14-years' follow-up. Cartilage. 2018 July 1:1947603518786545. https://doi.org/10.1177/1947603518786545. (Epub ahead of print).
12. Aichroth P. Osteochondritis dissecans of the knee. A clinical survey. J Bone Joint Surg Br. 1971;53(3):440–7.
13. DeLee JC, Drez D Jr, Miller MD. DeLee & Drez's orthopaedic sports medicine: principles and practice. 2nd ed. Philadelphia: Elsevier Science; 2003.
14. Obedian RS, Grelsamer RP. Osteochondritis dissecans of the distal femur and patel la. Clin Sports Med. 1997;16(1):157–74.
15. König F. Ueber freie Korper in den Glenken. Zeiteschr Chir. 1888;27:90–109.
16. Nagura S. The so-called osteochondritis dissecans of Konig. Clin Orthop. 1960;18:100–21.
17. Kothari A, Ponce P, Arriaza B, O'Connor-Read L. Osteochondritis dissecans of the knee in a mummy from Northern Chile. Knee. 2009;16(2):159–60.
18. Bauer KL. Osteochondral injuries of the knee in pediatric patients. Knee Surg. 2018;31(5):382–91.
19. Cruz AI Jr, Shea KG, Ganley TJ. Pediatric knee osteochondritis dissecans lesions. Orthop Clin North Am. 2016;47(4):763–75.
20. Schenck RC Jr, Goodnight JM. Osteochondritis dissecans. J Bone Joint Surg Am. 1996;78(3): 439–56.
21. Andriolo L, Crawford DC, Reale D, Zaffagnini S, Candrian C, Cavicchioli A, Filardo G. Osteochondritis dissecans of the knee: etiology and pathogenetic mechanisms. A systematic review. Cartilage. 2018 July 1:1947603518786557. https://doi.org/10.1177/1947603518786557. (Epub ahead of print).
22. Ribbing S. The hereditary multiple epiphyseal disturbance and its consequences for the aetiogenesis of local malacias--particularly the osteochondrosis dissecans. Acta Orthop Scand. 1955;24(4):286–99.
23. Stattin EL, Tegner Y, Domellof M, Dahl N. Familial osteochondritis dissecans associated with early osteoarthritis and disproportionate short stature. Osteoarthritis Cartilage. 2008;16(8):890–6.
24. Mubarak SJ, Carroll NC. Familial osteochondritis dissecans of the knee. Clin Orthop Relat Res. 1979;140:131–6.
25. Gornitzky AL, Mistovich RJ, Atuahuene B, Storey EP, Ganley TJ. Osteochondritis dissecans lesions in family members: does a positive family history impact phenotypic potency? Clin Orthop Relat Res. 2017;475(6):1573–80.
26. Petrie PW. Aetiology of osteochondritis dissecans. Failure to establish a familial background. J Bone Joint Surg Br. 1977;59(3):366–7.
27. Andrew TA, Spivey J, Lindebaum RH. Familial osteochondritis dissecans and dwarfism. Acta Orthop Scand. 1981;52(5):519–23.
28. Al Kaissi A, Klaushofer K, Grill F. Osteochondritis dissecans and Osgood Schlatter disease in a family with Stickler syndrome. Pediatr Rheumatol Online J. 2009;7:4.
29. Trepman E. Osteochondritis dissecans of the knee in an adult with Stickler syndrome. Orthop Rev. 1993;22(3):371–6.
30. Kubo H, Oommen PT, Hufeland M, Heusch P, Laws HJ, Krauspe R, Pilge H. Osteochondritis dissecans shows a severe course and poor outcome in patients with juvenile idiopathic arthritis: a matched pair study of 22 cases. Rheumatol Int. 2018; 38(9):1705–12.
31. Caffey J, Madell SH, Royer C, Morales P. Ossification of the distal femoral epiphysis. J Bone Joint Surg Am. 1958;40-A(3):647–54.
32. Enneking WF, Dunham WK. Resection and reconstruction for primary neoplasms involving the innominate bone. J Bone Joint Surg Am. 1978;60(6):731–46.
33 Reddy AS, Frederick RW. Evaluation of the intraosseous and extraosseous blood supply to the distal femoral condyles. Am J Sports Med. 1998;26(3):415–9.
34. Uozumi H, Sugita T, Aizawa T, Takahashi A, Ohnuma M, Itoi E. Histologic findings and possible causes of osteochondritis dissecans of the knee. Am J Sports Med. 2009;37(10):2003–8.
35 Koch S, Kampen WU, Laprell H. Cartilage and bone morphology in osteochondritis dissecans. Knee Surg Sports Traumatol Arthrosc. 1997;5(1):42–5.
36. Milgram JW. Radiological and pathological manifestations of osteochondritis dissecans of the distal femur. A study of 50 cases. Radiology. 1978;126(2):305–11.

37. Chiroff RT, Cooke CP 3rd. Osteochondritis dissecans: a histologic and microradiographic analysis of surgically excised lesions. J Trauma. 1975;15(8):689–96.
38. Linden B, Telhag H. Osteochondritis dissecans. A histologic and autoradiographic study in man. Acta Orthop Scand. 1977;48(6):682–6.
39. Kessler JI, Jacobs JC Jr, Cannamela PC, Shea KG, Weiss JM. Childhood obesity is associated with osteochondritis dissecans of the knee, ankle, and elbow in children and adolescents. J Pediatr Orthop. 2018;38(5):e296–9.
40. Fairbank HA. Osteochondritis dissecans. Br J Surg. 1933;21:67–82.
41. Nambu T, Gasser B, Schneider E, Bandi W, Perren SM. Deformation of the distal femur: a contribution towards the pathogenesis of osteochondrosis dissecans in the knee joint. J Biomech. 1991;24(6):421–33.
42. Wilson JNA. diagnostic sign in osteochondritis dissecans of the knee. J Bone Joint Surg Am. 1967;49(3):477–80.
43. Conrad JM, Stanitski CL. Osteochondritis dissecans: Wilson's sign revisited. Am J Sports Med. 2003;31(5):777–8.
44. Dirschl D, Cannada LK. Classification of fractures. In: Rockwood and green's fractures in adults, vol. 1. 6th ed. Philadelphia: Lippincott, Williams and Wilkins; 2006. p. 43–4.
45. Wall EJ, Vourazeris J, Myer GD, et al. The healing potential of stable juvenile osteochondritis dissecans knee lesions. J Bone Joint Surg Am. 2008;90(12):2655–64.
46. Pill SG, Ganley TJ, Milam RA, Lou JE, Meyer JS, Flynn JM. Role of magnetic resonance imaging and clinical criteria in predicting successful non-operative treatment of osteochondritis dissecans in children. J Pediatr Orthop. 2003;23(1):102–8.
47. Smillie IS. Treatment of osteochondritis dissecans. J Bone Joint Surg Br. 1957;39-B(2):248–60.
48. Cepero S, Ullot R, Sastre S. Osteochondritis of the femoral condyles in children and adolescents: our experience over the last 28 years. J Pediatr Orthop B. 2005;14(1):24–9.
49. Vangsness CT Jr, Kurzweil PR, Lieberman JR. Restoring articular cartilage in the knee. Am J Orthop (Belle Mead NJ). 2004;33(2 Suppl): 29–34.
50. Cahill BR, Berg BC. 99m-Technetium phosphate compound joint scintigraphy in the management of juvenile osteochondritis dissecans of the femoral condyles. Am J Sports Med. 1983;11(5):329–35.
51. Ramirez A, Abril JC, Chaparro M. Juvenile osteochondritis dissecans of the knee: perifocal sclerotic rim as a prognostic factor of healing. J Pediatr Orthop. 2010;30(2):180–5.
52. Jungesblut OD, Berger-Groch J, Meenen NM, Stuecker R, Rupprecht M. Validity of ultrasound compared with magnetic resonance imaging in evaluation of osteochondritis dissecans of the distal femur in children. Cartilage. 2019:1947603519828434. doi: 10.1177/1947603519828434. [Epub ahead of print].
53. Paletta GA Jr, Bednarz PA, Stanitski CL, Sandman GA, Stanitski DF, Kottamasu S. The prognostic value of quantitative bone scan in knee osteochondritis dissecans. A preliminary experience. Am J Sports Med. 1998;26(1):7–14.
54. Gorbachova T, Melenevsky Y, Cohen M, Cerniglia BW. Osteochondral lesions of the knee: differentiating the most common entities at MRI. Radiographics. 2018:38(5);1478–95.
55. Zbojniewicz AM, Stringer KF, Laor T, Wall EJ. Juvenile osteochondritis dissecans: correlation between histopathology and MRI. AJR Am J Roentgenol. 2015;205(1):W114–23.
56. Accadbled F, Vial J, Sales de Gauzy J. Osteochondritis dissecans of the knee. Orthop Traumatol Surg Res. 2018;104(1S):S97–S105.
57. De Smet AA, Fisher DR, Graf BK, Lange RH. Osteochondritis dissecans of the knee: value of MR imaging in determining lesion stability and the presence of articular cartilage defects. AJR Am J Roentgenol. 1990;155(3):549–53.
58. De Smet AA, Ilahi OA, Graf BK. Reassessment of the MR criteria for stability of osteochondritis dissecans in the knee and ankle. Skelet Radiol. 1996;25(2):159–63.
59. Haeri Hendy S, de Sa D, Ainsworth K, Ayeni OR, Simunovic N, Peterson D. Juvenile osteochondritis dissecans of the knee: does magnetic resonance imaging instability correlate with the need for surgical intervention? Orthop J Sports Med. 2017;5(11):2325967117738516. https://doi.org/10.1177/2325967117738516.
60. Uppstrom TJ, Gausden EB, Green DW. Classification and assessment of juvenile osteochondritis dissecans knee lesions. Curr Opin Pediatr. 2016;28(1):60–7.
61. Ishikawa M, Nakamae A, Nakasa T, Ikuta Y, Hayashi S, Ochi M, Deie M, Adachi N. Limitation of in-situ arthroscopic fixation for stable juvenile osteochondritis dissecans in the knee. J Pediatr Orthop B. 2018;27(6):516-21.
62. O'Connor MA, Palaniappan M, Khan N, Bruce CE. Osteochondritis dissecans of the knee in children. A comparison of MRI and arthroscopic findings. J Bone Joint Surg Br. 2002;84(2):258–62.
63. Samora WP, Chevillet J, Adler B, Young GS, Klingele KE. Juvenile osteochondritis dissecans of the knee: predictors of lesion stability. J Pediatr Orthop. 2012;32(1):1–4.
64. Yoshida S, Ikata T, Takai H, Kashiwaguchi S, Katoh S, Takeda Y. Osteochondritis dissecans of the femoral condyle in the growth stage. Clin Orthop Relat Res. 1998;346:162–70.
65. Kijowski R, Blankenbaker DG, Shinki K, Fine JP, Graf BK, De Smet AA. Juvenile versus adult osteochondritis dissecans of the knee: appropriate MR imaging criteria for instability. Radiology. 2008;248(2):571–8.

66. Guhl JF. Arthroscopic treatment of osteochondritis dissecans. Clin Orthop Relat Res. 1982;167: 65–74.
67. Ewing JW, Voto SJ. Arthroscopic surgical management of osteochondritis dissecans of the knee. Arthroscopy. 1988;4(1):37–40.
68. Gudas R, Simonaityte R, Cekanauskas E, Tamosiunas R. A prospective, randomized clinical study of osteochondral autologous transplantation versus microfracture for the treatment of osteochondritis dissecans in the knee joint in children. J Pediatr Orthop. 2009;29(7):741–8.
69. Gudas R, Kalesinskas RJ, Kimtys V, et al. A prospective randomized clinical study of mosaic osteochondral autologous transplantation versus microfracture for the treatment of osteochondral defects in the knee joint in young athletes. Arthroscopy. 2005;21(9):1066–75.
70. Chambers HG, Shea KG, Carey JLAAOS. Clinical practice guideline: diagnosis and treatment of osteochondritis dissecans. J Am Acad Orthop Surg. 2011;19(5):307–9.
71. Masquijo J, Kothari A. Juvenile osteochondritis dissecans (JOCD) of the knee: current concepts review. EFORT Open Rev. 2019;4(5):201–12.
72. Bauer KL, Polousky JD. Management of osteochondritis dissecans lesions of the knee, elbow and ankle. Clin Sports Med. 2017;36(3):469–87.
73. Gomoll AH, Farr J, Gillogly SD, Kercher J, Minas T. Surgical management of articular cartilage defects of the knee. J Bone Joint Surg Am. 2010;92(14):2470–90.
74. Zanon G, DIV G, Marullo M. Osteochondritis dissecans of the knee. Joints. 2014;2(1):29–36.
75. Cahill BR. Osteochondritis dissecans of the Knee: treatment of juvenile and adult forms. J Am Acad Orthop Surg. 1995;3(4):237–47.
76. Cahill BR, Phillips MR, Navarro R. The results of conservative management of juvenile osteochondritis dissecans using joint scintigraphy. A prospective study. Am J Sports Med. 1989;17(5):601–5. discussion 605-606
77. Sanders TL, Pareek A, Johnson NR, Carey JL, Maak TG, Stuart MJ, Krych AJ. Nonoperative management of osteochondritis dissecans of the knee: progression to 118. Osteoarthritis and Arthroplas ty at Mean 13-Year Follow-up. Orthop J Sports Med. 2017;5(7):2325967117704644. doi: 10.1177/2325967117704644.
78. Pare A. Oeuvres Completes, Paris: JB Balliere. 1840–1841;3:32.
79. Jones KJ, Cash BM, Arshi A, Williams RJ 3rd. Fresh osteochondral allograft transplantation for uncontained, elongated osteochondritis dissecans lesions of the medial femoral condyle. Arthrosc Tech. 2019;8(3):e267–e273.
80. Filardo G, Andriolo L, Soler F, Berruto M, Ferrua P, Verdonk P, Rongieras F, Crawford DC. Treatment of unstable knee osteochondritis dissecans in the young adult: results and limitations of surgical strategies-The advantages of allografts to address an osteochondral challenge. Knee Surg Sports Traumatol Arthrosc. 2019;27(6):1726–38.
81. Verdonk P, Dhollander A, Almqvist KF, Verdonk R, Victor J. Treatment of osteochondral lesions in the knee using a cell-free scaffold. Bone Joint J. 2015;97-B(3):318–23.
82. Delcogliano M, Menghi A, Placella G, Speziali A, Cerulli G, Carimati G, et al. Treatment of osteochondritis dissecans of the knee with a biomimetic scaffold. A prospective multicenter study. Joints. 2014;2(3):102–8.
83. Gobbi A, Karnatzikos G, Sankineani SR. One-step surgery with multipotent stem cells for the treatment of large full-thickness chondral defects of the knee. Am J Sports Med. 2014;42(3):648–57.
84. Vannini F, Battaglia M, Buda R, Cavallo M, Giannini S. "One step" treatment of juvenile osteochondritis dissecans in the knee: clinical results and T2 mapping characterization. Orthop Clin North Am. 2012;43(2):237–44.
85. Gunton MJ, Carey JL, Shaw CR, Murnaghan ML. Drilling juvenile osteochondritis dissecans: retro- or transarticular? Clin Orthop Relat Res. 2012;471(4):1144–51.
86. Kawasaki K, Uchio Y, Adachi N, Iwasa J, Ochi M. Drilling from the intercondylar area for treatment of osteochondritis dissecans of the knee joint. Knee. 2003;10(3):257–63.
87. Donaldson LD, Wojtys EM. Extraarticular drilling for stable osteochondritis dissecans in the skeletally immature knee. J Pediatr Orthop. 2008;28(8): 831–5.
88. Adachi N, Deie M, Nakamae A, Ishikawa M, Motoyama M, Ochi M. Functional and radiographic outcome of stable juvenile osteochondritis dissecans of the knee treated with retroarticular drilling without bone grafting. Arthroscopy. 2009;25(2):145–52.
89. Kocher MS, Micheli LJ, Yaniv M, Zurakowski D, Ames A, Adrignolo AA. Functional and radiographic outcome of juvenile osteochondritis dissecans of the knee treated with transarticular arthroscopic drilling. Am J Sports Med. 2001;29(5):562–6.
90. Gunton MJ, Carey JL, Shaw CR, Murnaghan ML. Drilling juvenile osteochondritis dissecans: retro- or transarticular? Clin Orthop Relat Res. 2013;471(4):1144–51.
91. Nuelle CW, Farr J. Internal fixation of osteochondritis dissecans lesions in the patellofemoral joint. J Knee Surg. 2018;31(3):206–11.
92. Johnson LL, Uitvlugt G, Austin MD, Detrisac DA, Johnson C. Osteochondritis dissecans of the knee: arthroscopic compression screw fixation. Arthroscopy. 1990;6(3):179–89.
93. Magnussen RA, Carey JL, Spindler KP. Does operative fixation of an osteochondritis dissecans loose body result in healing and long-term maintenance of knee function? Am J Sports Med. 2009;37(4):754–9.

94. Gomoll AH, Flik KR, Hayden JK, Cole BJ, Bush-Joseph CA, Bach BR Jr. Internal fixation of unstable Cahill Type-2C osteochondritis dissecans lesions of the knee in adolescent patients. Orthopedics. 2007;30(6):487–90.
95. Makino A, Muscolo DL, Puigdevall M, Costa-Paz M, Ayerza M. Arthroscopic fixation of osteochondritis dissecans of the knee: clinical, magnetic resonance imaging, and arthroscopic follow-up. Am J Sports Med. 2005;33(10):1499–504.
96. Rey Zuniga JJ, Sagastibelza J, Lopez Blasco JJ, Martinez Grande M. Arthroscopic use of the Herbert screw in osteochondritis dissecans of the knee. Arthroscopy. 1993;9(6):668–70.
97. Kouzelis A, Plessas S, Papadopoulos AX, Gliatis I, Lambiris E. Herbert screw fixation and reverse guided drillings, for treatment of types III and IV osteochondritis dissecans. Knee Surg Sports Traumatol Arthrosc. 2006;14(1):70–5.
98. Tabaddor RR, Banffy MB, Andersen JS, et al. Fixation of juvenile osteochondritis dissecans lesions of the knee using poly 96L/4D-lactide copolymer bioabsorbable implants. J Pediatr Orthop. 2010;30(1):14–20.
99. Kubota M, Ishijima M, Ikeda H, Takazawa Y, Saita Y, Kaneko H, Kurosawa H, Kaneko K. Mid and long term outcomes after fixation of osteochondritis dissecans. J Orthop. 2018;15(2):536–9.
100. Kocher MS, Czarnecki JJ, Andersen JS, Micheli LJ. Internal fixation of juvenile osteochondritis dissecans lesions of the knee. Am J Sports Med. 2007;35(5):712–8.
101. Din R, Annear P, Scaddan J. Internal fixation of undisplaced lesions of osteochondritis dissecans in the knee. J Bone Joint Surg Br. 2006;88(7):900–4.
102. Anderson AF, Pagnani MJ. Osteochondritis dissecans of the femoral condyles. Long-term results of excision of the fragment. Am J Sports Med. 1997;25(6):830–4.
103. Murray JR, Chitnavis J, Dixon P, et al. Osteochondritis dissecans of the knee; long-term clinical outcome following arthroscopic debridement. Knee. 2007;14(2):94–8.
104. Wright RW, McLean M, Matava MJ, Shively RA. Osteochondritis dissecans of the knee: long-term results of excision of the fragment. Clin Orthop Relat Res. 2004;424:239–43.
105. Kon E, Vannini F, Buda R, et al. How to treat osteochondritis dissecans of the knee: surgical techniques and new trends: AAOS exhibit selection. J Bone Joint Surg Am. 2012;94(1):e11–8.
106. Roffi A, Andriolo L, Di Martino A, Balboni F, Papio T, Zaffagnini S, Filardo G. Long-term results of matrix-assisted autologous chondrocyte transplantation combined with autologous bone grafting for the treatment of juvenile osteochondritis dissecans. J Pediatr Orthop. 2019. doi: 10.1097/BPO.0000000000001404. [Epub ahead of print].
107. Gwosdz J, Rosinski A, Chakrabarti M, Woodall BM, Elena N, McGahan PJ, Chen JL. Osteochondral allograft transplantation of the medial femoral condyle with orthobiologic augmentation and graft-recipient microfracture preparation. Arthrosc Tech. 2019:25;8(3):e321–e329.
108. Sánchez M, Delgado D, Garate A, Sánchez P, Padilla S, Azofra J. Platelet-rich plasma combined with allograft to treat osteochondritis dissecans of the knee: a case report. J Med Case Rep. 2019;13(1):105.
109. Hinzpeter J, Zamorano A, Barahona M, Campos P. Treatment of osteochondritis dissecans of the knee with autologous iliac bone graft and hyaluronic acid scaffold. Knee Surg Relat Res. 2019;31(2):143–6.
110. Steadman JR, Briggs KK, Rodrigo JJ, Kocher MS, Gill TJ, Rodkey WG. Outcomes of microfracture for traumatic chondral defects of the knee: average 11-year follow-up. Arthroscopy. 2003;19(5):477–84.
111. Polousky JD. Juvenile osteochondritis dissecans. Sports Med Arthrosc. 2011;19(1):56–63.
112. Kobayashi T, Fujikawa K, Oohashi M. Surgical fixation of massive osteochondritis dissecans lesion using cylindrical osteochondral plugs. Arthroscopy. 2004;20(9):981–6.
113. Fonseca F, Balaco I. Fixation with autogenous osteochondral grafts for the treatment of osteochondritis dissecans (stages III and IV). Int Orthop. 2009;33(1):139–44.
114. Miniaci A, Tytherleigh-Strong G. Fixation of unstable osteochondritis dissecans lesions of the knee using arthroscopic autogenous osteochondral grafting (mosaicplasty). Arthroscopy. 2007;23(8):845–51.
115. Miura K, Ishibashi Y, Tsuda E, Sato H, Toh S. Results of arthroscopic fixation of osteochondritis dissecans lesion of the knee with cylindrical autogenous osteochondral plugs. Am J Sports Med. 2007;35(2):216–22.
116. Emmerson BC, Gortz S, Jamali AA, Chung C, Amiel D, Bugbee WD. Fresh osteochondral allografting in the treatment of osteochondritis dissecans of the femoral condyle. Am J Sports Med. 2007;35(6):907–14.
117. Brittberg M, Lindahl A, Nilsson A, Ohlsson C, Isaksson O, Peterson L. Treatment of deep cartilage defects in the knee with autologous chondrocyte transplantation. N Engl J Med. 1994;331(14):889–95.
118. Peterson L, Minas T, Brittberg M, Lindahl A. Treatment of osteochondritis dissecans of the knee with autologous chondrocyte transplantation: results at two to ten years. J Bone Joint Surg Am. 2003;85-A (Suppl 2):17–24.
119. Mithofer K, Minas T, Peterson L, Yeon H, Micheli LJ. Functional outcome of knee articular cartilage repair in adolescent athletes. Am J Sports Med. 2005;33(8):1147–53.
120. Krishnan SP, Skinner JA, Carrington RW, Flanagan AM, Briggs TW, Bentley G. Collagen-covered

autologous chondrocyte implantation for osteochondritis dissecans of the knee: two- to seven-year results. J Bone Joint Surg Br. 2006;88(2):203–5.
121. Perdisa F, Kon E, Sessa A, Andriolo L, Busacca M, Marcacci M, Filardo G. Treatment of knee osteochondritis dissecans with a cell-free biomimetic osteochondral scaffold: clinical and imaging findings at midterm follow-up. Am J Sports Med. 2018;46(2):314–21.
122. Edmonds EW, Albright J, Bastrom T, Chambers HG. Outcomes of extra-articular, intra-epiphyseal drilling for osteochondritis dissecans of the knee. J Pediatr Orthop. 2010;30(8):870–8.
123. Yonetani Y, Tanaka Y, Shiozaki Y, et al. Transarticular drilling for stable juvenile osteochondritis dissecans of the medial femoral condyle. Knee Surg Sports Traumatol Arthrosc. 2011;20(8):1528–32.
124. Kramer DE, Yen YM, Simoni MK, Miller PE, Micheli LJ, Kocher MS, et al. Surgical management of osteochondritis dissecans lesions of the patella and trochlea in the pediatric and adolescent population. Am J Sports Med. 2015;43(3):654–62.
125. Mithoefer K, Hambly K, Della Villa S, Silvers H, Mandelbaum BR. Return to sports participation after articular cartilage repair in the knee: scientific evidence. Am J Sports Med. 2009;37(Suppl 1):167S–76S.

Surgical Approach to Articular Cartilage Repair

11

Jaskarndip Chahal, Benedict A. Rogers, and Allan E. Gross

11.1 Introduction

Articular cartilage defects of the knee are a common source of pain and/or loss of function in patients, frequently associated with meniscal and/or anterior cruciate ligament injuries [1]. In a consecutive series of over 31,000 arthroscopy procedures, one or more chondral lesions were found in 63% of patients with a symptomatic knee [2]. In detail, this study reported 41% Outerbridge grade III chondral injuries and 19.2% Outerbridge grade IV chondral injuries, with an estimated 3–4% of patients who had isolated chondral lesions greater than 2 cm^2.

Despite being common, it is important to emphasize that cartilage lesions can be incidental in nature and the decision to treat should be based on their confirmed contribution to patient symptomology. Furthermore, patients with knee pain often have multiple coexisting pathoanatomical findings. As such, it is important to consider global lower extremity function and take into consideration a patient's mechanical alignment, knee ligamentous instability, as well as the status of chondral and meniscal structures. In the end, cartilage repair should be offered to patients who have symptoms that are concordant with radiographic and magnetic resonance imaging (MRI) findings and whose activity or quality of life is limited by their physical impairment.

In regard to classification, cartilage injuries can be acute or chronic and can result from trauma, osteochondritis dissecans (OCD), and/or osteonecrosis (ON). With respect to pathogenesis, cartilage injuries that lie entirely within the hyaline cartilage and do not penetrate into the subchondral bone are referred to as *chondral defects*. In the adult, defects of this nature do not regenerate because of the lack of cells that could participate in the repair process. In contrast, *osteochondral (OC) defects* penetrate through the vascularized subchondral bone, and some spontaneous repair occurs as mesenchymal chondro-

J. Chahal, MD, FRCSC, MSc, MBA
Division of Orthopaedic Surgery, University of Toronto, Toronto, ON, Canada

University of Toronto Orthopaedic Sports Medicine and University Health Network Arthritis Program, Toronto, ON, Canada

Division of Orthopaedic Surgery, Toronto Western Hospital and Women's College Hospital, Toronto, ON, Canada

B. A. Rogers, MA, MSc, MRCGP, DipLMC, DipSEM, FRCS (Orth), PhD
Brighton and Sussex Medical School, Brighton, UK

Trauma and Orthopaedics Department, Brighton and Sussex University Hospitals NHS Trust, Brighton, UK

A. E. Gross, MD, FRCSC, O ONT (✉)
Division of Orthopaedic Surgery, University of Toronto, Toronto, ON, Canada

Gluskin Granovsky Division of Orthopaedics, Joseph and Wolf Lebovic Health Complex, Mount Sinai Hospital, Toronto, ON, Canada
e-mail: Allan.Gross@sinaihealthsystem.ca

H. K. Gahunia et al. (eds.), *Articular Cartilage of the Knee*,
https://doi.org/10.1007/978-1-4939-7587-7_11

progenitor cells invade the lesion and form cartilage. In the latter situation, full-thickness defect repair is only transient, and the novel tissue formed does not have the functional properties of native hyaline cartilage [3]. Finally, it is possible to have clinical scenarios where chondral lesions can have associated subchondral bone marrow edema without frank violation of the subchondral bone plate. These lesions should be treated as combined bone and cartilage lesions as opposed to partial-thickness chondral lesions, and treatment selection should reflect this distinction [4–6].

At the present time, there are a number of clinical algorithms that exist in order to guide surgeons to select the optimal cartilage restoration procedures for different patient subpopulations [4, 7–9]. In general, surgical options are guided by both *defect-specific* and *patient-specific* factors [4]. In keeping with these principles, the treatment algorithm should ideally consist of a graduated surgical plan. The least invasive treatment option necessary to alleviate the symptoms and restore joint function is performed first. In the event of treatment failure and the associated persistence of symptoms, future treatment should not be compromised by previous management [4, 6, 7].

11.2 Patient-Specific and Defect-Specific Considerations

Treatment selection should be guided by patient-specific and defect-specific factors, as well as global knee and lower extremity structure and function [4]. In regard to pertinent patient-specific factors, the type of treatment offered is influenced by patient expectations, the number and type of previous surgeries, body mass index (BMI), and activity level. Defect-specific factors which must be considered include defect aetiology (e.g. traumatic, OCD, ON), size, location, number of defects, and the presence of subchondral bone change. Of these factors, defect size is most often utilized by orthopedic surgeons to guide treatment recommendations. The caveat to remember is that MRI should not be used exclusively for predicting lesion size [4]. In a retrospective review, Gomoll et al. demonstrated that depending on defect location, the intraoperative defect measurements were larger than predicted by MRI in the range of 47– 377%, indicating that MRI is a poor predictor of defect size [10]. This suggests that while MRI may be effective in measuring the zone of full-thickness cartilage loss, most defects are surrounded by an area of degenerated or fissured cartilage that is less easily quantified. Given that most cartilage restoration treatments have upper size limit beyond which they are less successful, the importance of accurately quantifying defect size cannot be overstated. The use of computed tomography (CT) arthrogram and quantitative MRI techniques such as delayed gadolinium-enhanced MRI of cartilage (dGEMRIC) may prove to be better predictors of defect size in future studies. A preliminary staging arthroscopy is an alternative method to obtain accurate measurement of defect size [4]. Another defect-specific factor that must be taken into consideration is the presence of subchondral bone changes and edema as represented on preoperative MRI. The presence of subchondral change implies a bone and cartilage pathological process, whereas its absence signifies mainly a chondral origin. In the former situation, therapeutic options that address the cartilage and subchondral components (e.g. OC allograft) are preferred. In the latter, surface treatments such as microfracture, DeNovo Natural Tissue (NT) (Zimmer-Biomet, Warsaw, IN), and Autologous Chondrocyte Implantation (ACI) are more likely to be efficacious [4].

In a knee with multiple pathologies, each entity must be considered individually with respect to its influence on the overall status of the knee. Global knee and lower extremity factors that require careful consideration include the presence of varus or valgus malalignment (> 5°) ligamentous instability, and the degree of prior meniscal resection. In clinical scenarios where multiple comorbidities are present, there is an increasing support for addressing all pathoanatomical aberrations in a single surgery. A systematic review performed by Harris et al. analysed clinical outcomes in patients undergoing combined meniscal allograft transplantation with cartilage repair or restoration [11]. Out of the 6 studies included, 110 patients were identified as having undergone meniscal allograft transplantation and either ACI (n = 73), osteochondral allograft transplantation (n = 20), osteochondral autograft transplantation (OAT: n = 17), or microfracture (MXF: n = 3). Of note, 33% of patients (36/110) underwent other concomitant procedures including high tibial or distal femoral osteotomy, ligament reconstruction, and/or hardware removal. The authors noted improved outcomes in combined procedures compared to isolated surgery in four of the six studies. Overall, 12% of patients experienced failure of their combined procedure requiring revision surgery, and 85% of these failures were noted to be related to the meniscus procedure as opposed to the cartilage procedure [11]. These results emphasize the importance of a global knee and lower extremity assessment. Avoiding linear thinking and attributing the entirety of a patient's impairment and activity limitations to a focal defect without a comprehensive evaluation of all pertinent clinical factors are likely to compromise treatment outcomes and compromise patient recovery [4, 6].

11.3 Patient Evaluation

11.3.1 History

Patients often present with ipsilateral joint line tenderness, an effusion, and pain at the extremes of motion with an initial differential diagnosis of a meniscal tear. A specific traumatic event may be reported, but more commonly, there is an insidious onset that is aggravated by marching, running, or other repetitive impacts. Patients often have had numerous prior procedures, with Peterson et al. demonstrating patients had an average of 2.1 previous treatments before presenting for cartilage restoration [12]. Patients with chondral defects also commonly present with functional limitations. A full discussion should be undertaken with all patients to ensure they understand and are willing to undergo a prolonged rehabilitation regimen and that they have realistic expectations of outcome. Other pertinent points on history include the location of pain (medial, lateral, retropatellar), presence of side-to-side instability (cruciate ligament injury), linear instability (quadriceps weakness), mechanical symptoms, as well as the duration of symptoms. Finally, patients with such complex, combined knee pathologies (e.g. triad of meniscal deficiency, chondral pathology, malalignment) will typically complain of unilateral, single compartment knee pain. Often, their symptoms are chronic in nature, as it takes time for any one of these isolated injuries to have an additive effect on another [6].

11.3.2 Physical Examination

A complete standardized physical examination of both knees and lower extremities includes:

- Inspection
  - Sagittal, coronal, and transverse plane alignment
  - Muscle bulk
  - Prior incisions
- Palpation
  - Crepitus
  - Effusion
  - Joint line tenderness
- Active and passive range of motion (ROM)
  - Hip, knee, and ankle
- Strength
  - Core
  - Hamstrings
  - Quadriceps
- Hamstring flexibility and iliotibial (IT) band assessment (Ober's test)
- Patellar exam
  - Tilt
  - Apprehension
  - Tracking
  - J sign
  - Q angle
- Stability testing
- Ligamentous stability
  - Pivot shift, Lachman, and anterior drawer test
  - Posterior drawer test
  - Varus/valgus stress (0° and 30°)
  - Dial test
- Meniscal testing
  - McMurray and Appley's grind test
- Neurovascular exam

11.3.3 Diagnostic Imaging

Diagnostic imaging classification and assessment of chondral defect(s), other associated knee tissues, as well as post-cartilage repair remain an essential component of routine care and follow-up. Appropriate diagnostic imaging for patients includes plain radiographs, an MRI, and in certain situations a CT scan of the knee. Our preferred imaging protocol is as follows:

(a) *Plain radiographs*
- Non weight-bearing X-rays
  - Anteroposterior (AP)
  - 30° flexion lateral
  - Skyline view
- Weight-bearing X-rays
  - 45° flexion posteroanterior (PA)
  - 3 foot standing bilateral AP
- Sizing X-rays for meniscus transplantation and osteochondral allograft transplantation candidates (Fig. 11.1) [6]
  - *Standing bilateral 45 flexion P/A knee* with the *X-ray tube directed at 10° caudal*. The 10 cm marker should be placed on the lateral aspect of the affected knee at the level of the joint space.
  - *Lateral non-weight-bearing knee*. The 10 cm marker should be placed next to the knee cap at the level of the joint space.

(b) *Magnetic resonance imaging*

In general, MRI is useful for assessing chondral injuries of the knee, the involvement of the subchondral bone, and the structural integrity of knee ligaments and menisci. A minimum of 1.5 tesla MRI is required for adequate resolution to visualize cartilage abnormalities.

MR characteristics pertinent to chondral defects that requires repair include:
- Depth
  - Full or partial cartilage thickness
  - Involvement of tidemark

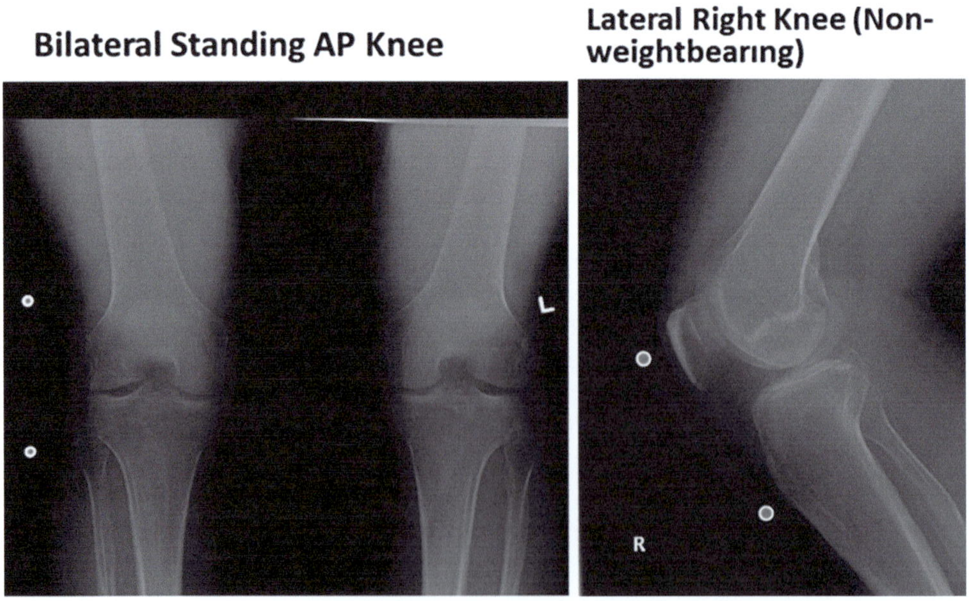

Fig. 11.1 Sizing radiographs. (**a**) Standing bilateral 45 flexion posteroanterior. (**b**) Lateral non-weight-bearing X-ray (Frank et al. [6])

- Size
- Location within the knee
  - Femur: condyle, trochlear
  - Tibia
  - Patella
  - Single or multiple lesions
  - Weight-bearing or non-weight-bearing region
  - Defined edge
- Contained
- Non-contained

(c) *Computed tomography*

Computed tomography provides a detailed morphology and measurement of the chondral defect(s) in certain situations as shown below:

- If a patellar or trochlear chondral defect is suspected, CT scan with patellofemoral views in 0°, 15°, and 30° of flexion to evaluate patellofemoral alignment may also be obtained. We calculate tilt and subluxation as described by Fulkerson [13].
- Assess tibial tuberosity-trochlear groove (TTTG) distance. Values greater than 20 mm are considered to be abnormal and can be corrected with an anteromedialization as described by Fulkerson.
- Assess bone tunnels in prior anterior cruciate ligament (ACL) reconstruction.

11.3.4 Arthroscopic Assessment and Classification

Various arthroscopic classification systems are available. The most commonly used clinical grading system is the Outerbridge classification, while the preferred classification for research purposes is the one put for by the International Cartilage Repair Society (ICRS). For details of arthroscopic assessment and classification of chondral lesions, refer to Chap. 7 and Appendix A.

11.4 Perioperative Decision-Making

As discussed above, treatment planning in patients with OC defects should be guided by defect- and patient-specific factors. In a systematic review of various articular cartilage repair procedures, lesion size, activity level, and age were the influencing parameters following surgery [14–19]. Lesions greater than 2.5 cm^2 had better outcomes with ACI or OAT, while microfracture was recommended to be the first-line treatment for smaller lesions [19]. Furthermore, patients who were active had better results with ACI or OAT compared with microfracture. Bekkers et al. also demonstrated that younger patients (< 30 years) seemed to benefit more from any cartilage repair surgery than older patients [19]. Harris et al. conducted a systematic review which is comprised of level I and II clinical studies to compare the efficacy of ACI with alternative treatments [20]. Defect size more than 4 cm^2 was the only factor predictive of better outcomes when ACI was compared to OATS or microfracture. None of the aforementioned studies included OC allografts as a study group. A recent systematic review of 19 clinical studies by Chahal et al. has demonstrated that at a mean follow-up of approximately 5 years (644 knees, average defect size 6.3 cm^2), the overall satisfaction rate was 86% [21]. The reported short-term complication rate was 2.4%, and the overall long-term failure rate was 18%.

Patient activity levels are another important consideration in the perioperative decision-making process. Mithoefer et al. conducted a systematic review to evaluate sports participation following articular cartilage surgery [22]. The authors demonstrated that the overall return to sport was 73% with highest return after OAT. Return to sports at the pre-injury level was 65%. The best durability with respect to sports participation was in patients with ACI. In the latter review, no studies assessing outcomes after fresh OC allografts were included. As such, Krych et al. evaluated return to activity following OC allografts in athletes [23]. They discovered that the return to sport was 88% with a return to previous level of sport at 79% (as defined by achieving the pre-injury level of the Cincinnati sports activity scale). In these individuals, the time to return to sport was 9.6 months (range, 7 to 13 months). In the athletes who returned to their previous level of competition, the postoperative International Knee Documentation Committee (IKDC), the activities of daily living (ADL), and the Marx activity rating scale scores were all significantly greater than in those athletes who did not return to sport. For the details of IKDC and Marx rating scale, please refer to Appendix B.

Patient compliance, motivation, expectations and goals, and overall patient health should also be taken into consideration. Furthermore, smoking has been shown to have an overall deleterious influence on basic science and clinical outcomes following articular cartilage surgery [24].

The treatment algorithms presented in Figs. 11.2 and 11.3 are based on the best available evidence, as well as on the experience of the senior author. For patients presenting with a failed index cartilage restoration procedure, an approach developed by Chahal and Cole is presented in Fig. 11.4 [4]. At Mount Sinai Hospital (Toronto, Ontario, Canada), the use of fresh OC allografts is the preferred treatment for large OC defects (> 3 cm^2) and for patients with failed prior cartilage surgery. For smaller defects (< 3 cm^2) undergoing initial cartilage repair surgery, microfracture is considered an acceptable first-line procedure.

Finally, it is critical to rule out the presence of malalignment, prior meniscal resection, and ligamentous instability. In the setting of varus and valgus malalignment, we prefer to treat this with a medial opening wedge high tibial osteotomy (MOW HTO) and a distal femoral varus (medial closing wedge) osteotomy (DFVO), respectively. Patients who have had a previous subtotal meniscectomy in the ipsilateral compartment are candidates for concomitant meniscal allograft transplantation, while patients with instability can be considered for a cruciate reconstruction (or medial patellofemoral ligament reconstruction +/− anteromedialization procedure in the setting of patellofemoral instability).

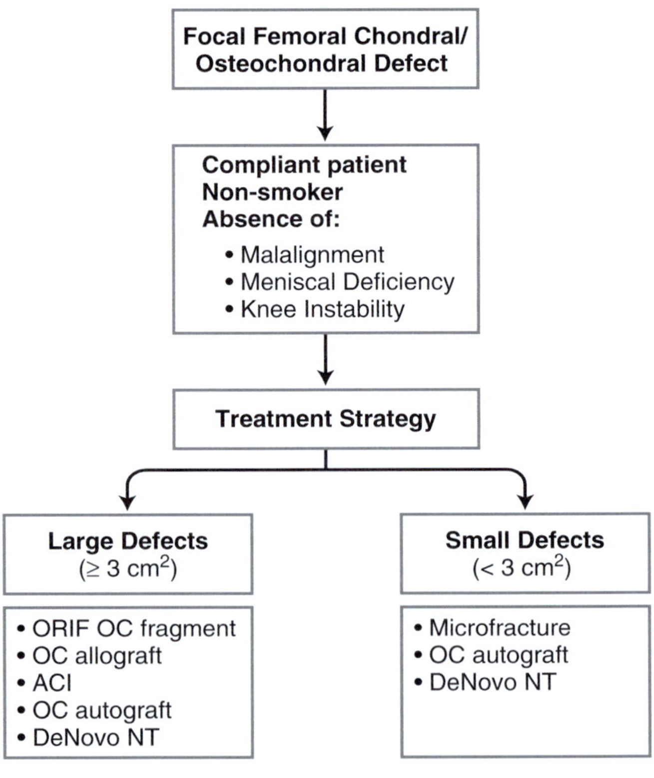

Fig. 11.2 Decision and treatment algorithm for focal chondral and osteochondral (OC) defects involving the femoral condyles. For larger defects, if there is an associated deformity then realignment osteotomy should be considered. Open reduction internal fixation (ORIF), OC allograft, OC autograft, autologous chondrocyte implantation (ACI), and DeNovo Natural Tissue (NT)

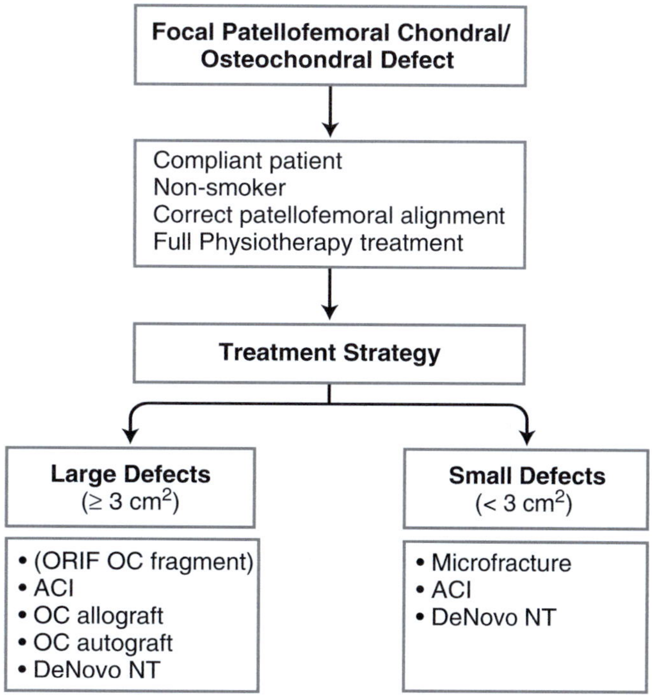

Fig. 11.3 Decision and treatment algorithm for focal chondral and osteochondral (OC) defects involving the patellofemoral joint. Open reduction internal fixation (ORIF), autologous chondrocyte implantation (ACI), OC allograft, OC autograft and DeNovo Natural Tissue (NT)

11.5 Osteochondral Defects Treatment Options

Prior to proceeding with one of the cartilage restoration algorithms highlighted in Figs. 11.2, 11.3, and 11.4, it is important to recognize when OC fragments can be fixed in situ or when displaced fragments can undergo fixation as opposed to removal. Table 11.1 highlights the indications for OC fragment fixation.

11.6 Fixation of Osteochondral Defects

The internal fixation of a traumatic OC defect is challenging for both the reduction and fixation of the fragment. The fragment(s) may be translated or rotated in either the axial, sagittal, or coronal planes and may be tethered to the chondral surface or entrapped anywhere within the joint. Osteochondral fractures are commonly reported in the distal femur of young adults, and the most common mechanism is acute patellar dislocation leading to either patellar or lateral femoral condyle defects [25–28]. If a substantial section of subchondral bone remains attached to the loose fragment, subsequent reduction and fixation of the OC fragment have been advocated [29]. However, there is a substantial body of historical evidence supporting the excision of such OC fragments [28–33]. The successful reduction and fixation of displaced lateral femoral condyle OC fragments have been described with a variety of techniques and devices. In young patients, every effort to obtain primary fixation of an OC fragment is made.

11.6.1 Screw Fixation

11.6.1.1 Countersunk Intra-Articular Screws

Osteochondral fractures of the lateral femoral condyle are not common and are often misdiagnosed. Taitsman et al. reported the use of countersunk cortical screws (2 mm or 2.4 mm, Synthes) for the fixation of large OC fragments in two cases [34]. These two patients presented following rotation injuries to the knee and patellar dislocation, with the OC fragments originating from the lateral femoral condyle. A direct lateral

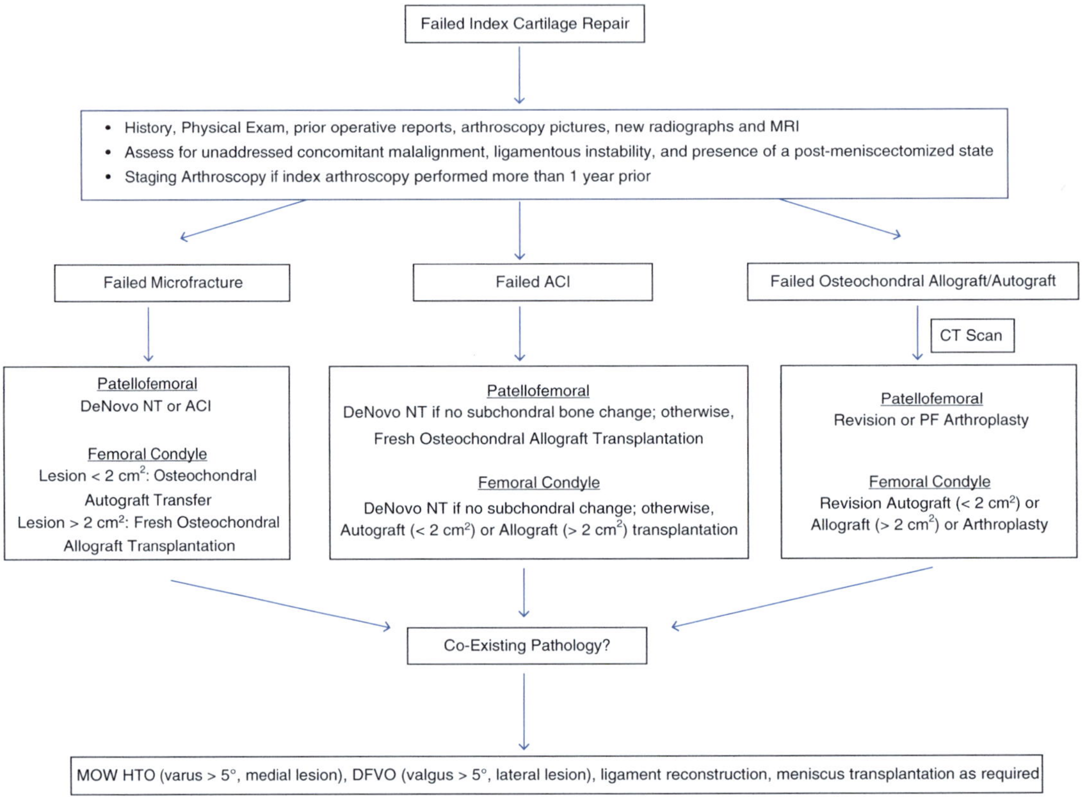

Fig. 11.4 Treatment algorithm for patients presenting with a failed index cartilage repair procedure [4]. Medial opening wedge high tibial osteotomy (MOW HTO), patellofemoral (PF), Distal femoral varus (closing wedge) osteotomy (DFVO), autologous chondrocyte implantation (ACI), DeNovo Natural Tissue (DeNovo NT). (Permission to use "Treatment algorithm Perioperative decision-making" for publication granted by Sports Medicine and Arthroscopy. "Managing the patient with failed cartilage restoration" [4]

Table 11.1 Indication for salvage of osteochondral (OC) fragments

Salvageable OC Fragments	Unsalvageable OC Fragments
Single OC fragment	Multifragmentary
Subchondral bone intact with OC fragment	None/little subchondral bone with OC fragment
Acute (< 2–3 weeks)[a]	Chronic (> 3–4 weeks)[a]
Non-smoker[a]	Smoker[a]
Compliant patient[a]	Noncompliant[a]

[a]*Relative indicator or contraindicator*

open approach was made to the knee joint, utilizing the interval between biceps femoris tendon and the peroneal nerve. After reduction and temporary K-wire fixation, the OC fragments were fixed with two screws. The authors advocate the preoperative use of Computed Tomography (CT) scanning to confirm the diagnosis and to clarify the location of the displaced fragment.

(a) *Mini-cancellous screws*

Binnet et al. reported a series of 13 adults with intercondylar eminence fractures that were treated with arthroscopic reduction and fixation using 40-mm-long mini cancellous screws designed following the techniques and principles of internal fixation developed by the Association for Osteosynthesis/Association for the Study of Internal Fixation (AO/ASIF) group [35]. Radiographic union was confirmed in all patients at a mean of 8.3 weeks. All the screws were removed by a second arthroscopic procedure after complete union was achieved. However, in a follow-up study by the same group evaluating the histological healing achieved with screw fixation, both cancellous screws and Herbert screws (see below), there was no correlation between the clinical results and the histologic findings [36]. Namely, after the treatment, there was no observable regeneration of normal articular cartilage in the junctional areas (i.e. between the adjacent native cartilage and that of the fixed OC fragment). The authors advocated an early motion for the recovery in OC fractures. The extracellular matrix (ECM) of articular cartilage, in particular chondroitin sulfate secretion, is stimulated by early passive motion [37–39].

(b) *Herbert screws*

The variable pitch design of a Herbert screw has been shown to afford a compressive force and resist shear that is similar to AO cortical screws [40]. It was designed for internal fixation of scaphoid fractures, for which there is substantial supporting evidence [41, 42]. Lewis and Foster reported eight cases that utilized the compression achieved with the variable pitch of a Herbert for the fixation of OC fractures of the patella or femoral condyle secondary to patella dislocation [43]. The study reported that normal knee function was regained 6 months after surgery and there were no further patella dislocations. Following a non-contact martial arts injury to a 16-year-old adolescent, Mbubaegbu and Percy reported substantial OC fracture of the lateral femoral condyle [44]. Dental screws and Herbert screws were used for fixation with the former requiring later arthroscopic removal due to protrusion from the chondral surface. Although not as common as OC injuries to the medial facet of the patella and the anterior lateral portion of the lateral femoral condyle, OC injury to the weight-bearing portion of the mid-lateral femoral condyle does occur with patella dislocation [45]. The recognition of this uncommon lesion by the surgeon who treats known patellofemoral dislocation should heighten suspicion of patellofemoral dislocation to ensure its detection and appropriate treatment.

(c) *Bioabsorbable screws*

Bioabsorbable screws are made from poly-∝ – hydroxy acids, for example, poly(glycolic acid) or poly(d- or l-lactic acid) [46, 47]. The biomechanical properties and degradation rates differ, thus leading to the development of copolymer bioabsorbable screws in an attempt to maximize mechanical strength while reducing the inflammatory reaction caused by these bioabsorbable screws [48–50]. An example of one such product is the SmartNail screw (ConMed Linvatec, Largo, FL), made from poly-96 L/4D–lactide copolymer. Tabaddor et al. reported a case series of 24 unstable OCD lesions treated with poly-96 L/4D–lactide copolymer implants [51]. Good functional outcome scores (Lysholm score and Tegner Activity Score, TAS) were reported, with 22 of the 24 having good-excellent outcomes. Larsen et al. reported a case series and biomechanical data from synthetic bone to characterize the mechanical strength and in vitro absorption properties of copolymer screw fixation [47]. Six of seven cases of OCD healed clinically and radiographically, with no evidence of adverse inflammatory reaction. In vitro testing demonstrated average pull-out and shear loads were 20.1 Kg and 22.3 Kg, respectively.

11.6.2 Bioabsorbable Pins

Bioabsorbable pins were designed to be embedded in the OC fragment to achieve fixation to the underlying subchondral bed [52–54]. Meniscus arrows (Bionx Implants, Tampere, Finland) have been used for the treatment of tears in the vascularized region of the meniscus. They are manufactured from polylactic acid polymer and have a smaller diameter (1.1 mm) than the smallest bioabsorbable screws (2.0 mm) or nails (1.5 mm), thus facilitating arthroscopic insertion. In an in vitro biomechanical testing study using meniscus arrows, Wouter et al. demonstrated that these bioabsorbable pins have sufficient strength to be used as fixation devices, and they further provided clinical evidence to support their use in the fixation of OC fragments [54, 55]. The quoted advantages of using bioabsorbable pins include ease of insertion, they do not need to be removed, lack of local allergic reactions, and no scatter with subsequent MRI or CT scanning or interference with radiation therapy [55].

11.6.3 Cyanoacrylate Glue

Cyanoacrylate glue was invented by Ardis in 1949 and was first used in surgery in 1959 by Coover [56]. A non-histotoxic form, N-butyl-2-cyanoacrylate, is frequently used for fixation in craniofacial surgery due to its strong tissue-binding properties [57]. Animal studies have supported the use of cyanoacrylate as an osseous adhesive [58]. Orthopedic use of N-butyl-2-cyanoacrylate initially included the fixation of OC fractures in the talus and in the knee [59, 60]. A fibrin glue (Tissucol©) has been used as an adjunct to the use of other forms of fixation of OC fragments [55].

11.6.4 Suture Bridge

Bowers and Huffman reported a "suture bridge" technique that was originally described for the fixation of shear fractures of the capitulum [61]. An anatomical reduction was reported, with sufficient rotational stability and compression to the underlying subchondral bone achieved to allow for immediate passive motion and stimulate healing. This technique was implemented in two cases of femoral condylar OC lesions (2 × 3 cm and 2 × 2 cm) [61]. Four retrograde osseous tunnels were drilled using a 1.5 mm drill bit to allow for two number 1 dyed, braided absorbable sutures (Ethicon Vicryl suture, Johnson & Johnson, Piscataway, NJ) to be passed over the OC fragment in a cruciform configuration. After the reduction of the fragment, the sutures were tensioned to assess the fragment conformity and stability through a full range of knee movement. In addition, fibrin glue was applied to the rim of the defect. A significant advantage of this technique is the use of biodegradable sutures that afforded the subsequent use of MRI evaluation. Both reported cases had a good clinical and MRI results with the authors concluding that this is a viable alternative technique to other accepted means of fixation for treatment of traumatic OC fragments in the knee [61].

11.7 Articular Cartilage Debridement, Repair, and Restoration

11.7.1 Debridement

The benefits of debridement of chondral lesions remain controversial, with the majority of results reported as part of the treatment of meniscal tears [62]. Chondral damage is associated with increased matrix metalloproteinase (MMP) activity in the cartilage surrounding the defect, which is thought to be the result of the increased mechanical load [63, 64]. The increased MMP activity is deleterious to both the opposing chondral surface and the surrounding cartilage (refer to Chap. 4 for articular cartilage degradation by proteinases).

Magnusson et al. first reported the debridement of unstable cartilage flaps, in addition to a washout and thorough debridement of any inflammatory tissue [65]. Removal of damaged cartilage by surgical excision has been reported to provide symptomatic improvement for up to 5 years [66]. Hubbard et al. selected 76 patients with symptomatic tenderness and an associated underlined chondral lesion for surgical debridement aiming to remove any unstable cartilage and to cause sufficient abrasion to the underlying subchondral bone to stimulate new tissue to form at the base of the defect [66]. In this study, only isolated medial femoral condylar lesions were considered, with simple arthroscopic lavage used as a control. When compared to the lavage group, those patients who had undergone debridement had a significant improvement using Lysholm and Gillquist score [67]. Thus, the evidence of beneficial outcomes of debridement per se is varied. Although the cleaning process may help to reduce symptoms, however, the effects are temporary. If the cartilage surface is unstable and not amenable to fixation or repair, the results of debridement and lavage are satisfactory [68].

In contrast, the results of debridement for non-focal cartilage pathology, in particular osteoarthritis (OA), are not conclusive [69, 70]. Good or excellent short-term results have been reported in 52% of patients following arthroscopic joint washout. This outcome enhanced the longevity of symptom improvement when combined with debridement [66, 71, 72]. In a level I randomized trial, Kirkley et al., however, demonstrated no benefit of arthroscopy and debridement compared to physical therapy and medical management in patients with OA [73].

11.7.2 Abrasion Arthroplasty

Abrasion arthroplasty is a surgical procedure where areas of chondral degeneration are roughened with a burr or shaver to stimulate repair of the articular surface. This technique has been advocated as a suitable treatment for OA of the knee associated with full-thickness chondral loss, eburnation, and osteophytes. In essence it is an extensive tissue debridement for patients that do not want to proceed with total knee arthroplasty (TKA).

Amongst the earliest reported studies in 1959, Pridie et al. used an open procedure for focal chondral lesions in patients with severe knee arthritis [74]. However, the recurrence of symptoms in patients treated with this surgical modality has been observed in 2 to 3 years, with the success rate for functional outcomes being only around 50% [75, 76].

An abrasion is produced deep enough to cause subchondral bleeding, hence forming a continuous clot over the treated region [77–80]. Since this surgery is commonly performed with multiple tissue debridements, including meniscal debridement and a varying amount of synovectomy, the exact amount of benefit attributable to the abrasion arthroplasty has not been quantified. No definitive prospective randomized clinical studies have been performed; in addition, there is considerable variation in indications, technique, and postoperative rehabilitation among surgeons. Finally, studies have shown that fibrocartilage, rather than hyaline cartilage, is formed at the abrasion site which is associated with inferior biomechanical properties [81].

Johnson stated that abrasion arthroplasty was beneficial for patients with rest or night pain and no significant change in coronal knee alignment (i.e. femoral tibial angle) [82]. Objective improvements in radiographic and histological findings were reported. However, Rand et al. provided clinical evidence to question the efficacy for this treatment modality, by comparing arthroscopic partial meniscectomy plus limited debridement with abrasion arthroplasty [83].

Bert and Maschka reviewed the outcome of 126 patients who had an arthroscopic diagnosis of unicompartmental Outerbridge stage IV OA and were treated with either abrasion arthroplasty with arthroscopic debridement or arthroscopic debridement alone. Using the Hospital for Special Surgery (HSS) Knee Scoring System, they reported that in the group treated with abrasion arthroplasty, there were 51% with good to excellent results, compared to 66% in the group treated with arthroscopic debridement. Further, the degree of articular repair was not related to the clinical outcome [84, 85].

11.7.3 Subchondral Bone Microfracture

The microfracture procedure is a form of bone marrow stimulation that enhances cartilage repair by taking advantage of the body's own healing potential (Fig. 11.5.) [86]. A sharp awl (i.e. pick)

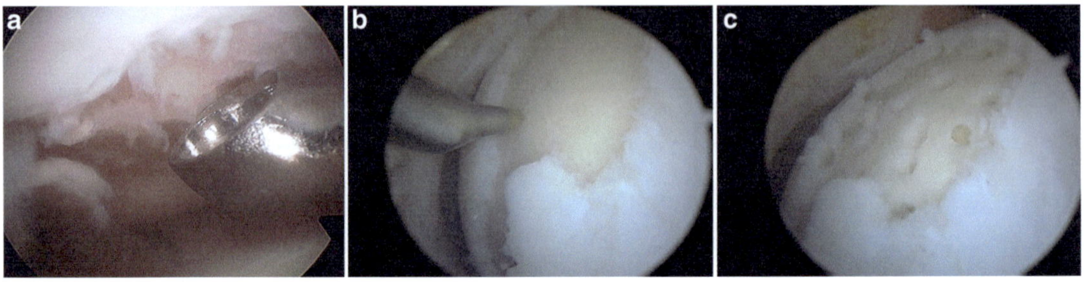

Fig. 11.5 Microfracture technique as described by Steadman [90]. (**a**) Debridement of unstable flaps of cartilage and removal of the calcified layer. (**b**) A microfracture awl is used to make holes 2 to 3 mm apart and at a depth of 1 to 2 mm. The awl penetrates the subchondral bone plate at an angle of 90°. (**c**) Microfractured defect created and there should be three to four holes per cm^2

is used arthroscopically through one of the arthroscopic skin portals, and a mallet is used to impact the awl into the subchondral bone to generate bleeding from the bone. Holes are created at regular intervals until the entire defect has been addressed. The penetration of the subchondral bone provides a passage for the mesenchymal stem cells and growth factors from the bone marrow to the OC defect; and this process eventually leads to the formation of fibrocartilaginous tissue that covers the defect [87]. The fibrocartilage produced by bone marrow stimulation techniques is comprised of varying amounts of type I, type II, and type III collagen, which been shown to have an inferior biomechanical properties compared to the adjacent native hyaline cartilage [88, 89]. In patients with isolated OC lesions, Steadman et al. reported good to excellent results based on patient-reported outcomes over an average follow-up period of approximately 11 years [90]. The success of this surgical intervention is inherently associated with the surgical technique and, according to Hurst et al., to a strict rehabilitation protocol employed postoperatively [86]. Early joint mobility with continuous passive motion and reduced weight-bearing is recommended to provide a suitable environment to stimulate clot maturation.

In an evidence-based systematic analysis on the efficacy of microfracture, several factors affecting functional outcomes were identified [91]. Positive prognostic factors included younger age (< 30 to 45 years), duration of symptoms < 12 months, lower body mass index, higher preoperative activity levels (TAS > 4), lesions less than 2 to 4 cm^2, and the use of microfracture as a first-line procedure. Mithoefer et al. concluded that while microfracture provides effective short-term improvement of knee function, there is insufficient data on its long-term results [91]. Additional shortcomings of the technique include limited hyaline repair tissue, variable repair cartilage volume, and possible functional deterioration over time [91].

Theoretical advantages of microfracture over drilling include reduced thermal damage to subchondral bone and the creation of a cartilage surface with a greater frictional coefficient, therefore allowing repair tissue to adhere more easily. In addition, it is technically easier to penetrate a defect perpendicularly with a curved awl during an arthroscopic procedure as compared with a drill. To our knowledge, there are currently no published studies which compare microfracture with drilling. In the case of both drilling and microfracture using awls, there is evidence that the use of smaller diameter drills and awls results in improved articular cartilage repair quality in animal models, respectively [92, 93]. One argument to be made in favour of subchondral bone drilling as opposed to using an awl is that deeper penetration of the subchondral bone results in improved quality and volume of cartilage repair tissue [94, 95].

11.7.4 Osteochondral Autograft Transplantation

The use of OC autografts to reconstruct knee articular cartilage defects was first described by Yamashita et al. [96] and further refined and popularized independently by Bobic and Hangody et al. [97, 98]. Osteochondral autograft transplantation involves using a cylindrical cutting device to harvest OC plugs, consisting of full-thickness articular cartilage and the underlying subchondral bone, from the donor site [99, 100]. These OC plugs are then used to fill an articular cartilage defect in the same patient (Fig. 11.6.).

Osteochondral plugs are usually taken from the peripheries of both femoral condyles at the level of the patellofemoral joint and introduced as a mosaic to fill the defect. Different sizes and numbers of plugs can be used in order to maximize filling of the defect. Biomechanical and topographic studies have shown that the medial and lateral trochleas are good donor sites for the femoral condyles and the intercondylar notch for the central trochlea [101, 102]. The gaps left behind fill-in with fibrocartilaginous tissue. Morelli et al. reported that when the grafts are less than 5 mm in diameter, degenerative changes do not present [103].

Although it is possible to perform OAT arthroscopically, it is usually undertaken as a single-stage open procedure [104]. Advantages of OAT include defects that can be filled immediately with native hyaline articular cartilage and also both chondral and OC defects that can be treated in the same way. However, donor site morbidity is a concern. Hangody et al. recom-

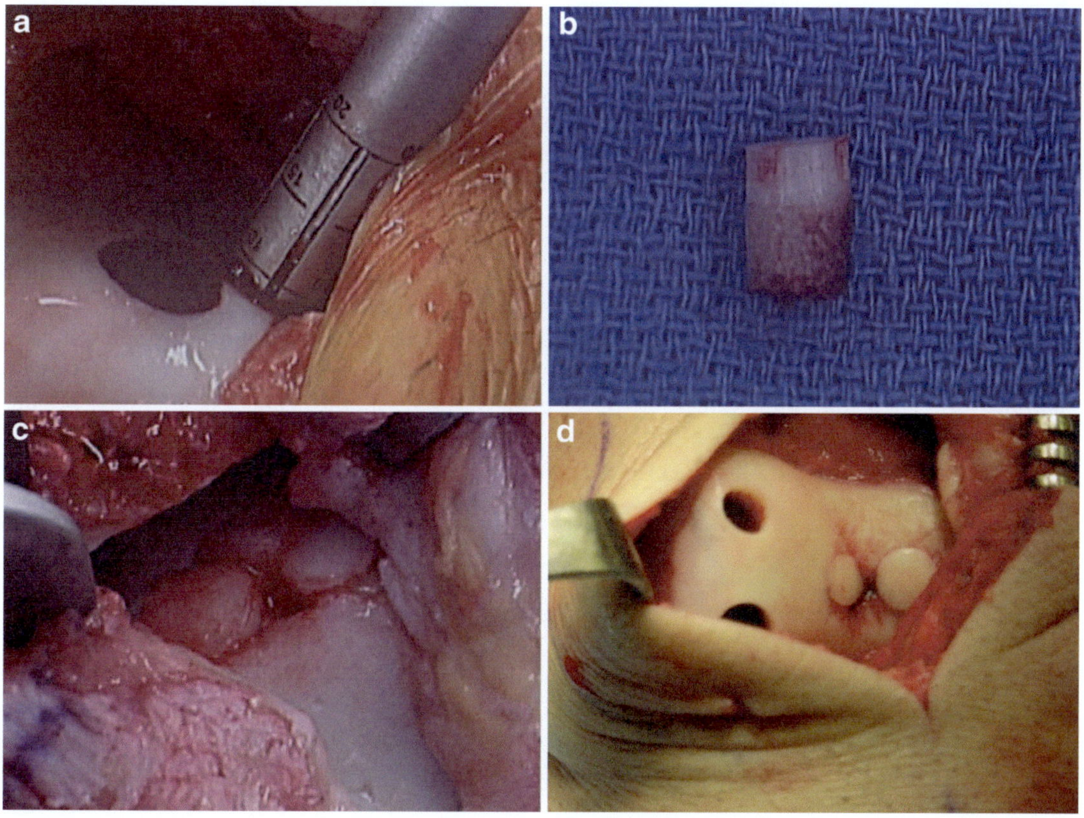

Fig. 11.6 An example of osteochondral autograft transplantation (OAT) used to treat a focal condylar defect of the knee. (**a**) Using a cylindrical cutting device, harvest of a donor OC plug from the non-weight-bearing portion of the lateral femoral condyle. (**b**) Harvested OC plug. (**c**) Implantation of autologous OC plugs into a focal defect in the knee. (**d**) Single image demonstrating donor and recipient sites following an OAT procedure (These figures were obtained with courtesy of Dr. Brian Cole MD MBA)

mend that the area to be treated is limited to between 1 and 4 cm^2 [105]. There are also technical difficulties in restoring the surfaces of both cartilage and bone to produce a smooth, convex joint surface. The thickness of the donor cartilage may differ from that of the area to be treated, and reconstitution of the important subchondral layer may not occur [104]. Perpendicular access to the cartilage surface by cylinder cutters is required for this technique, which makes it difficult to treat defects of the tibial plateau. Hangody and Fules documented the largest, single series of mosaicplasty to date [106]. They reported the results of surgery on 597 femoral condyle, 76 tibial plateau, and 118 patellofemoral surfaces followed up to 10 years postoperatively [106]. Good or excellent results were reported in 92%, 87%, and 79% of patients who underwent mosaicplasty of the femoral condyle, tibial plateau, and patellofemoral joint, respectively. Gudas et al. conducted a randomized controlled trial in 60 patients comparing OAT with microfracture [107]. At a mean follow-up of 10 years, patients in the OAT group had significantly better ICRS scores and a lower clinical failure rate (14% vs 38%). Furthermore, patients treated with OAT were more likely to have maintained pre-injury activity levels compared with microfracture controls at 10 years. Solheim et al. also conducted a long term follow-up of patients randomized to treatment with mosaicplasty or microfracture. At a minimum follow-up of 15 years in forty patients, patients treated with the osteochondral procedure had improved Lysholm scores compared to patients treated with microfracture [108–111].

11.7.5 Autologous Chondrocyte Implantation

Adult articular cartilage is avascular and lacks a source of mesenchymal stem cells; hence, it has a limited capacity for repair and regeneration. Therefore, transplantation of cells or tissue having chondrogenic potential into the chondral defect has been considered a valid approach [112–121]. One such technique is the ACI. Carticel is the brand name for the first Food and Drug Admistration (FDA)-approved cell therapy product involving autologous cultured chondrocytes. Recently, a third generation ACI referred to as matrix-induced autologous chondrocyte implantation (MACI, Verticel Corporation, Cambridge, MA) has also been FDA-approved. MACI is comprised of patient's autologous chondrocytes, which are cultured (expanded), placed on porcine collagen membrane and then implanted into the site of cartilage lesion. Patients eligible for ACI include those with clinically significant, symptomatic cartilage defects in the femoral condyle, trochlea, or patella caused by acute or repetitive trauma as well as those who have had inadequate response to a prior arthroscopic or other surgical cartilage repair procedures. ACI is appropriate for small and large defects and bipolar lesions, as well as in revision settings (albeit with inferior results following prior microfracture). Patients who are not eligible include those with OA and with extensive bone loss. These patients usually have joint pain, swelling, catching, or grinding.

(a) *Surgical Technique*

Autologous chondrocyte implantation is a two-stage procedure with an arthroscopic and open component (Figs. 11.7. and 11.8.). Stage I involves the confirmation, based on the criteria outlined above, that the chondral lesion is indeed suitable for an ACI procedure. This is followed by biopsy of the chondral margins of the intercondylar notch (non-weight-bearing area). Using an arthroscopic gouge or ring curet, two to three full-thickness chondral samples measuring 5 mm × 10 mm each (size of a tictac) is obtained [122]. During this initial stage, the defect is also sized and graded using the surgeon's preferred arthroscopic classification.

During stage II of ACI procedure, a standard medial or lateral parapatellar incision and arthrotomy are used for knee exposure. For patellofemoral defects, a midline incision can be utilized followed by a medial arthrotomy that allows for patellar eversion and exposure. During debridement of the defect, all damaged and calcified cartilage is removed using a No. 15 scalpel for sharp excision. Fissured edges also need to be debrided so that healthy, firm, vertical margins are achieved [122]. Any bleeding that is present

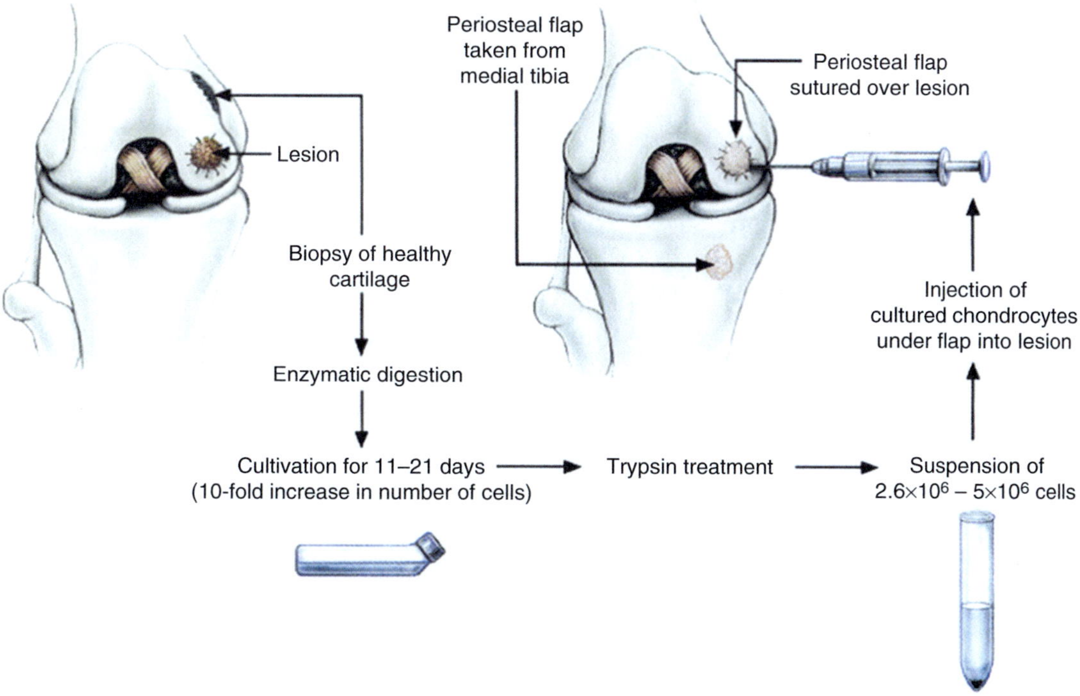

Fig. 11.7 Schematic illustration of autologous chondrocyte implantation technique for cartilage repair outlining procedures stages I and II (Permission granted by *New England Journal of Medicine* -Brittberg et al. [116])

at the base of the defect must be controlled using epinephrine-soaked pads and/or fibrin glue. The defect is then sized using metal foil paper or glove wrapping [122].

The original ACI technique involved debridement of the chondral defect, followed by suturing a membrane around the defect and then injecting a suspension of cultured chondrocytes into the defect under the membrane. The initial membrane used was a piece of periosteum, since it contains pluripotent mesenchymal stem cells with the potential for chondrogenic differentiation and it also produces bioactive factors that aid in chondrogenesis [122–125]. Both in vivo and in vitro data have demonstrated that periosteum-derived mesenchymal stem cells differentiate into neo-chondrocytes, and this has been the basis for using periosteal grafting (periosteal arthroplasty) for chondral defects [126–134]. When periosteum is used, the metal foil template is oversized by 1 to 1.5 mm around the circumference because the harvested periosteum tends to contract [122]. At the present time, it is more common to use a porcine-derived type I/III collagen bilayer membrane (ACI-C) [135, 136].

Following chondral defect preparation and sizing, the collagen bilayer membrane is aligned over the defect in the orientation matching the template. The membrane is sutured to the cartilage rim with multiple 6–0 dyed Vicryl interrupted sutures spaced every 2 to 3 mm [122]. If the defect is uncontained, suture anchors are used to attached the membrane on the uncontained side [122]. Knots are tied over the membrane, not over the articular cartilage. Next, the watertight integrity of the construct is tested using an 18-gauge catheter, and a saline-filled tuberculin syringe is placed deep to the membrane via a small residual opening [122]. After confirmation of a watertight seal, fibrin glue is placed over the margins of the repair. Sterile, viable cells are finally aspirated from the shipping vials and introduced through the tuberculin syringe with an 18-gauge angiocatheter. The injection site is closed with a simple Vicryl stich and sealed with fibrin glue [122].

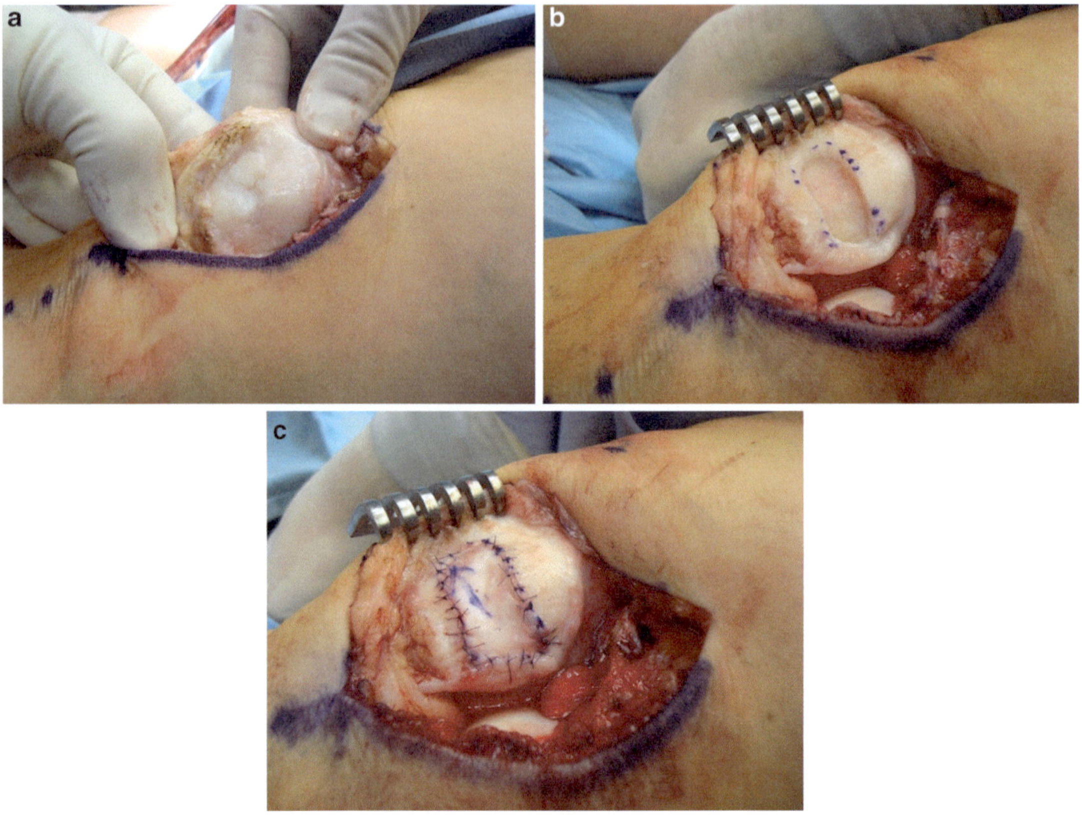

Fig. 11.8 Stage II of a Carticel procedure for the management of an isolated focal defect involving the patella. (**a**) Chondral defect assessment. (**b**) Defect sizing and creation of vertical walls at the margins. (**c**) Collagen type I/III bilayer membrane sutured onto the defect with 6–0 dyed Vicryl suture. Cultured chondrocytes were injected in a suspension through an opening in the construct which was subsequently closed (Arrow) (Images have been provided through the courtesy of Dr. Brian J Cole, MD, MBA)

An analysis of prospectively collected data from 199 patients that afford a favourable outcome following ACI was performed by the group at the Royal National Orthopaedic Hospital, London [137]. Patients were followed for up to 4 years following ACI surgery for symptomatic OC defects in the knee. Factors associated with a statistically superior outcome included younger patients with high preoperative function as assessed with modified Cincinnati score, symptoms for less than 2 years, mono-focal defects, defect(s) located on the lateral femoral condyle or trochlea, and fewer than two previous procedures on the index knee. The above findings corroborated the favourable outcome with respect to pain relief and significant improvement of function in adolescents post ACI treatment for symptomatic chondral and OC lesions [138]. Thirty-one symptomatic patients (age range, 14 to 18 years) were followed up for a period of 12 to 126 months. Excellent or good results were reported in 84% of patients with improvement in the modified Cincinnati rating system from 48 preoperatively to 92 postoperatively.

Harris et al. conducted a systematic review that is comprised of level I and II clinical studies to compare the efficacy of ACI with alternative cartilage repair treatments [20]. Based on this review, complications were reported to be higher with open, periosteal-covered, first-generation techniques. Furthermore, younger patients with a shorter duration of preoperative symptoms and fewer surgical procedures had the best outcomes following both microfracture and ACI. Defect size more than 4 cm^2 was the only factor predictive of better outcomes when ACI was compared to OATS or microfracture.

A level of evidence III retrospective cohort study was conducted by Jungmann et al. to investigate the patient's individual and environmental risk factors, which were predictive of re-intervention after an index ACI procedure [139]. Of the 413 patients who underwent an ACI procedure, 88 (21.3%) required re-intervention at a mean time of 1.8 years. The four prognostic factors associated with a significantly higher risk for repeat surgery were female gender, previous surgeries of the affected joint, previous bone marrow stimulation, and previous periosteal patch-covered ACI. Additional findings included lower re-intervention rates for the intermediate (overweight) BMI group (16.8%), suggesting that a BMI higher than 30 (obesity, 25.0%) and an increased physical activity of patients with low BMI (23.7%) are associated with an inferior outcome. Furthermore, the authors demonstrated that unlike that for microfracture, the defect size was not a predictor of re-intervention following ACI. The authors highlighted that these facts are easily obtainable in the preoperative period when considering an ACI procedure. Finally, a recent case-control study by Pestka et al. demonstrated that age- and defect-matched patients treated with ACI after a failed initial microfracture procedure were significantly more likely to have higher failure rates and lower Knee Injury and Osteoarthritis Outcome Score (KOOS) for pain and ADL scores compared with patients whose first-line treatment was with ACI [140]. Finally, Saris et al. conducted a level 1 randomized trial where patients were treated with either MACI or MFX. In this study of 144 patients, patients with defects larger or equal to 3 cm squared had improved KOOS scores and a similar safety profile in the group of patients treated with MACI. Mistry et al. have also demonstrated that in a survival analysis of studies comparing ACI to marrow stimularion, survival analysis suggests that long-term results are better with ACI. Further, economic modelling suggested that ACI was cost-effective compared with microfracture across a range of scenarios [141, 142].

11.7.6 Fresh Osteochondral Allografts

Gross et al. popularized the concept of OC allograft transplantation in the mid-1970s [143]. Since then an increased attention to this cartilage restoration technique for managing patients with both focal and diffuse OC defects in the knee has been seen [144]. Fresh OC allografts are indicated in patients who have large, deep, and extensive chondral or OC lesions, post-traumatic defects, ON, bone loss, or associated subchondral bone marrow edema and in patients with a failed index cartilage restoration procedure. The main advantage of using allograft is inherent to its bilayered structure comprising of full-thickness hyaline cartilage with viable chondrocytes and an underlying subchondral bone; while the articular cartilage component is fully developed at the time of implantation, the subchondral bone requires a substantial period of time to allow for creeping substitution [23].

The principle determinate for OC allograft selection is the chondrocyte viability. Historically, grafts were implanted within 24 h of procurement, but concerns for disease transmission have led to a minimum of 14 days required for aerobic, anaerobic, spore-forming bacterial and viral testing prior to release [23]. In addition, aseptically processed prolonged fresh grafts are most commonly used and maintained at 4°C as opposed to frozen or cryopreserved grafts [145]. Unfortunately, it is known that chondrocyte viability decreases in allografts stored for over 14 days and generally should be implanted by 24 days [146, 147]. Frozen grafts have demonstrated decreased cell viability with deterioration in graft quality in vivo exhibited in the form of fissures or fibrosis progressing to its eventual breakdown [148]. Frozen allografts have inferior biological and biomechanical properties compared with fresh allografts [149].

Articular cartilage is avascular and immunoprivileged; therefore, any failure of OC allograft tissue is not a result of immune reaction to the donor cartilage. Failure of cartilage and/or bone integration of the implanted graft with the corresponding host tissue is the most common mode of failure [150–153]. In a systematic review of 19 retrospective clinical studies, Chahal et al. documented that at a mean follow-up of 5 years, good clinical outcomes have been reported with a high satisfaction rate (86%) and a low short-term complication rate (2.4%). Furthermore, two studies included in this review also estimated that the survivorship of OC allografts was 75% at 15-year follow-up [21, 154, 155].

In the context of large uncontained OC defects, Gross et al. showed that patients undergoing concomitant osteotomy with OC allograft transplantation did better than patients with prior or delayed osteotomy [155–157]. Furthermore, concomitant meniscus transplantation was associated with improved long-term survivorship of bulk tibial OC allografts; whereas, patients with severe OA degeneration had poorer outcomes. Using data from the same group of patients, Ghazavi et al. stated that factors related to failure included age over 50 years, bipolar defects (femur and tibia), varus or valgus malalignment of the knee, and workers' compensation patients [158]. In regard to radiographic findings, graft collapse of more than 3 mm or joint space narrowing of 50% or more was likely to be associated with graft failure.

With respect to focal defects in an athletic population, Krych et al. investigated athletes' return to sport status post OC allograft transplantation [23]. Using a multiple logistic regression model for risk factors of failure, they reported that patients over 25 years old and with more than 12 months of preoperative symptoms were less likely to return to full athletic activity.

(a) *Surgical Technique*

Osteochondral allograft transplantation is an open surgical procedure which requires the use of an arthrotomy size to be consistent with the location and extent of the lesion [159]. For larger defects, an anterior midline incision is made from the proximal pole of the patella to the tibial tubercle. For smaller focal defects, a medial or lateral parapatellar skin incision and arthrotomy are made. Another alternative is to use the subvastus approach to allow for accelerated postoperative quadriceps rehabilitation. Subsequently, the patella is retracted with a Z-retractor placed into the notch [159].

For focal defects, a press-fit technique is utilized as shown in Fig. 11.9 [159]. After knee exposure, the chondral defect is identified. For more posterior chondral lesion, hyperflexion of the knee may be required. A cylindrical sizing guide is placed over the defect to determine the optimal diameter of the allograft plug. Following this, a guide pin is placed in the centre of the defect perpendicular to the surface at a depth of 2 to 3 cm [159]. A counterbore reamer is then used to make a recipient socket with a depth of 6 to 8 mm, and the depth of the recipient socket is then measured in four quadrants starting at the 12 o'clock position. Concomitantly, the donor graft is prepared at the back table. This requires careful matching of the size and surface contour of the donor and recipient sites using a proprietary allograft preparation system. Using light impaction forces to prevent chondrocyte injury and death, the graft is then press-fitted into the recipient site. An oversized tamp is used to make the graft flush with the surrounding native cartilage realizing that it is preferable to recess the graft rather than to leave it proud. When necessary, additional fixation can be achieved with absorbable polydioxanone pins [159].

For large uncontained OC defects, the transplantation of fresh OC allografts involves two surgical teams – one for the graft preparation and the other for the recipient surgery (Fig. 11.10). The recipient knee is approached through a midline incision, if possible. This is followed by exposure of the knee via a medial or lateral parapatellar arthrotomy, depending on the condyle to be replaced. Excision of the damaged area of the femoral condyle is accomplished by removing the least amount of bone required to reach a healthy, bleeding bed. Measurements of the defect and the excised fragment are taken [160].

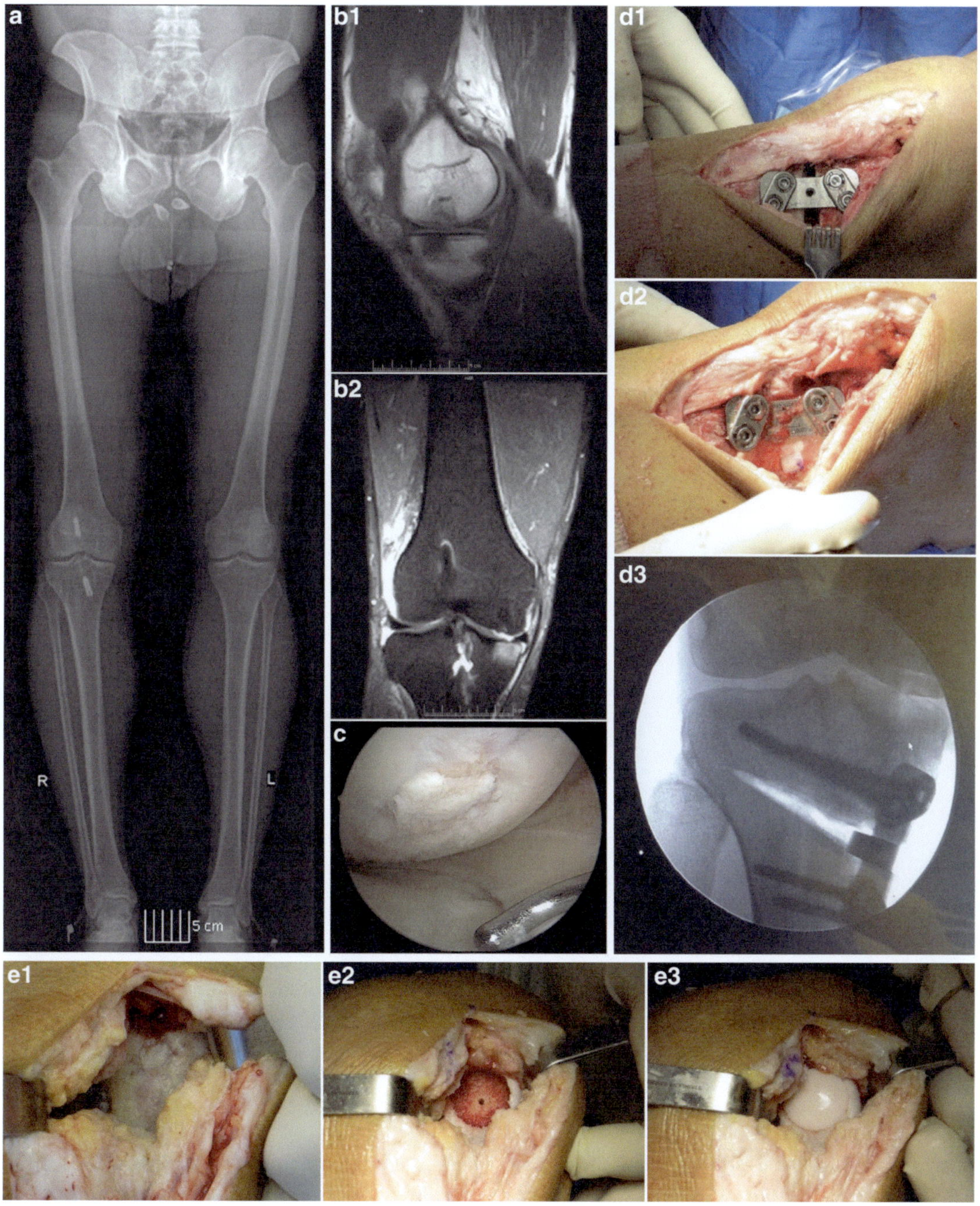

Fig. 11.9 Case presentation of a 47-year-old male with medial knee pain and swelling following a past history of osteochondral autograft transplantation. (**a**) Workup demonstrated varus alignment on X-ray. (**b**) Sagittal and coronal MR images revealed subchondral edema in the medial femoral condyle. (**c**) Corroborating arthroscopic view showed chondral pathology. (**d**) Definitive treatment consisted of a medial opening wedge high tibial osteotomy. (**e**) A fresh osteochondral allograft of the medial femoral condyle (**a**–**e** were obtained with permission from Dr. Brian Cole, MD, MBA)

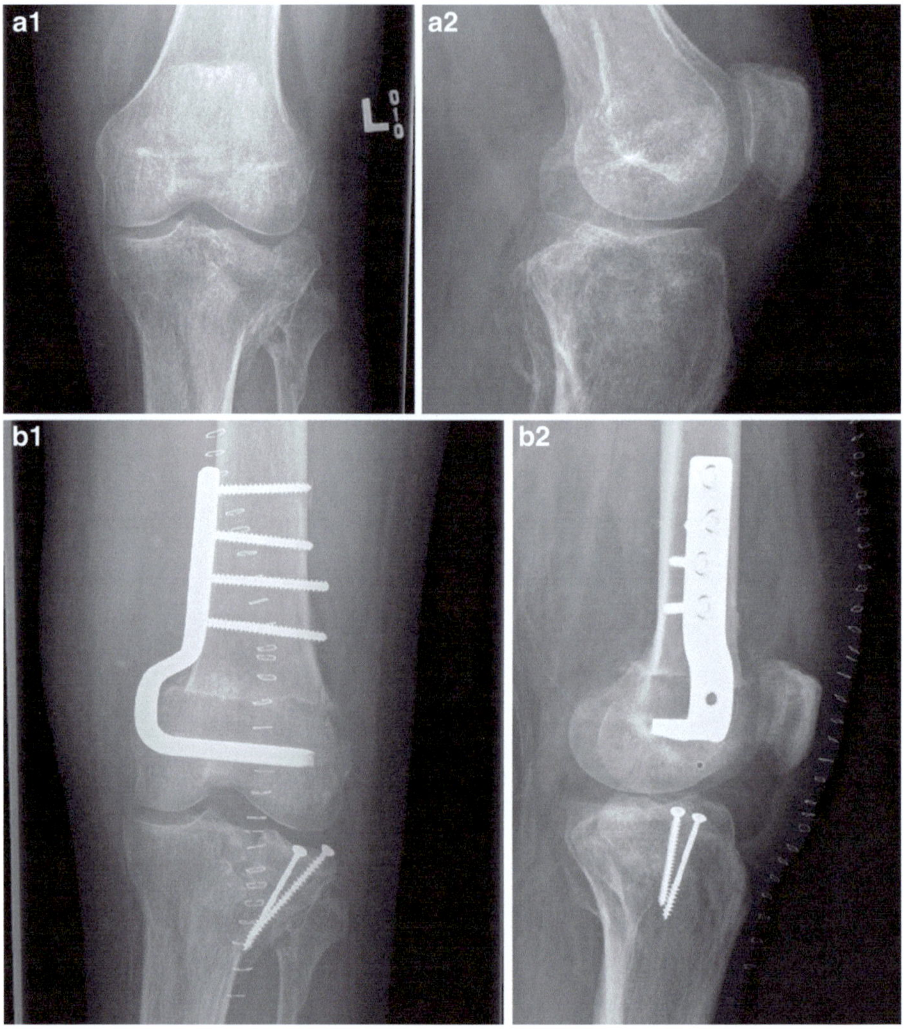

Fig. 11.10 Long-term follow-up after fresh osteochondral OC allograft transplantation for a large post-traumatic defect involving the lateral tibial plateau. (**a**) Anteroposterior and sagittal radiograph of the central defect in the lateral tibial plateau following a prior malunited tibial plateau fracture. (**b**) Treatment with a fresh OC allograft of the lateral tibial plateau in association with a distal femoral varus closing wedge osteotomy (Images obtained from Dr. Allan Gross MD, FRCSC, O ONT)

On a separate table, the harvested knee now has all soft tissue removed. Care is taken to preserve the meniscus if it is needed for transplantation [160]. Using an oscillating saw, an OC fragment equal in size to the excised fragment is removed. It is trimmed to fit well into the recipient's condylar defect. Two partially threaded small fragment cancellous screws with washers are used to hold the fragment in place [160]. According to the preoperative plan, a corrective valgus-producing high tibial osteotomy or varus-producing distal femoral osteotomy is performed.

Gross et al. conducted a long-term follow-up on 69 patients who have undergone revision surgery following a prior fresh OC allograft for focal post-traumatic defect [161]. The graft survival time ranged from 1 to 25 years. Histological features associated with long-term allograft survival included viable chondrocytes, functional preservation of the articular cartilage ECM, and complete replacement of the graft bone with the host bone. The authors concluded that given the chondrocyte viability, long-term survival of hyaline cartilage up to 25 years or more depends on graft stability by rigid fixation of host to graft bone (i.e. mechanical stability). Less stable host-graft interfaces tend to produce the replacement of the full-thickness hyaline cartilage with fibrocartilage. Thus, the fundamental cause of late fresh OC allograft failure appeared to be graft instability leading to nonunion and continued remodeling at the host-graft interface, both bony and cartilaginous. From a technical point of view, a precisely matched and fitted allograft into the prepared host bed is of paramount importance in ensuring the stability [161].

11.8 Conclusions

The surgical approach to treating patients with chondral and osteochondral defects is influenced by multiple patient- and defect-specific factors in the context of global lower extremity structure and function [162–164]. Not all cartilage lesions are symptomatic, and when they are, not all defects can be treated with a uniform treatment plan. The triad of meniscal deficiency, ligamentous instability, and malalignment must be taken into consideration, and when present, all existing pathoanatomical states should be addressed with staged or combined procedures. Patient selection is paramount, and decision-making should be guided by evidence-based recommendations. As new therapies using novel cell sources (e.g. minced cartilage, stem cells) and scaffolds are introduced into the market, an ongoing critical evaluation of the best available evidence should guide their incorporation into routine surgical practice.

References

1. Shelbourne KD, Jari S, Gray T. Outcome of untreated traumatic articular cartilage defects of the knee: a natural history study. J Bone Joint Surg Am. 2003;85-A(Suppl 2):8–16.
2. Curl WW, Krome J, Gordon ES, Rushing J, Smith BP, Poehling GG. Cartilage injuries: a review of 31,516 knee arthroscopies. Arthroscopy. 1997;13(4):456–60.
3. Shapiro F, Koide S, Glimcher MJ. Cell origin and differentiation in the repair of full-thickness defects of articular cartilage. J Bone Joint Surg Am. 1993;75(4):532–53.
4. Chahal J, Thiel GV, Hussey K, Cole BJ. Managing the patient with failed cartilage restoration. Sports Med Arthrosc. 2013;21(2):62–8.
5. Demange M, Gomoll AH. The use of osteochondral allografts in the management of cartilage defects. Curr Rev Musculoskelet Med. 2012;5(3):229–35.
6. Frank R, et al. Complex problems in knee articular cartilage. In: Cole BJ, Sekiya JK, editors. Surgical techniques of shoulder, elbow, and knee in sports medicine. 2nd ed. Saunders; 2013.
7. Cole BJ, Pascual-Garrido C, Grumet RC. Surgical management of articular cartilage defects in the knee. J Bone Joint Surg Am. 2009;91(7):1778–90.
8. Gomoll AH, et al. Surgical management of articular cartilage defects of the knee. J Bone Joint Surg Am. 2010;92(14):2470–90.
9. Redler LH, et al. Management of articular cartilage defects of the knee. Phys Sportsmed. 2012;40(1):20–35.
10. Gomoll AH, et al. Preoperative measurement of cartilage defects by MRI underestimates lesion size. Cartilage. 2011;2(4):389–93.
11. Harris JD, et al. Biological knee reconstruction: a systematic review of combined meniscal allograft transplantation and cartilage repair or restoration. Arthroscopy. 2011;27(3):409–18.
12. Peterson L, et al. Treatment of osteochondritis dissecans of the knee with autologous chondrocyte transplantation: results at two to ten years. J Bone Joint Surg Am. 2003;85-A(Suppl 2):17–24.
13. Fulkerson JP. Anteromedialization of the tibial tuberosity for patellofemoral malalignment. Clin Orthop Relat Res. 1983;177:176–81.
14. Buckwalter JA, Mankin HJ. Articular cartilage: tissue design and chondrocyte-matrix interactions. Instr Course Lect. 1998;47:477–86.
15. Caplan AI, et al. Principles of cartilage repair and regeneration. Clin Orthop Relat Res. 1997;342:254–69.
16. Buckwalter JA, Mankin HJ. Articular cartilage: degeneration and osteoarthritis, repair, regeneration, and transplantation. Instr Course Lect. 1998;47:487–504.
17. Meyers MH, Akeson W, Convery FR. Resurfacing of the knee with fresh osteochondral allograft. J Bone Joint Surg Am. 1989;71(5):704–13.
18. Noyes FR, Barber-Westin SD. Meniscus transplantation: indications, techniques, clinical outcomes. Instr Course Lect. 2005;54:341–53.
19. Bekkers JE, Inklaar M, Saris DB. Treatment selection in articular cartilage lesions of the knee: a sys-

tematic review. Am J Sports Med. 2009;37(Suppl 1):148S–55S.
20. Harris JD, et al. Autologous chondrocyte implantation: a systematic review. J Bone Joint Surg Am. 2010;92(12):2220–33.
21. Chahal J, Gross AE, Gross C, Mall N, Dwyer T. Chahal A, Whelan DB, Cole BJ. Outcomes of osteochondral allograft transplantation in the knee. Arthroscopy. 2013;29(3):575–88.
22. Mithoefer K, et al. Return to sports participation after articular cartilage repair in the knee: scientific evidence. Am J Sports Med. 2009;37(Suppl 1):167S–76S.
23. Krych AJ, Robertson CM, Williams RJ 3rd. Return to athletic activity after osteochondral allograft transplantation in the knee. Am J Sports Med. 2012;40(5):1053–9.
24. Kanneganti P, et al. The effect of smoking on ligament and cartilage surgery in the knee: a systematic review. Am J Sports Med. 2012;40(12):2872–8.
25. Cain EL, Clancy WG. Treatment algorithm for osteochondral injuries of the knee. Clin Sports Med. 2001;20(2):321–42.
26. Vaquero J, Vidal C, Cubillo A. Intra-articular traumatic disorders of the knee in children and adolescents. Clin Orthop Relat Res. 2005;432:97–106.
27. Kennedy JC, Grainger RW, McGraw RW. Osteochondral fractures of the femoral condyles. J Bone Joint Surg Br. 1966;48(3):436–40.
28. Rorabeck CH, Bobechko WP. Acute dislocation of the patella with osteochondral fracture: a review of eighteen cases. J Bone Joint Surg Br. 1976;58(2):237–40.
29. Rosenberg NJ. Osteochondral fractures of the lateral femoral condyle. J Bone Joint Surg Am. 1964;46:1013–26.
30. Ahstrom JP Jr. Osteochondral fracture in the knee joint associated with hypermobility and dislocation of the patella. Report of eighteen cases. J Bone Joint Surg Am. 1965;47(8):1491–502.
31. Makin M. Osteochondral fracture of the lateral femoral condyle. J Bone Joint Surg Am. 1951;**33**(A:1):262–4.
32. Matthewson MH, Dandy DJ. Osteochondral fractures of the lateral femoral condyle: a result of indirect violence to the knee. J Bone Joint Surg Br. 1978;60-B(2):199–202.
33. Sledge SL. Microfracture techniques in the treatment of osteochondral injuries. Clin Sports Med. 2001;20(2):365–77.
34. Taitsman LA, et al. Osteochondral fracture of the distal lateral femoral condyle: a report of two cases. J Orthop Trauma. 2006;20(5):358–62.
35. Binnet MS, et al. Arthroscopic fixation of intercondylar eminence fractures using a 4-portal technique. Arthroscopy. 2001;17(5):450–60.
36. Binnet MS, et al. Histopathologic assessment of healed osteochondral fractures. Arthroscopy. 2001;17(3):278–85.
37. O'Driscoll SW, Keeley FW, Salter RB. Durability of regenerated articular cartilage produced by free autogenous periosteal grafts in major full-thickness defects in joint surfaces under the influence of continuous passive motion. A follow-up report at one year. J Bone Joint Surg Am. 1988;70(4):595–606.
38. O'Driscoll SW, Salter RB. The repair of major osteochondral defects in joint surfaces by neochondrogenesis with autogenous osteoperiosteal grafts stimulated by continuous passive motion. An experimental investigation in the rabbit. Clin Orthop Relat Res. 1986;208:131–40.
39. Shimizu T, et al. Experimental study on the repair of full thickness articular cartilage defects: effects of varying periods of continuous passive motion, cage activity, and immobilization. J Orthop Res. 1987;5(2):187–97.
40. Murray RC, et al. Biomechanical comparison of the Herbert and AO cortical bone screws for compression of an equine third carpal bone dorsal plane slab osteotomy. Vet Surg. 1998;27(1):49–55.
41. Barton NJ. The Herbert screw for fractures of the scaphoid. J Bone Joint Surg Br. 1996;78(4):517–8.
42. Herbert TJ, Fisher WE, Leicester AW. The Herbert bone screw: a ten year perspective. J Hand Surg Br. 1992;17(4):415–9.
43. Lewis PL, Foster BK. Herbert screw fixation of osteochondral fractures about the knee. Aust N Z J Surg. 1990;60(7):511–3.
44. Mbubaegbu CE, Percy AJ. Femoral osteochondral fracture–a non-contact injury in martial arts? A case report. Br J Sports Med. 1994;28(3):203–5.
45. Mashoof AA, et al. Osteochondral injury to the mid-lateral weight-bearing portion of the lateral femoral condyle associated with patella dislocation. Arthroscopy. 2005;21(2):228–32.
46. Wouters DB, van Horn JR, Bos RR. The use of biodegradables in the treatment of osteochondritis dissecans of the knee: fiction or future? Acta Orthop Belg. 2003;69(2):175–81.
47. Larsen MW, Pietrzak WS, DeLee JC. Fixation of osteochondritis dissecans lesions using poly(l-lactic acid)/ poly(glycolic acid) copolymer bioabsorbable screws. Am J Sports Med. 2005;33(1):68–76.
48. Bostman OM. Osteolytic changes accompanying degradation of absorbable fracture fixation implants. J Bone Joint Surg Br. 1991;73(4):679–82.
49. Mainil-Varlet P, Rahn B, Gogolewski S. Long-term in vivo degradation and bone reaction to various polylactides. 1. One-year results. Biomaterials. 1997;18(3):257–66.
50. Wang X, et al. Tissue engineering of biphasic cartilage constructs using various biodegradable scaffolds: an in vitro study. Biomaterials. 2004;25(17):3681–8.
51. Tabaddor RR, et al. Fixation of juvenile osteochondritis dissecans lesions of the knee using poly 96L/4D-lactide copolymer bioabsorbable implants. J Pediatr Orthop. 2010;30(1):14–20.
52. Braune C, et al. Resorbable pin refixation of an osteochondral fracture of the lateral femoral con-

dyle due to traumatic patellar dislocation: case management, follow-up and strategy in adolescents. Z Orthop Ihre Grenzgeb. 2004;142(1):103–8.
53. Fuchs M, et al. Refixation of osteochondral fragments using absorbable implants. First results of a retrospective study. Chirurg. 2003;74(6):554–61.
54. Wouters DB, et al. The meniscus arrow or metal screw for treatment of osteochondritis dissecans? In vitro comparison of their effectiveness. Knee Surg Sports Traumatol Arthrosc. 2004;12(1):52–7.
55. Wouters DB, et al. Fixation of osteochondral fragments in the human knee using meniscus arrows. Knee Surg Sports Traumatol Arthrosc. 2011;19(2):183–8.
56. Shermak MA, et al. Fixation of the craniofacial skeleton with butyl-2-cyanoacrylate and its effects on histotoxicity and healing. Plast Reconstr Surg. 1998;102(2):309–18.
57. Shermak MA, et al. Butyl-2-cyanoacrylate fixation of mandibular osteotomies. Plast Reconstr Surg. 1998;102(2):319–24.
58. Harper MC. Viscous isoamyl 2-cyanoacrylate as an osseous adhesive in the repair of osteochondral osteotomies in rabbits. J Orthop Res. 1988;6(2):287–92.
59. Yilmaz C, Kuyurtar F. Fixation of a talar osteochondral fracture with cyanoacrylate glue. Arthroscopy. 2005;21(8):1009.
60. Gul R, et al. Osteochondral fractures in the knee treated with butyl-2-cyanoacrylate glue. A case report. Acta Orthop Belg. 2006;72(5):641–3.
61. Bowers AL, Huffman GR. Suture bridge fixation of a femoral condyle traumatic osteochondral defect. Clin Orthop Relat Res. 2008;466(9):2276–81.
62. Merchan EC, Galindo E. Arthroscope-guided surgery versus nonoperative treatment for limited degenerative osteoarthritis of the femorotibial joint in patients over 50 years of age: a prospective comparative study. Arthroscopy. 1993;9(6):663–7.
63. Blain EJ, et al. Up-regulation of matrix metalloproteinase expression and activation following cyclical compressive loading of articular cartilage in vitro. Arch Biochem Biophys. 2001;396(1):49–55.
64. Honda K, et al. The effects of high magnitude cyclic tensile load on cartilage matrix metabolism in cultured chondrocytes. Eur J Cell Biol. 2000;79(9):601–9.
65. Briggs KK, et al. Reliability, validity, and responsiveness of the Lysholm knee score and Tegner activity scale for patients with meniscal injury of the knee. J Bone Joint Surg Am. 2006;88(4):698–705.
66. Hubbard MJ. Articular debridement versus washout for degeneration of the medial femoral condyle. A five-year study. J Bone Joint Surg Br. 1996;78(2):217–9.
67. Lysholm J, Gillquist J. Evaluation of knee ligament surgery results with special emphasis on use of a scoring scale. Am J Sports Med. 1982;10(3):150–4.
68. Barber FA, Iwasko NG. Treatment of grade III femoral chondral lesions: mechanical chondroplasty versus monopolar radiofrequency probe. Arthroscopy. 2006;22(12):1312–7.
69. Moseley JB, et al. A controlled trial of arthroscopic surgery for osteoarthritis of the knee. N Engl J Med. 2002;347(2):81–8.
70. Jackson RW, Dieterichs C. The results of arthroscopic lavage and debridement of osteoarthritic knees based on the severity of degeneration: a 4- to 6-year symptomatic follow-up. Arthroscopy. 2003;19(1):13–20.
71. Harwin SF. Arthroscopic debridement for osteoarthritis of the knee: predictors of patient satisfaction. Arthroscopy. 1999;15(2):142–6.
72. Baumgaertner MR, et al. Arthroscopic debridement of the arthritic knee. Clin Orthop Relat Res. 1990;253:197–202.
73. Kirkley A, et al. A randomized trial of arthroscopic surgery for osteoarthritis of the knee. N Engl J Med. 2008;359(11):1097–107.
74. McNickle AG, Provencher MT, Cole BJ. Overview of existing cartilage repair technology. Sports Med Arthrosc. 2008;16(4):196–201.
75. O'Driscoll SW. The healing and regeneration of articular cartilage. J Bone Joint Surg Am. 1998;80(12):1795–812.
76. Friedman MJ, et al. Preliminary results with abrasion arthroplasty in the osteoarthritic knee. Clin Orthop Relat Res. 1984;182:200–5.
77. Convery FR, Akeson WH, Keown GH. The repair of large osteochondral defects. An experimental study in horses. Clin Orthop Relat Res. 1972;82:253–62.
78. Kim HK, Moran ME, Salter RB. The potential for regeneration of articular cartilage in defects created by chondral shaving and subchondral abrasion. An experimental investigation in rabbits. J Bone Joint Surg Am. 1991;73(9):1301–15.
79. Mitchell N, Shepard N. The resurfacing of adult rabbit articular cartilage by multiple perforations through the subchondral bone. J Bone Joint Surg Am. 1976;58(2):230–3.
80. Salter RB, et al. The biological effect of continuous passive motion on the healing of full-thickness defects in articular cartilage. An experimental investigation in the rabbit. J Bone Joint Surg Am. 1980;62(8):1232–51.
81. Hefti F, et al. Evaluation of knee ligament injuries with the IKDC form. Knee Surg Sports Traumatol Arthrosc. 1993;1(3–4):226–34.
82. Johnson LL. Arthroscopic abrasion arthroplasty historical and pathologic perspective: present status. Arthroscopy. 1986;2(1):54–69.
83. Rand JA. Role of arthroscopy in osteoarthritis of the knee. Arthroscopy. 1991;7(4):358–63.
84. Benthien JP, Schwaninger M, Behrens P. We do not have evidence based methods for the treatment of cartilage defects in the knee. Knee Surg Sports Traumatol Arthrosc. 2011;19(4):543–52.

85. Chen H, et al. Drilling and microfracture lead to different bone structure and necrosis during bone-marrow stimulation for cartilage repair. J Orthop Res. 2009;27(11):1432–8.
86. Hurst JM, et al. Rehabilitation following microfracture for chondral injury in the knee. Clin Sports Med. 2010;29(2):257–65.
87. Reinold MM, et al. Current concepts in the rehabilitation following articular cartilage repair procedures in the knee. J Orthop Sports Phys Ther. 2006;36(10):774–94.
88. Frisbie DD, et al. Arthroscopic subchondral bone plate microfracture technique augments healing of large chondral defects in the radial carpal bone and medial femoral condyle of horses. Vet Surg. 1999;28(4):242–55.
89. Bae DK, Yoon KH, Song SJ. Cartilage healing after microfracture in osteoarthritic knees. Arthroscopy. 2006;22(4):367–74.
90. Steadman JR, et al. Outcomes of microfracture for traumatic chondral defects of the knee: average 11-year follow-up. Arthroscopy. 2003;19(5):477–84.
91. Mithoefer K, et al. Clinical efficacy of the microfracture technique for articular cartilage repair in the knee: an evidence-based systematic analysis. Am J Sports Med. 2009;37(10):2053–63.
92. Orth P, et al. Small-diameter awls improve articular cartilage repair after microfracture treatment in a translational animal model. Am J Sports Med. 2016;44(1):209–19.
93. Eldracher M, et al. Small subchondral drill holes improve marrow stimulation of articular cartilage defects. Am J Sports Med. 2014;42(11):2741–50.
94. Chen H, et al. Depth of subchondral perforation influences the outcome of bone marrow stimulation cartilage repair. J Orthop Res. 2011;29(8):1178–84.
95. Pipino G, Risitano S, Alviano F, Wu EJ, Bonsi L, Vaccarisi DC, Indelli PF. Microfractures and hydrogel scaffolds in the treatment of osteochondral knee defects: A clinical and histological evaluation. J Clin Orthop Trauma. 2019;10(1):67–75.
96. Yamashita F, et al. The transplantation of an autogeneic osteochondral fragment for osteochondritis dissecans of the knee. Clin Orthop Relat Res. 1985;201:43–50.
97. Bobic V. Arthroscopic osteochondral autograft transplantation in anterior cruciate ligament reconstruction: a preliminary clinical study. Knee Surg Sports Traumatol Arthrosc. 1996;3(4):262–4.
98. Hangody L, Szigeti I, Karpati Z. A new method for the treatment of serious localized cartilage damage in the knee joint. Osteoporos Int. 1996;3:106–14.
99. Marcacci M, et al. Multiple osteochondral arthroscopic grafting (mosaicplasty) for cartilage defects of the knee: prospective study results at 2-year follow-up. Arthroscopy. 2005;21(4):462–70.
100. Hangody L, et al. Mosaicplasty for the treatment of articular defects of the knee and ankle. Clin Orthop Relat Res. 2001;391(Suppl):S328–36.
101. Ahmad CS, et al. Biomechanical and topographic considerations for autologous osteochondral grafting in the knee. Am J Sports Med. 2001;29(2):201–6.
102. Bartz RL, et al. Topographic matching of selected donor and recipient sites for osteochondral autografting of the articular surface of the femoral condyles. Am J Sports Med. 2001;29(2):207–12.
103. Morelli M, Nagamori J, Miniaci A. Management of chondral injuries of the knee by osteochondral autogenous transfer (mosaicplasty). J Knee Surg. 2002;15(3):185–90.
104. Hangody L, et al. Autologous osteochondral grafting–technique and long-term results. Injury. 2008;39(Suppl 1):S32–9.
105. Hangody L, et al. Clinical experiences with autologous osteochondral mosaicplasty in an athletic population: a 17-year prospective multicenter study. Am J Sports Med. 2010;38(6):1125–33.
106. Hangody L, Fules P. Autologous osteochondral mosaicplasty for the treatment of full-thickness defects of weight-bearing joints: ten years of experimental and clinical experience. J Bone Joint Surg Am. 2003;85-A(Suppl 2):25–32.
107. Gudas R, et al. Ten-year follow-up of a prospective, randomized clinical study of mosaic osteochondral autologous transplantation versus microfracture for the treatment of osteochondral defects in the knee joint of athletes. Am J Sports Med. 2012;40(11):2499–508.
108. Solheim E, Hegna J, Strand T, Harlem T, Inderhaug E. Randomized study of long-term (15–17 Years) outcome after microfracture versus mosaicplasty in knee articular cartilage defects. Am J Sports Med. 2018;46(4):826–31.
109. Solheim E, Hegna J, Inderhaug E. Clinical outcome after mosaicplasty of knee articular cartilage defects of patellofemoral joint versus tibiofemoral joint. J Orthop. 2019;18:36–40.
110. Solheim E, Hegna J, Inderhaug E. Long-term survival after microfracture and mosaicplasty for knee articular cartilage repair: a comparative study between two treatments cohorts. Cartilage. 2018:1947603518783482. https://doi.org/10.1177/1947603518783482. Epub ahead of print.
111. Viamont-Guerra MR, Bonin N, May O, Le Viguelloux A, Saffarini M, Laude F. Promising outcomes of hip mosaicplasty by minimally invasive anterior approach using osteochondral autografts from the ipsilateral femoral head. Knee Surg Sports Traumatol Arthrosc. 2019. https://doi.org/10.1007/s00167-019-05442-1. Epub ahead of print.
112. O'Driscoll SW, Salter RB. The induction of neochondrogenesis in free intra-articular periosteal autografts under the influence of continuous passive motion. An experimental investigation in the rabbit. J Bone Joint Surg Am. 1984;66(8):1248–57.

113. Asonuma K, Vacanti JP. Cell transplantation as replacement therapy for the future. Crit Care Nurs Clin North Am. 1992;4(2):249–54.
114. Cima LG, et al. Tissue engineering by cell transplantation using degradable polymer substrates. J Biomech Eng. 1991;113(2):143–51.
115. Goldberg VM, Caplan AI. Biological resurfacing: an alternative to total joint arthroplasty. Orthopedics. 1994;17(9):819–21.
116. Grandolfo M, et al. Culture and differentiation of chondrocytes entrapped in alginate gels. Calcif Tissue Int. 1993;52(1):42–8.
117. Hendrickson DA, et al. Chondrocyte-fibrin matrix transplants for resurfacing extensive articular cartilage defects. J Orthop Res. 1994;12(4):485–97.
118. Mow VC, et al. Experimental studies on repair of large osteochondral defects at a high weight bearing area of the knee joint: a tissue engineering study. J Biomech Eng. 1991;113(2):198–207.
119. Wakitani S, et al. Mesenchymal cell-based repair of large, full-thickness defects of articular cartilage. J Bone Joint Surg Am. 1994;76(4):579–92.
120. Mehl J, Huck J, Bode G, Hohloch L, Schmitt A, Südkamp NP, Niemeyer P. Clinical mid- to long-term outcome after autologous chondrocyte implantation for patellar cartilage lesions and its correlation with the geometry of the femoral trochlea. Knee. 2019;26(2):364–73.
121. Yoon KH, Kang SG, Kwon YB, Kim EJ, Kim SG. Clinical outcomes and survival rate of autologous chondrocyte implantation with and without concomitant meniscus allograft transplantation: 10- to 15-year follow-up study. Arch Orthop Trauma Surg. 2019. https://doi.org/10.1007/s00402-019-03148-0. Epub ahead of print.
122. Day JB, Gillogly SD. Autologous chondrocyte implantation in the knee. In: Cole BJ, Sekiya JK, editors. Surgical techniques of the shoulder, elbow, and knee in sports medicine. Philadelphia: Saunders Elsevier; 2008. p. 559–66.
123. Brittberg M, et al. Treatment of deep cartilage defects in the knee with autologous chondrocyte transplantation. N Engl J Med. 1994;331(14):889–95.
124. Peterson L, et al. Two- to 9-year outcome after autologous chondrocyte transplantation of the knee. Clin Orthop Relat Res. 2000;374:212–34.
125. O'Driscoll SW, Fitzsimmons JS. The role of periosteum in cartilage repair. Clin Orthop Relat Res. 2001;391(Suppl):S190–207.
126. Gallay SH, et al. Relationship of donor site to chondrogenic potential of periosteum in vitro. J Orthop Res. 1994;12(4):515–25.
127. Iwasaki M, et al. Regulation of proliferation and osteochondrogenic differentiation of periosteum-derived cells by transforming growth factor-beta and basic fibroblast growth factor. J Bone Joint Surg Am. 1995;77(4):543–54.
128. Nakahara H, et al. In vivo osteochondrogenic potential of cultured cells derived from the periosteum. Clin Orthop Relat Res. 1990;259:223–32.
129. O'Driscoll SW, Recklies AD, Poole AR. Chondrogenesis in periosteal explants. An organ culture model for in vitro study. J Bone Joint Surg Am. 1994;76(7):1042–51.
130. Poussa M, Rubak J, Ritsila V. Differentiation of the osteochondrogenic cells of the periosteum in chondrotrophic environment. Acta Orthop Scand. 1981;52(3):235–9.
131. Roush JK, Manley PA, Wilson JW. Effects of immobilization on cartilage formation after periosteal grafting in the rabbit stifle. Vet Surg. 1989;18(5):340–6.
132. Rubak JM, Poussa M, Ritsila V. Chondrogenesis in repair of articular cartilage defects by free periosteal grafts in rabbits. Acta Orthop Scand. 1982;53(2):181–6.
133. Vachon AM, et al. Morphologic study of repair of induced osteochondral defects of the distal portion of the radial carpal bone in horses by use of glued periosteal autografts [corrected]. Am J Vet Res. 1991;52(2):317–27.
134. Zarnett R, et al. Cellular origin and evolution of neochondrogenesis in major full-thickness defects of a joint surface treated by free autogenous periosteal grafts and subjected to continuous passive motion in rabbits. Clin Orthop Relat Res. 1987;222:267–74.
135. Bartlett W, et al. Autologous chondrocyte implantation at the knee using a bilayer collagen membrane with bone graft. A preliminary report. J Bone Joint Surg Br. 2005;87:330–2.
136. Haddo O, et al. The use of chondrogide membrane in autologous chondrocyte implantation. Knee. 2004;11:51–5.
137. Krishnan SP, et al. Who is the ideal candidate for autologous chondrocyte implantation? J Bone Joint Surg Br. 2006;88:61–4.
138. Macmull S, et al. Autologous chondrocyte implantation in the adolescent knee. Am J Sports Med. 2011;39(8):1723–30.
139. Jungmann PM, et al. Autologous chondrocyte implantation for treatment of cartilage defects of the knee: what predicts the need for reintervention? Am J Sports Med. 2012;40(1):58–67.
140. Pestka JM, et al. Clinical outcome of autologous chondrocyte implantation for failed microfracture treatment of full-thickness cartilage defects of the knee joint. Am J Sports Med. 2012;40(2):325–31.
141. Saris D, et al. Matrix-applied characterized autologous cultured chondrocytes versus microfracture: two-year follow-up of a prospective randomized trial. Am J Sports Med. 2014;42(6):1384–94.
142. Mistry H, et al. Autologous chondrocyte implantation in the knee: systematic review and economic evaluation. Health Technol Assess. 2017;21(6):1–294.
143. Gross AE, et al. The allotransplantation of partial joints in the treatment of osteoarthritis of the knee. Clin Orthop Relat Res. 1975;108:7–14.

144. Farr J, et al. Clinical cartilage restoration: evolution and overview. Clin Orthop Relat Res. 2011;469(10):2696–705.
145. Williams JM, et al. Prolonged-fresh preservation of intact whole canine femoral condyles for the potential use as osteochondral allografts. J Orthop Res. 2005;23(4):831–7.
146. Pearsall IAW, et al. Chondrocyte viability in refrigerated osteochondral allografts used for transplantation within the knee. Am J Sports Med. 2004;32(1):125–31.
147. Williams SK, et al. Prolonged storage effects on the articular cartilage of fresh human osteochondral allografts. J Bone Joint Surg Am. 2003;85-A(11):2111–20.
148. Garrett JC. Osteochondral allografts. Instr Course Lect. 1993;42:355–8.
149. Allen RT, et al. Analysis of stored osteochondral allografts at the time of surgical implantation. Am J Sports Med. 2005;33:1479–84.
150. Kandel RA, et al. Histopathology of failed osteoarticular shell allografts. Clin Orthop Relat Res. 1985;197:103–10.
151. Williams SK, et al. Analysis of cartilage tissue on a cellular level in fresh osteochondral allograft retrievals. Am J Sports Med. 2007;35(12):2022–32.
152. Czitrom AA, Keating S, Gross AE. The viability of articular cartilage in fresh osteochondral allografts after clinical transplantation. J Bone Joint Surg Am. 1990;72(4):574–81.
153. Langer F, Gross AE. Immunogenicity of allograft articular cartilage. J Bone Joint Surg Am. 1974;56(2):297–304.
154. Emmerson BC, et al. Fresh osteochondral allografting in the treatment of osteochondritis dissecans of the femoral condyle. Am J Sports Med. 2007;35(6):907–14.
155. Gross AE, Shasha N, Aubin P. Long-term followup of the use of fresh osteochondral allografts for posttraumatic knee defects. Clin Orthop Relat Res. 2005;435:79–87.
156. León SA, Mei XY, Safir OA, Gross AE, Kuzyk PR. Long-term results of fresh osteochondral allografts and realignment osteotomy for cartilage repair in the knee. Bone Joint J. 2019;101-B(1_Supple_A):46–52.
157. Abolghasemian M, León S, Lee PTH, Safir O, Backstein D, Gross AE, Kuzyk PRT. Long-term results of treating large posttraumatic tibial plateau lesions with fresh osteochondral allograft transplantation. J Bone Joint Surg Am. 2019;101(12):1102–08.
158. Ghazavi MT, et al. Fresh osteochondral allografts for post-traumatic osteochondral defects of the knee. J Bone Joint Surg Br. 1997;79(6):1008–13.
159. Kang RW, Gomoll AH, Cole BJ. Osteochondral allografting in the knee. In: Cole BJ, Sekiya JK, editors. Surgical techniques of the shoulder, elbow, and knee in sports medicine, vol. 549-557. Philadelphia: Saunders Elsevier; 2008.
160. Aubin PP, et al. Long-term followup of fresh femoral osteochondral allografts for posttraumatic knee defects. Clin Orthop Relat Res. 2001;391(Suppl):S318–27.
161. Gross AE, et al. Fresh osteochondral allografts for posttraumatic knee defects: long-term followup. Clin Orthop Relat Res. 2008;466(8):1863–70.
162. Medvedeva EV, Grebenik EA, Gornostaeva SN, Telpuhov VI, Lychagin AV, Timashev PS, Chagin AS. Repair of damaged articular cartilage: current approaches and future directions. Int J Mol Sci. 2018;19(8). pii: E2366. https://doi.org/10.3390/ijms19082366.
163. Frank RM, Cotter EJ, Hannon CP, Harrast JJ, Cole BJ. Cartilage restoration surgery: incidence rates, complications, and trends as reported by the American board of orthopaedic surgery part II candidates. Arthroscopy. 2019;35(1):171–8.
164. Jones KJ, Kelley BV, Arshi A, McAllister DR, Fabricant PD. Comparative effectiveness of cartilage repair with respect to the minimal clinically important difference. Am J Sports Med. 2019;13:363546518824552. https://doi.org/10.1177/0363546518824552. Epub ahead of print.

12 Clinical Outcome Assessment of Repaired Articular Cartilage

Benedict A. Rogers, Jaskarndip Chahal, and Allan E. Gross

12.1 Introduction

The ultimate goal of any articular cartilage repair technique is to generate or replace the cartilage defect with hyaline or hyaline-like tissue, to recreate normal articular congruity and to improve overall function, disability and health [1]. However, determining improvements in function, disability and health after an intervention in patients with articular cartilage injury of the knee can only be as effective as the measurement tools available to do so. The need for transparency of surgical outcome data and the drive for quality dictate the use of reliable, valid and responsive outcome measures following any surgical intervention, both clinician-reported and patient-reported.

Over the last two decades, there has been a paradigm shift in the outcome measures that have been developed and incorporated into clinical research. There has been an increasing emphasis on the patient's perspective attempting to measure outcomes from a biopsychosocial perspective. Whilst some instruments attempt to capture the overall function of the knee with a single score, other questionnaires have been developed to measure outcomes across different domains or "constructs" (i.e. physical symptoms, emotions, quality of life). The World Health Organization's International Classification of Functioning, Disability and Health (ICF) comprises a biopsychosocial model in which functioning and disability are conceived as a dynamic interaction between health conditions and environmental and personal factors (Fig. 12.1) [2]. According to the ICF, derangements in anatomic structures should lead to associated impairments as well as activity limitations and participation restrictions [3]. According to this model, the term "impairment" refers to problems in body function or structure such as a significant deviation or loss. "Activity limitation" refers to difficulty in the execution of a task or action by an individual, whilst "participation restrictions" refer to problems

B. A. Rogers, MA, MSc, MRCGP, DipLMC, DipSEM, FRCS (Orth), PhD
Brighton and Sussex Medical School, Brighton, UK

Trauma and Orthopaedics Department, Brighton and Sussex University Hospitals NHS Trust, Brighton, UK

J. Chahal, MD, FRCSC, MSc, MBA
Division of Orthopaedic Surgery, University of Toronto, Toronto, ON, Canada

University of Toronto Orthopaedic Sports Medicine and University Health Network Arthritis Program, Toronto, ON, Canada

Division of Orthopaedic Surgery, Toronto Western Hospital and Women's College Hospital, Toronto, ON, Canada

A. E. Gross, MD, FRCSC, O ONT (✉)
Division of Orthopaedic Surgery, University of Toronto, Toronto, ON, Canada

Gluskin Granovsky Division of Orthopaedics, Joseph and Wolf Lebovic Health Complex, Mount Sinai Hospital, Toronto, ON, Canada
e-mail: Allan.Gross@sinaihealthsystem.ca

H. K. Gahunia et al. (eds.), *Articular Cartilage of the Knee*,
https://doi.org/10.1007/978-1-4939-7587-7_12

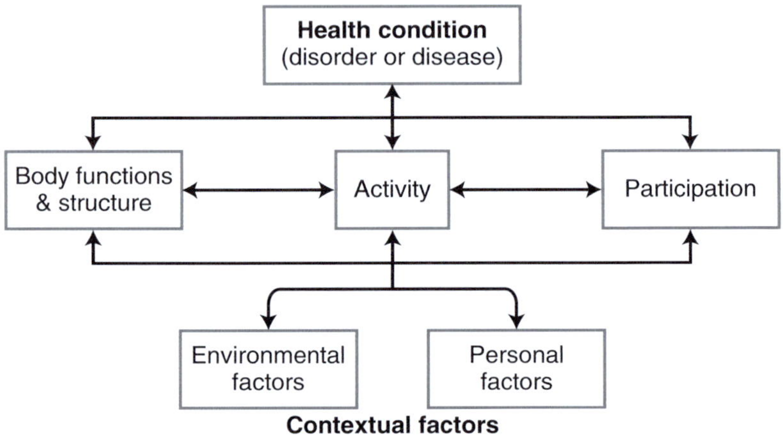

Fig. 12.1 The World Health Organization's International Classification of Functioning, Disability and Health

an individual may experience in involvement in life situations [3]. In the context of articular cartilage pathology, a focal osteochondral defect can result in pain and swelling (physical impairment), a lack of confidence in the knee (emotional impairment), an inability to run and pivot (activity limitation) and finally failure to work in a particular occupation (participation restriction). By selecting outcome instruments with items that emphasize the concerns and items across the three aforementioned constructs, investigators can truly get a sense of how an articular cartilage defect influences the overall well-being of a particular population.

12.2 Patient-Reported Outcome Measures

Patient-reported outcome measures (PROMs) are standardized, validated questionnaires that are completed by patients to measure their own functional status and general health. They were originally designed for use in clinical trials [4]. However, controversies exist regarding the widespread implementation, data collection and interpretation of PROMs [5].

12.2.1 Types of PROM Data

In general, there are two principal types of PROMs, firstly a measure of a patient's perception of their general health ("generic" health status) and secondly their perceptions of their health in relation to pathology ("specific" health status). Patients complete PROM questionnaires by rating their current health status in response to individual questions. Generic measures include a breadth of domains, often reflecting health-related quality of life (QoL), that are relevant across different diseases and populations. Examples of commonly used generic questionnaires include the 36-Item Short-Form Health Survey (SF-36), European Quality of Life-5 Dimensions (EQ-5D) and Perceived Impact of Problem Profile (PIPP). In contrast, specific measures include areas of importance in relation to a specific disease or organ [6]. Examples of commonly used specific questionnaires include the International Knee Documentation Committee (IKDC) Subjective Form, Knee Injury and Osteoarthritis Outcome Score (KOOS) and Western Ontario and McMaster Universities Osteoarthritis Index (WOMAC). In clinical research, both generic- and disease-specific instruments are usually chosen, with the latter as a secondary outcome.

The analysis of PROMs tends to focus on the amount of change that has occurred in the patients' condition or their general health-related QoL, as represented by a change in PROM score following an intervention. The collection of PROM data outside the remit of clinical research risks a lack of clarity and focus, which may in turn result in suboptimal data interpretation. Therefore, clinicians and managers should be aware that the quality of both processes and outcomes can be audited (see Box 12.1).

Box 12.1 Specific Examples of the Processes and Outcomes that May Be Quantified with PROM Data

Processes

1. Communication: improved communication between patient and health-care provider
2. Concordance: agreement between patient and health-care provider about problems and solutions
3. Provider behaviours: changes in health-care providers' diagnosis and treatment of patient conditions
4. Patient behaviours: patient self-efficacy, adherence and behavioural change

Outcomes

1. Patient satisfaction: patient-reported satisfaction with the consultation, treatment or care overall
2. Health status: patients' health and well-being as indicated by clinical measures or patient reports
3. Resource use: patients' subsequent use of health and other services

In order to minimize bias and systematic error, mechanisms need to be in place to ensure that only the patients are responding. Further, the means of patient recruitment need to be considered, for example, including only patients attending the outpatients' department risk selection bias, as there is likely to be a greater proportion of patients with problems attending. A mechanism should exist to reduce nonresponders' incomplete or duplicated data. Finally, as with all confidential patient information, data storage must be secure whilst remaining easily retrievable for analysis.

12.2.2 Collection of PROM Data

It is essential that there is a cogent reason for data collection and a defined duration of follow-up when no clear hypothesis or research question exists. As such, clearly stated inclusion and exclusion criteria will aid the standardization of data collection and interpretation. In addition, the data points need to be clearly specified, for example, the data patient-specific or pathology-specific (i.e. one patient may have two arthritic knees).

The logistics of data collection should be clarified prior to the widespread implementation of PROMs, preferably with the use of a pilot study. In essence, who, how, when and where is the data to be collected? In particular, has informed consent been obtained, is a written protocol available and is all the relevant documentation available in a variety of languages?

12.2.3 Potential Benefits of PROM Data

The appropriate implementation and interpretation of PROM data collection have several potential benefits. It can have a diverse role in altering how health problems are perceived and managed by patients and their health-care providers. Patients are stimulated to present problems that concern them in addition to symptoms elicited in traditional consultations. Health professionals are encouraged to think beyond the conventional limitations in identifying problems and selecting solutions jointly with patients. In addition, there is improved identification of goals and priorities over time between health professional and patients faced with complex, evolving and multifaceted problems. However, to date few academic studies have validated the use of the questionnaires currently used for PROM data against these potential benefits.

12.2.4 Potential Problems with PROM Data

The interpretation of PROM data has an inconsistent impact on health status depending on the actual questionnaire used. For any single condition, the choice of PROM questionnaire used will influence the study results. To increase provider understanding of patient needs, priorities and/or preferences, the most appropriate PROMs should be applied to accurately reflect these issues. However, the most commonly used PROMs currently only capture a single facet of patient health or were created without the involvement of patients. Therefore, they may not actually accurately reflect patients' needs, priorities and preferences [7]. For example, questions relating to sports activity are not relevant to most elderly patients. Whilst numerous measures are available (see MAPI Research Trust. Patient reported outcome and quality of life instruments database. 2009. http://www.proqolid.org), care is needed to ensure that the most appropriate choice of data capture is used.

The constraints on the number and focus of questions imposed by standardization may prevent PROM data from addressing the issues that are most important to patients. Furthermore, PROM data should be evaluated against potential impacts beyond provider actions and patient health status, for example, is there an impact on patient-clinician communication?

12.2.5 Psychometric Properties of PROMs

The quality and appropriateness of an outcome instrument are intrinsically related to its measurement properties and these include sensibility, reliability, validity and responsiveness. First, sensibility refers to an aggregate of properties that make up the "common sense" part of the instrument, including comprehensibility and face and content validity [8]. Content validity can be further assessed by determining floor effects and ceiling effects when administered to a larger group of patients. The concept of reliability refers to the repeatability or precision of an instrument. It is demonstrated when repeated administrations of an instrument to stable patients produce consistent results. Reliability can be measured by calculating test-retest reliability, which uses an intra-class correlation coefficient (ICC), representing the ratio of the between-subject variation to the total variation [9]. Acceptable reliability for a health-related QoL instrument for use in controlled clinical trials is generally agreed to be present when the ICC is greater than 0.80 [10, 11]. Acceptable reliability for tests used to make a decision about an individual is an ICC of 0.90 or greater [11]. Furthermore, internal consistency, an indication of how individual items correlate with one another and with the overall score, can also be used to assess the reliability of an instrument or its domains. Finally, "a measurement tool is valid if it is measuring what it is supposed to measure" [12]. Validation is clear when there is a gold standard to which the results can be compared (i.e. criterion validity) [8]. Since there is no gold standard for measuring "quality of life", this requires one to demonstrate that a measurement tool "behaves" in relation to other measures as one would predict if it were measuring QoL (i.e. construct validity) [8]. To evaluate the validity of an instrument as a discriminative tool, one examines the relationship between scores on the new instrument and other indices at a single point in time; hypotheses related to different categories of disease severity can also be tested.

12.3 Currently Available Knee-Specific Outcome Instruments

Tanner et al. described 11 commonly used measurement tools for patients with knee symptoms and divided them as 5 non-disease-specific and 6 disease-specific scales [13] as shown below:

The five general knee instruments include:

1. The American Academy of Orthopaedic Surgeons (AAOS) Sports Knee Rating Scale [14]
2. The Knee Injury and Osteoarthritis Outcome Score (KOOS) [15]
3. The 2000 International Knee Documentation Committee (IKDC) Standard Evaluation Form [16]

4. The Activities of Daily Living (ADL) of the Knee Outcome Survey [17]
5. The Knee Disorders Subjective Form of Visual Analog Scale (VAS, Hughston Sports Medicine Foundation) [18]

The ligament-specific knee instruments include:

1. The Cincinnati Knee Ligament Rating Scale [19, 20]
2. The Revised Hospital for Special Surgery (HSS) Knee Ligament Rating Form [21]
3. The Modified Lysholm Knee Scoring Scale [22]
4. The Mohtadi Quality of Life (QoL) Assessment in Anterior Cruciate Ligament Deficiency [23]

One of the instruments specific for osteoarthritis (OA) of the knee is the WOMAC Index [24].

The instrument specifically designed for meniscal tears is the Western Ontario Meniscal Evaluation Tool (WOMET) [8].

Given the large number of available choices for measuring outcomes in patients with articular cartilage injury, it is important to select instruments that contain the content most pertinent to the population of interest, as well as those that have demonstrated adequate psychometric properties.

12.4 Patient-Reported Versus Surgeon-Reported Outcome Measures in Articular Cartilage Repair Surgery

Historically, outcome measures were developed and completed by surgeons for assessment of knee function and symptoms. Examples of such instruments include the Knee Society Score (KSS), HSS Score and Lysholm Score. The content of the questionnaires reflects the surgeon's perspective and does not take into consideration the concerns, symptoms and limitations that are pertinent to patients [6]. As previously stated, the patients' perspective is the main driving force in determining outcomes. Refer to Appendix B for further details of the clinical outcome assessment tools used to assess patients with knee injuries to one or both knees.

According to the recommendation by the International Cartilage Repair Society (ICRS) in 2011, the IKDC Subjective Knee Form and KOOS represent two knee joint-specific outcome measures that both fulfil the basic requirements for reliability, validity and responsiveness in cartilage repair patients [6]. Whilst the former instrument provides a single global score, the latter outcome measure provides five separate subscale scores which allow for evaluation of separate constructs at all levels according to the World Health Organization's ICF [6]. This is pertinent because different constructs may change in a different manner over time as a result of an intervention. For example, in a 4-year follow-up of polymer-based ACI grafts, the KOOS Pain, ADL and knee-related QoL subscales showed significant improvements as early as 3 months, whereas the sports and recreation subscale did not show statistically significant improvement until 4 years [6, 25]. Finally, Hambly et al. [26] demonstrated that for the KOOS and IKDC, the majority of items contained within these instruments were important to and frequently experienced by patients who underwent articular cartilage repair. Whilst the IKDC performed better in this regard, this study demonstrates good content validity of both of these knee joint-specific outcome instruments in the cartilage repair population.

In addition to using the KOOS or IKDC, the ICRS also recommends the use of a generic health-related QoL questionnaire (e.g. SF-36 or EQ-5D) and an activity score (Tegner Activity Scale or Marx Activity Scale) among patients undergoing articular cartilage repair (see Box 12.2).

Box 12.2 Scoring Systems Recommended by the ICRS for the Assessment of PROMs Following Articular Cartilage Surgery of the Knee

Generic (select one)

1. Medical Outcome Study 36-Item Short-Form Health Survey (SF-36)
2. EuroQoL 5-Dimension Health Questionnaire (EQ-5D)

Knee-specific (select one)

Patient reported

1. Knee Injury and Osteoarthritis Outcome Score (KOOS)
2. International Knee Documentation Committee (IKDC) Subjective Knee Form

Activity scale (select one)

1. Marx Activity Rating Scale
2. Tegner Activity Scale (TAS)

12.5 Commonly Used Knee Outcome Instruments in the Current Articular Cartilage Literature

Knee-specific patient outcome self-reporting tools are used to follow patients after traumatic knee injuries, knee cartilage repair surgical procedure, disease progression or pharmacological clinical trials to gain insight into the patient's changing symptoms and function over time. These scoring tools were developed for patients to assess their view about their knee health, which are used to assess one or more of the following criteria: pain, symptoms, sports, ADL, QOL and physical health value. Refer to Appendix B for details of the clinical outcome scoring systems.

12.5.1 Tegner and Lysholm Knee Scores

The Lysholm Scoring Scale was first described in 1982 and then modified in 1985 [22, 27] . The score was designed to be physician administered and measure outcomes after knee ligament surgery. The Lysholm Score consists of 8 items assessing pain (25 points), instability (25 points), locking (15 points), swelling (10 points), limp (5 points), stair climbing (10 points), squatting (5 points) and need for support (5 points). The total score is from 0 to 100, worst to best. The score emphasized the evaluation of instability and was intended to correspond with the patient's own opinion of function and signs of instability [27]. Although some studies have demonstrated adequate reliability, validity and responsiveness in cartilage repair patients [28], Smith et al. demonstrated that the arbitrary weighing system of the Lysholm was not supported using Rasch analysis.

The Tegner Activity Scale (TAS) was developed to complement the Lysholm Score [22]. This new scale graded activity based on work and sports activities [22]. The TAS activity levels (0 to 10) are described in detail in Appendix B. It was important to the authors to measure both function and activity level; however, due to differences in the recovery process, they thought it was important that this was done in two different scores. The TAS scores a person's activity level between 0 and 10, where 0 is "on sick leave/disability" and 10 is "participation in competitive sport such as soccer at a national or international elite level". Scores of 6 to 10 can only be achieved if a person takes part in recreational or competitive sports. This instrument separates recreational and competitive sporting activities because the risk and injury incidence are higher in competitive sports. Work activities are also classified on the TAS. The maximum level for a work activity is 5 (e.g. firefighter or military). Moreover, the ability to perform in running and walking and the participation in recreational sports were different levels on the International Classification of Impairments, Disabilities and Handicaps (ICIDH).

The TAS is a commonly used scale for post-operative knee patients, due to its ease of use. It has been cited as being the most widely used activity scoring instrument for knee disorders. Although frequently used as a patient-reported scale, it was initially developed as a clinician-administered tool. The psychometric parameters of the TAS for a range of knee disorders demonstrate good test-retest reliability and ceiling and floor effects [29–33]. There is moderate correlation with the IKDC score ranging from 0.22 to 0.54 [30, 32]. The normative knee function TAS score, from a sample population of 488 people who considered their knee function to be normal, was 5.7 (range 1–10). Further, the TAS is inversely correlated to age, and the average TAS for men (6.0) was higher than for women (5.4) [34].

TAS was one of the first scores used to quantify the outcome following articular cartilage repair procedures, as return to sports is one of the principal reasons given by individuals to elect to undergo cartilage repair surgery. Mithoefer et al. reported that the mean post-operative TAS score following articular cartilage repair in the knee for studies with mixed ages and gender was 6.1 [35]. McNickle et al. have also demonstrated an effect size of 0.67 four years following autologous chondrocyte implantation [36].

12.5.2 Western Ontario and McMaster Universities Osteoarthritis Index

The WOMAC was extensively evaluated with regard to psychometric parameters prior to its introduction and needs licensees' agreement from the copyright holders before it is used [37]. It is commonly used and easy to implement consisting of three main domains (refer to Appendix B):

1. Pain (5 questions)
2. Stiffness (2 questions)
3. Physical function (17 questions)

The index was designed for degenerative joint disease of the knee and has been shown to be sensitive to change and has a greater efficiency than most other instruments in the assessment of knee OA [38, 39]. Although commonly used, caution should prevail if it is used in the assessment of chondral lesions as this was not its intended use. Both the WOMAC and Oxford Knee Score (OKS) appear to be the most reliable and valid assessments of outcome after total knee arthroplasty; however their use in segmental or biological knee arthroplasty remains to be fully evaluated.

12.5.3 Knee Injury and Osteoarthritis Outcome Score

The KOOS was developed as an extension of the WOMAC OA index to evaluate short-term and long-term symptoms and function in patients with knee injuries and OA. The reasoning to develop a single instrument for different types of knee pathology was that traumatic knee injury frequently leads to damage in multiple structures within the knee joint, in particular ligaments, meniscus and cartilage. Furthermore, OA is a common later consequence of these injuries.

The Lysholm knee scoring system considered short-term functioning, whereas the WOMAC OA index viewed only longer-term consequences, and the KOOS was developed to account for both acute injuries in younger patients and more chronic symptoms in older patients.

The KOOS is knee specific with 42 individual items, each of which is divided into 5 separate score subscales (refer to Appendix B):

1. Pain
2. Other symptoms
3. Activities of daily living (ADL)
4. Function in sports and recreational activities
5. Knee-related quality of life (QoL)

Each subscale is scored from 0 to 100, worst to best. As other scoring systems for acute knee injury aggregate items measuring different aspects into one score, they tend to "flatten" the results, making interpretation more difficult. The self-administered KOOS takes approximately 10 min to complete, and evidence shows that less than 4% of subjects failed to complete the entire questionnaire when administered by mail [40, 41]. The KOOS has been validated in several patient populations that have undergone surgical procedures, including varying diseases, durations, ages and activity levels. Published evidence has validated the KOOS following ACL surgery [15, 42], knee arthroscopy [40, 43], post meniscectomy [44, 45], total knee arthroplasty [41, 46] and articular cartilage repair [47].

The KOOS has demonstrated adequate test-retest reliability (ICC 0.87–0.95 for the five subscales), construct validity and responsiveness in patients undergoing articular cartilage repair [47]. The effect size 3 years following autologous chondrocyte implantation or microfracture was similar and considered moderate to large (effect sizes range from 0.70 to 1.32 across domains) [6, 47]. An advantage of using the KOOS for studies of the long-term consequences of joint injury is that it assesses sports and recreational function and knee-related QoL and demonstrates a superior responsiveness compared to more generic instruments such as the WOMAC and SF-36.

12.5.4 International Knee Documentation Committee Subjective Knee Form

The IKDC is a patient-focused instrument that has been developed to assess knee disability and function before and after treatment [16, 48]. With the aim of standardizing the assessment of outcomes following knee surgery or treatment, the American Orthopaedic Society for Sports Medicine (AOSSM) and the European Society of Sports Traumatology, Knee Surgery and Arthroscopy (ESSKA) developed the IKDC for patients with a wide variety of knee problems. They were concerned that the available scoring systems had assigned numerical values to factors that were not actually quantifiable, and therefore arbitrary scores were summated for noncomparable parameters [49].

The IKDC Subjective Knee Form can be obtained from Irrgang et al. [16]. The IKDC is a knee-specific (rather than disease-specific) 18-item score designed to measure symptoms, function and sports activity as follows (refer to Appendix B):

1. Symptoms: pain, stiffness, swelling, joint locking and instability.
2. Function and sports activity: ability to run, jump and land, stop and start quickly, ascend and descend stairs, stand and kneel on the front of a chair.

Responses are quantified using 5-point Likert scales, 11-point Likert scales and dichotomous yes/no. The responses to the 18 items are summed and expressed as a percentage of the maximum total possible scores. Scores range from 0 to 100, with 100 indicating the absence of symptoms and higher levels of functioning. The score has been validated in several languages and shows no gender or age differentiation or differences across diagnoses [16, 50, 51]. The IKDC score has shown significant concurrent validity with the SF-36 physical function subscales (r = 0.44–0.66), but not to the emotional SF-36 subscale (r = 0.16–0.26) [52]. Additional information including knee compartment findings, donor site pathology, radiographic findings and functional abilities are recorded but do not contribute to the final evaluation.

Although originally designed for the assessment of ligament disruption, the IKDC has been evaluated in individuals with articular cartilage lesions and OA [53]. The test-retest reliability at 6 and 12 months following articular cartilage repair is greater than 0.90. The effect size at 12 months following a variety of articular cartilage procedures was 0.76 and considered to be moderate. The minimal clinical important difference for the IKDC 12 months following cartilage repair was demonstrated to be 16.7 [53].

12.5.5 Marx Activity Rating Scale

The Marx Activity Scale assesses the activity levels of patients with knee disorders to determine the outcome for a variety of knee injuries and operations. It is derived from patient and expert input that contains functional activity of specific motions rather than sports-specific questions, both of which are in contrast to the TAS [54, 55]. The Marx Activity Scale consists of four questions assessing running, cutting, decelerating and pivoting (refer to Appendix B). Items are scored from 0 to 4, depending on frequency and intensity of activity. The frequency of participation for each activity is classified from "none" to "4 or more times a week". The overall score ranges from 0 to 16 (worst to best). The Marx Activity Scale correlates well with the TAS and has demonstrated responsiveness following cartilage repair (effect size 0.76) [47].

12.5.6 Medical Outcome Study 36-Item Short-Form Health Survey

The SF-36 is a set of generic, coherent and easily implemented QoL measure (refer to Appendix B). SF-36 consists of eight subscales (physical functioning, role limitations due to physical health problems, bodily pain, general health perceptions, vitality as measure of energy/fatigue, social functioning, role limitations due to personal or emotional problems and mental health) and two summary scores (physical component summary, emotional component summary). Standardized scores range from 0 to 100, with higher scores indicating better health status [6, 56, 57]. The SF-36 has been widely used as a general health status measure in clinical trials of cartilage repair and has demonstrated sensitivity to change (effect sizes range from 0.06 to 0.67 across domains) [53]. The SF-36 scores can be mapped to utility scores which in turn can be converted to quality-adjusted life years (QALYs) for cost-effectiveness analyses. From a government and societal perspective, cost-effectiveness studies will become increasingly important in the future as new cell-based cartilage repair therapies are introduced into the marketplace for articular cartilage regeneration.

12.6 Conclusions

Measuring outcomes following articular cartilage repair should be performed using instruments that have demonstrated content validity as well as adequate psychometric properties including reliability, construct validity and responsiveness in this population of interest. As per the ICRS recommendation, the primary outcome for articular cartilage surgery should be either the KOOS or the IKDC. Secondary outcomes should include an activity scale as well as a measure of generic health-related QoL which can concomitantly allow for an evaluation of the cost-effectiveness of a group of interventions. Such a biopsychosocial approach towards outcome measurement will allow for a comprehensive understanding of how patients experience articular cartilage pathology and how they respond to treatment over time.

References

1. Nho SJ, et al. Rehabilitation after autologous chondrocyte implantation in athletes. Clin Sports Med. 2010;29(2):267–82.
2. Badley EM. Enhancing the conceptual clarity of the activity and participation components of the international classification of functioning, disability, and health. Soc Sci Med. 2008;66(11):2335–45.
3. World Health Organization. International classification of functioning, disability, and health: ICF. Geneva: World Health Organization; 2001.
4. Fitzpatrick R, et al. Evaluating patient-based outcome measures for use in clinical trials. Health Technol Assess. 1998;2(14):i-iv, 1–74.
5. Dawson J, Doll H, Fitzpatrick R, Jenkinson C, Carr AJ. The routine use of patient reported outcome measures in healthcare settings. BMJ. 2010;340:c186.
6. Roos EM, et al. ICRS recommendation document: patient-reported outcome instruments for use in patients with articular cartilage defects. Cartilage. 2011;2(2):122–36.
7. Higginson IJ, Carr AJ. Measuring quality of life: using quality of life measures in the clinical setting. BMJ. 2001;322(7297):1297–300.
8. Kirkley A, Griffin S, Whelan D. The development and validation of a quality of life-measurement tool for patients with meniscal pathology: the Western Ontario Meniscal Evaluation Tool (WOMET). Clin J Sport Med. 2007;17(5):349–56.
9. Bartko JJ. The intraclass correlation coefficient as a measure of reliability. Psychol Rep. 1966;19(1):3–11.
10. Streiner DL, Norman GR. Health measurement scales: a practical guide to their development and use. Oxford: Oxford University Press; 1989.
11. Nunnally JC. Psychometric Theory (2nd ed.). New York: McGraw-Hill; 1978.
12. Guyatt G. Measuring health-related quality of life: general issues. Can Respir J. 1997;4(3):123–30.

13. Tanner SM, et al. Knee-specific quality-of-life instruments: which ones measure symptoms and disabilities most important to patients? [see comment]. Am J Sports Med. 2007;35(9):1450–8.
14. American Academy of Orthopaedic Surgeons. Scoring algorithms for the lower limb: outcomes data collection instrument: 2. In: Rosemont. Illinois: American Academy of Orthopaedic Surgeons; 1998.
15. Roos EM, et al. Knee injury and osteoarthritis outcome score (KOOS)–development of a self-administered outcome measure. J Orthop Sports Phys Ther. 1998;28(2):88–96.
16. Irrgang JJ, et al. Development and validation of the international knee documentation committee subjective knee form. Am J Sports Med. 2001;29(5):600–13.
17. Irrgang JJ, et al. Development of a patient-reported measure of function of the knee. J Bone Joint Surg Am. 1998;80(8):1132–45.
18. Flandry F, et al. Analysis of subjective knee complaints using visual analog scales. Am J Sports Med. 1991;19(2):112–8.
19. Noyes FR, et al. The symptomatic anterior cruciate-deficient knee. Part II: the results of rehabilitation, activity modification, and counseling on functional disability. J Bone Joint Surg Am. 1983;65(2):163–74.
20. Noyes FR, et al. The symptomatic anterior cruciate-deficient knee. Part I: the long-term functional disability in athletically active individuals. J Bone Joint Surg Am. 1983;65(2):154–62.
21. Windsor RE, et al. The hospital for special surgery knee ligament rating form. Am J Knee Surg. 1988;1:140–5.
22. Tegner Y, Lysholm J. Rating systems in the evaluation of knee ligament injuries. Clin Orthop Relat Res. 1985;198:43–9.
23. Mohtadi N. Development and validation of the quality of life outcome measure (questionnaire) for chronic anterior cruciate ligament deficiency. Am J Sports Med. 1998;26(3):350–9.
24. Bellamy N, et al. Validation study of WOMAC: a health status instrument for measuring clinically important patient relevant outcomes to antirheumatic drug therapy in patients with osteoarthritis of the hip or knee. J Rheumatol. 1988;15(12):1833–40.
25. Kreuz PC, et al. Treatment of focal degenerative cartilage defects with polymer-based autologous chondrocyte grafts: four-year clinical results. Arthritis Res Ther. 2009;11(2):R33.
26. Hambly K, Griva K. IKDC or KOOS? Which measures symptoms and disabilities most important to postoperative articular cartilage repair patients? Am J Sports Med. 2008;36(9):1695–704.
27. Lysholm J, Gillquist J. Evaluation of knee ligament surgery results with special emphasis on use of a scoring scale. Am J Sports Med. 1982;10(3):150–4.
28. Kocher MS, et al. Reliability, validity, and responsiveness of the Lysholm knee scale for various chondral disorders of the knee. J Bone Joint Surg Am. 2004;86-A(6):1139–45.
29. Briggs KK, et al. Reliability, validity, and responsiveness of the Lysholm knee score and Tegner activity scale for patients with meniscal injury of the knee. J Bone Joint Surg Am. 2006;88(4):698–705.
30. Briggs KK, et al. The reliability, validity, and responsiveness of the Lysholm score and Tegner activity scale for anterior cruciate ligament injuries of the knee: 25 years later. Am J Sports Med. 2009;37(5):890–7.
31. Gobbi A, Francisco R. Factors affecting return to sports after anterior cruciate ligament reconstruction with patellar tendon and hamstring graft: a prospective clinical investigation. Knee Surg Sports Traumatol Arthrosc. 2006;14(10):1021–8.
32. Paxton EW, et al. The reliability and validity of knee-specific and general health instruments in assessing acute patellar dislocation outcomes. Am J Sports Med. 2003;31(4):487–92.
33. Smith TO, et al. An evaluation of the clinical tests and outcome measures used to assess patellar instability. Knee. 2008;15(4):255–62.
34. Briggs KK, et al. Lysholm score and Tegner activity level in individuals with normal knees. Am J Sports Med. 2009;37(5):898–901.
35. Mithoefer K, et al. Return to sports participation after articular cartilage repair in the knee: scientific evidence. Am J Sports Med. 2009;37(Suppl 1):167S–76S.
36. McNickle AG, et al. Outcomes of autologous chondrocyte implantation in a diverse patient population. Am J Sports Med. 2009;37(7):1344–50.
37. Davies AP. Rating systems for total knee replacement. Knee. 2002;9(4):261–6.
38. Patt JC, Mauerhan DR. Outcomes research in total joint replacement: a critical review and commentary. Am J Orthop (Belle Mead NJ). 2005;34(4):167–72.
39. Whitehouse SL, Crawford RW, Learmonth ID. Validation for the reduced Western Ontario and McMaster universities osteoarthritis index function scale. J Orthop Surg (Hong Kong). 2008;16(1):50–3.
40. Roos EM, et al. Knee injury and Osteoarthritis Outcome Score (KOOS)–validation of a Swedish version. Scand J Med Sci Sports. 1998;8(6):439–48.
41. Roos EM, Toksvig-Larsen S. Knee injury and Osteoarthritis Outcome Score (KOOS) – validation and comparison to the WOMAC in total knee replacement. Health Qual Life Outcomes. 2003;1:17.
42. Lansdown DA, Xiao W, Zhang AL, Allen CR, Feeley BT, et al. Quantitative imaging of anterior cruciate ligament (ACL) graft demonstrates longitudinal compositional changes and relationships with clinical outcomes at 2 years after ACL reconstruction. J Orthop Res. 2019. https://doi.org/10.1002/jor.24572. [Epub ahead of print].
43. Hashimoto Y, Nishida Y, Takahashi S, Nakamura H, Mera H, et al. Transplantation of autologous bone marrow-derived mesenchymal stem cells under arthroscopic surgery with microfracture versus microfracture alone for articular cartilage lesions in the

knee: a multicenter prospective randomized control clinical trial. Regen Ther. 2019;11:106–13.
44. Roos EM, Roos HP, Lohmander LS. WOMAC osteoarthritis index–additional dimensions for use in subjects with post-traumatic osteoarthritis of the knee. Western Ontario and MacMaster universities. Osteoarthritis Cartilage. 1999;7(2):216–21.
45. Lamplot JD, Tompkins WP, Friedman MV, Nguyen JT, Rai MF, et al. Radiographic and clinical evidence for osteoarthritis at medium-term follow-up after arthroscopic partial medial meniscectomy. Cartilage. 2019:1947603519892315. https://doi.org/10.1177/1947603519892315. [Epub ahead of print]
46. Toguchi K, Nakajima A, Akatsu Y, Sonobe M, Yamada M, et al. Predicting clinical outcomes after total knee arthroplasty from preoperative radiographic factors of the knee osteoarthritis. BMC Musculoskelet Disord. 2020;21(1):9.
47. Bekkers JE, et al. Validation of the Knee Injury and Osteoarthritis Outcome Score (KOOS) for the treatment of focal cartilage lesions. Osteoarthritis Cartilage. 2009;17(11):1434–9.
48. Anderson AF, et al. The international knee documentation committee subjective knee evaluation form: normative data. Am J Sports Med. 2006;34(1):128–35.
49. Hefti F, et al. Evaluation of knee ligament injuries with the IKDC form. Knee Surg Sports Traumatol Arthrosc. 1993;1(3–4):226–34.
50. Haverkamp D, et al. Translation and validation of the Dutch version of the international knee documentation committee subjective knee form. Am J Sports Med. 2006;34(10):1680–4.
51. Padua R, et al. Italian version of the international knee documentation committee subjective knee form: cross-cultural adaptation and validation. Arthroscopy. 2004;20(8):819–23.
52. Ware JE Jr, Sherbourne CD. The MOS 36-item short-form health survey (SF-36). I. Conceptual framework and item selection. Med Care. 1992;30(6):473–83.
53. Greco NJ, et al. Responsiveness of the international knee documentation committee subjective knee form in comparison to the Western Ontario and McMaster universities osteoarthritis index, modified Cincinnati knee rating system, and short form 36 in patients with focal articular cartilage defects. Am J Sports Med. 2010;38(5):891–902.
54. Marx RG, et al. Development and evaluation of an activity rating scale for disorders of the knee. Am J Sports Med. 2001;29(2):213–8.
55. Wright RW. Knee injury outcomes measures. J Am Acad Orthop Surg. 2009;17(1):31–9.
56. McHorney CA, et al. The MOS 36-item short-form health survey (SF-36): III. Tests of data quality, scaling assumptions, and reliability across diverse patient groups. Med Care. 1994;32(1):40–66.
57. McHorney CA, Ware JE Jr, Raczek AE. The MOS 36-item short-form health survey (SF-36): II. Psychometric and clinical tests of validity in measuring physical and mental health constructs. Med Care. 1993;31(3):247–63.

Part VI

Qualitative and Quantitative Assessment of Articular Cartilage Repair

Pre- and Postoperative Imaging of Knee Articular Cartilage

13

Avneesh B. Chhabra, Gaurav K. Thawait, and Gustav Andreisek

13.1 Introduction

Adult articular cartilage is avascular resulting in limited transport of inflammatory mediators and cells to the injured site; thus, cartilage damaged by trauma or degeneration has no intrinsic capacity to heal itself [1, 2]. Chondral injury, a frequent cause of pain and knee function limitation, poses a serious problem for orthopedic surgeons. The associated pain and physical disability can restrict an individual's ability to perform activities of daily living, which, in athletes, can even have career-ending consequences. Further, in the young population, cartilage lesions predispose to the development of precocious osteoarthritis.

Cartilage repair surgery is a highly dynamic research field. Over the past two decades, there have been several exciting, sophisticated surgical repair procedures for the treatment of focal traumatic or degenerative cartilage lesions, which in turn has created the need for an accurate, noninvasive assessment of the repair tissue. With its excellent soft tissue contrast and precise morphological evaluation of articular cartilage and repair tissue, magnetic resonance imaging (MRI) is the method of choice as a noninvasive and objective outcome measure [3–13].

Within the past decade, evolution of MRI technology has significantly improved the image quality. The cartilage-specific pulse sequences have enhanced the ability of qualitative (morphological) and quantitative (biochemical/functional) assessment of cartilage injury and repair. Higher magnetic field strengths have substantially increased the signal-to-noise ratio, spatial resolution, and speed of image acquisition; however, limitations to the increased field strength include greater amount of noise, imaging contrast issues, and safety concerns.

A. B. Chhabra, MBBS, MD (✉)
Department of Radiology and Orthopedic Surgery, University of Texas Southwestern Medical Center, Dallas, TX, USA

Department of Musculoskeletal Radiology, Parkland Health and Hospital System, Dallas, TX, USA
e-mail: avneesh.chhabra@utsouthwestern.edu

G. K. Thawait, MBBS, MD
Russell H. Morgan Department of Radiology and Radiological Science, Johns Hopkins University, Baltimore, MD, USA

Department of Biomedical Engineering, Johns Hopkins University, Baltimore, MD, USA

G. Andreisek, MD, MBA
Department of Radiology, University Hospital Zurich, University of Zurich, Zurich, Switzerland

Swiss Center for Musculoskeletal Imaging, Balgrist Campus AG, Zurich, Switzerland

Department of Radiology, St Claraspital, Basel, Switzerland

Department of Radiology, Spital Thurgau AG, Cantonal Hospital, Munsterlingen, Switzerland
e-mail: gustav@andreisek.de

H. K. Gahunia et al. (eds.), *Articular Cartilage of the Knee*,
https://doi.org/10.1007/978-1-4939-7587-7_13

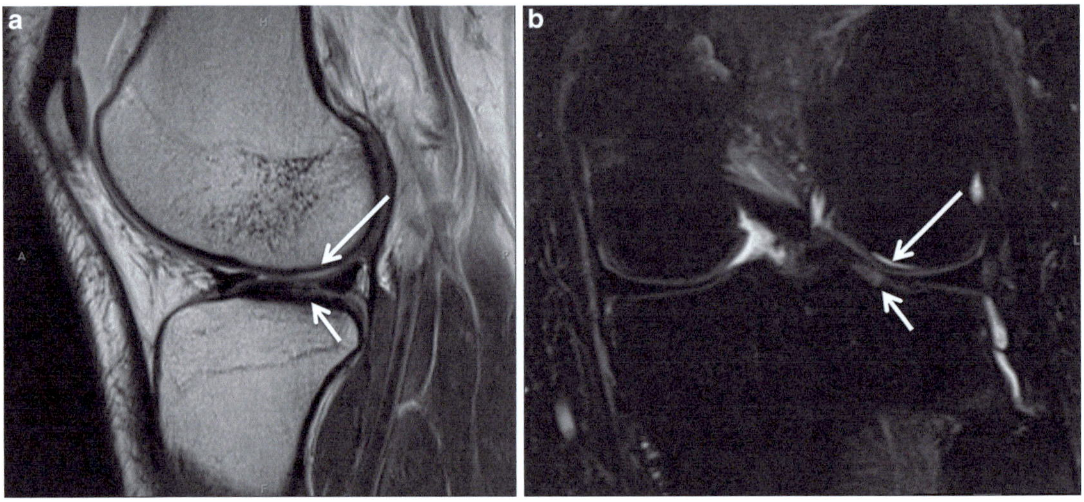

Fig. 13.1 Sagittal proton density (**a**) and coronal fat-saturated proton density (**b**) MR images in a 33-year-old woman with knee pain. Note a focal area of articular cartilage delamination (large arrow) over the lateral femoral condyle and an irregular partial-thickness defect on the corresponding tibial surface (small arrows)

MR imaging of the knee is the method of choice to identify articular cartilage injuries and disease progression [14–17]. In order to evaluate the effectiveness or compare various therapeutic intervention and surgical treatments for chondral repair, an appropriate, reliable, and objective cartilage repair assessment system or combination of systems is necessary. MR imaging has been shown to be a reliable tool in the preoperative diagnosis of cartilage injury and postoperative evaluation of cartilage repair tissue [18–22]. During the postsurgical follow-up, MR imaging aids in assessing the surgical success or potential complications of cartilage repair procedures. In contrast to arthroscopy, MR imaging can assess the morphology, width, and depth of the repair tissue and evaluate the subchondral bone, as well as other internal derangements noninvasively. Although various biochemical techniques, such as T2 mapping, post-contrast T1 mapping, T1rho imaging, and sodium MR, enable the assessment of cartilage architecture, conventional anatomic and morphologic imaging remain the mainstay for pre- and postoperative assessment of the articular cartilage (Fig. 13.1).

In this chapter, we describe the role of MRI in the preoperative diagnosis of knee cartilage injury and postoperative follow-up as it relates to the visualization, assessment, and characterization of cartilage repair tissue. The cartilage repair tissue-specific MR techniques and the morphological/biochemical outcome of a given cartilage repair treatment procedure are reviewed in Chap. 14, whereas this chapter briefly summarizes the routinely used techniques and their advantages; provides an overview of the available treatment options, including their indications, technique, and clinical results; and illustrates the MR morphology of repair sites as well as postoperative complications. Further, we also discuss the two-dimensional (2D) and three-dimensional (3D) Magnetic Resonance Observation of Cartilage Repair Tissue (MOCART) scoring system, which has been well validated in studies of cartilage regeneration techniques.

13.2 Preoperative Assessment of Articular Cartilage Injury

Articular cartilage contributes to a large component of the load-bearing capability of the joint that is subjected to repetitive mechanical forces. In the event of an abnormal mechanical load or high impaction force, there may be focal carti-

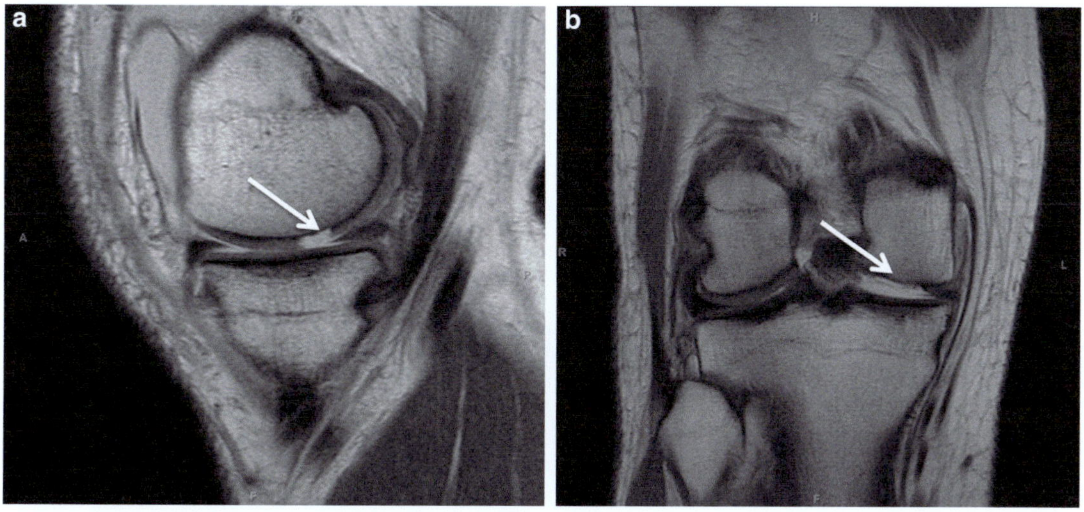

Fig. 13.2 Sagittal (**a**) and coronal (**b**) proton density MR images of a 51-year-old man with recent knee injury. An area with shouldered cartilage defect over the medial femoral condyle can be seen (arrows)

lage injury. The acute trauma-related defect is usually focal and isolated and shows a shouldered margin (Fig. 13.2). The knowledge of such a defect, especially in young patient, is particularly important because articular cartilage has a limited capacity for spontaneous repair. Cartilage loss can further result in stress changes in the underlying bone, causing pain and decreased range of motion in the affected joint. Finally, cartilage injury can lead to premature joint degeneration in young adults leading to significant morbidity. A normal adult loses 1–3% of knee articular cartilage with aging, which further worsens with onset of osteoarthritis. The arthritis-related defects show irregular and obtuse margins due to repetitive wear and tear.

13.2.1 Role of Magnetic Resonance Imaging

The direct visualization of articular cartilage, multiplanar capabilities, and high soft tissue contrast provided by MRI enables the accurate and reproducible assessment of the morphologic features of injured articular cartilage. By using a cartilage-sensitive MR sequence, the adjacent joint fluid and subchondral bone can be distinguished from cartilage MR signal characteristics. The most commonly used clinical MR imaging techniques to assess the status of articular cartilage are fat-suppressed T2-weighted (fs T2W) or proton density-weighted (PDW) sequences. These MR images delineate the intermediate signal intensity of articular cartilage from the high signal intensity of joint fluid (Figs. 13.1 and 13.2). These images are also useful for accurate grading of the cartilage loss (low- or high-grade) and full-thickness defects, as well as for the detection of subchondral bone marrow edema and cyst formation, which shows increased signal intensity [23–25]. Fat-suppressed 3D sequences, such as fast spin echo (FSE) or spoiled gradient-recalled (SPGR) sequences and double-echo steady-state (DESS) sequences, provide excellent morphological depiction of the cartilage in multiple planes, thus, avoiding partial volume effects [26–29]. Higher spatial resolution and accuracy for individual cartilage lesions have been shown using 3D over 2D sequences in knee joint [30] and other smaller joints in accordance with the author's experience (Fig. 13.3). However, 3D gradient data sets are often more susceptible to metal artifacts and may be less sensitive to meniscal and ligament pathologies as well as subchondral bone marrow edema.

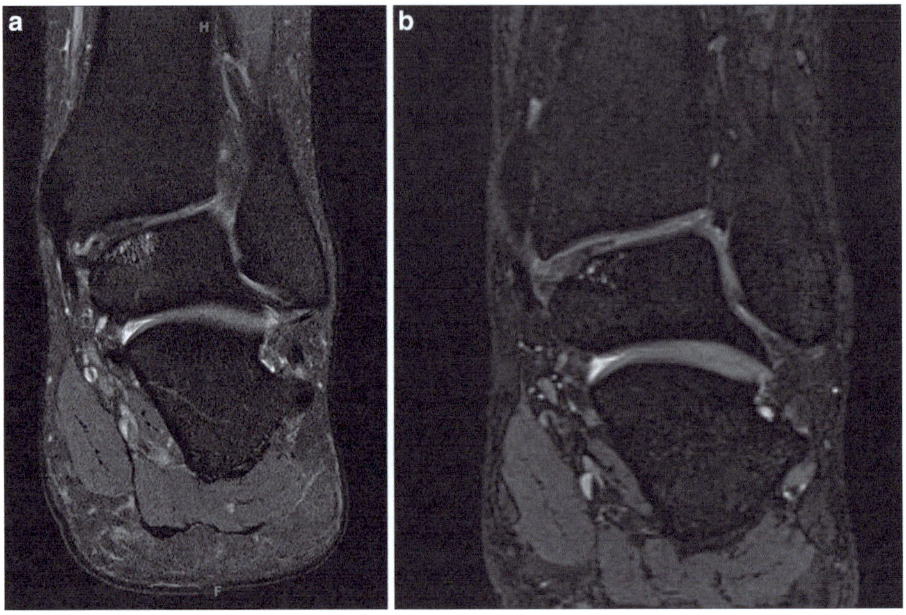

Fig. 13.3 Coronal fat-saturated proton density (**a**) and coronal DESS (**b**) MR images of a 25-year-old woman with osteochondral lesion of the posteromedial talar dome. Note better depiction of bone marrow edema and cystic changes on fat-saturated proton density; however, the cartilage evaluation is limited on 2D sequence due to partial volume artifacts. Corresponding DESS imaging shows better cartilage demarcation and separates the tibial and talar articular cartilages

13.2.2 Treatment of Injured Articular Cartilage

Cartilage repair and regeneration is a treatment recommended for patients with knee cartilage damage or deterioration caused by:

- Injury or trauma, including sports injuries
- Repetitive use of the joint
- Congenital abnormalities affecting normal joint structure
- Hormonal disorders that affect bone and joint development, such as osteochondritis dissecans (OCD)

To determine the best cartilage repair approach for the patient, MRI is used to determine the severity, size, and location of cartilage injuries. The commonly used surgical techniques for the treatment of injured cartilage can be prudently classified into repair, reconstruction, and regeneration techniques [31]. For details of surgical procedure, refer to Chap. 11.

13.2.2.1 Repair Techniques

The simplest treatment for displaced, multi-fragmented, avascular, or deformed chondral lesions is removal of the lesion and debridement of its bony base. The principal indication for such an arthroscopic debridement is during the treatment of concurrent meniscal tears in patients with minimal malalignment [32]. Microfracture is a related older technique for the treatment of chondral lesions. Multiple perforations are arthroscopically created using an angulated ice pick crossing the subchondral bone to induce bleeding in the damaged site. Bleeding, which gradually creates a clot, brings various bone marrow elements including progenitor cells, cytokines, and growth factors that have the ability to form repair tissue. The hematopoietic and mesenchymal stem cells are stimulated to form the fibrocartilage composed of collagen types I and II, which is of inferior quality and not as resilient in dealing with stress when compared to the native articular cartilage. Microfractures are effective in small injuries/areas of cartilage defects (less than 2 cm^2) with an intact subchondral plate [33, 34].

13.2.2.2 Reconstruction Techniques

Osteochondral autograft transplantation (OAT) provides a structure that integrates well with the surrounding bone. An osteochondral (OC) graft is taken from a non-weight-bearing area of the knee and is transplanted into the cartilage defect site. The OC grafts are press fitted into the defect and flushed with the adjacent native cartilage to provide good contact with the healthy tissue. This can be achieved by placing the plugs perpendicular to the articular surface. The area of coverage is limited with a single OAT procedure. Alternatively, mosaicplasty is a procedure where multiple OC autografts cover a larger area.

Allografts are more adaptable and can be designed for any defect shape or size. The main limitations of this technique include risk of immune reaction and transmission of disease. Additionally, these allografts have to be used within a short period of time because of reduction in cell viability with time [35]. Allografts are indicated in young active patients with injuries greater than 2.5 cm in diameter [36].

Bioabsorbable devices have gained popularity because of the technical ease to arthroscopically implant them without the risk of blood-borne disease transmission or the requirement for removal of the implanted device. Also, the appropriate dimensions (thickness and length) can be chosen to fit the entire articular cartilage lesion.

13.2.2.3 Regeneration Techniques

Autologous chondrocyte implantation (ACI) is a two-step technique that involves harvesting the articular cartilage from a non-weight-bearing area of the knee. The harvested chondrocytes are cultured to increase the chondrocyte count to two to five million cells, which are then reimplanted in the host knee cartilage defect site with an overlying periosteal patch. The main indication for this technique is failure of other techniques in patients less than 50 years of age with cartilage lesions between 1 and 10 cm^2 [15, 37]. The second- and third-generation ACI techniques have been subsequently developed to include the use of seeded membranes and biomaterials such as collagen type I or the chondro-inductive/chondro-conductive matrices. However, the comparison of first and second generation of ACI has not shown any significant clinical differences [38, 39].

13.3 Postoperative Assessment of Articular Cartilage Repair

MRI is used for the assessment of graft incorporation, graft congruity, and examination of the repair tissue characteristics. Postsurgical MRI is used for follow-up of patients after cartilage repair surgery in order to determine the success of surgical treatment and to assess the morphology and composition of the repair tissue. In the first 4 weeks after the procedure, the plugs and surrounding marrow have altered marrow signal. By 12 months, the plugs and the surrounding marrow return to normal fatty marrow signal. Persistent edema visualized as high signal intensity in the subchondral bone marrow and cyst formation indicates graft failure and poor incorporation.

13.3.1 Morphological Assessment of Articular Cartilage Repair: Qualitative

To successfully assess the graft morphology and integration to native tissue, it is essential to obtain a high spatial resolution, which in turn can be achieved either by using a surface coil (at 1.5 T scanner) or a knee coil (at 3 T scanner) [40–42]. Cartilage-sensitive MR sequences that allow excellent visualization of the articular cartilage with good signal-to-noise ratio (SNR) and contrast-to-noise ratio (CNR) within reasonable imaging times includes: fs PDW, T2 FSE and 3D gradient recalled echo (GRE) sequences [24, 30, 43–45]. Using a combination of these morphologic imaging sequences has provided excellent soft tissue contrast.

Several proposals for the morphological analysis of the repair tissue include evaluations of the structure and MR signal intensity of the repair tissue (at its surface, the defect filling and integration with adjacent native cartilage); degree of defect filling; morphology of repair tissue with respect to native cartilage (flush, proud, or depressed); delamination (in the setting of ACI); integration with the adjacent native cartilage; nature of the interface with the adjacent surface (presence or absence and size of fissures); integrity of cartilage on the opposite articular surface; as well as the assessment of the status of the subchondral bone and bone marrow [40, 42, 46, 47].

13.3.1.1 Two-Dimensional Magnetic Resonance Observation of Cartilage Repair Tissue Score

Among various MR scoring systems, the MOCART proposed by Marlovits et al. [40] is an efficient scoring system that has shown to have proven validity, reliability, and clinical usefulness with excellent interobserver reproducibility [40, 48, 49]. The MR assessment of the MOCART score is based on standard 2D MR sequences. Depending on the anatomic site of the cartilage repair, the MR evaluation of the cartilage repair tissue is performed on sagittal, axial, or coronal 2D planes using high spatial resolution together with a slice thickness of 2–4 mm. See Appendix C for details of 2D MOCART assessment criteria.

The 2D MOCART scoring system involved the analysis of the following nine variables:

1. Degree of defect repair and filling
2. Integration of cartilage repair tissue to border zone
3. Structure of repair tissue on surface
4. Structure of whole volume of repair tissue
5. Signal intensity of repair tissue
6. Constitution to subchondral lamina
7. Status of the subchondral bone
8. Possible adhesions
9. Possible joint effusion (Fig. 13.4)

13.3.1.2 Three-Dimensional Magnetic Resonance Observation of Cartilage Repair Tissue Score

With improvement of MR technology, pulse sequences, and development of 3D sequences, Welsch et al. proposed a new 3D MOCART score by using the isotropic 3D TrueFISP sequence and its multiplanar reconstruction (MPR) [49]. The new isovoxel 3D sequences have the potential for high-resolution isotropic imaging with a voxel size down to 0.4 mm^3, which can then be reformatted in arbitrary planes without any loss of spatial resolution. Building on the capabilities of MPR, the cartilage repair 3D visualization and subsequent development of the 3D MOCART scoring system were feasible.

The 3D MOCART score was based on the standard 2D MOCART score by including variables and subcategories. The 3D MOCART included 11 variables as follows (see Appendix C for details of 3D MOCART assessment criteria):

1. Defect fill relative to adjacent native articular cartilage
2. Repair tissue interface with native cartilage
3. Bone interface
4. Surface of repair tissue
5. Structure of repair tissue
6. Signal intensity of repair tissue
7. Subchondral lamina
8. Chondral osteophyte
9. Bone marrow edema
10. Subchondral bone integrity
11. Effusion (Figs. 13.5 and 13.6)

A pertinent discussion of the variables in 3D MOCART score is as follows:

1. *Defect Fill*

   Defect fill is evaluated in comparison to the adjacent native cartilage. Defect fill is described as 100% (flush with the native cartilage), when the repair tissue is of comparable thickness to the adjacent cartilage. If

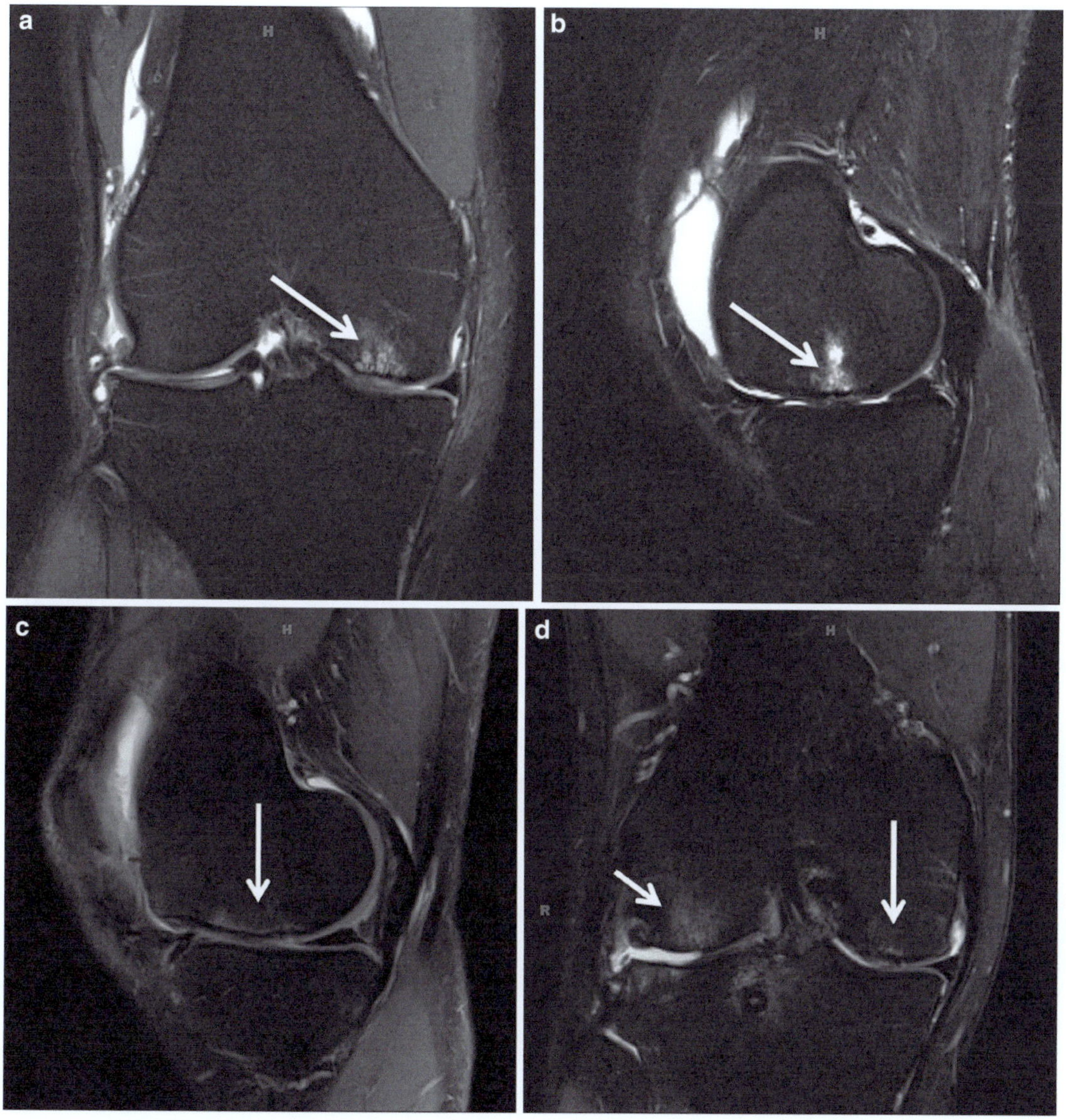

Fig. 13.4 Coronal (**a**) and sagittal (**b**) fat-saturated proton density MR images of a 47-year-old woman with history of right knee pain. She had a prior lateral meniscectomy as well as microfracture surgery within the medial femoral condyle (arrows). 2D MOCART (Magnetic Resonance Observation of Cartilage Repair Tissue) staging for medial femoral condyle: (1) degree of defect repair and filling: complete (at the level of the adjacent cartilage); (2) integration to the border zone, complete (complete integration with adjacent cartilage) demarcating border visible, no; (3) surface of the repair tissue, surface intact; (4) structure of the repair tissue, fairly homogenous; (5) signal intensity of the repair tissue, dual T2-FSE isointense; (6) constitution to subchondral lamina, good; (7) subchondral bone, subchondral cysts and bone marrow edema; (8) adhesions, no; (9) joint effusion, yes. After a 2-year follow-up, sagittal (**c**) and coronal (**d**) fat-saturated proton density MR show decreased bone marrow edema and cystic changes on medial femoral condyle (large arrows). However, coronal image also shows worsening lateral compartment cartilage loss with developing bone marrow edema (small arrow)

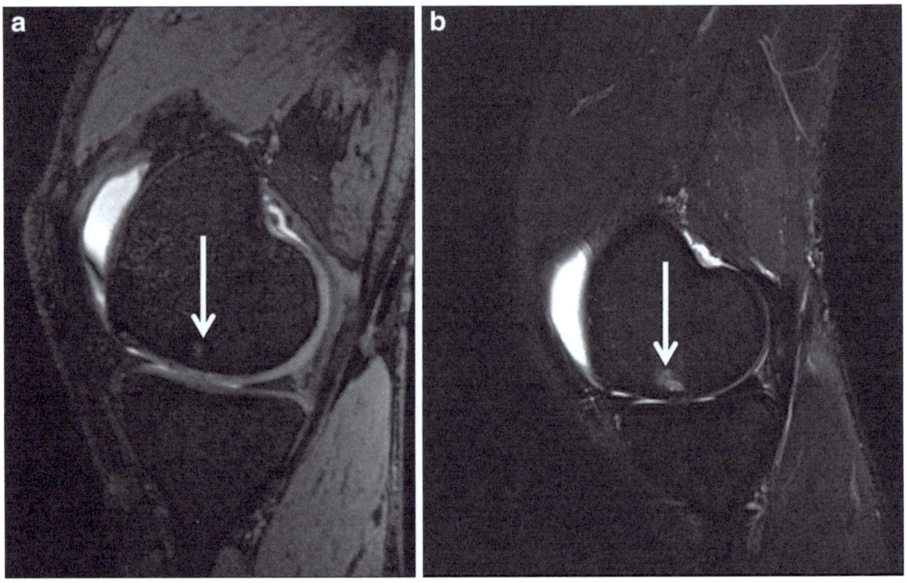

Fig. 13.5 Sagittal 3D DESS (**a**) and sagittal fat-saturated proton density (**b**) MR images of a 47-year-old woman with a prior microfracture surgery within the medial femoral condyle (arrows). Notice better depiction of cartilage definition on 3D image (**a**) and reactive bone marrow changes in the medial femoral condyle on 2D image (**b**), respectively

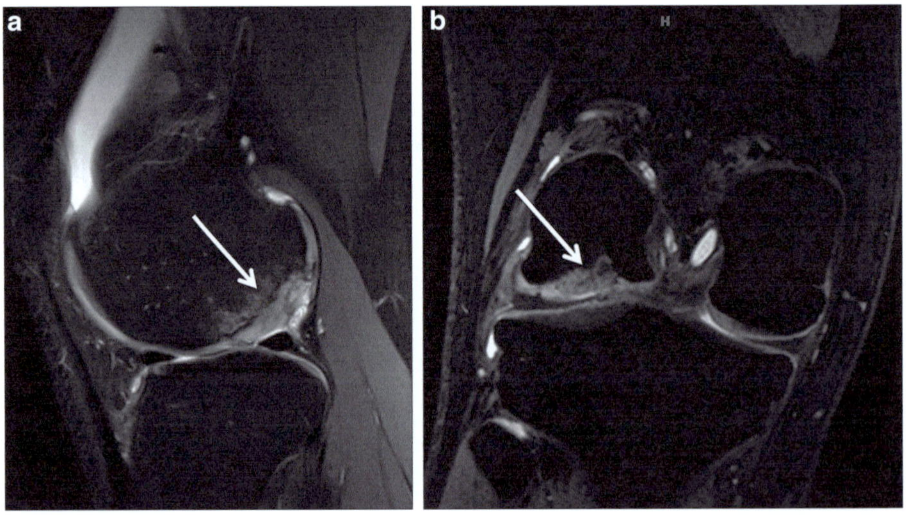

Fig. 13.6 Sagittal fat-saturated proton density (**a**) and coronal (**b**) 3D TrueFISP MR images of a 15-year-old boy with history of prior ACI within the lateral femoral condyle (arrows). 3D MOCART (Magnetic Resonance Observation of Cartilage Repair Tissue) staging for medial femoral condyle: (1) degree of defect repair and filling, complete and hypertrophy (75–100% above the level of the adjacent cartilage); (2) cartilage interface (integration to the border zone), complete; (3) surface of the repair tissue, surface irregular; (4) structure of the whole repair tissue, fairly homogeneous; (5) signal intensity, dual T2-FSE isointense; 3D TrueFISP, isointense; (6) constitution to subchondral lamina, good; (7) subchondral lamina, irregular; (8) chondral osteophyte, no; (9) bone marrow edema, yes, medium; (10) subchondral bone, cysts; joint effusion, yes, medium

the value is below 100%, it is referred to as a cartilage defect underfilling, and if it is above 100% (proud relative to the native cartilage), it is termed as hypertrophy. Further, it can be classified on the basis of localization in the weight-bearing areas or elsewhere.

2. *Cartilage Interface*

   It refers to the integration of the repair tissue to the native cartilage border zone. It is stated as complete or incomplete, depending upon the presence or absence of gap at the interface between the repair tissue and the adjacent cartilage.

3. *Bone Interface*

   This evaluates integration of the repair tissue to the subchondral bone or the integration to a possible periosteal flap depending on surgical technique. It is reported as completely attached, partially detached, or complete detached.

4. *Repair Tissue Surface*

   The cartilage surface may be damaged with the appearance of fibrillations, fissures, or ulcerations above or below 50% of repair tissue depth, or there may be a total degeneration. Further, any signs of adhesions are also recorded at the site of damage.

5. *Repair Tissue Structure*

   The architecture of the repaired cartilage is reported as homogeneous when there is typical cartilage layering over the entire repair tissue or inhomogeneous if it shows cleft formation.

6. *MR Signal Intensity*

   The signal intensity of the repair tissue is compared to the adjacent native cartilage. It can be evaluated as nearly normal or abnormal, depending on the amount of the signal alterations. The abnormal signal intensity can be higher (hyperintense) or lower (hypointense) relative to native articular cartilage.

7. *Subchondral Lamina*

   The subchondral lamina between the repair tissue and the bone is reported as either intact or irregular and broken.

8. *Chondral Osteophyte*

   Osteophytes can emerge in the region of the cartilage transplant. Further, they can be found in different sizes, which can be classified based on their thickness of above or below 50% of the thickness of the cartilage transplant.

9. *Bone Marrow Edema*

   Subchondral bone marrow edema size can be classified as small (diameter, < 1 cm), medium (< 2 cm), large (< 4 cm), or diffuse.

10. *Subchondral Bone*

    Excluding the bone marrow edema, the subchondral bone criteria evaluate the changes in the subchondral bone adjacent to the area of repair tissue such as the presence of granulation tissue, sclerosis, or cysts.

11. *Effusion*

    Based on the extent, joint effusion is classified as absent, small, medium, or large.

In the clinical routine follow-up after cartilage repair, the 2D evaluation with the standard 2D MOCART scoring system obtained by using three standard MR sequences provided comparable information to the 3D MOCART scoring system assessed by using only one high-resolution isotropic 3D TrueFISP sequence. However, artifacts were more frequently visible within the 3D TrueFISP sequence.

Another MRI scoring system, the cartilage repair osteoarthritis knee score (CROAKS) was developed for follow-up of knee cartilage repair procedures integrating assessment of the repair site and the whole joint [50]. This semiquantitative assessment system combined the assessment of the cartilage repair site using features of MOCART scores and for the whole the joint based on experiences with the Magnetic Resonance Imaging Osteoarthritis Knee Score (MOAKS). MRI examinations of 20 patients at 12 months post matrix-associated autologous chondrocyte transplantation (MACT) of the knee showed good to excellent reliability with the combined, established semiquantitative scoring systems (MOCART and MOAKS) [50].

13.3.2 Magnetic Resonance Imaging Assessment of Repair Tissue

Recently, there has been a great interest in developing MR imaging techniques to evaluate the biochemical composition of the cartilage repair procedure. The proteoglycan content MR specific sequences include delayed gadolinium-enhanced MR imaging of cartilage (dGEMRIC), T1rho mapping, and sodium MR imaging, whereas the collagen content-sensitive techniques include T2 mapping and magnetization transfer [51–53].

Chondrocytes usually repair by formation of fibrocartilage composed of collagen types I and II, which is not as resilient in dealing with stress as the compressive, native hyaline cartilage primarily composed of collagen type II. On MR imaging, initially the tissue may be indistinct; however, by 1–2 years, repair tissue is expected to fill the defect with a smooth contour. The signal intensity may be similar, although more commonly, less than the native cartilage related to predominant fibrocartilage formation [14]. Following surgical treatment, underlying bone marrow edema often regresses but may not resolve completely. Surface fissures and flaps may be present (Fig. 13.7).

MRI has been proven to be highly accurate in assessing the repair tissue with good correlation to the lesion fill and tissue quality and its integration with the adjacent native cartilage [54]. Further, at post-surgery and during follow-up, MR imaging facilitates accurate assessment of complications of repair surgery including graft/periosteal hypertrophy and delamination, adhesions, surface incongruence, and reactive/inflammatory changes (such as effusions and synovitis). Based on the treatment procedure, the nature of the repair tissue is outlined below:

13.3.2.1 Abrasion Arthroplasty/Debridement

Removal of few millimeters of subchondral bone causes local bleeding, fibrin clot formation, and subsequent development of a fibrocartilage-like tissue composed of collagen type I and type III. Fibrocartilage is stronger against tension rather than compression forces and is therefore not a durable long-lasting substitute for hyaline cartilage. Although early results and symptom relief from this procedure were promising, long-term results have not been satisfactory [55].

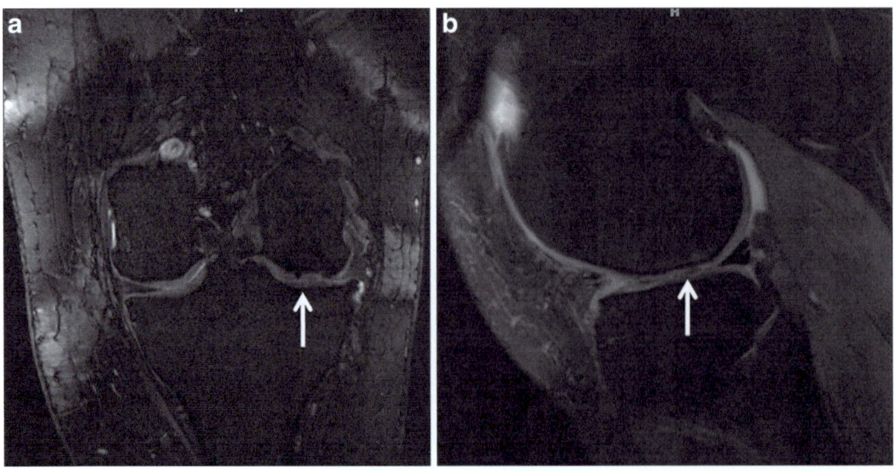

Fig. 13.7 Coronal 3D DESS (**a**) and sagittal fat-saturated proton density (**b**) MR images of a young woman with a prior microfracture surgery within the lateral femoral condyle (arrows). Notice good cartilage fill and better depiction of cartilage definition on the 3D image (**a**) with minimal surface irregularities

13.3.2.2 Autologous Osteochondral Grafts

The repaired tissue is better when OAT is used in the femoral condyles rather than in the tibial plateau or in the patella [56]. The problems of lack of integration or fibrocartilage formation at the border zone with native cartilage may occur. MRI after the mosaicplasty procedure involves assessment of graft incorporation, graft congruity, and examination of the repair tissue characteristics. In the first 4 weeks after the procedure, the plugs and surrounding marrow have altered marrow signal. By 12 months, the plugs and the surrounding marrow return to normal fatty marrow signal. Persistent edema like subchondral bone marrow signal and cyst formation indicates graft failure and poor incorporation.

13.3.2.3 Allogenic Osteochondral Transplants

MRI is useful in determining the surface congruity between graft and the native cartilage [14]. Usually, the bony plug margin is also visible indicating the type of repair. Bone marrow edema can be prominent for up to 12 months post-surgery. Graft-host reactions can be seen as persistent signal abnormalities within the graft marrow or at the graft-host interface [57].

13.3.2.4 Synthetic Grafts, Scaffolds, and Osteochondral Plugs

The synthetic plugs are radiolucent but can be visualized on MR imaging with varying signal intensity depending on the biomaterial used. Frequently, during the first few months, these plugs appear as low signal intensity tracts on T1W and T2W MR images. However, by the end of the first year, the grafts with repair tissue become hyperintense on T2W MR images. Most of them are not visible after 2 years [58].

13.3.2.5 Autologous Chondrocyte Implants

During the follow-up of post ACI cartilage repair, MRI can accurately detect and classify the defect fill as flush, underfilling, or hypertrophy as well as the graft integration [59]. Surface irregularity is commonly seen on MR imaging (Fig. 13.6) [15]. The signal intensity of repair cartilage decreases after the first 12 months. Persistent bone marrow edema, chondral osteophytes, and cartilage delamination are adverse outcome indicative of ACI failure (Fig. 13.8). The common complications of ACI technique are symptomatic graft hypertrophy, perturbed fusion or integration, delamination, and fibrosis, which may require re-intervention [60–62]. Among

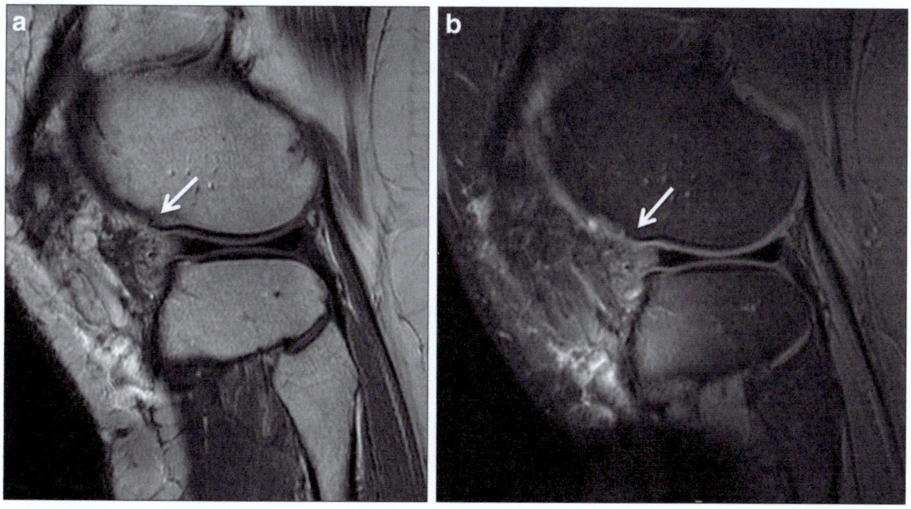

Fig. 13.8 Sagittal proton density (**a**) and sagittal fat-saturated proton density (**b**) MR images of a young man with a prior ACI repair surgery within the lateral femoral condyle 1 year ago (arrows). Notice failure of ACI repair with visible chondral osteophytes (large arrow) and overlying cartilage delamination (small arrow)

those, the overall complication rate and incidence of hypertrophy of the transplant were higher for periosteum-covered ACI. Graft hypertrophy may occur 3–7 months post ACI and has been reported as a complication in 10–63% of cases [16–18]. Furthermore, an increased rate of symptomatic hypertrophy was found for patellar defects. Delamination occurs when the graft separates from the parent bone, which is visualized in MR as a linear fluid high signal intensity undermining the graft. When significant, both delamination and graft hypertrophy may require repeat surgery, either debridement in the case of hypertrophy or repeat ACI in both cases.

13.4 Conclusions

Cartilage injuries are common and a variety of repair procedures have been developed for their treatment. MR imaging has proven to be an excellent tool for presurgical mapping and post-surgical assessment of these lesions.

References

1. Mankin HJ. The response of articular cartilage to mechanical injury. J Bone Joint Surg Am. 1982;64(3):460–6. Epub 1982/03/01.
2. Newman AP. Articular cartilage repair. Am J Sports Med. 1998;26(2):309–24. Epub 1998/04/21.
3. Ebert JR, Fallon M, Ackland TR, Janes GC, Wood DJ. Minimum 10-year clinical and radiological outcomes of a randomized controlled trial evaluating 2 different approaches to full weight bearing after matrix-induced autologous chondrocyte implantation. Am J Sports Med. 2020;48(1):133–42.
4. Donoso R, Figueroa D, Espinoza J, Yañez C, Saavedra J. Osteochondral autologous transplantation for treating patellar high-grade chondral defects: a systematic review. Orthop J Sports Med. 2019;7(10):2325967119876618.
5. Zhao X, Ruan J, Tang H, Li J, Shi Y, et al. Multi-compositional MRI evaluation of repair cartilage in knee osteoarthritis with treatment of allogeneic human adipose-derived mesenchymal progenitor cells. Stem Cell Res Ther. 2019;10(1):308.
6. Kyriakidis T, Iosifidis M, Michalopoulos E, Melas I, Stavropoulos-Giokas C, et al. Good mid-term outcomes after adipose-derived culture-expanded mesenchymal stem cells implantation in knee focal cartilage defects. Knee Surg Sports Traumatol Arthrosc. 2019. https://doi.org/10.1007/s00167-019-05688-9. [Epub ahead of print].
7. Schreiner MM, Raudner M, Marlovits S, Bohndorf K, Weber M, et al. The MOCART (Magnetic Resonance Observation of Cartilage Repair Tissue) 2.0 knee score and atlas. Cartilage. 2019:1947603519865308. https://doi.org/10.1177/1947603519865308. [Epub ahead of print].
8. Ackermann J, Mestriner AB, Shah N, Gomoll AH. Effect of autogenous bone marrow aspirate treatment on magnetic resonance imaging integration of osteochondral allografts in the knee: a matched comparative imaging analysis. Arthroscopy. 2019;35(8):2436–44.
9. Liu YW, Tran MD, Skalski MR, Patel DB, White EA, et al. MR imaging of cartilage repair surgery of the knee. Clin Imaging. 2019;58:129–39.
10. Ogura T, Merkely G, Bryant T, Winalski CS, Minas T. Autologous chondrocyte implantation "Segmental-sandwich" technique for deep osteochondral defects in the knee: clinical outcomes and correlation with magnetic resonance imaging findings. Orthop J Sports Med. 2019;7(5):2325967119847173.
11. Trattnig S, Raudner M, Schreiner M, Roemer F, Bohndorf K. Biochemical cartilage imaging-update 2019. Radiologe. 2019;59(8):742–9.
12. de Girolamo L, Schönhuber H, Viganò M, Bait C, Quaglia A, et al. Autologous Matrix-Induced Chondrogenesis (AMIC) and AMIC enhanced by autologous concentrated Bone Marrow Aspirate (BMAC) allow for stable clinical and functional improvements at up to 9 years follow-up: results from a randomized controlled study. J Clin Med. 2019;8(3). pii: E392. https://doi.org/10.3390/jcm8030392.
13. Kreuz PC, Kalkreuth RH, Niemeyer P, Uhl M, Erggelet C. Long-term clinical and MRI results of matrix-assisted autologous chondrocyte implantation for articular cartilage defects of the knee. Cartilage. 2019;10(3):305–13.
14. Alparslan L, Winalski CS, Boutin RD, Minas T. Postoperative magnetic resonance imaging of articular cartilage repair. Semin Musculoskelet Radiol. 2001;5(4):345–63.
15. Brittberg M, Winalski CS. Evaluation of cartilage injuries and repair. J Bone Joint Surg Am. 2003;85-A(Suppl 2):58–69.
16. Potter HG, Foo LF. Magnetic resonance imaging of articular cartilage: trauma, degeneration, and repair. Am J Sports Med. 2006;34(4):661–77.
17. Welsch GH, Mamisch TC, Hughes T, Domayer S, Marlovits S, Trattnig S. Advanced morphological and biochemical magnetic resonance imaging of cartilage repair procedures in the knee joint at 3 tesla. Semin Musculoskelet Radiol. 2008;12(3):196–211.
18. Disler DG. Fat-suppressed three-dimensional spoiled gradient-recalled MR imaging: assessment of articular and physeal hyaline cartilage. AJR Am J Roentgenol. 1997;169(4):1117–23.
19. Kawahara Y, Uetani M, Nakahara N, Doiguchi Y, Nishiguchi M, Futagawa S, et al. Fast spin-echo MR of the articular cartilage in the osteoarthrotic knee.

Correlation of MR and arthroscopic findings. Acta Radiol. 1998;39(2):120–5.
20. Yoshioka H, Stevens K, Hargreaves BA, Steines D, Genovese M, Dillingham MF, et al. Magnetic resonance imaging of articular cartilage of the knee: comparison between fat-suppressed three-dimensional SPGR imaging, fat-suppressed FSE imaging, and fat-suppressed three-dimensional DEFT imaging, and correlation with arthroscopy. J Magn Reson Imaging. 2004;20(5):857–64.
21. Hede K, Christensen BB, Jensen J, Foldager CB, Lind M. Combined bone marrow aspirate and platelet-rich plasma for cartilage repair: two-year clinical results. Cartilage. 2019:1947603519876329. https://doi.org/10.1177/1947603519876329. [Epub ahead of print].
22. Monckeberg JE, Rafols C, Apablaza F, Gerhard P, Rosales J. Intra-articular administration of peripheral blood stem cells with platelet-rich plasma regenerated articular cartilage and improved clinical outcomes for knee chondral lesions. Knee. 2019;26(4):824–31.
23. Bredella MA, Tirman PF, Peterfy CG, Zarlingo M, Feller JF, Bost FW, et al. Accuracy of T2-weighted fast spin-echo MR imaging with fat saturation in detecting cartilage defects in the knee: comparison with arthroscopy in 130 patients. AJR Am J Roentgenol. 1999;172(4):1073–80.
24. Potter HG, Linklater JM, Allen AA, Hannafin JA, Haas SB. Magnetic resonance imaging of articular cartilage in the knee. An evaluation with use of fast-spin-echo imaging. J Bone Joint Surg Am. 1998;80(9):1276–84.
25. Ebert JR, Smith A, Fallon M, Wood DJ, Ackland TR. Degree of preoperative subchondral bone edema is not associated with pain and graft outcomes after matrix-induced autologous chondrocyte implantation. Am J Sports Med. 2014;42(11):2689–98. Epub 2014/09/13.
26. Yang X, Li Z, Cao Y, Xu Y, Wang H, et al. Efficacy of magnetic resonance imaging with an SPGR sequence for the early evaluation of knee cartilage degeneration and the relationship between cartilage and other tissues. J Orthop Surg Res. 2019;14(1):152.
27. Chaudhari AS, Stevens KJ, Sveinsson B, Wood JP, Beaulieu CF, et al. Combined 5-minute double-echo in steady-state with separated echoes and 2-minute proton-density-weighted 2D FSE sequence for comprehensive whole-joint knee MRI assessment. J Magn Reson Imaging. 2019;49(7):e183–94.
28. Hayashi D, Roemer FW, Guermazi A. Magnetic resonance imaging assessment of knee osteoarthritis: current and developing new concepts and techniques. Clin Exp Rheumatol. 2019;37 Suppl 120(5):88–95.
29. Hayashi D, Li X, Murakami AM, Roemer FW, Trattnig S, et al. Understanding magnetic resonance imaging of knee cartilage repair: a focus on clinical relevance. Cartilage. 2018;9(3):223–36.
30. Disler DG, McCauley TR, Kelman CG, Fuchs MD, Ratner LM, Wirth CR, et al. Fat-suppressed three-dimensional spoiled gradient-echo MR imaging of hyaline cartilage defects in the knee: comparison with standard MR imaging and arthroscopy. AJR Am J Roentgenol. 1996;167(1):127–32.
31. Forriol F. Growth factors in cartilage and meniscus repair. Injury. 2009;40(Suppl 3):S12–6.
32. Merchan EC, Galindo E. Arthroscope-guided surgery versus nonoperative treatment for limited degenerative osteoarthritis of the femorotibial joint in patients over 50 years of age: a prospective comparative study. Arthroscopy. 1993;9(6):663–7.
33. Steadman JR, Miller BS, Karas SG, Schlegel TF, Briggs KK, Hawkins RJ. The microfracture technique in the treatment of full-thickness chondral lesions of the knee in National Football League players. J Knee Surg. 2003;16(2):83–6.
34. Steadman JR, Briggs KK, Rodrigo JJ, Kocher MS, Gill TJ, Rodkey WG. Outcomes of microfracture for traumatic chondral defects of the knee: average 11-year follow-up. Arthroscopy. 2003;19(5):477–84.
35. McGoveran BM, Pritzker KP, Shasha N, Price J, Gross AE. Long-term chondrocyte viability in a fresh osteochondral allograft. J Knee Surg 2002 Spring;15(2):97–100.
36. Gross AE, Kim W, Las Heras F, Backstein D, Safir O, Pritzker KP. Fresh osteochondral allografts for posttraumatic knee defects: long-term followup. Clin Orthop Relat Res. 2008;466(8):1863–70.
37. Vaquero J, Forriol F. Knee chondral injuries: clinical treatment strategies and experimental models. Injury. 2011;43:694–705.
38. Bartlett W, Skinner JA, Gooding CR, Carrington RW, Flanagan AM, Briggs TW, et al. Autologous chondrocyte implantation versus matrix-induced autologous chondrocyte implantation for osteochondral defects of the knee: a prospective, randomised study. J Bone Joint Surg Br. 2005;87(5):640–5.
39. Manfredini M, Zerbinati F, Gildone A, Faccini R. Autologous chondrocyte implantation: a comparison between an open periosteal-covered and an arthroscopic matrix-guided technique. Acta Orthop Belg. 2007;73(2):207–18.
40. Marlovits S, Striessnig G, Resinger CT, Aldrian SM, Vecsei V, Imhof H, et al. Definition of pertinent parameters for the evaluation of articular cartilage repair tissue with high-resolution magnetic resonance imaging. Eur J Radiol. 2004;52(3):310–9. Epub 2004/11/17.
41. Qian Y, Williams AA, Chu CR, Boada FE. High-resolution ultrashort echo time (UTE) imaging on human knee with AWSOS sequence at 3.0 T. J Magn Reson Imaging. 2012;35(1):204–10. Epub 2011/10/18.
42. Trattnig S, Millington SA, Szomolanyi P, Marlovits S. MR imaging of osteochondral grafts and autologous chondrocyte implantation. Eur Radiol. 2007;17(1):103–18. Epub 2006/06/28.
43. Recht M, White LM, Winalski CS, Miniaci A, Minas T, Parker RD. MR imaging of cartilage repair procedures. Skelet Radiol. 2003;32(4):185–200. Epub 2003/03/26.

44. Recht MP, Piraino DW, Paletta GA, Schils JP, Belhobek GH. Accuracy of fat-suppressed three-dimensional spoiled gradient-echo FLASH MR imaging in the detection of patellofemoral articular cartilage abnormalities. Radiology. 1996;198(1):209–12. Epub 1996/01/01.
45. Trattnig S, Mlynarik V, Huber M, Ba-Ssalamah A, Puig S, Imhof H. Magnetic resonance imaging of articular cartilage and evaluation of cartilage disease. Invest Radiol. 2000;35(10):595–601. Epub 2000/10/21.
46. Trattnig S, Ba-Ssalamah A, Pinker K, Plank C, Vecsei V, Marlovits S. Matrix-based autologous chondrocyte implantation for cartilage repair: noninvasive monitoring by high-resolution magnetic resonance imaging. Magn Reson Imaging. 2005;23(7):779–87. Epub 2005/10/11.
47. Roberts S, McCall IW, Darby AJ, Menage J, Evans H, Harrison PE, et al. Autologous chondrocyte implantation for cartilage repair: monitoring its success by magnetic resonance imaging and histology. Arthritis Res Ther. 2003;5(1):R60–73. Epub 2003/04/30.
48. van den Borne MP, Raijmakers NJ, Vanlauwe J, Victor J, de Jong SN, Bellemans J, et al. International Cartilage Repair Society (ICRS) and Oswestry macroscopic cartilage evaluation scores validated for use in Autologous Chondrocyte Implantation (ACI) and microfracture. Osteoarthritis Cartilage. 2007;15(12):1397–402.
49. Welsch GH, Zak L, Mamisch TC, Resinger C, Marlovits S, Trattnig S. Three-dimensional magnetic resonance observation of cartilage repair tissue (MOCART) score assessed with an isotropic three-dimensional true fast imaging with steady-state precession sequence at 3.0 tesla. Invest Radiol. 2009;44(9):603–12.
50. Roemer FW, Guermazi A, Trattnig S, Apprich S, Marlovits S, Niu J, et al. Whole joint MRI assessment of surgical cartilage repair of the knee: cartilage repair osteoarthritis knee score (CROAKS). Osteoarthritis Cartilage. 2014;22(6):779–99. Epub 2014/04/02.
51. Krusche-Mandl I, Schmitt B, Zak L, Apprich S, Aldrian S, Juras V, et al. Long-term results 8 years after autologous osteochondral transplantation: 7 T gagCEST and sodium magnetic resonance imaging with morphological and clinical correlation. Osteoarthritis Cartilage. 2012;20(5):357–63. Epub 2012/02/23.
52. Eshed I, Trattnig S, Sharon M, Arbel R, Nierenberg G, Konen E, et al. Assessment of cartilage repair after chondrocyte transplantation with a fibrin-hyaluronan matrix–correlation of morphological MRI, biochemical T2 mapping and clinical outcome. Eur J Radiol. 2012;81(6):1216–23. Epub 2011/04/05.
53. Collins AT, Hatcher CC, Kim SY, Ziemian SN, Spritzer CE, et al. Selective enzymatic digestion of proteoglycans and collagens alters cartilage T1rho and T2 relaxation times. Ann Biomed Eng. 2019;47(1):190–201.
54. Ramappa AJ, Gill TJ, Bradford CH, Ho CP, Steadman JR. Magnetic resonance imaging to assess knee cartilage repair tissue after microfracture of chondral defects. J Knee Surg. 2007;20(3):228–34.
55. Bert JM, Maschka K. The arthroscopic treatment of unicompartmental gonarthrosis: a five-year follow-up study of abrasion arthroplasty plus arthroscopic debridement and arthroscopic debridement alone. Arthroscopy. 1989;5(1):25–32.
56. Bentley G, Biant LC, Carrington RW, Akmal M, Goldberg A, Williams AM, et al. A prospective, randomised comparison of autologous chondrocyte implantation versus mosaicplasty for osteochondral defects in the knee. J Bone Joint Surg Br. 2003;85(2):223–30.
57. Sirlin CB, Brossmann J, Boutin RD, Pathria MN, Convery FR, Bugbee W, et al. Shell osteochondral allografts of the knee: comparison of mr imaging findings and immunologic responses. Radiology. 2001;219(1):35–43.
58. Furukawa T, Eyre DR, Koide S, Glimcher MJ. Biochemical studies on repair cartilage resurfacing experimental defects in the rabbit knee. J Bone Joint Surg Am. 1980;62(1):79–89.
59. Ho YY, Stanley AJ, Hui JH, Wang SC. Postoperative evaluation of the knee after autologous chondrocyte implantation: what radiologists need to know. Radiographics. 2007;27(1):207–20. discussion 221-2.
60. Brown WE, Potter HG, Marx RG, Wickiewicz TL, Warren RF. Magnetic resonance imaging appearance of cartilage repair in the knee. Clin Orthop Relat Res. 2004;422(422):214–23.
61. Henderson I, Gui J, Lavigne P. Autologous chondrocyte implantation: natural history of postimplantation periosteal hypertrophy and effects of repair-site debridement on outcome. Arthroscopy. 2006 Dec;22(12):1318–1324.e1.
62. Recht MP, Goodwin DW, Winalski CS, White LM. MRI of articular cartilage: revisiting current status and future directions. AJR Am J Roentgenol. 2005;185(4):899–914.

14 Magnetic Resonance Imaging of the Ultrastructural Composition of Articular Cartilage in Disease and Repair

Siegfried Trattnig, Götz H. Welsch, Sebastian Röhrich, Markus M. Schreiner, and Martin Zalaudek

14.1 Introduction

Articular cartilage injuries are commonly seen in orthopedic practice. In a retrospective review of 31,510 knee arthroscopies, the incidence of chondral lesions was 63%. Full-thickness articular cartilage lesions with exposed subchondral bone were found in 20% of patients, with 5% of all arthroscopy in patients less than 40 years of age with grade IV chondral lesions [1].

The treatment of articular cartilage damage after traumatic insult or due to degenerative joint disease remains a challenge because of the limited capacity of adult cartilage for spontaneous repair [2]. Knee cartilage defects that exceed a critical size heal poorly and usually lead to osteoarthritis (OA). Several surgical and nonsurgical strategies have been developed in an attempt to repair articular cartilage lesions. The surgical techniques may be arthroscopic or open and include marrow stimulation techniques, such as drilling and microfracturing, osteochondral (OC) grafts, and cell-based techniques [3]. Refer to Chaps. 7, 11, 12, and 17 for in-depth information pertaining to the arthroscopic and surgical techniques for cartilage repair.

The high prevalence of knee cartilage lesions and disease created a strong demand for a noninvasive diagnostic tool that is reliable and reproducible. Likewise, with the variety of treatment

S. Trattnig, MD (✉)
High Field MR Center, Department of Biomedical Imaging and Image-Guided Therapy, Medical University of Vienna, Vienna, Austria

Austrian Cluster for Tissue Regeneration, Vienna, Austria

Christian Doppler Laboratory for Clinical Molecular MR Imaging, Vienna, Austria
e-mail: siegfried.trattnig@meduniwien.ac.at

G. H. Welsch, MD
Department of Athletics and Sports Medicine, University Medical Center Hamburg-Eppendorf, Hamburg, Germany

UKE Athleticum, Division of Orthopaedic Sports Medicine, University Hospital of Hamburg-Eppendorf, Hamburg, Germany

S. Röhrich, MD
High Field MR Centre, Department of Biomedical Imaging and Image-Guided Therapy, Computational Imaging Research Laboratory, Medical University of Vienna, Vienna, Austria

M. M. Schreiner, MD · M. Zalaudek, MD
Department of Orthopaedics and Trauma Surgery, Medical University of Vienna, Vienna, Austria

High Field MR Center, Department of Biomedical Imaging and Image-Guided Therapy, Medical University of Vienna, Vienna, Austria

H. K. Gahunia et al. (eds.), *Articular Cartilage of the Knee*,
https://doi.org/10.1007/978-1-4939-7587-7_14

options available to address the chondral and osteochondral lesions, there is a need for an imaging modality that offers the most sensitive and safe, noninvasive way to monitor and assess repair tissue and its integration to native cartilage following regenerative cartilage treatment. Magnetic resonance imaging (MRI) has advanced tremendously over the last several years and has offered the opportunity to fulfill this demand. Cartilage-sensitive sequences, high-resolution three-dimensional (3D) isotropic sequences, semiquantitative MR-based scores, and volumetric assessments provide invaluable information. Morphologic sequences allow diagnostic cartilage imaging with increased precision; and, in combination with volumetry and semiquantitative scores, it also allows the reproducible and repetitive MR assessment of repair tissue. However, morphological MRI is limited to the cartilage structure and does not provide any information about cartilage molecular composition. The recent development of biochemical MR imaging has filled this void by providing information about the ultrastructural elements of cartilage, such as water, collagen, and proteoglycans. In the following pages, we outline the basic principles of morphological and biochemical MRI and the current state-of-the-art clinical practice for applying these techniques to the articular cartilage of the knee.

14.2 Morphological Magnetic Resonance Imaging of Articular Cartilage

Postsurgical follow-up protocols vary and involve assessment of clinical symptoms, direct visualization of grafts with arthroscopy, or indirect visualization of grafts with MRI. For long-term follow-up of these procedures, clinical scores and the morphological and biochemical evaluation of biopsies taken during control arthroscopies remain the standard of reference [4–6]. However, considering the invasive character of arthroscopic procedures and the risk for associated morbidity, objective noninvasive measures of the properties of the grafted regions after biological cartilage repair is highly desirable and very helpful to facilitate the evaluation of longitudinal repair tissue follow-up. The purpose of cartilage imaging is to visualize the integrity of cartilage surface and its matrix; to evaluate cartilage thickness, volume, and – once cartilage repair is performed – the integration of the repair tissue to surrounding native cartilage and underlying bone. Providing these informations, morphological MRI is playing an important role in pre- and postoperative imaging as well as follow-up assessment of repair tissue throughout the postoperative period. Hence, MRI is the current standard imaging method for the noninvasive assessment of articular cartilage [5, 7–15].

In a clinical setting, the evolution of MRI technology has provided excellent contrast between articular cartilage and adjacent structures within reasonable imaging times. MR evaluation of cartilage repair can be performed using the same acquisition techniques as those used for native cartilage. In 2000, the Articular Cartilage Imaging Group (ACIG) of the International Cartilage Repair Society (ICRS) compiled an MR acquisition protocol for cartilage imaging, which has not been updated since. The most commonly used MR imaging techniques on 1.5 tesla (T), 3.0 T, and research 7 T scanners are fluid-sensitive sequences, such as two-dimensional (2D) fat-suppressed (fs), intermediate and T2-weighted (T2W) fast spin echo (FSE), as well as 3D gradient-recalled echo (GRE) techniques with fat suppression or water excitation, all in combination with dedicated extremity coils [9, 11–15, 16–18]. A minimal in-plane resolution of 0.3 mm was found to be necessary to show early signs of superficial fraying of the articular cartilage surface, which was also substantial for the detection of cartilage fissures and insufficient repair-tissue integration to native cartilage [19]. Compared to 2D, the 3D acquisition is advantageous with regard to higher contrast- and signal-to-noise ratios which also yields higher and isotropic resolutions for multi-planar reconstructions that enables 3D visualizations and volume measurements [10, 11, 16, 20].

14.2.1 Cartilage-Specific MR Sequences

Magnetic resonance imaging is the most important modality for the detection and evaluation of traumatic or degenerative cartilaginous lesions in the knee as well as for monitoring the effects of pharmacological and surgical therapy. To date, several cartilage-specific MR imaging techniques have been developed to assess the morphological integrity of knee cartilage such as FSE, 3D spin echo, and gradient echo as well as isotropic imaging.

14.2.1.1 Fast Spin Echo Technique

Fast spin echo imaging combines strong T2 weighting, magnetization transfer effects, and relative preservation of high signal intensity in the marrow fat and free water (Fig. 14.1). With FSE technique, articular cartilage is visualized as low signal intensity (dark) hence producing high contrast between cartilage and the adjacent synovial fluid and bone marrow [21, 22]. Intermediate-weighted FSE sequences are useful for both the detection of cartilage surface lesions and intrachondral extracellular matrix lesions. The FSE technique is relatively insensitive to magnetic susceptibility artifacts, which is advantageous in patients who have undergone previous surgery of the joint. FSE sequences are normally included in the clinical standard MR imaging protocol for the knee, as high-resolution images can be acquired in a relatively short scan time [12, 13, 23]. Apart from the usual 2D FSE imaging, a 3D FSE sequence has also been developed and is available if subsequent reconstructions or semiquantitative assessments are desired [24].

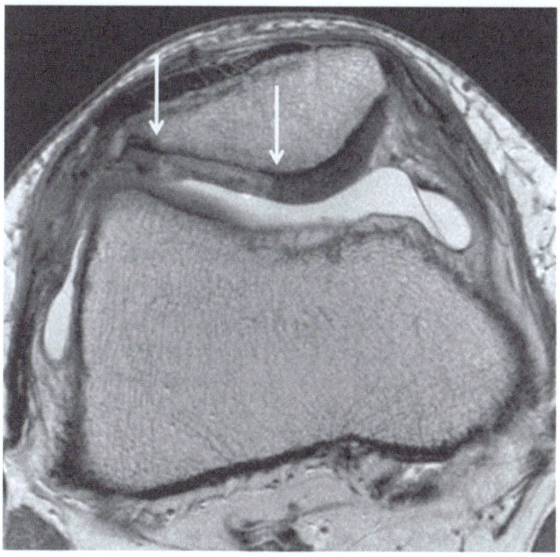

Fig. 14.1 Conventional axial proton-density-weighted (PDW) high-resolution turbo-spin-echo (TSE) MRI of a 30-year-old female patient at early follow-up of 3 months after matrix-associated chondrocyte transplantation. The arrows show inhomogeneous MR signal intensity of the repair tissue matrix. (Acquisition parameters: TR: 2400 ms; TE: 28 ms; flip angle: 160°; in-plane resolution: 0.23 × 0.23 mm; matrix: 512 × 512; slice thickness: 2 mm; slices: 34; TA: 6:01 min)

14.2.1.2 Three-Dimensional Gradient Echo Technique

Three-dimensional spoiled GRE imaging with fs or water excitation is widely available and easy to perform. This technique yield images with higher resolution and contrast-to-noise ratio (CNR) than 2D acquisitions. Contrary to other cartilage imaging techniques, 3D-GRE does not require data post-processing and avoids misregistration artifacts [9, 11, 13, 14, 16]. It exhibits a relatively high signal intensity (bright) articular cartilage in contrast to low signal intensity (dark) adjacent fat-suppressed tissue. The 3D dataset can subsequently be reformatted in any other plane for further 3D visualization and volume measurements [10, 11, 16]. However, GRE sequences are especially prone to susceptibility artifacts caused by metal abrasion which may hamper accurate cartilage evaluation in patients who have undergone arthroscopy.

14.2.1.3 Isotropic Imaging

Isotropic imaging requires 3D acquisitions of voxels with uniform length in any dimension. This isotropic dataset allows the sequence to be performed in one plane, for example, in the sagittal plane; and subsequently, it can be reformatted in all other planes, even oblique planes, without any loss of resolution. Many isotropic 3D gradient echo sequences, such as dual echo steady state (DESS), true fast imaging with steady-state precession (True-FISP), fast low angle shot (FLASH), balanced fast field echo (Balanced

FFE), volumetric interpolated breath-hold examination (VIBE), and multiple echo data image combination (MEDIC), have been developed. A voxel size down to 0.5 cm for 1.5 T with a high gradient strength has great potential for cartilage imaging.

The 3D DESS sequence has proved to be valuable for first-stage cartilage assessment [25–27]. This sequence provides an intermediate cartilage signal intensity, high cartilage-to-fluid contrast, and is suitable for quantitative volumetric measurements [28, 29]. The 3D-True-FISP sequence provides substantially higher signal-to-noise ratio (SNR) and contrast-to-noise ratio (CNR) than the 3D-FLASH sequence [30]. This advantage in signal intensity allows for higher spatial resolution and, thus, potential improvement in the accuracy of the segmentation process, especially at the articular surface [30]. With high-field MRI, this advantage might also be used to perform isotropic MR measurements in a minimal amount of time (Fig. 14.2). With the use of a dedicated, eight-channel knee coil, an isotropic (0.6 mm^3), 3D-True-FISP dataset can be assessed in approximately 3 min. The potential of 3D-True-FISP to diagnose cartilage defects and other knee soft tissue aberrations (such as anterior cruciate ligament (ACL) abnormalities and meniscal tears) can be expected to be higher than with a set of standard 2D sequences [31].

Another exciting 3D FSE sequence development is the "3D sampling perfection with application of optimized contrasts using different flip angle evolution" sequence (3D SPACE), which features isotropic voxels and consecutive reformatting in any plane without loss of resolution, and the advantages of the FSE approach (Fig. 14.3). Steady-state free precession (SSFP)-based techniques have increased SNR and CNR efficiency at 3 T MRI [32]. The True-FISP sequence, an SSFP-based sequence, was studied in detail at 1.5 T and is clinically available for morphological evaluation of cartilage [31, 33]. Compared to a 3D-FLASH and a 3D-DESS sequence, the preoperative detection of cartilage defects is possible with similar sensitivity, specificity, and accuracy for the water-excitation True-FISP sequence; however, the SSFP-based sequences show the highest SNR and CNR efficiency.

14.2.2 Quantitative Morphological Magnetic Resonance Imaging

Quantitative morphological cartilage parameters (e.g., cartilage thickness) provide more specific information and are less observer-dependent when compared to a qualitative approach. Given sufficient refinement, they may act as markers for the prediction of disease onset, progression of cartilage degeneration, or monitoring of therapeutic interventions. Quantitative morphological parameters encompass, for example, the volume of cartilage, the total area of subchondral bone,

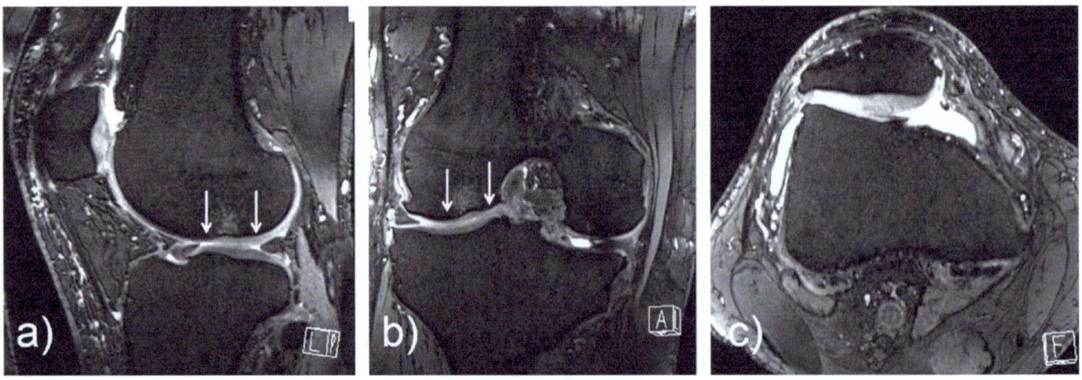

Fig. 14.2 MR images of the lateral femoral condyle of a 48-year-old male patient obtained with a 3D True FISP sequence 24 months after matrix-associated chondrocyte transplantation. Image acquisition was performed in the sagittal plane (**a**) and reconstructed in the coronal (**b**) as well as in the transversal (**c**) plane. (Acquisition parameters: TR: 8.9 ms; TE: 3.8 ms; in-plane-resolution: 0.4 × 0.4 mm; slice thickness: 0.4 mm; slices: 320; TA: 6:46 min)

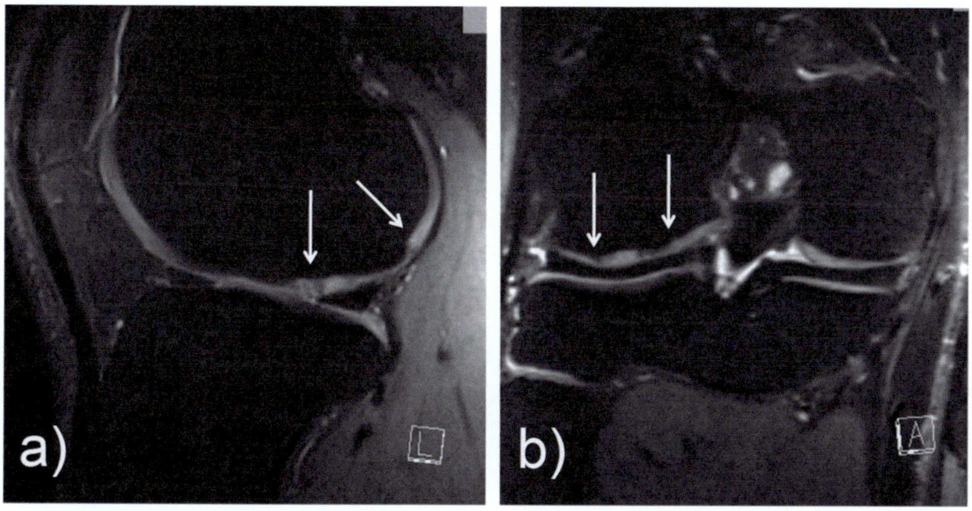

Fig. 14.3 Sagittal (**a**) and coronal (**b**) MR images acquired with a 3D-SPACE of the femoral condyle of a patient were obtained 36 months after microfracture therapy. Inhomogeneous cartilage repair tissue can be appreciated (arrows). (Acquisition parameters: TR: 1500 ms; TE: 34 ms; Resolution: 0.5 × 0.5 × 0.5 mm; slices: 192; TA: 7:53 min)

and the denuded part thereof, ratios between the aforementioned measures, and many others [34]. Clinical utility of MR pulse sequences for accurate and precise quantitative analysis of cartilage morphology in cross-sectional and longitudinal studies involving healthy subjects and OA patients has been reported [35]. Using quantitative MRI technique, the investigators examined the 4-year trajectory of femoro-tibial cartilage thickness loss (measured annually, longitudinal data) in OA patients prior to knee replacement and compared the data with that of matched controls by age, sex, and baseline radiographic stage. Accelerated cartilage loss, in particular the 2 years prior to knee replacement in OA patients compared to control subjects, was reported [35]. Other authors have investigated the possibility of quantifying bone marrow lesion volume, as well as denuded bone area, and have shown an association with the Boston Leeds Osteoarthritis Knee Score (BLOKS) [36, 37]. In a phase III clinical trial, cartilage volume loss and bone marrow lesions were used to demonstrate a beneficial effect of strontium ranelate on structural alterations in patients with symptomatic OA [38].

However, to achieve a qualified and validated imaging biomarker, many preconditions need to be fulfilled as follows:

First, the standardization in image acquisition must be ascertained. Different vendors of scanners, MR pulse sequences, and patient-specific factors contribute to a large variance in data, making it difficult to evaluate small changes in quantitative parameters. As an example, one study found that in a healthy population with a mean knee cartilage thickness of 3.8 mm, a change of 1 mm already puts an individual two standard deviations away from the mean indicating the necessity of accurate procedures to avoid losing a relevant change in the abovementioned variance [39]. A prominent project that provides a large body of standardized longitudinal data is the Osteoarthritis Initiative [40].

Second, the region or volume of interest needs to be defined. Semiquantitative scores, such as the Whole-organ Magnetic Resonance Imaging Score (WORMS) [41], suggest that knee compartments and subregions are relevant features to be evaluated. This is important, as different regions in the knee joint vary in morphological appearance [39], as well as exhibit different functional behavior [42] and dynamics in disease [43].

Third, the chosen volume of interest must be segmented. An accurate, automated approach would be preferable; however, the current consensus is that, although time-consuming, expert segmentation with the aid of segmentation assistance is superior to the purely computational variant [44].

Finally, the further development of quantitative MR imaging biomarkers can be described by three distinctive steps [45]. *Analytical validation* leads to the demonstration of the feasible, accurate, and precise measurement of a biomarker. *Qualification* of a biomarker means the demonstration of an association with a clinical outcome. *Utilization* involves an evaluation of the practicability in clinical routine. This includes its efficient (i.e., automatic) extraction, integration into existent radiology information systems, usefulness in decision-making, and cost-effectiveness.

14.2.3 High-Resolution Magnetic Resonance Imaging

Several studies on articular cartilage have tried to optimize MR pulse sequences for the assessment of articular cartilage by selecting imaging parameters that accentuate the CNR for cartilage. However, these studies did not focus on optimizing the image resolution. Fat-suppressed, 3D GRE imaging provides a high CNR between cartilage and surrounding tissue, and 3D acquisition produces smaller voxels by decreasing the slice thickness. Still, in all sequences, a trade-off has to be made between signal-to-noise ratio, voxel size, and acquisition time. By accepting longer scan times, an in-plane resolution of 0.27– 0.31 mm could be achieved at 3 T [42]. However, the image resolution of standard MR sequences reported in the literature is inadequate to reveal fraying of the articular cartilage surface or to discriminate the smooth surface of healthy cartilage from early superficial changes in degenerative cartilage [9, 11, 13, 14, 46, 47]. Thus, an increase in in-plane resolution is necessary to reliably depict changes in the integrity of the superficial zone of articular cartilage, which is critical in the assessment of early stage of cartilage degeneration in OA. In particular, the optimal definition of the morphology of cartilage repair following matrix-based autologous cartilage implantation (ACI) benefits from high-resolution MRI (Fig. 14.4). Indeed, the thin zonal layering of cartilage necessitates high-resolution MRI and, therefore, also the implementation of specialized technical equipment.

Previously, a 1.0 or 1.5 T MR scanner with a high-performance gradient system and a dedicated extremity coil (quadrature/phased array coil) were the minimum requirements. Then, the availability of 3 T clinical MR systems for routine examinations enabled high signal-to-noise ratios and high-resolution imaging, which was subsequently surpassed by 7 T scanners [48]. In 2003, the US Food and Drug Administration (FDA) approved field strengths lower than 8 T in adults as a "nonsignificant risk" [49], facilitating the use of 7 T scanners for certain routine clinical imaging indications, and thus, the next important step in achieving even higher resolutions in MRI (Fig. 14.5a, b). For the newest generation of 7 T scanners, an isotropic spatial resolution of 0.2 mm is expected. Analogous to the advancement from 1.5 T to 3 T, qualitative and quantitative cartilage imaging will continue to be the most important aspect of 7 T MR in musculoskeletal imaging. This statement is supported by a recent study which compared the diagnostic confidence of readers between 3 T and 7 T MRI of patellar cartilage and found a significant improvement in diagnostic confidence for low-grade cartilage lesions at 7 T [50].

The MRI SNR can be partially improved by the use of dedicated extremity coils with the optimal pulse sequence to increase resolution within a given imaging time [51]. In most cases, these coils act as receive coils that offer a high SNR, which allows the application of a small field of view (FOV) and a large matrix size, resulting in an increased in-plane resolution that can be achieved within a clinically acceptable scan time.

14.2.4 Magnetic Resonance Morphologic Imaging of Repair Tissue

Since the past two decades, there has been a significant progress in the field of cartilage repair procedures. Innovative surgical techniques are

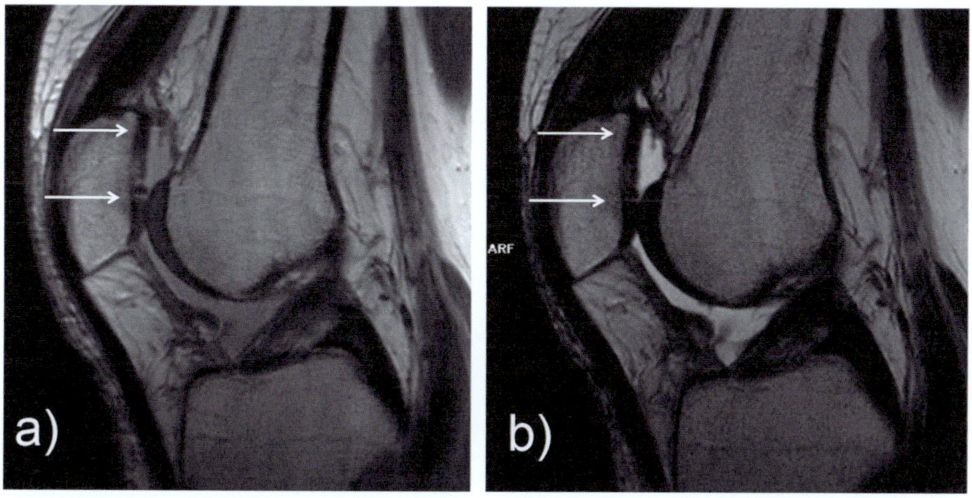

Fig. 14.4 Conventional high-resolution sagittal T2-weighted dual FSE MRI of the patello-femoral joint of a 30-year-old female patient (same patient as in Fig. 14.1) in an early follow-up three months after matrix-associated chondrocyte transplantation. (Acquisition parameters: TR: 5120 ms; TE: 9.5 ms (image **a**) and 124 ms (image **b**); flip angle: 160°; matrix size: 448 × 448; FOV: 18cm; slice thickness: 3mm; slices: 32; TA: 6:35 min). The depicted hyperintense or inhomogeneous cartilage repair tissue, and even the questionable split-like lesions of the repair tissue surface (arrows, **a**) usually disappear after 6–12 months (**b**)

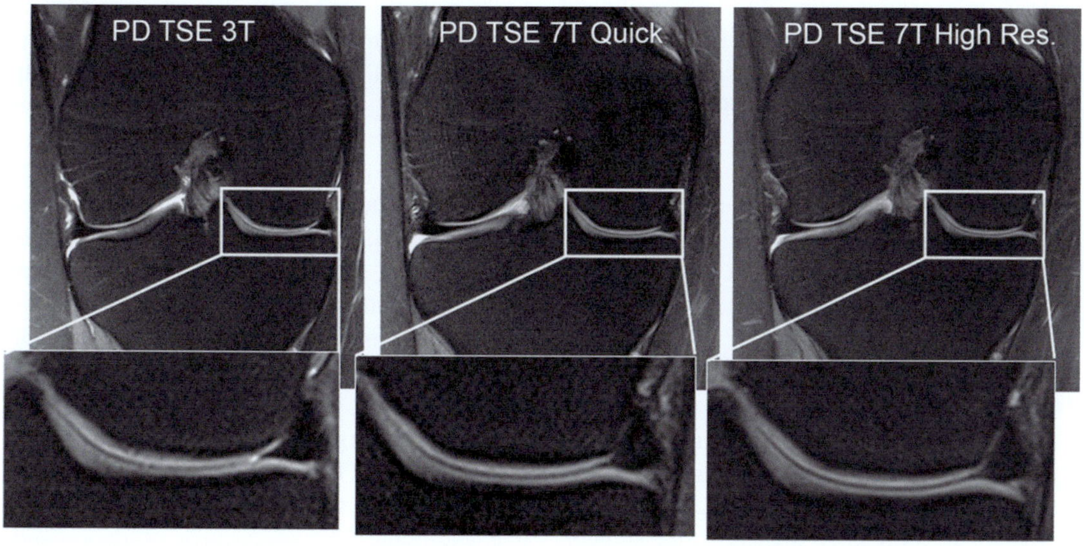

Fig. 14.5 Comparison of 3 T (left) and 7 T (middle and right) coronal MR images of the knee of a healthy volunteer acquired with a fat-saturated (fs) 2D proton-density turbo-spin-echo (PD TSE) sequence. The magnified picture detail of the medial knee compartment allows for better visualization of the image quality of the articular cartilage. The gain in SNR at 7T can be invested in faster acquisition (middle) or higher resolution at similar acquisition time (right). (Image obtained with permission from the Ref. [51])

currently available to treat patients with symptomatic, focal cartilage defect due to injury or disease. These surgical techniques include microfracture, OC auto- or allografting, matrix-induced autologous chondrocyte implantation (MACI), juvenile cartilage cell implantation, and non-cell-seeded biocompatible matrix implantation. To date, the choice of knee cartilage treatment is guided by patient age, goal, and expectations, the association of other joint tissue injuries, history of prior treatment, and the cartilage defect dimension (extent, size, and depth) and location. Although not routinely performed, arthroscopic biopsy is still considered the gold standard to assess cartilage repair tissue quality in cartilage repair. However, due to the associated morbidity of arthroscopy, MRI became the most widely used tool to assess the status of repair tissue. The radiologist must be aware of "normal" findings associated with these procedures, as well as "abnormal" findings, which may require short-term follow-up or therapeutic intervention.

Repair tissue morphology on MRI strongly depends on the surgical technique. Hence, concise clinical information from the referring physician is critical for a comprehensive and accurate radiological assessment. Generally, MR imaging of cartilage repair in the knee should be performed with dedicated extremity coils. While examinations during the clinical routine are usually performed on 1.5 T and 3 T systems, a considerable number of studies have already been carried out on 7 T systems. The higher SNR that is offered by high-field and ultrahigh-field MR is invested in faster acquisitions or higher spatial resolution which is crucial in cartilage imaging [50, 51]. Generally, an in-plane resolution of 0.3 mm or less is favored to enable an adequate and reliable display of the fraying of cartilage [19].

14.2.4.1 Marrow Stimulation

Post bone marrow stimulation surgical procedure, the repair tissue undergoes a gradual maturation process that is well reflected by MR morphology. Soon after microfracture surgery, the creation of tiny fractures in the underlying subchondral bone results in the development of a super-clot, which fills the defect region. This initial phase involving genesis of repair tissue appears hyperintense on T2W images compared to adjacent healthy cartilage. In this early phase, even differentiation from fluid can be challenging [52], which emphasizes the importance of additional clinical information for adequate radiological assessment. As the pluripotent bone marrow cells infiltrate to the defect site and differentiate, the repair tissue consolidates. Usually, the clot takes about 8–15 weeks to be replaced by fibrous-like tissue and about 4 months postsurgery to form fibrous or fibrocartilage repair tissue. Concomitantly, the MR signal intensity decreases continuously until it is similar to or even lower than that of healthy cartilage [53, 54]. The higher the fibrous component of the repair tissue, the lower the MR signal compared to the adjacent native articular cartilage. This maturation process should normally be completed after 1–2 years, with the repair tissue filling the former defect and developing an even surface. In the early postoperative phase, bone marrow edema is frequently observed but should gradually resolve over time. However, persistent bone marrow edema may be a sign of treatment failure [52, 53].

14.2.4.2 Osteochondral Autograft and Allograft Transfer

Osteochondral auto- and allograft transfers are valuable treatment alternatives to address cartilage injury [3]. In osteochondral autograft transplant (OAT), OC plugs are harvested from low-weight-bearing areas of the knee and transferred into the cartilage lesion site. Naturally, the size of treatable defects (usually up to 2.5 cm^2) is limited by the amount of available OC donor tissue [55]. In comparison, allograft procedure involve obtaining OC plugs from donor knee with the advantage that it does not create additional OC lesions at the donor site of the patients knee. Therefore, allograft procedure can also be used to cover larger cartilage defects. Regarding the radiological follow-up, the main difference between the two techniques relates to an imperative additional MR assessment of donor sites after osteochondral autograft.

MR Image analysis should include the evaluation of the number and size of the OC graft, the contour of the bone and cartilage interface, as well as an assessment of the MR signal of the graft, the donor site, and the adjacent bone marrow. Furthermore, contrast enhancement patterns and soft tissue abnormalities in the joint, such as joint effusion and synovitis, should be investigated. The OC grafts usually show solid, osseous incorporation between 6 and 14 weeks. Initially, postsurgical subchondral bone marrow edema is often present but is expected to resolve as the graft incorporates into the subchondral bone. Normal fatty marrow MR signal is seen within and around the plugs when solid bony incorporation occurs. Poor integration of the graft with the adjacent native tissue may be suggested by cystic cavities shown as fluid-like high MR signal intensity on T2W images and persistent edema-like high MR signal within the subchondral bone marrow.

Several investigators have extensively described the postsurgical MR findings of the OC graft and the adjacent native tissue [56–58]. From these studies, the following normal findings and possible complications post OC graft can be derived: *normal* MR findings associated with OC autograft procedure include bone marrow edema in and around the grafts, which was noted in more than 50% of the subjects within the first 12 months [56]. The bone marrow edema persisted for up to 3 years in a small number of patients. Also of note was joint effusion and synovitis, which sometimes persisted for more than 2 years. Incongruities at the bone-bone interface were frequently found, while incongruities at the cartilage-cartilage interface were uncommon findings. These frequently observed substantial incongruities of the bone-bone interface might seem pathological at first; however, they should not be considered a complication. It is rather an inherent side effect of the technique due to the fact that the plugs are harvested in areas where the cartilage thickness may differ from the implant site. Since the surgeon aims for a smooth articular surface, the bone-bone interface may often be incongruent.

Complications of OC grafting may include graft loosening or migration, incongruency of the cartilage-cartilage interface and gaps between OC plugs and adjacent native cartilage. Although partial or complete necrosis of the grafts was noted, these represented relatively rare findings. In the study by Link et al. [56], OATS procedure in the knee was performed in 45 patients with one or more OATS cylinder implanted in each patient. Second-look arthroscopies and MRI findings consistent with osteonecroses were detected in six OATS cylinders. The osteonecrotic graft cylinders did not lead to the collapse of the bone or pathological changes of the cartilage. Interestingly, only two of these cases were associated with clinical abnormalities. An explanation might be that cartilage derives its nutrition almost exclusively from the synovial membrane, thus rendering its viability less interconnected with changes of this nature.

14.2.4.3 Cell-Based Repair Techniques

Similar to bone marrow stimulation techniques, the repair tissue matures over time after ACI, and matrix-associated chondrocyte transplantation (MACT) procedures. The maturation of repair tissue is documented by a decrease in MR signal intensity on T2W images. Initially the repair tissue appears hyperintense, but, over time, it develops a comparable MR signal intensity to that of healthy cartilage reference [52, 59, 60]. In the early postoperative phase, subchondral bone marrow edema is a normal finding, which should, however, gradually resolve during follow-up. Persistent bone marrow edema after 1 year might be indicative of (pending) treatment failure [52]. Similarly, incomplete integration on the border zones, as seen by thin fissure-like hyperintensities, is commonly observed at early stages but should also eventually resolve. What should be considered to be a defective fill in the early postoperative stage depends on the applied method. While slight underfill can be anticipated for MACT, complete fill or even overfill is commonly observed after ACI. However, both techniques should foster complete fill within 1–2 years. Subsequent graft hypertrophy is particularly associated with the use of periosteal flaps and might necessitate surgical debridement in symptomatic cases. Delamination is also more commonly observed with a periosteal cover than with synthetic collagen [61]. Graft delamination is best appreciated on T2W images and is characterized by a linear hyperintense signal that extends between repair tissue and underlying subchondral bone [52]. In most cases, the subchondral lamina should remain intact after ACI and MACT surgery.

14.2.5 Semiquantitative Scoring Systems of Cartilage Repair Based on Morphological Magnetic Resonance Imaging

Semiquantitative scoring systems play an important role in the postoperative evaluation of cartilage repair, as they allow for a standardized, reproducible, and objective assessment of defined parameters. This provides a mean to compare the outcome between different cartilage repair procedures and also compare results obtained from different studies. In particular, the Magnetic Resonance Observation of Cartilage Repair Tissue (MOCART) scoring system, in its original 2D design and in the updated 3D version, has been widely applied in research since its introduction in 2004 (refer to Chap. 13 and Appendix C). To facilitate the best repair tissue outcome for comparison between studies, the MOCART scores should be obtained at set time intervals. However, particularly in the early postoperative phase, these intervals may depend on the applied cartilage repair surgical technique. Despite their extensive use in research, the MOCART scoring system has not yet been fully integrated into the daily clinical routine. Since it is reasonable to hypothesize that this way of standardized reporting might also improve patient care in the daily routine, the integration of MOCART scoring system is highly encouraged.

14.2.5.1 Magnetic Resonance Observation of Cartilage Repair Tissue

The original MOCART [62] assessed and scored [59] nine different variables: filling of the defect, integration with adjacent cartilage and bone, surface of the repair tissue, structure of the repair tissue, signal characteristics of the repair tissue, subchondral lamina at the repair site, subchondral bone at the repair site, the presence of adhesions, and synovitis. These variables were evaluated on the basis of several 2D sequences acquired with a circular polarized knee coil and a high-resolution sagittal dual FSE sequence acquired with a surface coil [62]. In the MOCART, zero to a hundred points may be reached, with zero representing the worst and one hundred the best radiological outcome possible [59]. The MOCART can be employed for the assessment of any type of cartilage repair technique and its versatility is evidenced by its extensive use in research in both cross-sectional and longitudinal studies [63].

14.2.5.2 Three-Dimensional Magnetic Resonance Observation of Cartilage Repair Tissue

Subsequently, high-resolution, isotropic 3D sequences were developed, which enabled isotropic image acquisitions with a voxel size down to 0.4 mm. Using multi-planar reconstruction, these data sets can be reconstructed in every plane without a loss of resolution. Welsch et al. used this new possibility to establish and introduce the 3D-MOCART, a variation of the original MOCART which is based on the acquisition of a single, isotropic 3D sequence [64]. For that purpose, the authors chose the 3D True-FISP, a gradient echo-based sequence. Taking advantage of the smaller slice thickness and the possibility of reformatting any desired image plane, the authors extended the score to a total of 11 variables. The 3D MOCART also assesses the three-dimensional position of the repair tissue and its borders with healthy cartilage reference in every plane. Furthermore, the authors introduced the possibility to denote the relative 3D position of some features. The nine variables that were assessed in the original 2D-MOCART showed good correlation with the 3D-MOCART [64]; however, there was a larger number of artifacts in the 3D-True-FISP compared to the 2D sequences. Subsequently, a different 3D sequence, the turbo spin echo-based 3D-SPACE, was evaluated for its usability in assessing the 3D-MOCART [65]. In this study, the 3D-SPACE sequence was compared to the 3D True-FISP, as well as the 2D sequences. The authors concluded that, although different 3D sequences may be used to determine the 3D-MOCART score, the 3D-SPACE yielded the best results. However, despite the creation of the 3D MOCART, the traditional MOCART based on 2D sequences is still widely used.

14.2.5.3 Cartilage Repair Osteoarthritis Knee Score

The MOCART scoring system allows for objective and reproducible assessment of repair tissue and its surrounding structures. However, it does not take into account the condition of other structures of the knee such as meniscus, ligament, tendon, etc. The condition of these structures might have a profound impact on the clinical presentation and outcome. In addition, their assessment is a prerequisite for an investigation of whether it is possible to delay or prevent OA development after cartilage injury. The Cartilage Repair OA Knee Score (CROAKS) [66] combines the features assessed in the MOCART with features from the Magnetic Resonance Imaging Osteoarthritis Knee Score (MOAKS) [67], with the goal of assessing not only the repair site but also the joint in its entirety, to foster a more holistic view. The CROAKS can be used for the assessment of all different types of repair procedures.

14.2.6 Summary of Magnetic Resonance Morphological Imaging of Cartilage Repair

Fast spin echo and GRE sequences are the cornerstone of knee MRI. For quantitative imaging, isotropic 3D-GRE sequences, such as 3D-FLASH or 3D-DESS, are utilized. Whereas morphological MRI for cartilage evaluation has focused on qualitative features thus far, a quantitative approach may yield even more information. For this purpose, standardization is important both during the acquisition of images (i.e., scanners, sequences, and patient-specific factors) and during the further processing of images (i.e., volume of interest identification, segmentation, and definition, extraction, and qualification of parameters).

For cartilage repair, high-resolution MRI provides an accurate, noninvasive evaluation of the repair site and provides the basis for the use of scoring systems, such as the MOCART score, which enables an evaluation of the development of the cartilage repair site over time and facilitates interindividual comparison. Particularly in patients after matrix-associated autologous chondrocyte transplantation, dynamic processes with biological cartilage repair can be observed over time. Thus, post cartilage repair surgical procedure, two follow-up MR examinations in the patient without clinical symptoms seem to be appropriate, the initial MR assessment after the first year and subsequently after the second year. Whenever clinical symptoms develop or a new trauma occurs, follow-up MR examination should be performed immediately.

14.3 Biochemical Magnetic Resonance Assessment of Cartilage Repair Tissue

To visualize the constitution of articular cartilage and cartilage repair tissue, a variety of different methodologies are available. These methodologies should depict either one or a combination of the different components of healthy hyaline articular cartilage. Chapter 1 describes in depth the structure, morphology, and composition of articular cartilage at the macro- and microlevel.

Articular cartilage is a complex, dense, specialized connective tissue that relies on the diffusion of solutes for its nutrition [68]. Responsible for the biomechanical properties of articular cartilage is the extracellular matrix, mainly composed of water (~75%), collagen (~20%), and proteoglycan aggregates (~5%) [68, 69]. Water either freely moves throughout the matrix or is bound to macromolecules. Collagen is largely represented by type II, which creates a stable network throughout the cartilage. Proteoglycans are composed of a central core protein with glycosaminoglycan (GAG) side chains which carry up to two anionic groups on its disaccharide units, which contribute to a negative charge of the cartilage matrix. As these ionic groups are fixed to the extracellular matrix components, they are referred to as *fixed charge*, and their distribution within the tissue is described as *fixed charge density (FCD)* [70–72]. This negative FCD attracts positive ions and water molecules, which strongly contribute to the unique mechanical properties of articular cartilage. Articular cartilage architecture is stratified primarily according to the orientation of collagen within a three-dimensional network [69, 73]. The superficial/tangential zone is characterized by flattened chondrocytes, relatively low quantities of proteoglycans, and high quantities of collagen fibrils arranged parallel to the articular surface. The middle/transitional zone has round chondrocytes, a high level of proteoglycans, and a random arrangement of collagen fibers. The deep/radial zone is characterized by low cell density, thick collagen fibrils that are perpendicular to the bone, and columns of chondrocytes. After the "tidemark," the underlying calcified cartilage layer is partly mineralized and acts as the transition zone between cartilage and the subchondral bone.

The structure and the components of healthy hyaline cartilage form the basis for the different biochemical MR methodologies and their use in the evaluation of articular cartilage in disease and repair. Many of these approaches have already been successfully applied for the assessment of cartilage repair. Depending on the different cartilage repair techniques, the cartilage repair tissue in histological studies has appeared to be hyaline-like cartilage, mixed hyaline-like and fibrocartilage, fibrocartilage or fibrous. Nevertheless, these histological studies show different results for these different cartilage repair procedures [74–81].

Since changes in GAG content generally take place before changes in collagen architecture occur, depiction of the ultrastructure of the repair tissue, using biochemical MRI, may be important not only to detect different stages of cartilage degeneration (GAG decrease) but also to detect different stages of cartilage repair (GAG increase). Negatively charged proteoglycans, composed of a central core protein with bound GAG chains, have been visualized by delayed gadolinium-enhanced MRI of cartilage (dGEMRIC) [82], sodium MR imaging [83, 84], and more recently, chemical exchange-dependent saturation transfer (CEST) [85, 86]. To date, only dGEMRIC was introduced into clinics for cartilage repair imaging; however, recently linear gadolinium contrast agents have been withdrawn from the market due to the deposition of gadolinium in the brain [87]. As such, based on the decision of the European Medical Agency, the clinical use of dGEMRIC is now severely restricted.

Although, also reflective of water content, the classic biochemical MR method that focuses on the collagen content and architecture of articular cartilage is transverse relaxation time (T2) mapping [86, 88, 89]. In addition to the T2 of articular cartilage, recently, T2* relaxation was shown to reflect collagen architecture and could be a promising tool for faster detection of tissue degeneration and repair tissue assessment within shorter acquisition times and higher resolutions [89–95]. Furthermore, magnetization transfer contrast (MTC) might also play a more important role in future cartilage imaging approaches. Another MR technique reported to reflect a combination of cartilage macromolecules, namely the proteoglycan [96] plus collagen content of articular cartilage [97], might be $T1\rho$ relaxometry.

14.3.1 T2 Relaxation Time Mapping

The T2 of articular cartilage is a sensitive parameter for the evaluation of changes in water and collagen content, as well as tissue anisotropy [88]. Cartilage T2 reflects the interaction of water and the extracellular matrix on a molecular level, with the collagen fiber orientation defining the layers of articular cartilage. The 3D organization and the "gothic" arch-like curvature of the collagen network, influenced by water mobility, the proteoglycan orientation, and the resulting magic angle at 55° (with respect to the static magnetic field), influence the appearance of T2 [73, 98]. In healthy articular cartilage, an increase in T2 values from deep to superficial cartilage layers can be observed, based on the anisotropy of collagen fibers running perpendicular to cortical bone in the deep layer of cartilage [99]. Latter orientation reduces the mobility of water protons with consecutive lower T2 relaxation times. Histologically validated animal studies have shown this zonal increase in T2 values to be a marker of hyaline or hyaline-like cartilage structure after cartilage repair procedures in the knee [100, 101]. To visu-

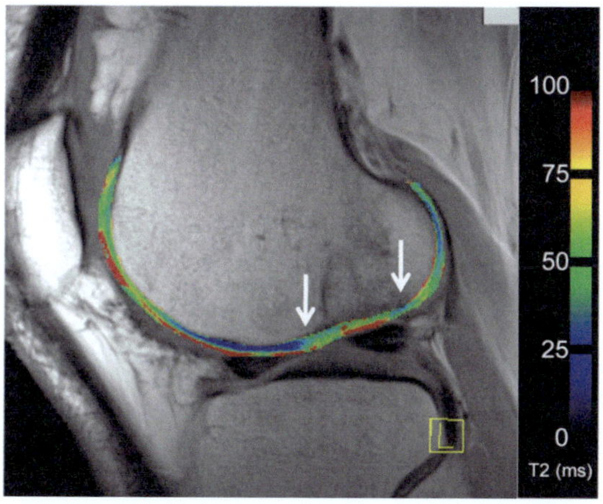

Fig. 14.6 Sagittal multi-echo spin-echo MR image with a color-coded T2 map overlay of the lateral femoral condyle of a 32-year-old male, 6 months after matrix-associated chondrocyte transplantation. Higher T2 values within the repair tissue (arrows) can be appreciated, when compared to the surrounding native articular cartilage. (Acquisition parameters: TR: 1650 ms; TE: 12.9, 25.8, 38.7, 51.6, 65.5, 77.4; flip angle 180°; matrix size: 384 × 384; FOV: 16 cm; slice thickness: 3 mm; slices: 6; TA: 5:37 min)

alize this zonal variation in vivo, high spatial resolution is essential, which can already be achieved at high-field MR, together with dedicated multichannel coils in clinical approaches [102] (Fig. 14.6). In addition, as shown in a comparison of T2 mapping at 3 T and 7 T, the SNR also benefits from the increased field strength [103]. As a result, with the appropriate technological setup, even in joints with thin cartilage layers such as the ankle, a zonal evaluation of cartilage is possible [102], and also the differences in cartilage T2 values of distinct anatomical regions, such as between the ankle and knee, can be quantified [104].

Recently, it has been observed that T2 mapping may provide valuable information about the development and progression of OA [105–108]. In a study with data from the OA Initiative, the authors found increased T2 values in knees, which progressed from a Kellgren-Lawrence (KL) score of 0 to a KL of 2 within 4 years compared to controls without progression [109]. Another study found a positive correlation between the ICRS grade of cartilage and increased T2 values next to the defect [110]. Further applications of T2 mapping may include the monitoring of cartilage alterations in the course of ACL injury and reconstruction, as higher T2 values prior to ACL reconstruction correlate positively with the clinical outcome 1-year postsurgery, according to the Knee Injury and OA Outcome Score [111]. In 2016, an initial randomized controlled trial used T2 values to evaluate the effects of a physical exercise intervention in early OA [112]; there was a decrease of T2 values after 4 months of aquatic training in postmenopausal women with early OA. This promising research must be further analyzed to determine the specific role of T2 as an absolute quantification parameter.

In cartilage repair tissue, global (bulk) T2 values, as well as line profiles, have shown an increase in the early postoperative follow-up, which might enable visualization of cartilage repair maturation [113]. Furthermore, another study has shown the ability of zonal T2 evaluation to differentiate cartilage repair tissue after microfracture (MFX) and MACT [27]. Whereas cartilage repair tissue after MFX, histologically seen as fibrocartilage, has shown no zonal T2 value increase from deep to superficial cartilage aspects in the mentioned study, repair tissue after MACT, histologically reported as hyaline-like, has shown a significant cartilage stratification.

The advance of ultrahigh magnetic field strengths enables the application of higher spatial resolution and, thus, an improvement in T2 mapping through better visualization of zonal variations in cartilage [103]. However, higher field strengths introduce disadvantages, such as a higher specific absorption rate (SAR) and B1 inhomogeneity. This affects common sequences for the derivation of T2 maps (e.g., Carr-Purcell-Meiboom-Gill or CPMG) and renders their application challenging. An alternative is to compensate for these issues by using single-echo spin echo (SE) sequences but with the disadvantage of an increase in acquisition time [114]. A possible solution is provided by the triple-echo steady-state (TESS) sequence [115] (Fig. 14.7). This new SSFP sequence acquires three echoes in one repetition time (TR) and has an inherent sta-

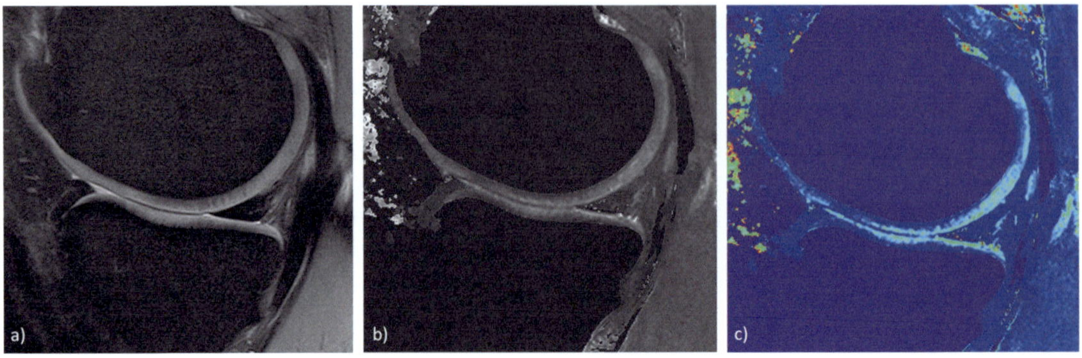

Fig. 14.7 Proton density-weighted 7 T MRI of the medial compartment femoro-tibial articular cartilage of a 26-year-old healthy male volunteer. Three cartilage layers can be seen from the bone-cartilage interface to the cartilage surface. The hypointense lines perpendicular to the bone seem to resemble the effects of the underlying collagenous architecture (**a**). T2-map calculated from a 3D triple-echo steady state (3D–TESS) sequence at 7 T (acquisition time = 1:48 min) from the same subject, where hyperintense voxels highlight the distribution of T2 values throughout the cartilage. Again, three layers can be differentiated (**b**). The same T2-map with different coloring scheme to better visualize the T2 value distribution within articular cartilage revealed brighter voxels having a higher T2 value (**c**)

bility against B1 inhomogeneity. In addition, due to low flip angles, TESS makes it easier to adhere to the SAR limit, thus further increasing the synergistic value of TESS and ultrahigh-field strengths. In total, the image acquisition can be accelerated by a factor of 4 to 5 compared to conventional multi-echo, multi-slice spin echo sequences (CPMG) used for T2 mapping [116, 117].

14.3.2 T2*(Star) Relaxation Time Mapping

Compared to T2 values, T2* additionally reflects very short transverse de-phasing effects caused by local field heterogeneities due to static magnetic field inhomogeneities, applied gradients, chemical shift, and magnetic susceptibility – at the macroscopic level, at the cartilage bone interface, or at the microscopic level within the cartilage ultrastructure [90, 118, 119]. Since SE sequences eliminate these de-phasing effects by applying refocusing pulses, T2* acquisition is exclusive to GRE sequences because refocusing is performed by magnetic gradients instead [118, 119]. Moreover, T2* relaxation is less influenced by stimulated echoes and magnetization transfer [120].

T2* maps are created similar to T2 maps: for each slice, several images are acquired with multi-echo sequence protocols at set echo times and are used to fit the signal levels to the corresponding echo time (TE) by applying a mono- or bi-exponential decay equation [121]. No special hardware components are needed for T2* mapping and further featured benefits are a biochemical approach with high-resolution 3D acquisition within short scan times [122]. Because the deep and calcified zone of articular cartilage consists of highly organized, dense collagen fibrils, sequences that are able to acquire short TEs provide more information and are more sensitive to pathological changes at this specific location [93, 118, 122]. With ultrashort TE (UTE) T2* mapping, acquisition of echo times on the order of 0.3 ms is possible. This allows the evaluation of higher organized tissues more sensitively, especially by omitting longer TEs that are related to cartilage bulk water content, underlining the potential ability and robustness of this method to improve the assessment of articular degeneration [91, 118, 123].

Due to its sensitivity to changes in collagen architecture, T2* mapping was investigated as another possible modality for cartilage repair tissue evaluation. Studies have demonstrated and histologically validated a decrease in T2* relax-

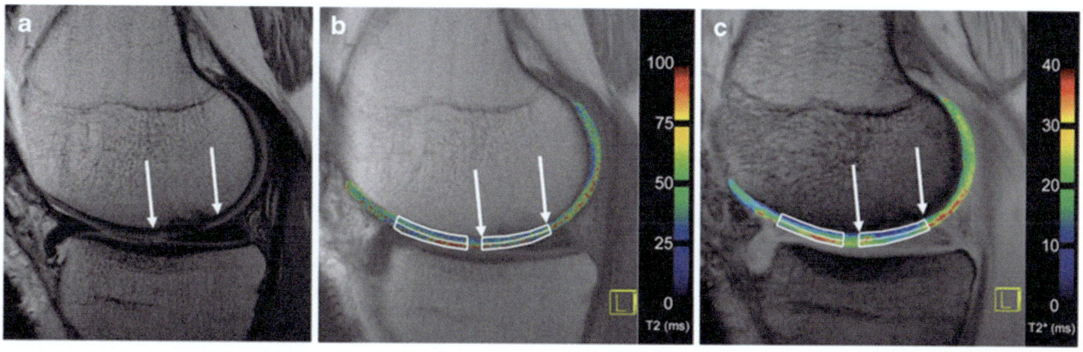

Fig. 14.8 MRI of the medial femoral condyle of a patient obtained at 60 months after matrix-associated chondrocyte transplantation. MR images were obtained using morphological proton density Turbo Spin Echo (PD-TSE) sequence (**a**), matched quantitative T2 map (**b**), and T2* (**c**) maps. Arrows mark the area of cartilage repair. The rectangular regions of interest (ROIs), considering a possible zonal variation, provided information on the mean (full-thickness) as well as the deep and superficial aspects of control native cartilage (left) and cartilage repair tissue (right, arrows). Zonal stratification is visible for both T2 and T2* images in most parts of the cartilage. A possible "magic angle" effect occurs within the posterior aspect of the femoral condyle. Lower T2* values and similar T2 values within the cartilage repair tissue are apparent, compared with the adjacent cartilage (These images are reproduced with permission from: Welsch et al. [125])

ation time measurements with increasing grades of cartilage degeneration and its sensitivity to mild and severe degradation [91, 94, 124]. In a retrospective study, the initial in vivo measurements in patients who previously underwent MACT were also successful at 2.5 years postsurgery in depicting similar global T2 and T2* values in the superficial and deep layer of healthy, native cartilage as well as repair tissue. Furthermore, a zonal stratification of signal intensity values, with values increasing from the depth to the surface, was shown for healthy cartilage, but not within the MACT repair tissue [90]. A prospective follow-up with examinations at 3, 6, 12, 24, 36/42, and 60 months post-MACT demonstrated comparable T2 values between repair tissue and healthy cartilage but lower T2* in repair tissue. The zonal differences in T2* values were also more pronounced compared to T2 (Fig. 14.8) [125]. Another study that evaluated MFX at 1.9 years after surgery found higher and positively correlated T2 and T2* values in healthy cartilage compared to repair tissue. Spatial variation from deep to more superficial layers was again demonstrated within healthy cartilage but not in MFX repair tissue [93].

Although these results suggest promising future applications for a faster isotropic, biochemical imaging modality, more studies need to be performed to create normative data and establish standardized acquisition protocols.

14.3.3 T1rho Magnetic Resonance Imaging

Relaxation time in the rotating frame (T1rho also called T1ρ) is a time constant with elements of both T1 and T2 weighting, and it characterizes magnetic relaxation of spins under the influence of a radiofrequency field that is parallel to the magnetization. The resulting contrast is sensitive to the low-frequency interactions between water molecules and their local macromolecular environment, such as collagen and GAGs. The amount of their respective macromolecular contribution, however, is still under discussion. Regatte et al. observed changes in T1ρ in cartilage plugs that were chemically or enzymatically depleted of GAG, but not in collagenase-treated tissue [126], suggesting a sensitivity to GAG content. However, Menezes et al. found no correlation between the cartilage $T_1\rho$ and GAG concentration [127]. In addition, it has been reported that the dominant T1ρ and T2 relaxation mechanism at B_0 (=static magnetic field) < 3 T is a dipolar interaction due to slow anisotropic motion of the water molecules in the collagen matrix [97]. This fits the observation that, similar to T2 measurements, T1ρ is also influenced by collagen orientation, as evidenced by the presence of the magic angle effect. These findings were reinforced by a study that compared T1ρ and dGEMRIC with histology and concluded that T1ρ is not suitable to accurately measure GAG content in vivo in OA patients [128]. However, even though T1ρ does not seem to reflect a specific macromolecular component of the extracellular matrix exclusively, it has been demonstrated to be a predictive marker for the development of morphologic lesions in articular cartilage [129]. T1ρ has also been used in addition to T2 relaxation time measurements to monitor repair tissue maturation after MFX and mosaicplasty by Holtzman et al. [130]. The authors concluded that T1ρ and T2 relaxation time measurements are complementary methods. A study investigating patients after MFX [131] noted a significant difference in both T1ρ and T2 between repair tissue and healthy reference cartilage after 3–6 months. At the 1-year follow-up, only T1ρ still demonstrated a significant difference. Based on these results, the authors concluded that T1ρ is also suited for the noninvasive evaluation of cartilage repair tissue.

14.3.4 Magnetization Transfer Contrast

The use of MTC imaging for articular cartilage was first described by Wolff et al. [132]. MT effects are based on the interaction of two different water pools, a free (unbound) bulk water pool, which is visible by MRI, and a bound water pool, with water molecules bound to macromolecules. The mobility of these bound water molecules is decreased to such an extent that, with standard MRI, protons of these water molecules do not provide a measureable MR signal. In certain tissues of the human body, such as the liver, thyroid, muscle, and cartilage, however, there is an interaction between the two pools: either chemical exchange or exchange of magnetization due to a dipolar interaction (so-called cross-relaxation). After saturation of bound water protons by off-resonance pulses, the magnetization of the free water pool is also affected, resulting in a reduction of the observable magnetization, which is reflected on MR image as reduced signal intensity. Thus, MT is tissue-specific and may provide a quantitative method for tissue characterization of basic macromolecular dynamics and chemistry [132–137]. Nevertheless, to date, MT has rarely been used for the quantitative in vivo evaluation of articular cartilage. However, one study demonstrated initial, and promising, results for cartilage repair [138]. Using a magnetization transfer-sensitized, SSFP MRI sequence introduced by Scheffler and Bieri [139], MTC was compared to T2 mapping for the assessment of global mean values, as well as for zonal variations of healthy, native articular cartilage and repair tissue after MACT and MFX [140]. Significant differences in global mean MT ratio (MTR) values were observed between sites of healthy cartilage and that of cartilage repair. The decrease in MTR was more pronounced in post-MFX repair tissue compared to post-MACT repair tissue. However, in contrast to T2 relaxation, MTC showed lower values for both MFX and MACT, whereas T2 showed lower values only for MFX, when the repair tissue was compared to surrounding healthy, native cartilage. Hence, both biochemical methods do not measure exactly the same properties of native cartilage and repair tissue. Considering the results of in vitro studies [141, 142], it seems that collagen concentration and collagen orientation may possibly play the most important role for both MTC and T2 relaxation. The latter, nevertheless, might also be influenced by hydration, to which MTC might be less sensitive.

When using these (and other) biochemical MR techniques in cartilage repair, one of the most important things is to either (i) use an area of healthy cartilage as an internal reference or (ii) perform longitudinal studies and compare the same subject at the same time of day. Furthermore, histologically validated studies might help to further clarify the impact of biochemical MR techniques in the visualization of cartilage ultrastructure and specific macromolecular components of articular cartilage.

14.3.5 Glycosaminoglycan Chemical Exchange Saturation Transfer

Glycosaminoglycan chemical exchange saturation transfer (gagCEST) is another promising technique for the noninvasive evaluation of glycosaminoglycan (GAG) content in articular cartilage in vivo [85]. GagCEST imaging exploits the fact that, in articular cartilage, labile protons from the OH groups of GAGs are in constant exchange with the protons of water molecules. Similar to MTC experiment, these labile protons on GAGs can be saturated using radiofrequency-selective saturation pulses. When these protons are then subsequently transferred to the bulk water pool by chemical exchange, they reduce the bulk water signal, which can, in turn, be measured. By applying this saturation over a longer period, saturated protons accumulate in the water pool, thus providing a significant contrast enhancement [143]. Due to the intricacy of the method, however, the quality of gagCEST maps is prone to error by a variety of factors, such as B0 and B1 inhomogeneities, motion artifacts, varying labeling efficiency, as well as insufficiently accurate definition of the z-spectra. In 2011, Schmitt et al. [144] investigated patients after MFX and MACT using gagCEST, at a mean follow-up time of 21 months, and compared the results to those reported with sodium imaging at 7 Tesla (Fig. 14.9) [144]. These investigators found lower asymmetric magnetization transfer ratio (MTR_{asym}) values in repair tissue than in healthy reference cartilage and observed a strong correlation between gagCEST and sodium imaging, indicative of the specificity of gagCEST for GAGs. GagCEST was also used to assess the outcome of autologous OC transplantation in nine patients after a mean follow-up of 7.9 years, along with sodium imaging at 7 T and T2-mapping at 3 T [145]. The clinical patient outcome was good, as demonstrated by a median, modified Lysholm score of 90. The strongest correlation was observed between gagCEST and sodium imaging ($\rho = 0.952$ with a 95% confidence interval of [0.753; 0.992]). However, only T2-mapping showed a correlation with the modified Lysholm score.

Due to rather long measurement times, patient motion is an important issue that should be addressed both mechanically, via good fixation and via post-processing, with registration tools [146]. Currently, the best results are obtained on ultrahigh-field systems [147] because of the

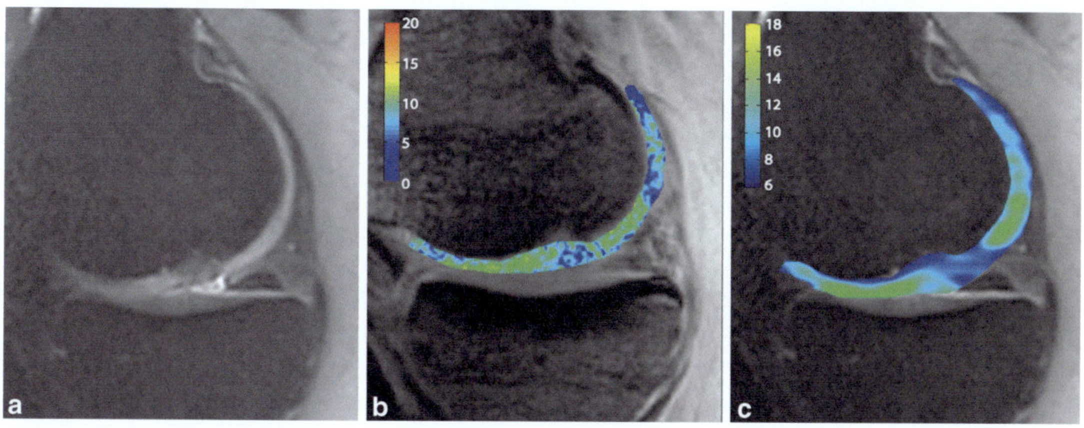

Fig. 14.9 A 30-year-old patient after microfracturing in the medial femoral condyle was examined using high-resolution (**a**) morphological, (**b**) gagCEST, and (**c**) 23Na MR imaging. Color bars on (**b**) and (**c**) represent MTR asym values summed over offsets from 0 to 1.3 ppm (gagCEST) and sodium SNRs, respectively. Both techniques show decreased signal intensity in repair tissue compared with surrounding native tissue (With permission from Ref. [144])

higher signal-to-noise ratio and spectral resolution compared to routine 3 T systems [148]. Conversely, B_0 (static magnetic field) and B_1 (radiofrequency field strength) inhomogeneities, as well as SAR limitations, are more pronounced at ultrahigh fields. In particular, accurate B_0 correction has been shown to be crucial for accurate gagCEST measurements [147]. For that purpose, water saturation shift referencing (WASSR) [149] was introduced and was shown to further improve the quality of gagCEST maps [150]. Despite these challenges, gagCEST has valuable advantages. Unlike dGEMRIC, the gagCEST imaging does not require the administration of a contrast agent but rather employs the endogenous contrast provided by chemical exchange. In addition, gagCEST does not rely on special multinuclear hardware as does sodium imaging. Furthermore, gagCEST combines GAG specificity with favorable spatial resolution. However, additional refinement will be necessary to make this technique applicable for routine clinical assessment.

14.3.6 Delayed Gadolinium-Enhanced Magnetic Resonance Imaging

Glycosaminoglycans are important for the biochemical and biomechanical behavior of cartilage tissue. GAGs are the main source of fixed charge density in cartilage and are often decreased in the early stages of cartilage degeneration [151] or in cartilage repair tissue [152]. Intravenously administered gadolinium diethylenetriamine pentaacetate anion ($Gd\text{-}DTPA^{2-}$) penetrates the cartilage through both the articular surface and the subchondral bone. The contrast equilibrates in inverse relation to the FCD, which is, in turn, directly related to the GAG concentration. Therefore, T1, which correlates inversely with the $Gd\text{-}DTPA^{2-}$ concentration, becomes a specific measure of tissue GAG concentration, suggesting that $Gd\text{-}DTPA^{2}$-enhanced MRI has the potential to monitor the GAG content of cartilage in vivo [153]. Thus, T1 mapping, enhanced by delayed administration of $Gd\text{-}DTPA^{2-}$ (T1 dGEMRIC), was considered the most widely used methodology to detect proteoglycan depletion in articular cartilage (especially in the knee) and has shown promising results [154, 155]. However, there are several drawbacks that hamper the clinical applicability of dGEMRIC due to a costly protocol in terms of time. Further, there are risks in the form of nephrogenic systemic fibrosis, as well as the not-yet-completely-understood retention of gadolinium deposits in tissue [156]. Considering the necessary double dose of $Gd\text{-}DTPA^{2-}$ for dGEMRIC [82], special caution is warranted.

As differences in pre-contrast values between repair tissue and normal hyaline cartilage are larger compared to early cartilage degeneration, the pre-contrast T1 values must be calculated in cartilage repair tissue as well [152]. The concentration of GAG is represented by delta $\Delta R1$, i.e., the difference in relaxation rate ($R1 = 1/T1$) between $T1_{precontrast}$ and $T1_{postcontrast.}$ Thus, the sequence must be performed twice, for pre-contrast and delayed post-contrast T1 mapping. This increases the total scan time and requires a break between the two MR scans, in which the contrast agent must be administered. A delay of at least 90 min after injection is then required for penetration of the contrast agent into the cartilage. Scan time reduction, compared to the standard inversion recovery (IR) evaluation, has been achieved with a different approach using fast T1 mapping [157]. Although the 90-min delay is still required, this might increase the clinical applicability of the dGEMRIC technique.

Using dGEMRIC, one study was able to differentiate between different postsurgical technique repair tissues with higher delta $\Delta R1$ values, and thus, lower GAG content, in cartilage repair tissue after MFX, compared to MACT [158]. Furthermore, dGEMRIC may help to determine alterations associated with the development of OA, both in hip dysplasia and femoroacetabular impingement [159, 160], as well as in the longitudinal evaluation of knee cartilage [161, 162]. The applicability of this technique has also been shown in regions other than the knee and hip joint [163–165].

14.3.7 Sodium Magnetic Resonance Imaging

In articular cartilage, positive sodium ions are the naturally distributed counterions to the negative fixed charged density, which is mainly caused by negatively charged side chains of GAGs. This direct proportionality allows indirect estimation of the concentrations and distributions of GAGs in articular cartilage through the assessment of relative sodium concentrations [166–169]. Although sodium (^{23}Na) is the second best detectable nucleus in living systems, sodium imaging is challenging due to short T2 relaxation times and the significantly lower concentration of sodium as compared to water protons in articular cartilage. These properties result in low intrinsic SNR, which makes sodium MRI a technically challenging, especially in a clinical environment with limited scan times [170–174]. These challenges were addressed with the development and introduction of dedicated coils and new sequences that made sodium measurements more feasible, even in a clinical setting [174]. Moreover, it was reported that sodium imaging is comparable to T2 mapping with regard to repeatability and, in addition, might provide sufficient sensitivity for the in vivo evaluation of OA [175]. However, compared to proton imaging, sodium imaging is still limited by resolutions between 2–4 mm and longer scan times (15–30 min), the requirement for special hardware with a multinuclear setup, the need for dedicated coils – as well as favorable 3D sequences with very short TEs – and, especially, by the need for higher field strengths (3 T or, better, 7 T) [176, 177].

Since GAG depletion precedes collagen deterioration and the resultant gross morphological damage, one of the great potentials sodium imaging carries is its ability to detect pathological changes early, before they become visible on morphological MR images [178–180]. Early clinical trials for OA evaluation concluded that sodium imaging may be useful for diagnosing and monitoring early changes in the GAG content of OA cartilage [181, 182]. As partial volume effects play an important role because of the previously mentioned limited resolutions, the sodium signal may be contaminated by synovial fluid or joint effusion [182]. With further technical refinements, such as IR preparation-based fluid suppression, it was possible to report that sodium was a reliable and reproducible biomarker for the prediction of OA [183, 184]. The sensitivity of this method was demonstrated in a clinical trial on patients suffering from type 1 diabetes mellitus (DM1) without any pathological findings based on clinical examination or morphological MR imaging in the knee. Sodium imaging, however, already revealed slight biochemical changes in articular cartilage composition in these DM1 patients compared to healthy volunteers [185].

The first sodium imaging studies on characteristics of repair tissue demonstrated the ability of this technique to successfully discriminate repair tissue from native cartilage after MACT or MFX surgical techniques for treatment cartilage repair. Furthermore, high correlations of these particular findings to dGEMRIC, as well as to gagCEST values, were also shown (see also Fig. 14.9) [144, 186]. Based on these results, the assessment of the value of sodium imaging in evaluating the quality of repair tissue in bone marrow stimulation (BMS) and MACT was performed. Although the morphological appearance of the repair tissue evaluated by the MOCART score showed no significant difference, higher sodium MR signal intensities, indicative of higher GAG concentration, and thus a higher quality of repair tissue were observed in patients who underwent MACT. This suggests that sodium MRI could be used not only as a marker for postsurgical follow-up but also as a possible noninvasive method for performance evaluation of new cartilage repair surgical techniques, at least in the knee [187].

Overall, sodium imaging is a promising, reproducible, and sensitive approach for the noninvasive assessment of cartilage composition. However, in order to confirm the clinical feasibility, hardware and software optimization must be performed to ameliorate current limitations, such as limited spatial resolution, relatively long scan times, and restriction to higher field strengths.

14.4 Conclusions

Magnetic resonance imaging has made tremendous advances over the last several years and has matured into the most commonly used noninvasive tool for the assessment of cartilage injury, degeneration, and repair. Both morphological imaging (with the use of semiquantitative scores or volumetric measurements) and biochemical imaging can provide quantitative, reproducible data. These data have been shown to have the potential for the early diagnosis of degeneration and injury, as well as for treatment monitoring. Thus, both morphological and biochemical imaging form one of the cornerstones in the current attempts aimed at the success of surgical cartilage repair techniques and improving OA therapy.

References

1. Curl WW, Krome J, Gordon ES, Rushing J, Smith BP, Poehling GG. Cartilage injuries: a review of 31,516 knee arthroscopies. Arthroscopy. 1997;13(4):456–60.
2. Buckwalter JA, Mankin HJ. Articular cartilage .2. Degeneration and osteoarthrosis, repair, regeneration, and transplantation. J Bone Joint Surg Am. 1997;79A(4):612–32.
3. Hunziker EB, Lippuner K, Keel MJ, Shintani N. An educational review of cartilage repair: precepts & practice–myths & misconceptions–progress & prospects. Osteoarthritis Cartilage. 2015;23(3):334–50.
4. Buckwalter JA. Evaluating methods of restoring cartilaginous articular surfaces. Clin Orthop Relat Res. 1999;367:S224–S38.
5. Roberts S, McCall IW, Darby AJ, Menage J, Evans H, Harrison PE, et al. Autologous chondrocyte implantation for cartilage repair: monitoring its success by magnetic resonance imaging and histology. Arthritis Res Ther. 2003;5(1):R60–73.
6. Gersoff WK. Considerations prior to surgical repair of articular cartilage injuries of the knee. Oper Tech Sports Med. 2000;8(2):86–9.
7. Alparslan L, Minas T, Winalski CS. Magnetic resonance imaging of autologous chondrocyte implantation. Semin Ultrasound CT MR. 2001;22(4):341–51.
8. Winalski CS, Minas T. Evaluation of chondral injuries by magnetic resonance imaging: repair assessments. Oper Tech Sports Med. 2000;8(2):108–19.
9. Peterfy CG, Majumdar S, Lang P, Vandijke CF, Sack K, Genant HK. Mr-imaging of the arthritic knee – improved discrimination of cartilage, synovium, and effusion with pulsed saturation-transfer and fat-suppressed T1-weighted sequences. Radiology. 1994;191(2):413–9.
10. Peterfy CG, Vandijke CF, Lu Y, Nguyen A, Connick TJ, Kneeland JB, et al. Quantification of the volume of articular-cartilage in the metacarpophalangeal joints of the hand – accuracy and precision of 3-dimensional Mr-imaging. Am J Roentgenol. 1995;165(2):371–5.
11. Disler DG, McCauley TR, Kelman CG, Fuchs MD, Ratner LM, Wirth CR, et al. Fat-suppressed three-dimensional spoiled gradient-echo MR imaging of hyaline cartilage defects in the knee: comparison with standard MR imaging and arthroscopy. Am J Roentgenol. 1996;167(1):127–32.
12. Potter HG, Linklater JM, Allen AA, Hannafin JA, Haas SB. Magnetic resonance imaging of articular cartilage in the knee – an evaluation with use of fast-spin-echo imaging. J Bone Joint Surg Am. 1998;80A(9):1276–84.
13. Kawahara Y, Uetani M, Nakahara N, Doiguchi Y, Nishiguchi M, Futagawa S, et al. Fast spin-echo MR of the articular cartilage in the osteoarthrotic knee – correlation of MR and arthroscopic findings. Acta Radiol. 1998;39(2):120–5.
14. Trattnig S, Huber M, Breitenseher MJ, Trnka HJ, Rand T, Kaider A, et al. Imaging articular cartilage defects with 3D fat-suppressed echo planar imaging: comparison with conventional 3D fat-suppressed gradient echo sequence and correlation with histology. J Comput Assist Tomogr. 1998;22(1):8–14.
15. Recht M, Bobic V, Burstein D, Disler D, Gold G, Gray M, et al. Magnetic resonance imaging of articular cartilage. Clin Orthop Relat Res. 2001;391:S379–S96.
16. Recht MP, Piraino DW, Paletta GA, Schils JP, Belhobek GH. Accuracy of fat-suppressed three-dimensional spoiled gradient-echo FLASH MR imaging in the detection of patellofemoral articular cartilage abnormalities. Radiology. 1996;198(1):209–12.
17. Roemer FW, Kwoh CK, Hannon MJ, Crema MD, Moore CE, Jakicic JM, et al. Semiquantitative assessment of focal cartilage damage at 3T MRI: a comparative study of dual echo at steady state (DESS) and intermediate-weighted (IW) fat suppressed fast spin echo sequences. Eur J Radiol. 2011;80(2):e126–31.
18. Mohr A. The value of water-excitation 3D FLASH and fat-saturated PDw TSE MR imaging for detecting and grading articular cartilage lesions of the knee. Skeletal Radiol. 2003;32(7):396–402.
19. Rubenstein JD, Li JG, Majumdar S, Henkelman RM. Image resolution and signal-to-noise ratio requirements for MR imaging of degenerative cartilage. AJR Am J Roentgenol. 1997;169(4):1089–96.
20. Notohamiprodjo M, Horng A, Pietschmann MF, Muller PE, Horger W, Park J, et al. MRI of the knee at 3T: first clinical results with an isotropic PDfs-weighted 3D-TSE-sequence. Invest Radiol. 2009;44(9):585–97.
21. Constable RT, Anderson AW, Zhong J, Gore JC. Factors influencing contrast in fast spin-Echo Mr imaging. Magn Reson Imaging. 1992;10(4):497–511.

22. Yao L, Gentili A, Thomas A. Incidental magnetization transfer contrast in fast spin-echo imaging of cartilage. J Magn Reson Imaging. 1996;6(1):180–4.
23. Bredella MA, Tirman PFJ, Peterfy CG, Zarlingo M, Feller JF, Bost FW, et al. Accuracy of T2-weighted fast spin-echo MR imaging with fat saturation in detecting cartilage defects in the knee: comparison with arthroscopy in 130 patients. Am J Roentgenol. 1999;172(4):1073–80.
24. Lichy MP, Wietek BM, Mugler JP 3rd, Horger W, Menzel MI, Anastasiadis A, et al. Magnetic resonance imaging of the body trunk using a single-slab, 3-dimensional, T2-weighted turbo-spin-echo sequence with high sampling efficiency (SPACE) for high spatial resolution imaging: initial clinical experiences. Invest Radiol. 2005;40(12):754–60.
25. Hardy PA, Recht MP, Piraino D, Thomasson D. Optimization of a dual echo in the steady state (DESS) free-precession sequence for imaging cartilage. J Magn Reson Imaging. 1996;6(2):329–35.
26. Domayer SE, Kutscha-Lissberg F, Welsch G, Dorotka R, Nehrer S, Gabler C, et al. T2 mapping in the knee after microfracture at 3.0 T: correlation of global T2 values and clinical outcome - preliminary results. Osteoarthritis Cartilage. 2008;16(8):903–8.
27. Welsch GH, Mamisch TC, Domayer SE, Dorotka R, Kutscha-Lissberg F, Marlovits S, et al. Cartilage T2 assessment at 3-T MR imaging: in vivo differentiation of normal hyaline cartilage from reparative tissue after two cartilage repair procedures – initial experience. Radiology. 2008;247(1):154–61.
28. Eckstein F, Hudelmaier M, Wirth W, Kiefer B, Jackson R, Yu J, et al. Double echo steady state magnetic resonance imaging of knee articular cartilage at 3 tesla: a pilot study for the osteoarthritis initiative. Ann Rheum Dis. 2006;65(4):433–41.
29. Moriya S, Miki Y, Kanagaki M, Matsuno Y, Miyati T. 90 degrees -flip-angle three-dimensional double-echo steady-state (3D-DESS) magnetic resonance imaging of the knee: isovoxel cartilage imaging at 3T. Eur J Radiol. 2014;83(8):1429–32.
30. Weckbach S, Mendlik T, Horger W, Wagner S, Reiser MF, Glaser C. Quantitative assessment of patellar cartilage volume and thickness at 3.0 tesla comparing a 3D-fast low angle shot versus a 3D-true fast imaging with steady-state precession sequence for reproducibility. Invest Radiol. 2006;41(2):189–97.
31. Duc SR, Pfirrmann CWA, Koch PP, Zanetti M, Hodler J. Internal knee derangement assessed with 3-minute three-dimensional isovoxel true FISP MR sequence: preliminary study. Radiology. 2008;246(2):526–35.
32. Kornaat PR, Reeder SB, Koo S, Brittain JH, Yu H, Andriacchi TP, et al. MR imaging of articular cartilage at 1.5T and 3.0T: comparison of SPGR and SSFP sequences. Osteoarthritis Cartilage. 2005;13(4):338–44.
33. Duc SR, Koch P, Schmid MR, Horger W, Hodler J, Pfirrmann CWA. Diagnosis of articular cartilage abnormalities of the knee: prospective clinical evaluation of a 3D water-excitation true FISP sequence. Radiology. 2007;243(2):475–82.
34. Eckstein F, Wirth W. Quantitative cartilage imaging in knee osteoarthritis. Arthritis. 2011;2011:475684.
35. Eckstein F, Boudreau RM, Wang Z, Hannon MJ, Wirth W, Cotofana S, et al. Trajectory of cartilage loss within 4 years of knee replacement--a nested case-control study from the osteoarthritis initiative. Osteoarthritis Cartilage. 2014;22(10):1542–9.
36. Hunter DJ, Lo GH, Gale D, Grainger AJ, Guermazi A, Conaghan PG. The reliability of a new scoring system for knee osteoarthritis MRI and the validity of bone marrow lesion assessment: BLOKS (Boston Leeds osteoarthritis knee score). Ann Rheum Dis. 2008;67(2):206–11.
37. Pang J, Driban JB, Destenaves G, Miller E, Lo GH, Ward RJ, et al. Quantification of bone marrow lesion volume and volume change using semi-automated segmentation: data from the osteoarthritis initiative. BMC Musculoskelet Disord. 2013;14:3.
38. Pelletier JP, Roubille C, Raynauld JP, Abram F, Dorais M, Delorme P, et al. Disease-modifying effect of strontium ranelate in a subset of patients from the phase III knee osteoarthritis study SEKOIA using quantitative MRI: reduction in bone marrow lesions protects against cartilage loss. Ann Rheum Dis. 2015;74(2):422–9.
39. Eckstein F, Yang M, Guermazi A, Roemer FW, Hudelmaier M, Picha K, et al. Reference values and Z-scores for subregional femorotibial cartilage thickness–results from a large population-based sample (Framingham) and comparison with the non-exposed osteoarthritis initiative reference cohort. Osteoarthritis Cartilage. 2010;18(10):1275–83.
40. Sommer FG, Jeffrey RB Jr, Rubin GD, Napel S, Rimmer SA, Benford J, et al. Detection of ureteral calculi in patients with suspected renal colic: value of reformatted noncontrast helical CT. AJR Am J Roentgenol. 1995;165(3):509–13. Epub 1995/09/01.
41. Peterfy CG, Guermazi A, Zaim S, Tirman PF, Miaux Y, White D, et al. Whole-Organ Magnetic Resonance Imaging Score (WORMS) of the knee in osteoarthritis. Osteoarthritis Cartilage. 2004;12(3):177–90.
42. Horng A, Raya JG, Stockinger M, Notohamiprodjo M, Pietschmann M, Hoehne-Hueckstaedt U, et al. Topographic deformation patterns of knee cartilage after exercises with high knee flexion: an in vivo 3D MRI study using voxel-based analysis at 3T. Eur Radiol. 2015;25(6):1731–41.
43. Frobell RB, Nevitt MC, Hudelmaier M, Wirth W, Wyman BT, Benichou O, et al. Femorotibial subchondral bone area and regional cartilage thickness: a cross-sectional description in healthy reference cases and various radiographic stages of osteoarthritis in 1,003 knees from the osteoarthritis initiative. Arthritis Care Res (Hoboken). 2010;62(11):1612–23.
44. Eckstein F, Cicuttini F, Raynauld JP, Waterton JC, Peterfy C. Magnetic resonance imaging (MRI) of articular cartilage in knee osteoarthritis (OA): mor-

phological assessment. Osteoarthritis Cartilage. 2006;14(Suppl A):A46–75.
45. Micheel CM, Ball JR, editors. Evaluation of biomarkers and surrogate endpoints in chronic disease. Washington, DC: National Academies Press; 2010.
46. Rubenstein JD, Li JG, Majumdar S, Henkelman RM. Image resolution and signal-to-noise ratio requirements for MR imaging of degenerative cartilage. Am J Roentgenol. 1997;169(4):1089–96.
47. Gagliardi JA, Chung EM, Chandnani VP, Kesling KL, Christensen KP, Null RN, et al. Detection and staging of chondromalacia patellae – relative efficacies of conventional Nir imaging, Mr arthrography, and Ct arthrography. Am J Roentgenol. 1994;163(3):629–36.
48. Juras V, Welsch G, Bar P, Kronnerwetter C, Fujita H, Trattnig S. Comparison of 3T and 7T MRI clinical sequences for ankle imaging. Eur J Radiol. 2012;81(8):1846–50.
49. Rubin GD, Napel S. Increased scan pitch for vascular and thoracic spiral CT. Radiology. 1995;197(1):316–7. Epub 1995/10/01.
50. Springer E, Bohndorf K, Juras V, Szomolanyi P, Zbyn S, Schreiner MM, Schmitt B and Trattnig S. Comparison of Routine Knee Magnetic Resonance Imaging at 3 T and 7 T. Invest Radiol. 2017;52:42–54.
51. Welsch GH, Juras V, Szomolanyi P, Mamisch TC, Baer P, Kronnerwetter C, et al. Magnetic resonance imaging of the knee at 3 and 7 tesla: a comparison using dedicated multi-channel coils and optimised 2D and 3D protocols. Eur Radiol. 2012;22(9):1852–9.
52. Alparslan L, Winalski CS, Boutin RD, Minas T. Postoperative magnetic resonance imaging of articular cartilage repair. Semin Musculoskelet Radiol. 2001;5(4):345–63.
53. Choi YS, Potter HG, Chun TJMR. Imaging of cartilage repair in the knee and ankle. Radiographics. 2008;28(4):1043–59.
54. Guermazi A, Roemer FW, Alizai H, Winalski CS, Welsch G, Brittberg M, et al. State of the art: MR imaging after knee cartilage repair surgery. Radiology. 2015;277(1):23–43.
55. Farr J, Cole B, Dhawan A, Kercher J, Sherman S. Clinical cartilage restoration: evolution and overview. Clin Orthop Relat Res. 2011;469(10):2696–705.
56. Link TM, Mischung J, Wortler K, Burkart A, Rummeny EJ, Imhoff AB. Normal and pathological MR findings in osteochondral autografts with longitudinal follow-up. Eur Radiol. 2006;16(1):88–96.
57. Sanders TG, Mentzer KD, Miller MD, Morrison WB, Campbell SE, Penrod BJ. Autogenous osteochondral "plug" transfer for the treatment of focal chondral defects: postoperative MR appearance with clinical correlation. Skelet Radiol. 2001;30(10):570–8.
58. Herber S, Runkel M, Pitton MB, Kalden P, Thelen M, Kreitner KF. Indirect MR-arthrography in the follow up of autologous osteochondral transplantation. Rofo. 2003;175(2):226–33. Indirekte MR-Arthrographie zur Verlaufskontrolle nach autologer osteochondraler Transplantation.
59. Trattnig S, Ba-Ssalamah A, Pinker K, Plank C, Vecsei V, Marlovits S. Matrix-based autologous chondrocyte implantation for cartilage repair: noninvasive monitoring by high-resolution magnetic resonance imaging. Magn Reson Imaging. 2005;23(7):779–87. Epub 2005/10/11.
60. Trattnig S, Pinker K, Krestan C, Plank C, Millington S, Marlovits S. Matrix-based autologous chondrocyte implantation for cartilage repair with HyalograftC: two-year follow-up by magnetic resonance imaging. Eur J Radiol. 2006;57(1):9–15. Epub 2005/09/27.
61. Trattnig S, Millington SA, Szomolanyi P, Marlovits S. MR imaging of osteochondral grafts and autologous chondrocyte implantation. Eur Radiol. 2007;17(1):103–18. Epub 2006/06/28.
62. Marlovits S, Striessnig G, Resinger CT, Aldrian SM, Vecsei V, Imhof H, et al. Definition of pertinent parameters for the evaluation of articular cartilage repair tissue with high-resolution magnetic resonance imaging. Eur J Radiol. 2004;52(3):310–9. Epub 2004/11/17.
63. Trattnig S, Ohel K, Mlynarik V, Juras V, Zbyn S, Korner A. Morphological and compositional monitoring of a new cell-free cartilage repair hydrogel technology – GelrinC by MR using semi-quantitative MOCART scoring and quantitative T2 index and new zonal T2 index calculation. Osteoarthritis Cartilage. 2015;23(12):2224–32.
64. Welsch GH, Zak L, Mamisch TC, Resinger C, Marlovits S, Trattnig S. Three-dimensional magnetic resonance observation of cartilage repair tissue (MOCART) score assessed with an isotropic three-dimensional true fast imaging with steady-state precession sequence at 3.0 tesla. Invest Radiol. 2009;44(9):603–12. Epub 2009/08/21.
65. Welsch GH, Zak L, Mamisch TC, Paul D, Lauer L, Mauerer A, et al. Advanced morphological 3D magnetic resonance observation of cartilage repair tissue (MOCART) scoring using a new isotropic 3D proton-density, turbo spin echo sequence with variable flip angle distribution (PD-SPACE) compared to an isotropic 3D steady-state free precession sequence (true-FISP) and standard 2D sequences. J Magn Reson Imaging. 2011;33(1):180–8. Epub 2010/12/25.
66. Roemer FW, Guermazi A, Trattnig S, Apprich S, Marlovits S, Niu J, et al. Whole joint MRI assessment of surgical cartilage repair of the knee: cartilage repair osteoarthritis knee score (CROAKS). Osteoarthritis Cartilage. 2014;22(6):779–99.
67. Hunter DJ, Guermazi A, Lo GH, Grainger AJ, Conaghan PG, Boudreau RM, et al. Evolution of semi-quantitative whole joint assessment of knee OA: MOAKS (MRI osteoarthritis knee score). Osteoarthritis Cartilage. 2011;19(8):990–1002.
68. Buckwalter JA, Mankin HJ. Articular cartilage: degeneration and osteoarthritis, repair, regeneration, and transplantation. Instr Course Lect. 1998;47:487–504.

69. Poole AR, Kojima T, Yasuda T, Mwale F, Kobayashi M, Laverty S. Composition and structure of articular cartilage – a template for tissue repair. Clin Orthop Relat Res. 2001;391:S26–33.
70. Maroudas A. Physicochemical properties of cartilage in the light of ion exchange theory. Biophys J. 1968;8(5):575–95.
71. Maroudas A, Muir H, Wingham J. The correlation of fixed negative charge with glycosaminoglycan content of human articular cartilage. Biochim Biophys Acta. 1969;177(3):492–500.
72. Grodzinsky AJ. Electromechanical and physicochemical properties of connective tissue. Crit Rev Biomed Eng. 1983;9(2):133–99.
73. Goodwin DW, Zhu HQ, Dunn JF. In vitro MR imaging of hyaline cartilage: correlation with scanning electron microscopy. Am J Roentgenol. 2000;174(2):405–9.
74. Bachmann G, Basad E, Lommel D, Steinmeyer J. MRI in the follow-up after MACI((R)) or microfracture. Radiologe. 2004;44(8):773–82.
75. Bentley G, Biant LC, Carrington RWJ, Akmal M, Goldberg A, Williams AM, et al. A prospective, randomised comparison of autologous chondrocyte implantation versus mosaicplasty for osteochondral defects in the knee. J Bone Joint Surg. 2003;85B(2):223–30.
76. Brittberg M, Lindahl A, Nilsson A, Ohlsson C, Isaksson O, Peterson L. Treatment of deep cartilage defects in the knee with autologous chondrocyte transplantation. N Engl J Med. 1994;331(14):889–95.
77. Gudas R, Kalesinskas RJ, Kimtys V, Stankevicius E, Toliusis V, Bernotavicius G, et al. A prospective randomized clinical study of mosaic osteochondral autologous transplantation versus microfracture for the treatment of osteochondral defects in the knee joint in young athletes. Arthroscopy. 2005;21(9):1066–75.
78. Gudas R, Stankevicius E, Monastyreckiene E, Pranys D, Kalesinskas RJ. Osteochondral autologous transplantation versus microfracture for the treatment of articular cartilage defects in the knee joint in athletes. Knee surgery sports traumatology. Arthroscopy. 2006;14(9):834–42.
79. Knutsen G, Drogset JO, Engebretsen L, Grontvedt T, Isaksen V, Ludvigsen TC, et al. A randomized trial comparing autologous chondrocyte implantation with microfracture. J Bone Joint Surg Am. 2007;89A(10):2105–12.
80. Knutsen G, Engebretsen L, Ludvigsen TC, Drogset JO, Grontvedt T, Solheim E, et al. Autologous chondrocyte implantation compared with microfracture in the knee – a randomized trial. J Bone Joint Surg Am. 2004;86A(3):455–64.
81. Nieminen MT, Nissi MJ, Mattila L, Kiviranta I. Evaluation of chondral repair using quantitative MRI. J Magn Reson Imaging. 2012;36(6):1287–99.
82. Burstein D, Velyvis J, Scott KT, Stock KW, Kim YJ, Jaramillo D, et al. Protocol issues for delayed Gd(DTPA)(2-)-enhanced MRI: (dGEMRIC) for clinical evaluation of articular cartilage. Magn Reson Med. 2001;45(1):36–41.
83. Bashir A, Gray ML, Burstein D. Gd-DTPA(2-) as a measure of cartilage degradation. Magn Reson Med. 1996;36(5):665–73.
84. Borthakur A, Shapiro EM, Beers J, Kudchodkar S, Kneeland JB, Reddy R. Sensitivity of MRI to proteoglycan depletion in cartilage: comparison of sodium and proton MRI. Osteoarthritis Cartilage. 2000;8(4):288–93.
85. Ling W, Regatte RR, Navon G, Jerschow A. Assessment of glycosaminoglycan concentration in vivo by chemical exchange-dependent saturation transfer (gagCEST). Proc Natl Acad Sci U S A. 2008;105(7):2266–70. Epub 2008/02/13.
86. Windschuh J, Zaiss M, Ehses P, Lee JS, Jerschow A, et al. Assessment of frequency drift on CEST MRI and dynamic correction: application to gagCEST at 7 T. Magn Reson Med. 2019;81(1):573–82.
87. Trattnig S, Raudner M, Schreiner M, Roemer F, Bohndorf K. Biochemical cartilage imaging-update 2019. Radiologe. 2019;59(8):742–49.
88. Mosher TJ, Dardzinski BJ. Cartilage MRI T2 relaxation time mapping: overview and applications. Semin Musculoskelet Radiol. 2004;8(4):355–68.
89. Nebelung S, Post M, Knobe M, Tingart M, Emans P, et al. Detection of early-stage degeneration in human articular cartilage by multiparametric MR imaging mapping of tissue functionality. Sci Rep. 2019;9(1):5895.
90. Welsch GH, Mamisch TC, Hughes T, Zilkens C, Quirbach S, Scheffler K, et al. In vivo biochemical 7.0 tesla magnetic resonance – preliminary results of dGEMRIC, zonal T2, and T2 * mapping of articular cartilage. Invest Radiol. 2008;43(9):619–26.
91. Williams A, Qian Y, Bear D, Chu CR. Assessing degeneration of human articular cartilage with ultra-short echo time (UTE) T2* mapping. Osteoarthritis Cartilage. 2010;18(4):539–46.
92. Pauli C, Bae WC, Lee M, Lotz M, Bydder GM, D'Lima DL, et al. Ultrashort-echo time MR imaging of the patella with bicomponent analysis: correlation with histopathologic and polarized light microscopic findings. Radiology. 2012;264(2):484–93.
93. Mamisch TC, Hughes T, Mosher TJ, Mueller C, Trattnig S, Boesch C, et al. T2 star relaxation times for assessment of articular cartilage at 3 T: a feasibility study. Skelet Radiol. 2012;41(3):287–92.
94. Bittersohl B, Hosalkar HS, Miese FR, Schibensky J, Konig DP, Herten M, et al. Zonal T2* and T1Gd assessment of knee joint cartilage in various histological grades of cartilage degeneration: an observational in vitro study. BMJ Open. 2015;5(2):e006895.
95. Juras V, Mlynarik V, Szomolanyi P, Valkovič L, Trattnig S. Magnetic resonance imaging of the musculoskeletal system at 7T: morphological imaging and beyond. Top Magn Reson Imaging. 2019;28(3):125–35.
96. Regatte RR, Akella SVS, Lonner JH, Kneeland JB, Reddy R. T-1p relaxation mapping in human osteo-

arthritis (OA) cartilage: comparison of T-1p with T-2. J Magn Reson Imaging. 2006;23(4):547–53.
97. Mlynarik V, Szomolanyi P, Toffanin R, Vittur F, Trattnig S. Transverse relaxation mechanisms in articular cartilage. J Magn Reson. 2004;169(2):300–7. Epub 2004/07/21.
98. Goodwin DW, Wadghiri YZ, Dunn JF. Micro-imaging of articular cartilage: T2, proton density, and the magic angle effect. Acad Radiol. 1998;5(11):790–8.
99. Smith HE, Mosher TJ, Dardzinski BJ, Collins BG, Collins CM, Yang QX, et al. Spatial variation in cartilage T2 of the knee. J Magn Reson Imaging. 2001;14(1):50–5.
100. Watrin-Pinzano A, Ruaud JP, Cheli Y, Gonord P, Grossin L, Bettembourg-Brault I, et al. Evaluation of cartilage repair tissue after biomaterial implantation in rat patella by using T2 mapping. Magn Reson Mater Phys Biol Med. 2004;17(3–6):219–28.
101. White LM, Sussman MS, Hurtig M, Probyn L, Tomlinson G, Kandel R. Cartilage T2 assessment: differentiation of normal hyaline cartilage and reparative tissue after arthroscopic cartilage repair in equine subjects. Radiology. 2006;241(2):407–14.
102. Domayer SE, Apprich S, Stelzeneder D, Hirschfeld C, Sokolowski M, Kronnerwetter C, et al. Cartilage repair of the ankle: first results of T2 mapping at 7.0 T after microfracture and matrix associated autologous cartilage transplantation. Osteoarthritis Cartilage. 2012;20(8):829–36.
103. Welsch GH, Apprich S, Zbyn S, Mamisch TC, Mlynarik V, Scheffler K, et al. Biochemical (T2, T2* and magnetisation transfer ratio) MRI of knee cartilage: feasibility at ultra-high field (7T) compared with high field (3T) strength. Eur Radiol. 2011;21(6):1136–43.
104. Juras V, Zbyn S, Mlynarik V, Szomolanyi P, Hager B, Baer P, et al. The compositional difference between ankle and knee cartilage demonstrated by T2 mapping at 7 tesla MR. Eur J Radiol. 2016;85(4):771–7.
105. Martín Noguerol T, Raya JG, Wessell DE, Vilanova JC, Rossi I, et al. Functional MRI for evaluation of hyaline cartilage extracelullar matrix, a physiopathological-based approach. Br J Radiol. 2019;92(1103):20190443. https://doi.org/10.1259/bjr.20190443.
106. Li Z, Wang H, Lu Y, Jiang M, Chen Z, et al. Diagnostic value of T1ρ and T2 mapping sequences of 3D fat-suppressed spoiled gradient (FS SPGR-3D) 3.0-T magnetic resonance imaging for osteoarthritis. Medicine (Baltimore). 2019;98(1):e13834.
107. Colotti R, Omoumi P, Bonanno G, Ledoux JB, van Heeswijk RB. Isotropic three-dimensional T2 mapping of knee cartilage: Development and validation. J Magn Reson Imaging. 2018;47(2):362–71.
108. Joseph GB, Nevitt MC, McCulloch CE, Neumann J, Lynch JA, et al. Associations between molecular biomarkers and MR-based cartilage composition and knee joint morphology: data from the Osteoarthritis Initiative. Osteoarthritis Cartilage. 2018;26(8):1070–77.
109. Liebl H, Joseph G, Nevitt MC, Singh N, Heilmeier U, Subburaj K, et al. Early T2 changes predict onset of radiographic knee osteoarthritis: data from the osteoarthritis initiative. Ann Rheum Dis. 2015;74(7):1353–9.
110. Apprich S, Mamisch TC, Welsch GH, Stelzeneder D, Albers C, Totzke U, et al. Quantitative T2 mapping of the patella at 3.0T is sensitive to early cartilage degeneration, but also to loading of the knee. Eur J Radiol. 2012;81(4):e438–43.
111. Su F, Pedoia V, Teng HL, Kretzschmar M, Lau BC, McCulloch CE, et al. The association between MR T1rho and T2 of cartilage and patient-reported outcomes after ACL injury and reconstruction. Osteoarthritis Cartilage. 2016;24(7):1180–9.
112. Munukka M, Waller B, Rantalainen T, Hakkinen A, Nieminen MT, Lammentausta E, et al. Efficacy of progressive aquatic resistance training for tibiofemoral cartilage in postmenopausal women with mild knee osteoarthritis: a randomised controlled trial. Osteoarthritis Cartilage. 2016;24(10):1708–17.
113. Trattnig S, Mamisch TC, Welsch GH, Glaser C, Szomolanyi P, Gebetsroither S, et al. Quantitative T-2 mapping of matrix-associated autologous chondrocyte transplantcation at 3 tesla – an in vivo cross-sectional study. Invest Radiol. 2007;42(6):442–8.
114. Liney GP, Knowles AJ, Manton DJ, Turnbull LW, Blackband SJ, Horsman A. Comparison of conventional single echo and multi-echo sequences with a fast spin-echo sequence for quantitative T2 mapping: application to the prostate. J Magn Reson Imaging. 1996;6(4):603–7.
115. Heule R, Ganter C, Bieri O. Triple echo steady-state (TESS) relaxometry. Magn Reson Med. 2014;71(1):230–7.
116. Juras V, Bohndorf K, Heule R, Kronnerwetter C, Szomolanyi P, Hager B, Bieri O, Zbyn S and Trattnig S. A comparison of multi-echo spin-echo and triple-echo steady-state T2 mapping for in vivo evaluation of articular cartilage. Eur Radiol. 2016;26:1905–12.
117. Schoenbauer E, Szomolanyi P, Shiomi T, Juras V, Zbyn S, Zak L, et al. Cartilage evaluation with biochemical MR imaging using in vivo knee compression at 3T-comparison of patients after cartilage repair with healthy volunteers. J Biomech. 2015;48(12):3349–55.
118. Du J, Takahashi AM, Chung CB. Ultrashort TE spectroscopic imaging (UTESI): application to the imaging of short T2 relaxation tissues in the musculoskeletal system. J Magn Reson Imaging. 2009;29(2):412–21.
119. Chavhan GB, Babyn PS, Thomas B, Shroff MM, Haacke EM. Principles, techniques, and applications of T2*-based MR imaging and its special applications. Radiographics. 2009;29(5):1433–49.
120. Maier CF, Tan SG, Hariharan H, Potter HG. T2 quantitation of articular cartilage at 1.5 T. J Magn Reson Imaging. 2003;17(3):358–64.

121. Lusse S, Claassen H, Gehrke T, Hassenpflug J, Schunke M, Heller M, et al. Evaluation of water content by spatially resolved transverse relaxation times of human articular cartilage. Magn Reson Imaging. 2000;18(4):423–30.
122. Bittersohl B, Miese FR, Hosalkar HS, Mamisch TC, Antoch G, Krauspe R, et al. T2* mapping of acetabular and femoral hip joint cartilage at 3 T: a prospective controlled study. Invest Radiol. 2012;47(7):392–7.
123. Robson MD, Gatehouse PD, Bydder M, Bydder GM. Magnetic resonance: an introduction to ultrashort TE (UTE) imaging. J Comput Assist Tomogr. 2003;27(6):825–46.
124. Bittersohl B, Miese FR, Hosalkar HS, Herten M, Antoch G, Krauspe R, et al. T2* mapping of hip joint cartilage in various histological grades of degeneration. Osteoarthritis Cartilage. 2012;20(7):653–60.
125. Welsch GH, Trattnig S, Hughes T, Quirbach S, Olk A, Blanke M, et al. T2 and T2* mapping in patients after matrix-associated autologous chondrocyte transplantation: initial results on clinical use with 3.0-tesla MRI. Eur Radiol. 2010;20(6):1515–23.
126. Regatte RR, Akella SVS, Wheaton AJ, Borthakur A, Kneeland JB, Reddy R. T-1 rho-relaxation mapping of human femoral-tibial cartilage in vivo. J Magn Reson Imaging. 2003;18(3):336–41.
127. Menezes NM, Gray ML, Hartke JR, Burstein D. T-2 and T-1, MRI in articular cartilage systems. Magn Reson Med. 2004;51(3):503–9.
128. van Tiel J, Kotek G, Reijman M, Bos PK, Bron EE, Klein S, et al. Is T1rho mapping an alternative to delayed gadolinium-enhanced MR imaging of cartilage in the assessment of Sulphated glycosaminoglycan content in human osteoarthritic knees? An in vivo validation study. Radiology. 2016;279(2):523–31.
129. Prasad AP, Nardo L, Schooler J, Joseph GB, Link TM. T(1)rho and T(2) relaxation times predict progression of knee osteoarthritis. Osteoarthritis Cartilage. 2013;21(1):69–76.
130. Holtzman DJ, Theologis AA, Carballido-Gamio J, Majumdar S, Li X, Benjamin C. T(1rho) and T(2) quantitative magnetic resonance imaging analysis of cartilage regeneration following microfracture and mosaicplasty cartilage resurfacing procedures. J Magn Reson Imaging. 2010;32(4):914–23.
131. Theologis AA, Schairer WW, Carballido-Gamio J, Majumdar S, Li X, Ma CB. Longitudinal analysis of T1rho and T2 quantitative MRI of knee cartilage laminar organization following microfracture surgery. Knee. 2012;19(5):652–7.
132. Wolff SD, Chesnick S, Frank JA, Lim KO, Balaban RS. Magnetization transfer contrast – Mr-imaging of the knee. Radiology. 1991;179(3):623–8.
133. Gray ML, Burstein D, Lesperance LM, Gehrke L. Magnetization-transfer in cartilage and its constituent macromolecules. Magn Reson Med. 1995;34(3):319–25.
134. Kim DK, Ceckler TL, Hascall VC, Calabro A, Balaban RS. Analysis of water-macromolecule proton magnetization transfer in articular-cartilage. Magn Reson Med. 1993;29(2):211–5.
135. Seo GS, Aoki J, Moriya H, Karakida O, Sone S, Hidaka H, et al. Hyaline cartilage: in vivo and in vitro assessment with magnetization transfer imaging. Radiology. 1996;201(2):525–30.
136. Wolff SD, Balaban RS. Magnetization transfer contrast (Mtc) and tissue water proton relaxation Invivo. Magn Reson Med. 1989;10(1):135–44.
137. Wolff SD, Eng J, Balaban RS. Magnetization transfer contrast – method for improving contrast in gradient-recalled-Echo images. Radiology. 1991;179(1):133–7.
138. Palmieri F, De Keyzer F, Maes F, Van Breuseghem I. Magnetization transfer analysis of cartilage repair tissue: a preliminary study. Skelet Radiol. 2006;35(12):903–8.
139. Bieri O, Scheffler K. Optimized balanced steady-state free precession magnetization transfer imaging. Magn Reson Med. 2007;58(3):511–8.
140. Welsch GH, Trattnig S, Scheffler K, Szomonanyi P, Quirbach S, Marlovits S, et al. Magnetization transfer contrast and T2 mapping in the evaluation of cartilage repair tissue with 3T MRI. J Magn Reson Imaging. 2008;28(4):979–86.
141. Potter K, Butler JJ, Horton WE, Spencer RGS. Response of engineered cartilage tissue to biochemical agents as studied by proton magnetic resonance microscopy. Arthritis Rheum. 2000;43(7):1580–90.
142. Vahlensieck M, Dombrowski F, Leutner C, Wagner U, Reiser M. Magnetization-Transfer Contrast (Mtc) and Mtc-subtraction – enhancement of cartilage lesions and Intracartilaginous degeneration in-vitro. Skelet Radiol. 1994;23(7):535–9.
143. Kogan F, Hariharan H, Reddy R. Chemical Exchange Saturation Transfer (CEST) imaging: description of technique and potential clinical applications. Curr Radiol Rep. 2013;1(2):102–14. Epub 2013/06/05.
144. Schmitt B, Zbyn S, Stelzeneder D, Jellus V, Paul D, Lauer L, et al. Cartilage quality assessment by using glycosaminoglycan chemical exchange saturation transfer and (23)Na MR imaging at 7 T. Radiology. 2011;260(1):257–64.
145. Krusche-Mandl I, Schmitt B, Zak L, Apprich S, Aldrian S, Juras V, et al. Long-term results 8 years after autologous osteochondral transplantation: 7 T gagCEST and sodium magnetic resonance imaging with morphological and clinical correlation. Osteoarthritis Cartilage. 2012;20(5):357–63.
146. Schreiner MM, Zbyn S, Schmitt B, Weber M, Domayer S, Windhager R, et al. Reproducibility and regional variations of an improved gagCEST protocol for the in vivo evaluation of knee cartilage at 7 T. MAGMA. 2016;29(3):513–21.
147. Singh A, Haris M, Cai K, Kassey VB, Kogan F, Reddy D, et al. Chemical exchange saturation transfer magnetic resonance imaging of human knee cartilage at 3 T and 7 T. Magn Reson Med. 2012;68(2):588–94. Epub 2012/01/04.

148. Zaiss M, Bachert P. Chemical exchange saturation transfer (CEST) and MR Z-spectroscopy in vivo: a review of theoretical approaches and methods. Phys Med Biol. 2013;58(22):R221–69. Epub 2013/11/10.
149. Kim M, Gillen J, Landman BA, Zhou J, van Zijl PC. Water saturation shift referencing (WASSR) for chemical exchange saturation transfer (CEST) experiments. Magn Reson Med. 2009;61(6):1441–50. Epub 2009/04/10.
150. Krishnamoorthy G, Nanga RPR, Bagga P, Hariharan H and Reddy R. High quality three-dimensional gagCEST imaging of in vivo human knee cartilage at 7 Tesla. Magn Reson Med. 2017;77:1866–73.
151. Burstein D, Bashir A, Gray ML. MRI techniques in early stages of cartilage disease. Invest Radiol. 2000;35(10):622–38.
152. Watanabe A, Wada Y, Obata T, Ueda T, Tamura M, Ikehira H, et al. Delayed gadolinium-enhanced MR to determine glycosaminoglycan concentration in reparative cartilage after autologous chondrocyte implantation: preliminary results. Radiology. 2006;239(1):201–8.
153. Bashir A, Gray ML, Boutin RD, Burstein D. Glycosaminoglycan in articular cartilage: in vivo assessment with delayed Gd(DTPA)(2-)-enhanced MR imaging. Radiology. 1997;205(2):551–8.
154. Tiderius CJ, Olsson LE, Leander P, Ekberg O, Dahlberg L. Delayed gadolinium-enhanced MRI of cartilage (dGEMRIC) in early knee osteoarthritis. Magn Reson Med. 2003;49(3):488–92.
155. Williams A, Gillis A, McKenzie C, Po B, Sharma L, Micheli L, et al. Glycosaminoglycan distribution in cartilage as determined by delayed gadolinium-enhanced MRI of cartilage (dGEMRIC): potential clinical applications. Am J Roentgenol. 2004;182(1):167–72.
156. Rubin GD, Napel S. Helical CT angiography of renal artery stenosis. AJR Am J Roentgenol. 1997;168(4):1109–11. Epub 1997/04/01.
157. Trattnig S, Marlovits S, Gebetsroither S, Szomolanyi P, Welsch GH, Salomonowitz E, et al. Three-dimensional delayed gadolinium-enhanced MRI of cartilage (dGEMRIC) for in vivo evaluation of reparative cartilage after matrix-associated autologous chondrocyte transplantation at 3.0T: preliminary results. J Magn Reson Imaging. 2007;26(4):974–82.
158. Trattnig S, Mamisch TC, Pinker K, Domayer S, Szomolanyi P, Marlovits S, et al. Differentiating normal hyaline cartilage from post-surgical repair tissue using fast gradient echo imaging in delayed gadolinium-enhanced MRI (dGEMRIC) at 3 tesla. Eur Radiol. 2008;18(6):1251–9.
159. Kim YJ, Jaramillo D, Millis MB, Gray ML, Burstein D. Assessment of early osteoarthritis in hip dysplasia with delayed gadolinium-enhanced magnetic resonance imaging of cartilage. J Bone Joint Surg Am. 2003;85A(10):1987–92.
160. Lattanzi R, Petchprapa C, Ascani D, Babb JS, Chu D, Davidovitch RI, et al. Detection of cartilage damage in femoroacetabular impingement with standardized dGEMRIC at 3 T. Osteoarthritis Cartilage. 2014;22(3):447–56.
161. Owman H, Ericsson YB, Englund M, Tiderius CJ, Tjornstrand J, Roos EM, et al. Association between delayed gadolinium-enhanced MRI of cartilage (dGEMRIC) and joint space narrowing and osteophytes: a cohort study in patients with partial meniscectomy with 11 years of follow-up. Osteoarthritis Cartilage. 2014;22(10):1537–41.
162. Crema MD, Hunter DJ, Burstein D, Roemer FW, Li L, Eckstein F, et al. Association of changes in delayed gadolinium-enhanced MRI of cartilage (dGEMRIC) with changes in cartilage thickness in the medial tibiofemoral compartment of the knee: a 2 year follow-up study using 3.0 T MRI. Ann Rheum Dis. 2014;73(11):1935–41.
163. Vaga S, Raimondi MT, Caiani EG, Costa F, Giordano C, Perona F, et al. Quantitative assessment of intervertebral disc glycosaminoglycan distribution by gadolinium-enhanced MRI in orthopedic patients. Magn Reson Med. 2008;59(1):85–95.
164. Williams A, Shetty SK, Burstein D, Day CS, McKenzie C. Delayed gadolinium enhanced MRI of cartilage (dGEMRIC) of the first carpometacarpal (1CMC) joint: a feasibility study. Osteoarthritis Cartilage. 2008;16(4):530–2.
165. Pittschieler E, Szomolanyi P, Schmid-Schwap M, Weber M, Egerbacher M, Traxler H, et al. Delayed gadolinium-enhanced MRI of the fibrocartilage disc of the temporomandibular joint–a feasibility study. Magn Reson Imaging. 2014;32(10):1223–9.
166. Lesperance LM, Gray ML, Burstein D. Determination of fixed charge density in cartilage using nuclear magnetic resonance. J Orthop Res. 1992;10(1):1–13.
167. Reddy R, Insko EK, Noyszewski EA, Dandora R, Kneeland JB, Leigh JS. Sodium MRI of human articular cartilage in vivo. Magn Reson Med. 1998;39(5):697–701.
168. Shapiro EM, Borthakur A, Dandora R, Kriss A, Leigh JS, Reddy R. Sodium visibility and quantitation in intact bovine articular cartilage using high field (23)Na MRI and MRS. J Magn Reson. 2000;142(1):24–31.
169. Shapiro EM, Borthakur A, Gougoutas A, Reddy R. 23Na MRI accurately measures fixed charge density in articular cartilage. Magn Reson Med. 2002;47(2):284–91.
170. Pabst T, Sandstede J, Beer M, Kenn W, Neubauer S, Hahn D. Sodium T2* relaxation times in human heart muscle. J Magn Reson Imaging. 2002;15(2):215–8.
171. Jerecic R, Bock M, Nielles-Vallespin S, Wacker C, Bauer W, Schad LR. ECG-gated 23Na-MRI of the human heart using a 3D-radial projection technique with ultra-short echo times. MAGMA. 2004;16(6):297–302.
172. Borthakur A, Mellon E, Niyogi S, Witschey W, Kneeland JB, Reddy R. Sodium and T1rho MRI for molecular and diagnostic imaging of articular

cartilage. NMR Biomed. 2006;19(7):781–821. Epub 2006/11/01.
173. Rahmer J, Bornert P, Groen J, Bos C. Three-dimensional radial ultrashort echo-time imaging with T2 adapted sampling. Magn Reson Med. 2006;55(5):1075–82.
174. Nielles-Vallespin S, Weber MA, Bock M, Bongers A, Speier P, Combs SE, et al. 3D radial projection technique with ultrashort echo times for sodium MRI: clinical applications in human brain and skeletal muscle. Magn Reson Med. 2007;57(1):74–81.
175. Jordan CD, McWalter EJ, Monu UD, Watkins RD, Chen W, Bangerter NK, et al. Variability of CubeQuant T1rho, quantitative DESS T2, and cones sodium MRI in knee cartilage. Osteoarthritis Cartilage. 2014;22(10):1559–67.
176. Trattnig S, Zbyn S, Schmitt B, Friedrich K, Juras V, Szomolanyi P, et al. Advanced MR methods at ultra-high field (7 tesla) for clinical musculoskeletal applications. Eur Radiol. 2012;22(11):2338–46.
177. Madelin G, Regatte RR. Biomedical applications of sodium MRI in vivo. J Magn Reson Imaging. 2013;38(3):511–29.
178. Grushko G, Schneiderman R, Maroudas A. Some biochemical and biophysical parameters for the study of the pathogenesis of osteoarthritis: a comparison between the processes of ageing and degeneration in human hip cartilage. Connect Tissue Res. 1989;19(2–4):149–76.
179. Lohmander LS. Articular cartilage and osteoarthrosis. The role of molecular markers to monitor breakdown, repair and disease. J Anat. 1994;184(Pt 3):477–92.
180. Wheaton AJ, Borthakur A, Dodge GR, Kneeland JB, Schumacher HR, Reddy R. Sodium magnetic resonance imaging of proteoglycan depletion in an in vivo model of osteoarthritis. Acad Radiol. 2004;11(1):21–8.
181. Wheaton AJ, Borthakur A, Shapiro EM, Regatte RR, Akella SV, Kneeland JB, et al. Proteoglycan loss in human knee cartilage: quantitation with sodium MR imaging–feasibility study. Radiology. 2004;231(3):900–5.
182. Wang L, Wu Y, Chang G, Oesingmann N, Schweitzer ME, Jerschow A, et al. Rapid isotropic 3D-sodium MRI of the knee joint in vivo at 7T. J Magn Reson Imaging. 2009;30(3):606–14.
183. Madelin G, Babb J, Xia D, Chang G, Krasnokutsky S, Abramson SB, et al. Articular cartilage: evaluation with fluid-suppressed 7.0-T sodium MR imaging in subjects with and subjects without osteoarthritis. Radiology. 2013;268(2):481–91.
184. Newbould RD, Miller SR, Tielbeek JA, Toms LD, Rao AW, Gold GE, et al. Reproducibility of sodium MRI measures of articular cartilage of the knee in osteoarthritis. Osteoarthritis Cartilage. 2012;20(1):29–35.
185. Marik W, Nemec SF, Zbyn S, Zalaudek M, Ludvik B, Riegler G, et al. Changes in cartilage and tendon composition of patients with type I diabetes mellitus: identification by quantitative sodium magnetic resonance imaging at 7 T. Invest Radiol. 2016;51(4):266–72.
186. Trattnig S, Welsch GH, Juras V, Szomolanyi P, Mayerhoefer ME, Stelzeneder D, et al. 23Na MR imaging at 7 T after knee matrix-associated autologous chondrocyte transplantation preliminary results. Radiology. 2010;257(1):175–84.
187. Zbyn S, Stelzeneder D, Welsch GH, Negrin LL, Juras V, Mayerhoefer ME, et al. Evaluation of native hyaline cartilage and repair tissue after two cartilage repair surgery techniques with 23Na MR imaging at 7 T: initial experience. Osteoarthritis Cartilage. 2012;20(8):837–45.

15 Histopathology Evaluation of Cartilage Disease and Repair

Kenneth P. H. Pritzker and Harpal K. Gahunia

15.1 Introduction

Histological changes in articular cartilage pathology have been reported for more than 125 years [1]. Using the light microscope, the avascular and aneural nature of articular cartilage was known by the beginning of the twentieth century [2]. With advancement in technology (electron microscopy, isotopic tracer techniques, biochemistry) and discoveries, by the middle of the twentieth century, our understanding of articular cartilage structure, collagen architecture (gothic arcade model), and macromolecular constitution was much enhanced [3, 4]. Throughout the second half of the twentieth century, major advances in technological innovation in articular cartilage imaging (magnetic resonance imaging – MRI, ultrasound, enhanced microscopy), surgical repair procedures, biochemistry, and immunology (enzymology, immunologic assays, etc.) coupled with the extensive collaboration among clinicians, scientists, and engineers have accelerated our understanding of articular cartilage structure and function at the cellular, macromolecular, and organ level [5–48]. Since the beginning of the twenty-first century, continued technological innovation and scientific progress has provided us with the understanding of articular cartilage as a very dynamic tissue in health, aging, injury, and disease [49–73]. To illustrate the range of disease affecting articular cartilage, cartilage pathomorphology in chondromalacia, rheumatoid arthritis (RA), and osteoarthritis (OA) are discussed briefly as follows.

Although chondromalacia is a condition common among young, athletic individuals, it also affects people of all activity levels and ages including older adults who have arthritis of the knee [74, 75]. It is often recognized as involving the extensor mechanism of the knee and accordingly also referred to as chondromalacia patella, patellofemoral syndrome, or runner's knee [76, 77]. Chondromalacia involves macroscopic softening of the articular cartilage usually focally and commonly presents in patella articular cartilage. In young individuals, chondromalacia is most likely a consequence of an acute injury such as a trauma, repetitive overuse, knee malalignment, or even muscle weakness. Cartilage softness is related to cartilage matrix edema (swelling) and if limited can resolve without residual damage. However, repeated injury where

K. P. H. Pritzker, MD, FRCPC
Department of Laboratory Medicine and Pathobiology, Department of Surgery, and Institute of Biomaterials and Biomedical Engineering, University of Toronto, Toronto, ON, Canada

Department of Pathology and Laboratory Medicine, Mount Sinai Hospital, Toronto, ON, Canada

H. K. Gahunia, MSc, PhD (✉)
Orthopaedic Science Consulting Services, Oakville, ON, Canada
e-mail: harpal.gahunia@utoronto.ca

H. K. Gahunia et al. (eds.), *Articular Cartilage of the Knee*,
https://doi.org/10.1007/978-1-4939-7587-7_15

mechanical forces are highest can result in erosion of the cartilage, which in chronic phase may be manifested as vertical clefts from the extracellular matrix (ECM) surface and edema or even cysts within the cartilage of middle zone (MZ). With complete cartilage erosion, the articular surface may become bone (due to exposure of subchondral bone) in which there is a shiny surface (referred as eburnation) and beneath this, increased bone density within the articular plate (osteosclerosis). In contrast, RA is an autoimmune, chronic systemic inflammatory disorder that affects primarily synovium but not the cartilage [78]. The initial pathologic event within the joint in RA appears to be immune-mediated activation of synovial cells, eventually progressing to a more chronic stage resulting from the extensively hyperplastic synovium. Cartilage injury is passive in RA. In response to proteolytic enzymes, e.g., metalloproteases elaborated by synovial cells, degradation of cartilage ECM macromolecules ensues. Similarly increased cytokines from synovial cells act on chondrocytes to decrease collagen and proteoglycan (PG) synthesis [79]. Subsequently, progressive thinning and loss of cartilage matrix occur over the entire surface of the joint starting peripherally at the synovium-cartilage interface.

Osteoarthritis, occurring in older population (> 65 years; affecting about 60% men and 70% women), is the leading cause of global musculoskeletal disability [80–82]. Nevertheless, OA can also affect children and younger adults [83–89]. The key risk factors for the accelerated development of OA in young adults include obesity and a history of sport-related traumatic knee injury such as anterior cruciate ligament rupture and/or meniscal tear [83, 90, 91]. Knee OA usually affects articular cartilage where mechanical forces are maximum. The etiology of OA is multifactorial, and the associated pathophysiological events involve the inflammatory cytokines, such as interleukin-1 beta (Il-1β) and tumor necrosis factor-alpha (TNF-α), which can be involved in initiating a cycle of catabolic and matrix degradative events in cartilage [63, 65–71, 92–94]. Production of cartilage-degrading enzymes and pro-inflammatory cytokines can also result from intra-articular deposition of endogenous particulates, such as OA-associated basic calcium phosphate crystals [95]. Metalloproteinases from chondrocytes mediate articular cartilage ECM degradation and remodeling of the underlying subchondral bone. Nitric oxide exerts pro-inflammatory effects, and cartilage from RA and OA patients has shown to spontaneously produce nitric oxide in vitro [96, 97]. In experimental OA, nitric oxide has been shown to exert pro-inflammatory effects by inducing chondrocyte programmed cell death, apoptosis [63]. The percentage of chondrocytes with nitric oxide–induced apoptosis is known to increase in cartilage obtained from trauma patients, and the subsequent number of apoptotic chondrocytes decreased with increasing time from injury [98, 99]. Chondrocyte apoptosis can be inferred by observing nuclear fragmentation in a ladder pattern. A recent study showed that the presence and severity of chronic synovitis characterized by slight increased synovial lining cells with subjacent fibrosis can assist in identifying distinct histopathological OA subgroups [100]. This chronic synovitis is less in extent and different morphologically than that observed in chronic inflammatory arthritis such as RA. Further, this study also documented that the infiltration of blood vessels through the tidemark referred to as "tidemark breaching" was greater in the OA group compared with the "non-arthritic" group. See Appendix D for OsteoArthritis Research Society International (OARSI) histopathological grading system for OA cartilage.

15.2 Early Changes in Articular Cartilage Injury and Disease

Normal hyaline cartilage, as a material, is isotropic; cartilage matrix has similar material properties in three dimensions both on a microscopic and macroscopic scale (Fig. 15.1). A direct correlation exists between the histological changes of articular cartilage and its altered biomechanics during the progression of OA [102]. With disease, the cartilage matrix becomes more heterogeneous, with adverse biomechanical consequences. Through early therapeutic intervention, the damaged cartilage can heal and repair

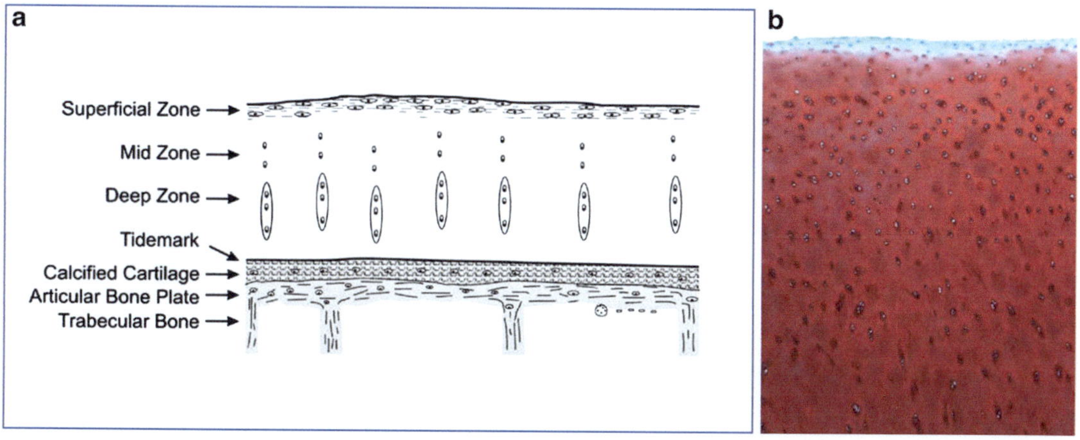

Fig. 15.1 (**a**) Schematic diagram of normal articular cartilage showing smooth knee cartilage surface. The uncalcified articular cartilage extracellular matrix and chondrocytes are organized into superficial, mid, and deep zones. Subjacent, the tidemark separates the deep zone from the calcified cartilage. (**b**) 5 μm section of normal articular cartilage reveals the smooth surface (Safranin O stain, Magnification, 5×) (Permission is granted to reprint these figures from Osteoarthritis And Cartilage, Elsevier [101])

better to prevent progression to degenerative arthritis. Identification and diagnosis of the early stage of cartilage lesions in disease as chondromalacia patellae, OA, RA, or other processes is the key to the success of devising strategies for articular cartilage repair and timely treatment resulting in favorable outcomes for patients [64]. Softening of articular cartilage regularly noted as the earliest morphological change (Grade 1 and II lesions) in chondromalacia patella has been associated with PG depletion and reduction in the size of aggrecans [103]. The earliest abnormalities in RA involve proliferation of the synovium and soft tissue swelling, which is followed by pannus (inflamed synovial tissue) overlying across the articular cartilage surface resulting in disorganization of collagen, decreased PG content, and subjacent chondrocyte death. Typically, focal chondrocyte death is seen as well in the cartilage superficial zone (SZ) and upper MZ adjacent to cartilage surface covered by pannus. In contrast, the earliest focal degeneration in OA knee articular cartilage occurs in the more central weight-bearing area within an intact SZ and is associated with increased collagenase cleavage of collagen type II which may be accompanied by subjacent focal chondrocyte hypertrophy, clustering, and/or disorganization (Fig. 15.2) [104]. Chondrocyte hypertrophy can be recognized by the relative increase of chondrocyte cytoplasm compared to other chondrocytes. The breakdown of collagen fibers results in matrix edema due to net increase in water content [105–109]. The earliest nonreversible OA changes are perichondronal collagen formation, microscars from previous injury. This leads to cartilage matrix heterogeneity, which in turn leads to asymmetric responses to mechanical forces furthering progressive cycles of injury and collagenous repair tissue. Recently, using an experimental OA model and also noted in patients with OA, an interesting association between synovitis and collagen structural damage was observed in early OA [110, 111]. Further, using Second Harmonic Generation (SHG) imaging, a decrease in collagen fiber thickness in the deep zone (DZ) and an increase in collagen fiber disorganization in the SZ was detected very early in OA development.

15.3 Histopathology of Articular Cartilage Lesions

Histopathological techniques and assessment criteria of articular cartilage lesions due to injury or disease have been evolving over the past 40 years [101, 112–124]. The evaluation of the reproducibility, validity, and reliability (intra- and interobserver) of the histological assessment of the

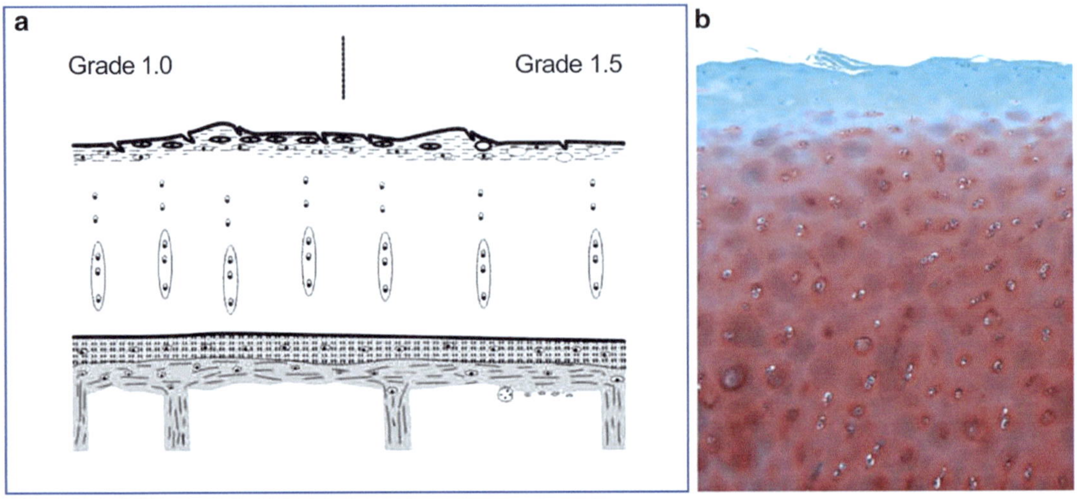

Fig. 15.2 (**a**) Schematic diagram of early (Grade 1) osteoarthritic lesions of knee articular cartilage surface demonstrating uneven cartilage surface with superficial zone fibrillation. (**b**) Histologically, these surface lesions are characterized by proteoglycan depletion, exhibited by slight reduction of Safranin O staining intensity, which extends to the upper 5% of the mid-zone (Safranin O stain, Magnification, 5×) (Permission is granted to reprint these figures from Osteoarthritis And Cartilage, Elsevier [101])

extent of cartilage lesion and nature of repair as well as its utility as the gold standard for comparison with other imaging modality has been extensively reported [52, 53, 101, 114, 115, 117–120, 122, 124–137]. Histologic methods were developed first to assess OA activity and progression and to assess cartilage injury in experimental arthritis [101, 113, 124, 138–142]. More recently, specific models for cartilage repair have been developed in animals ranging in size from mice to horses [143–146]. Histologic methods to evaluate cartilage repair were developed modeled on methods to assess cartilage injury [122]. Histologic assessment continues to be the most integrative method for assessing the reparative response of cartilage chondrocytes and matrix. Figures 15.3, 15.4, 15.5, 15.6, and 15.7 show the schematic diagrams with its corresponding histologic assessment for OA Grades 2–6.

The principles of simplicity, utility, scalability, extendability, and comparability, operative in histopathologic systems to evaluate OA [101], also need to be applied to systems of cartilage repair. Paramount considerations for histopathology evaluation of cartilage repair include addressing the following key questions:

1. Does the classification system reflect the capacity of cartilage as a living system to continue repair and subsequently maintain cartilage integrity? Crucially this would include the capacity of the reparative cartilage to adapt to a changing biomechanical environment.
2. Does the classification system reflect the biomechanical integrity of articular cartilage? Ideally, reparative cartilage would have identical cell distribution and matrix architecture as is found in pristine hyaline cartilage. This presupposes that cartilage adjacent to the reparative cartilage has normal properties, a situation that does apply after acute cartilage injury but may not be present with disease such as advanced OA. In practice, reparative cartilage that has similar functional properties but differs in matrix architecture from normal cartilage may be seen. This means that adequacy of cartilage repair needs to be assessed not purely on architecture arrangement of cells and matrix components but on how well the reparative tissue reflects the intact functional state.
3. Does the classification system reflect the volume of reparative cartilage, the location, and the extent of cartilage repair within the joint? This is the question of sample adequacy and representativeness.

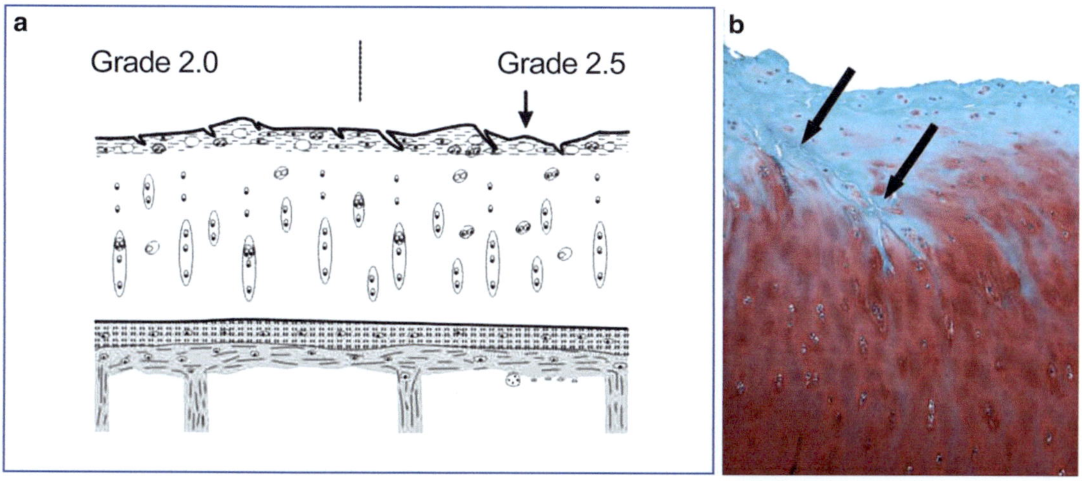

Fig. 15.3 (**a**) Schematic diagram of Grade 2 osteoarthritic lesions showing marked surface discontinuity of the knee articular cartilage. Fibrillation extends through the superficial zone to the mid-zone. (**b**) Histologically, the fibrillation (indicated by arrow) may be accompanied by hypercellularity or small chondrocyte clusters and/or cell death along with increased or decreased extracellular matrix Safranin O staining that may extend to the upper third of the mid-zone. Initiation of matrix disorganization may also be seen (Magnification, 5×) (Permission is granted to reprint these figures from Osteoarthritis And Cartilage, Elsevier [101])

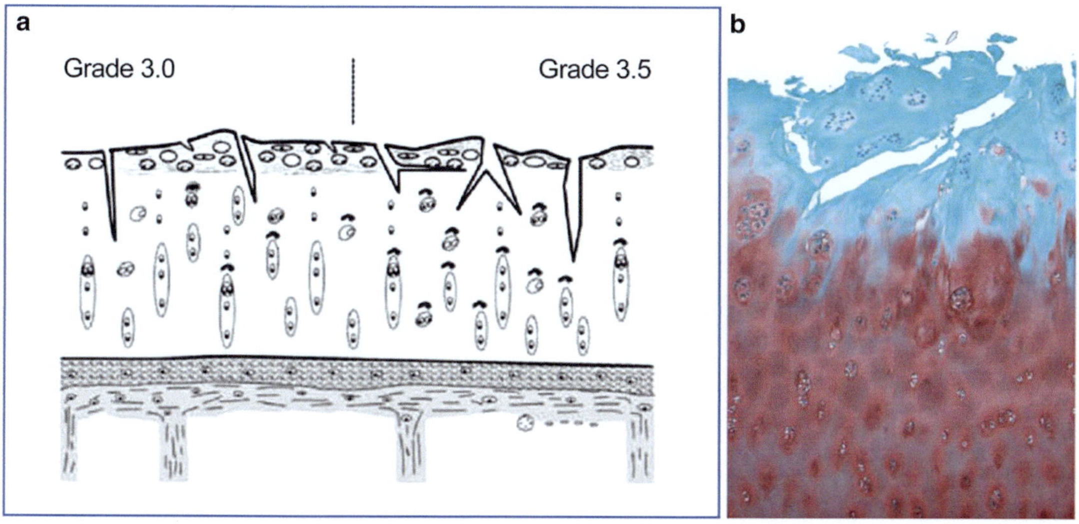

Fig. 15.4 (**a**) Schematic diagram of Grade 3 osteoarthritic lesions of the knee articular cartilage illustrating vertical fissures that extend well within the mid-zone. The cartilage surface integrity is disrupted with fibrillation that extends vertically downward into the mid-zone. Cell death and/or proliferation as well as chondrocyte clustering may be observed, most prominently adjacent to fissures. (**b**) Fissures are present that branch and extend into the deep zone. Cell death and large chondrocyte clusters depicting active repair response are observed most prominently adjacent to the fissures and extend well within the mid-zone. Note the chondrocyte hypertrophy demonstrating intrinsic cellular response to cartilage repair and varying Safranin O staining intensity (Magnification, 5×) (Permission is granted to reprint these figures from Osteoarthritis And Cartilage, Elsevier [101])

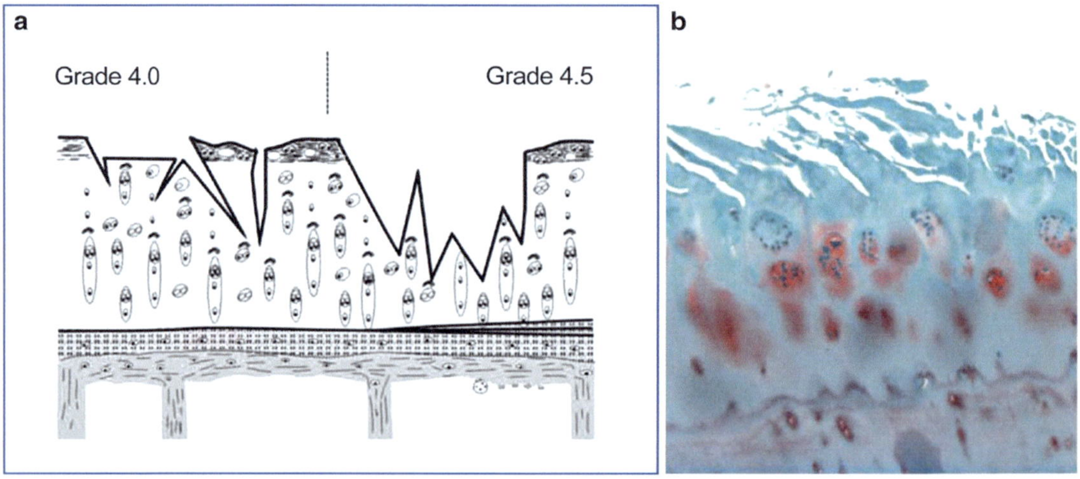

Fig. 15.5 (**a**) Schematic diagram of Grade 4 osteoarthritic lesions of the knee articular cartilage illustrating fissures and matrix erosion that may extend into the upper part of the deep zone. Reduplication of the tidemark may be present. (**b**) Cartilage matrix loss with deep fissures is seen. Hypocellularity and chondrocyte clusters with markedly decreased Safranin O staining are noted. Duplication of tidemark is prominent (Safranin O stain, Magnification, 5×) (Permission is granted to reprint these figures from Osteoarthritis And Cartilage, Elsevier [101])

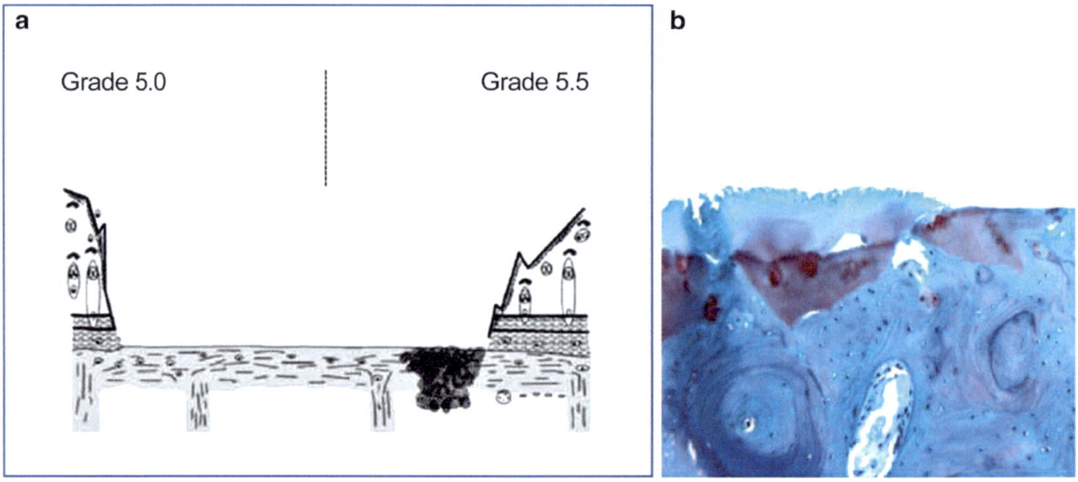

Fig. 15.6 (**a**) Schematic diagram of Grade 5 osteoarthritic lesions of the knee articular cartilage illustrating large extent of cartilage denudation or focal areas of total uncalcified cartilage loss. (**b**) Full-thickness erosion of unmineralized hyaline cartilage. The articular surface consists of the calcified cartilage or bone (Safranin O stain, Magnification, 5×) (Permission is granted to reprint these figures from Osteoarthritis And Cartilage, Elsevier [101])

4. Can the histopathology classification system reflect functional state of cartilage repair as visualized by imaging techniques? Ideally, noninvasive imaging would reflect the cartilage repair by same or better criteria as histology, but presently, this is a goal rather than reality. Accordingly, it is necessary to map the status of functional repair as seen by histology to that as observed by imaging. Cluster formation is a sign of repair in early OA, and in cartilage repair, cluster formation may be interpreted as a positive phenomenon as cell proliferation is central to new tissue formation [147, 148].

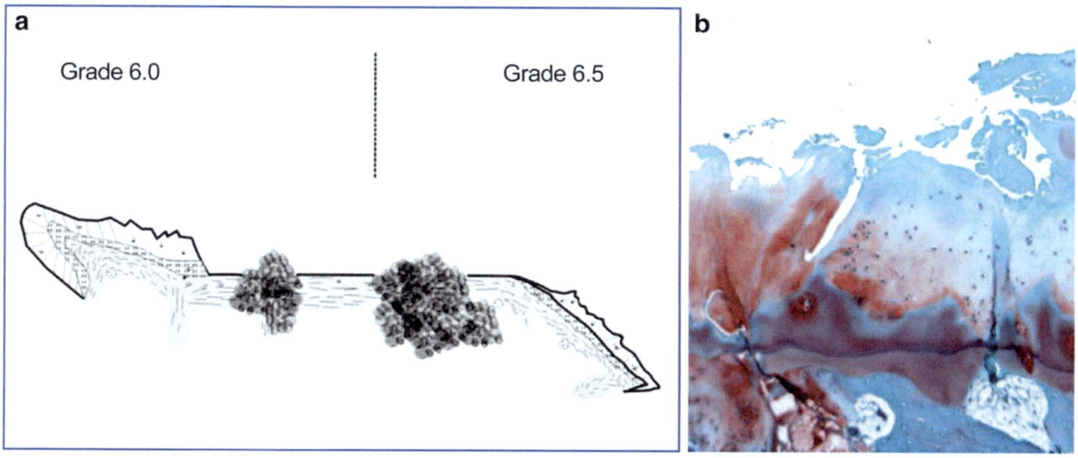

Fig. 15.7 (**a**) and (**b**) Schematic diagram and Safranin O stained photomicrograph of Grade 6 osteoarthritic lesions of the knee articular cartilage showing eburnation and articular contour deformation. The articular surface contour is altered through the processes of microfracture, repair, and bone remodeling (Magnification, 5×) (Permission is granted to reprint these figures from Osteoarthritis And Cartilage, Elsevier [101])

15.4 Articular Cartilage Repair Versus Regeneration

The common vision of cartilage *repair* refers to the restoration of a histologic defect in articular cartilage ranging in size from superficial fibrillation over a small area through cleft formation, erosion, or alternately repair of a fracture vertically through the articular plate or horizontally through mid-cartilage. Similar concepts can be extended to meniscal fibrocartilage with repair usually associated with restoration of tissue following a soft tissue fracture, commonly termed "tear." When the repair is effected by tissue with cell and matrix histologic characteristics of normal cartilage, this is termed *regeneration.*

In fact, cartilage repair should be more broadly defined to include restoration of the normal cartilage functional state from a state of lesser function. This broader definition can be assessed by cartilage tissue texture and would include repair from cartilage edema where the cartilage is softer and weaker and from cartilage sclerosis where the cartilage is firmer and more brittle. Knee cartilage edema, at least of superficial cartilage follows commonly in professional athletes and from acute traumatic injury [149, 150]. As noted above, in the patella where it may affect a broad domain within mid-cartilage, this is commonly termed "chondromalacia." In OA, cartilage matrix "sclerosis" may follow formation of excess collagen as microscar tissue in defects and around chondrons. Alternatively, cartilage may be firmer as a result of amyloid infiltration or calcium pyrophosphate dihydrate (CPPD) or apatite crystal deposition or very rarely, ochronosis [151–154].

A decreased functional state may be associated with chondrocyte death (necrosis) as commonly occurs in RA or superficial cartilage in OA. An age-related imbalance in reactive oxygen species (ROS includes superoxide, hydrogen peroxide, the reactive nitrogen species nitric oxide, and the nitric oxide derived product peroxynitrite) production relative to the anti-oxidant capacity of chondrocytes plays a role in cartilage degradation as well as chondrocyte cell death [155]. Excess levels of these ROS cause oxidative damage and, more importantly, disruption in cell signaling pathways. Chondrocyte death is identified by the absence of chondrocytes within the chondron or, prior to cell resorption, by the presence of chondrocytes with a cell membrane "ghost" and with nucleus devoid of basophilic staining [101]. Chondrocyte death has the effect of changing cartilage matrix into a nonadaptive less functional material subject to development of cracks (including fibrillation, cleft formation), fragmentation, and erosion by usual mechanical forces. More subtle loss of cartilage function may be associated with pigment deposition related to oxidized lipids or dehydration both commonly but not inevitably associated with cartilage aging [156, 157]. Cartilage dysfunction related to dehydration or endogenous infiltrates and deposits such as amyloid and calcium crystals are not yet amenable to repair, but reparative strategies are possible. The successful example is monosodium urate crystal deposition (gout) where following removal of urate crystals by drug therapy, cartilage repair can ensue [158, 159].

It was commonly taught that hyaline articular cartilage is incapable of repair and that injured cartilage cannot be restored to hyaline cartilage (regeneration). Both concepts are demonstrably wrong. Cartilage repair takes place by one or more of three processes, each with its own features and limitations: repair from adjacent native cartilage, repair from subjacent bone or adjacent soft tissue, and, more recently, repair from graft tissue inserted into cartilage defects. Under some conditions, OA cartilage after an extended period of passive motion exercise such as on a stationary bicycle or experimentally under insulin-like growth factor-1 (IGF-1) stimulation can show chondrocyte replication at the edge of the defect and hyaline matrix regeneration with collagen type II [160]. This process rarely is extensive and therefore repair is incomplete. This limitation arises because cartilage matrix is impermeable to large molecules. Accordingly, enzyme inhibitors formed on the chondrocyte surfaces can migrate only slightly into the surrounding matrix [161]. These inhibitors protect the cartilage matrix from proteolytic enzyme degradation, a process necessary for chondrocytes to activate replication and extensive new collagenous matrix formation. This reparative cartilage may be hyaline or fibrocartilage depending on local ambient conditions. Similarly, connective tissue can generate hyaline cartilage under some conditions, the most well-known human example being synovial chondrometaplasia (synovial chondromatosis) [162, 163].

Cartilage repair derived from subjacent bone is the most common repair process observed. This process begins with migration of less differentiated fibroblastic connective tissue cells from the marrow into the defect. These cells are capable of producing proteolytic enzymes that degrade cartilage matrix at the edge of the defect rendering it capable of adhesion to the matrix generated by the incoming cells. These cells can replicate giving rise to chondrons often containing several small cells and synthesize the ECM usually composed principally of collagen type I and PG. Because collagen type I fibers contain less water than collagen type II, and can form thicker fibers, this reparative tissue is termed fibrocartilage [164]. While fibrocartilage can be easily distinguished from hyaline cartilage using polarized light microscopy, nonetheless its functional properties under some conditions can be adequate. It should be noted that reparative fibrocartilage formation can be facilitated surgically by drilling and microfracture from the base of a cartilage defect into the subchondral bone.

Cartilage repair can be facilitated or accelerated by surgical insertion of grafts containing autologous or allogenic chondrocytes (refer to Chap. 11 for detail of these procedures). Allogenic cartilage grafts now have a clinical practice history of more than 40 years and are known to survive with viable chondrocytes for more than 25 years [165–168]. In these grafts, repair takes place in the subchondral bone, essentially the process of fracture repair and by generation of fibrocartilage at the graft-host cartilage interface. As well chondrocyte replication and PG matrix production organized around existing chondrons can be seen within the hyaline cartilage graft. Typically, graft chondrons containing multiple replicated chondrocytes demonstrate loss of chondron polarity. Similar changes on a smaller scale can be seen with the insertion of cartilage plug grafts as performed during Mosaicplasty or osteochondral autograft transfer system (OATS) [169–173].

More recently, autologous or allogenic chondrocytes embedded in endogenous matrix generated by the cells or placed in exogenous matrices (scaffolds) have been used to repair cartilage defects [62, 173–177]. For details of these procedures, refer to Chaps. 17 and 18. With these grafts, features of successful repair include differentiation and/or maintenance of chondrocyte phenotype, elaboration of matrix with collagen and PG architecture, composition and functional properties similar to normal articular cartilage, orderly replacement of scaffold if present by chondroid matrix, and integration of the graft with the adjacent native cartilage and subchondral bone.

In general, the time for complete graft repair will vary with the size of the graft. In cases of large osteoarticular shell allografts, repair time may extend > 2 years. Graft failure is manifest by graft disruption, graft resorption, neovascularization of adjacent tissues, and extrusion of graft particulates (matrix, scaffold) into the synovial and/or marrow spaces sometimes inciting acute or chronic inflammation. In graft techniques, where the matrix is doped with growth or other regulatory factors, graft failure is sometimes accompanied by excess or insufficiency of reparative tissue or the presence of fibrocytic metaplasia of the graft chondrocytes [178, 179].

15.5 Histologic Evaluation of Cartilage Repair Tissue

In 2003, the International Cartilage Repair Society (ICRS), using consensus methods, developed a Visual Histologic Assessment Scale (VHAS) to evaluate cartilage repair in hyaline cartilage [122]. Following the assessment method of Mankin et al. for OA, VHAS evaluates the following histologic features on a scale of 0–3: surface continuity/discontinuity, matrix tissue composition (hyaline cartilage vs fibrocartilage vs fibrous tissue), chondrocyte organization/distribution, chondrocyte population viability, calcified cartilage mineralization and subchondral bone integrity [113, 122, 123]. While useful for assessing extent of graft failure within grafts, this classification had limited utility to assess graft integration with host cartilage or the biomechanical competence of the graft in vivo. A study was reported pertaining to the relationship of mechanical compression on knee cartilage plugs correlating Young's modulus with ICRS VHAS Grade [135]. Cartilage with ICRS VHAS Grade 3 had 50% less compression resistance as measured by Young's modulus than Grade 1 cartilage. However, these results were not confirmed using dynamic biomechanical testing methods [180]. See Appendix D for ICRS histological assessment of cartilage repair.

Further extensive histologic studies with biochemical and biomechanical correlation using human knee articular cartilage demonstrated that tensile strength and biochemical properties were decreased even with minor histologic change such as SZ fibrillation [181]. This suggests that even slight morphologic changes can represent significant deterioration of mechanical properties. Cell viability, apoptosis, and necrosis play an important role in understanding various processes including early development to aging, acute injury, and in disease [182]. Including these criteria in the assessment of healthy and diseased cartilage as well as post surgical repair tissue is essential.

15.5.1 Meniscal Fibrocartilage

The architecture of meniscal fibrocartilage differs from hyaline cartilage in three important aspects. First, the matrix is composed of collagen type I, which is more fibrillar and less hydrated than collagen type II of hyaline cartilage. Second, the outer portions of the meniscus are vascularized. Third, meniscal fibrocartilage is innervated and contains proprioceptors. Therefore, the meniscus is intrinsically more capable of repair than hyaline articular cartilage. However, in practice, this is not usually the case probably related to mechanical instability of portions of the injured meniscus. As with hyaline cartilage, numerous techniques are available to promote endogenous repair or supply graft cells/tissue [183–190]. Histologic evaluation of meniscal repair involves assessment of the integrity of the repaired meniscus, for example, the graft-host interface, the viability of meniscal cells, and the anchoring of the meniscus to the edge of the joint. Further, completeness of repair can be assessed by the absence of chronic inflammation and by observation that meniscal blood vessel lumina are comparable in diameter to those in normal meniscus. Differentiating distinct types of meniscal pathology, such as MR assessment of meniscal morphologic deformity/extrusion and maceration rather than intrameniscal tear, were shown to be important in determining OA severity and progression [100].

As histologic assessment of cartilage repair is invasive, and under clinical circumstances at best only a portion of a viable graft can be biopsied, it would be desirable to image cartilage repair using radiologic techniques [132, 133, 191, 192]. Presently conventional imaging including MRI cannot distinguish reparative cartilage [133]. Sodium MRI and gadolinium MRI, techniques for imaging fixed ion density as a surrogate for matrix PGs, show promise to distinguish early cartilage repair [193, 194]. However, at present to achieve sufficient resolution of reparative cartilaginous tissue, arthroscopic techniques such as optical coherence tomography and high-frequency ultrasound are required [61, 138].

15.5.2 Cartilage Repair Tissue Evaluation Methods: Problems and Prospects

Presently, although histology is the gold standard to evaluate articular cartilage integrity in injury, disease, and repair, because of clinical reluctance to biopsy articular cartilage, histologic technique has had limited application for evaluation of cartilage repair. This statement also applies to biomechanical studies. Beside insufficient resolution, current imaging modalities cannot reflect the functional state of the reparative tissue compared to normal cartilage. To address this problem, two steps are required.

First, matrix morphologic features need to be identified that are closely associated with cartilage mechanical properties. The architecture, type, and density of collagen is one such feature and might be ultimately assessed by examining intrinsic cartilage fluorescence [72, 195]. Perhaps more promising is quantitative assessment of PG matrix domain density and distribution. Detection of change in fixed charge density by itself is unlikely to provide sufficient resolution. Also promising but farther in the future would be assessment of matrix domains that include volume/density of particular domains in cartilage territorial and interterritorial matrix. Second, noninvasive imaging techniques are required at histologic resolution scales < 30 μm in length. High contrast, high resolution microcomputer tomography is now showing experimentally that imaging of this type is possible [196]. Future work is needed to demonstrate the association of biomechanical properties with microimaging features. In this regard, the close correlation of articular plate bone properties with OA grade and the association of OA cartilage histopathological grade with biomechanical properties are promising [197–199]. When this is achieved, functional imaging and functional histology of cartilage repair will be united as one modality. As this goal is approached, the clinical applications for these techniques not only to visualize but also to monitor cartilage repair will be realized.

15.6 Conclusions

Histologic analysis of knee articular cartilage structure whether by conventional histopathology or by advanced imaging techniques has been the most useful surrogate technique for assessment of the basal functional state of cartilage and the potentiality for repair and regeneration. As much of the mechanical force on the joint is absorbed by bone, this analysis should include the structural state of the subchondral bone plate. While to date, most analyses have been based on two dimensions and usually restricted to one joint surface, to be most useful, future studies should endeavor to develop a quantitative three-dimensional "picture" of the joint including the apposing articular plates. Of necessity, this "picture" will not only involve visualization but also algorithmic mathematical analysis. With these developments, future histopathological evaluation of the health status of knee articular cartilage will be even more clinically useful to determine strategies for cartilage repair that will result in functional improvement or even restoration up to the normal functional state.

References

1. Weichselbaum A. Die senilen Veranderungen der Gelenke und deren Zusammenhang mit der Arthritis deformans. Sit Akad W Math Nat. 1877;75:193–243.
2. Benedek TG. A history of the understanding of cartilage. Osteoarthritis Cartilage. 2006;14(3):203–9.
3. Benninghoff A. Form und Bau der Gelenkknorpel in ihren Beziehungen zur Funktion. Zweiter teil: Der aufbau des gelenkknorpels in seinin beziehungen zur fuction. Z Anat Entwicklungsgesch. 1925;76(1):43–63.
4. Benninghoff A. Form und Bau der Gelenkknorpel in ihren Beziehungen zur Funktion. Z Zellforsch. 1925;2(5):783–862.
5. Bland JH, Cooper SM. Osteoarthritis: a review of the cell biology involved and evidence for reversibility. Management rationally related to known genesis and pathophysiology. Semin Arthritis Rheum. 1984;14(2):106–33.
6. Bland JH. The reversibility of osteoarthritis: a review. Am J Med. 1983;74:16–26.
7. Poole AR. Proteoglycans in health and disease: structures and functions. Biochem J. 1986;236:1–14.
8. Goldring MB, Birkhead J, Sandell LJ, Kimura T, Krane SM. Interleukin 1 suppresses expression of cartilage-specific types II and IX collagens and increases types I and III collagens in human chondrocytes. J Clin Invest. 1988;82:2026–37.
9. Choi HU, Tang LH, Johnson TL, Pal S, Rosenberg LC, Reiner A, Poole AR. Isolation and characterization of a 35,000 molecular weight subunit fetal cartilage matrix protein. J Biol Chem. 1983;258:655–61.
10. Rosenberg LC, Choi HU, Tang LH, Johnson TL, Pal S, Webber C, Reiner A, Poole AR. Isolation of dermatan sulfate proteoglycans from mature bovine articular cartilages. J Biol Chem. 1985;260:6304–13.
11. Dean DD, Woessner JF Jr. Extracts of human articular cartilage contain an inhibitor of tissue metalloproteinases. Biochem J. 1984;218:277–80.
12. Murphy G, Cawston TE, Galloway WA, Barnes MJ, Bunning RA, Mercer E, Reynolds JJ, Burgeson RE. Metalloproteinases from rabbit bone culture medium degrade types IV and V collagens, laminin and fibronectin. Biochem J. 1981;199:807–11.
13. Sellers A, Reynolds JJ, Meikle MC. Neutral metalloproteinases of rabbit bone. Separation in latent forms of distinct enzymes that when activated degrade collagen, gelatin and proteoglycans. Biochem J. 1978;171:493–6.
14. Rhodes RK, Miller EJ. Physicochemical characterization and molecular organization of the collagen A and B chains. Biochemistry. 1978;17:3442–8.
15. Ehrlich MG, Mankin HJ, Jones H, Wright R, Crispen C, Vigliani G. Collagenase and collagenase inhibitors in osteoarthritic and normal cartilage. J Clin Invest. 1977;59:226–33.
16. Sapolsky AI, Keiser H, Howell DS, Woessner JF Jr. Metalloproteases of human articular cartilage that digest cartilage proteoglycan at neutral and acid pH. J Clin Invest. 1976;58:1030–41.
17. Keiser H, DeVito J. Immunochemical studies of fragments of bovine nasal cartilage proteoglycan subunit. Connect Tissue Res. 1974;2:273–82.
18. Hardingham TE, Muir H. The specific interaction of hyaluronic acid with cartilage proteoglycans. Biochim Biophys Acta. 1972;279:401–5.
19. Hardingham TE, Muir H. Binding of oligosaccharides of hyaluronic acid to proteoglycans. Biochem J. 1973;135:905–8.
20. Hardingham TE, Muir H. Hyaluronic acid in cartilage and proteoglycan aggregation. Biochem J. 1974;139:565–81.
21. Atkins ED, Hardingham TE, Isaac DH, Muir H. X-ray fibre diffraction of cartilage proteoglycan aggregates containing hyaluronic acid. Biochem J. 1974;141:919–21.
22. Hardingham TE, Ewins RJ, Muir H. Cartilage proteoglycans. Structure and heterogeneity of the protein core and the effects of specific protein modifications on the binding to hyaluronate. Biochem J. 1976;157:127–43.
23. Nieduszynski IA, Sheehan JK, Phelps CF, Hardingham TE, Muir H. Equilibrium-binding studies of pig laryngeal cartilage proteoglycans with hyaluronate oligosaccharide fractions. Biochem J. 1980;185:107–14.
24. Perkins SJ, Miller A, Hardingham TE, Muir H. Physical properties of the hyaluronate binding region of proteoglycan from pig laryngeal cartilage. Densitometric and small-angle neutron scattering studies of carbohydrates and carbohydrate-protein macromolecules. J Mol Biol. 1981;150:69–95.
25. Hardingham TE, Perkins SJ, Muir H. Molecular conformations in proteoglycan aggregation. Biochem Soc Trans. 1983;11(Pt 2):128–30.
26. Carney SL, Billingham ME, Caterson B, Ratcliffe A, Bayliss MT, Hardingham TE, Muir H. Changes in proteoglycan turnover in experimental canine osteoarthritic cartilage. Matrix. 1992;12:137–47.
27. Strawich E, Nimni ME. Properties of a collagen molecule containing three identical compo-

nents extracted from bovine articular cartilage. Biochemistry. 1971;10:3905–11.
28. Mankin HJ, Lippiello L. The turnover of adult rabbit articular cartilage. J Bone Joint Surg Am. 1969;51:1591–600.
29. McElligott TF, Collins DH. Chondrocyte function of human articular and costal cartilage compared by measuring the in vitro uptake of labelled (35S) sulphate. Ann Rheum Dis. 1960;19:31–41.
30. Little K, Pimm LH, Trueta J. Osteoarthritis of the hip: an electron microscope study. J Bone Joint Surg. 1958;40-B:123–31.
31. Fawns HT, Landells JW. Histochemical studies of rheumatic conditions. I. Observations on the fine structures of the matrix of normal bone and cartilage. Ann Rheum Dis. 1953;12:105–13.
32. Mac CM. The movements of bones and joints; the mechanical structure of articulating cartilage. J Bone Joint Surg. 1951;33B:251–7.
33. Takada N, Wada I, Sugimura I, Sakuma E, Maruyama H, Matsui N. A possible barrier function of the articular surface, Kaibogaku zasshi. J Anat. 1999;74:631–7.
34. Asari A, Miyauchi S, Kuriyama S, Machida A, Kohno K, Uchiyama Y. Localization of hyaluronic acid in human articular cartilage. J Histochem Cytochem. 1994;42:513–22.
35. Jeffery AK, Blunn GW, Archer CW, Bentley G. Three-dimensional collagen architecture in bovine articular cartilage. J Bone Joint Surg. 1991;73:795–801.
36. Duance VC. Surface of articular cartilage: immunohistological studies. Cell Biochem Funct. 1983;1:143–4.
37. Lane JM, Weiss C. Review of articular cartilage collagen research. Arthritis Rheum. 1975;18:553–62.
38. Mankin HJ. The reaction of articular cartilage to injury and osteoarthritis (second of two parts). N Engl J Med. 1974;291:1335–40.
39. Mankin HJ. The reaction of articular cartilage to injury and osteoarthritis (first of two parts). N Engl J Med. 1974;291:1285–92.
40. McDevitt CA. Biochemistry of articular cartilage. Nature of proteoglycans and collagen of articular cartilage and their role in ageing and in osteoarthrosis. Ann Rheum Dis. 1973;32:364–78.
41. Clarke IC. Articular cartilage: a review and scanning electron microscope study. 1. The interterritorial fibrillar architecture. J Bone Joint Surg. 1971;53:732–50.
42. Clarke IC. Articular cartilage: a review and scanning electron microscope study. II. The territorial fibrillar architecture. J Anat. 1974;118:261–80.
43. Silberberg R. Ultrastructure of articular cartilage in health and disease. Clin Orthop Relat Res. 1968;57:233–57.
44. Hamerman D, Rosenberg LC, Schubert M. Diarthrodial joints revisited. J Bone Joint Surg Am. 1970;52:725–74.
45. Hamerman D, Schubert M. Diarthrodial joints, an essay. Am J Med. 1962;33:555–90.
46. Slack HG. Some notes on the composition and metabolism of connective tissue. Am J Med. 1959;26:113–24.
47. Davidson E, Hoffman P, Linker A, Meyer K. The acid mucopolysaccharides of connective tissue. Biochim Biophys Acta. 1956;21:506–18.
48. de Bont LG, Liem RS, Havinga P, Boering G, van der Korst J. Collagenous network in cartilage of human femoral condyles. A light microscopic and scanning electron microscopic study. Acta Anat. 1986;126:41–7.
49. Miyatake K, Iwasa K, McNary SM, Peng G, Reddi AH. Modulation of superficial zone protein/lubricin/PRG4 by kartogenin and transforming growth factor-beta1 in surface zone chondrocytes in bovine articular cartilage. Cartilage. 2016;7:388–97.
50. Engen CN, Loken S, Aroen A, Ho C, Engebretsen L. No degeneration found in focal cartilage defects evaluated with dGEMRIC at 12-year follow-up. Acta Orthop. 2017;88:82–9.
51. Stone KR, Pelsis JR, Na K, Walgenbach AW, Turek TJ. Articular cartilage paste graft for severe osteochondral lesions of the knee: a 10- to 23-year follow-up study. Knee Surg Sports Traumatol Arthrosc. 2017;25:3824–33.
52. Anderson DE, Williams RJ 3rd, DeBerardino TM, Taylor DC, Ma CB, Kane MS, Crawford DC. Magnetic resonance imaging characterization and clinical outcomes after NeoCart surgical therapy as a primary reparative treatment for knee cartilage injuries. Am J Sports Med. 2017;45:875–83.
53. Van Rossom S, Smith CR, Zevenbergen L, Thelen DG, Vanwanseele B, Van Assche D, Jonkers I. Knee cartilage thickness, T1rho and T2 relaxation time are related to articular cartilage loading in healthy adults. PLoS One 2017;12(1):e0170002. eCollection 2017.
54. Garnero P, Rousseau JC, Delmas PD. Molecular basis and clinical use of biochemical markers of bone, cartilage, and synovium in joint diseases. Arthritis Rheum. 2000;43(5):953–68.
55. Lee SY, Nakagawa T, Reddi AH. Mesenchymal progenitor cells derived from synovium and infrapatellar fat pad as a source for superficial zone cartilage tissue engineering: analysis of superficial zone protein/lubricin expression. Tissue Eng Part A. 2010;16(1):317–25.
56. Wu JP, Kirk TB, Zheng MH. Study of the collagen structure in the superficial zone and physiological state of articular cartilage using a 3D confocal imaging technique. J Orthop Surg Res. 2008;3:29.
57. Hollander AP, Dickinson SC, Kafienah W. Stem cells and cartilage development: complexities of a simple tissue. Stem Cells. 2010;28:1992–6.
58. Kumar P, Oka M, Toguchida J, Kobayashi M, Uchida E, Nakamura T, Tanaka K. Role of uppermost super-

ficial surface layer of articular cartilage in the lubrication mechanism of joints. J Anat. 2001;199:241–50.
59. Fujioka R, Aoyama T, Takakuwa T. The layered structure of the articular surface. Osteoarthritis Cartilage. 2013;21:1092–8.
60. Nagel T, Kelly DJ. The composition of engineered cartilage at the time of implantation determines the likelihood of regenerating tissue with a normal collagen architecture. Tissue Eng Part A. 2013;19:824–33.
61. Chu CR, Izzo NJ, Irrgang JJ, Ferretti M, Studer RK. Clinical diagnosis of potentially treatable early articular cartilage degeneration using optical coherence tomography. J Biomed Opt. 2007;12:051703.
62. Ahmed TA, Hincke MT. Mesenchymal stem cell-based tissue engineering strategies for repair of articular cartilage. Histol Histopathol. 2014;29:669–89.
63. Charlier E, Relic B, Deroyer C, Malaise O, Neuville S, Collee J, Malaise MG, De Seny D. Insights on molecular mechanisms of chondrocytes death in osteoarthritis. Int J Mol Sci. 2016;17:pii: E2146.
64. Speziali A, Delcogliano M, Tei M, Placella G, Chillemi M, Tiribuzi R, Cerulli G. Chondropenia: current concept review. Musculoskelet Surg. 2015;99:189–200.
65. Spector TD, MacGregor AJ. Risk factors for osteoarthritis: genetics. Osteoarthritis Cartilage. 2004;12(Suppl A):S39–44.
66. Corti MC, Rigon C. Epidemiology of osteoarthritis: prevalence, risk factors and functional impact. Aging Clin Exp Res. 2003;15:359–63.
67. Loughlin J. The genetic epidemiology of human primary osteoarthritis: current status. Expert Rev Mol Med. 2005;7:1–12.
68. Zhang Y, Jordan JM. Epidemiology of osteoarthritis. Clin Geriatr Med. 2010;26:355–69.
69. Papavasiliou KA, Kenanidis EI, Potoupnis ME, Kapetanou A, Sayegh FE. Participation in athletic activities may be associated with later development of hip and knee osteoarthritis. Phys Sportsmed. 2011;39:51–9.
70. Panoutsopoulou K, Zeggini E. Advances in osteoarthritis genetics. J Med Genet. 2013;50:715–24.
71. Yucesoy B, Charles LE, Baker B, Burchfiel CM. Occupational and genetic risk factors for osteoarthritis: a review. Work. 2015;50:261–73.
72. Kutsuna T, Sato M, Ishihara M, Furukawa KS, Nagai T, Kikuchi M, Ushida T, Mochida J. Noninvasive evaluation of tissue-engineered cartilage with time-resolved laser-induced fluorescence spectroscopy. Tissue Eng Part C Methods. 2010;16:365–73.
73. Zbyn S, Mlynarik V, Juras V, Szomolanyi P, Trattnig S. Evaluation of cartilage repair and osteoarthritis with sodium MRI. NMR Biomed. 2016;29:206–15.
74. Crossley KM, Callaghan MJ, van Linschoten R. Patellofemoral pain. Br J Sports Med 2016;50(4):247–250.
75. Habusta SF, Griffin EE. Chondromalacia patella. StatPearls [Internet]. Treasure Island (FL): StatPearls Publishing; 2019.
76. Habusta SF, Griffin EE. Chondromalacia Patella. StatPearls [Internet]. StatPearls Publishing, Treasure Island (FL). 2018.
77. Hong E, Kraft MC. Evaluating anterior knee pain. Med Clin North Am. 2014;98(4):697–717.
78. Harris ED Jr. Rheumatoid arthritis. Pathophysiology and implications for therapy. N Engl J Med. 1990;322:1277–89.
79. Mitchell DM. Rheumatoid arthritis. In: Utsinger PD, Zvaifler NJ, Ehrlich GE, editors. Rheumatoid arthritis: etiology, diagnosis and treatment. Philadelphia: JB Lippincott; 1985. p. 133–50.
80. Sangha O. Epidemiology of rheumatic diseases. Rheumatology (Oxford). 2000;39(Suppl 2):3–12.
81. Cross M, Smith E, Hoy D, Nolte S, Ackerman I, Fransen M, Bridgett L, Williams S, Guillemin F, Hill CL, Laslett LL, Jones G, Cicuttini F, Osborne R, Vos T, Buchbinder R, Woolf A, March L. The global burden of hip and knee osteoarthritis: estimates from the global burden of disease 2010 study. Ann Rheum Dis. 2014;73:1323–30.
82. Jeon OH, David N, Campisi J, Elisseeff JH. Senescent cells and osteoarthritis: a painful connection. J Clin Invest. 2018;128(4):1229–37.
83. Ackerman IN, Kemp JL, Crossley KM, Culvenor AG, Hinman RS. Hip and knee osteoarthritis affects younger people, too. J Orthop Sports Phys Ther. 2017;47:67–79.
84. Gushue DL, Houck J, Lerner AL. Effects of childhood obesity on three-dimensional knee joint biomechanics during walking. J Pediatr Orthop. 2005;25:763–8.
85. Johnson VL, Roe JP, Salmon LJ, Pinczewski LA, Hunter DJ. Does age influence the risk of incident knee osteoarthritis after a traumatic anterior cruciate ligament injury? Am J Sports Med. 2016;44:2399–405.
86. Lattermann C, Jacobs CA, Proffitt Bunnell M, Huston LJ, Gammon LG, Johnson DL, Reinke EK, Huebner JL, Kraus VB, Spindler KP. A multicenter study of early anti-inflammatory treatment in patients with acute anterior cruciate ligament tear. Am J Sports Med. 2017;45:325–33.
87. Pamukoff DN, Lewek MD, Blackburn JT. Greater vertical loading rate in obese compared to normal weight young adults. Clin Biomech (Bristol, Avon). 2016;33:61–5.
88. Toomey CM, Whittaker JL, Nettel-Aguirre A, Reimer RA, Woodhouse LJ, Ghali B, Doyle-Baker PK, Emery CA. Higher fat mass is associated with a history of knee injury in youth sport. J Orthop Sports Phys Ther. 2017;47:80–7.
89. Whittaker JL, Woodhouse LJ, Nettel-Aguirre A, Emery CA. Outcomes associated with early post-traumatic osteoarthritis and other negative health consequences 3-10 years following knee joint

injury in youth sport. Osteoarthritis Cartilage. 2015;23:1122–9.
90. Pihl K, Englund M, Lohmander LS, Jorgensen U, Nissen N, Schjerning J, Thorlund JB. Signs of knee osteoarthritis common in 620 patients undergoing arthroscopic surgery for meniscal tear. Acta Orthop. 2017;88:90–5.
91. Francisco V, Pérez T, Pino J, López V, Franco E, Alonso A, Gonzalez-Gay MA, Mera A, Lago F, Gómez R, Gualillo O. Biomechanics, obesity, and osteoarthritis. The role of adipokines: When the levee breaks. J Orthop Res. 2018;36(2):594–604.
92. Hunter DJ, March L, Sambrook PN. Knee osteoarthritis: the influence of environmental factors. Clin Exp Rheumatol. 2002;20:93–100.
93. Wearing SC, Hennig EM, Byrne NM, Steele JR, Hills AP. Musculoskeletal disorders associated with obesity: a biomechanical perspective. Obes Rev. 2006;7:239–50.
94. Wang ZW, Chen L, Hao XR, Qu ZA, Huang SB, et al. Elevated levels of interleukin-1β, interleukin-6, tumor necrosis factor-α and vascular endothelial growth factor in patients with knee articular cartilage injury. World J Clin Cases. 2019;7(11):1262–69.
95. Mahon OR, Dunne A. Disease-Associated Particulates and Joint Inflammation; Mechanistic Insights and Potential Therapeutic Targets. Front Immunol. 2018;9:1145. https://doi.org/10.3389/fimmu.2018.01145. eCollection 2018.
96. Zhou Y, Liu SQ, Yu L, He B, SH W, Zhao Q, Xia SQ, Mei HJ. Berberine prevents nitric oxide-induced rat chondrocyte apoptosis and cartilage degeneration in a rat osteoarthritis model via AMPK and p38 MAPK signaling. Apoptosis. 2015;20:1187–99.
97. Jang D, Murrell GAC. Nitric oxide in arthritis. Free Radic Biol Med. 1998;24(9):1511–9.
98. Prince DE, Greisberg JK. Nitric oxide-associated chondrocyte apoptosis in trauma patients after high-energy lower extremity intraarticular fractures. J Orthop Traumatol. 2015;16(4):335–41.
99. Kurz B, Lemke AK, Fay J, Pufe T, Grodzinsky AJ, Schünke M. Pathomechanisms of cartilage destruction by mechanical injury. Ann Anat. 2005;187(5-6):473–85.
100. Wyatt LA, Moreton BJ, Mapp PI, Wilson D, Hill R, Ferguson E, Scammell BE, Walsh DA. Histopathological subgroups in knee osteoarthritis. Osteoarthritis Cartilage. 2017;25:14–22.
101. Pritzker KP, Gay S, Jimenez SA, Ostergaard K, Pelletier JP, Revell PA, Salter D, van den Berg WB. Osteoarthritis cartilage histopathology: grading and staging. Osteoarthritis Cartilage. 2006;14:13–29.
102. Seidenstuecker M, Watrinet J, Bernstein A, Suedkamp NP, Latorre SH, et al. Viscoelasticity and histology of the human cartilage in healthy and degenerated conditions of the knee. J Orthop Surg Res. 2019;14(1):256.
103. Vaatainen U, Hakkinen T, Kiviranta I, Jaroma H, Inkinen R, Tammi M. Proteoglycan depletion and size reduction in lesions of early grade chondromalacia of the patella. Ann Rheum Dis. 1995;54:831–5.
104. Tchetina EV, Squires G, Poole AR. Increased type II collagen degradation and very early focal cartilage degeneration is associated with upregulation of chondrocyte differentiation related genes in early human articular cartilage lesions. J Rheumatol. 2005;32:876–86.
105. Bollet AJ, Nance JL. Biochemical findings in normal and osteoarthritic articular cartilage. II. Chondroitin sulfate concentration and chain length, water, and ash content. J Clin Invest. 1966;45:1170–7.
106. Brocklehurst R, Bayliss MT, Maroudas A, Coysh HL, Freeman MA, Revell PA, Ali SY. The composition of normal and osteoarthritic articular cartilage from human knee joints. With special reference to unicompartmental replacement and osteotomy of the knee. J Bone Joint Surg Am. 1984;66:95–106.
107. Grushko G, Schneiderman R, Maroudas A. Some biochemical and biophysical parameters for the study of the pathogenesis of osteoarthritis: a comparison between the processes of ageing and degeneration in human hip cartilage. Connect Tissue Res. 1989;19:149–76.
108. Mankin HJ, Thrasher AZ. Water content and binding in normal and osteoarthritic human cartilage. J Bone Joint Surg Am. 1975;57:76–80.
109. Maroudas A, Venn M. Chemical composition and swelling of normal and osteoarthrotic femoral head cartilage. II. Swelling. Ann Rheum Dis. 1977;36:399–406.
110. Hui Mingalone CK, Liu Z, Hollander JM, Garvey KD, Gibson AL, Banks RE, Zhang M, McAlindon TE, Nielsen HC, Georgakoudi I, Zeng L. Bioluminescence and second harmonic generation imaging reveal dynamic changes in the inflammatory and collagen landscape in early osteoarthritis. Lab Invest. 2018;98(5):656–69.
111. MacFarlane LA, Yang H, Collins JE, Jarraya M, Guermazi A, et al. Association of changes in effusion-synovitis with progression of cartilage damage over eighteen months in patients with osteoarthritis and meniscal tear. Arthritis Rheumatol. 2019;71(1):73–81.
112. Ito Y, Sanyal A, Fitzsimmons JS, Mello MA, O'Driscoll SW. Histomorphological and proliferative characterization of developing periosteal neochondrocytes in vitro. J Orthop Res. 2001;19:405–13.
113. Mankin HJ, Dorfman H, Lippiello L, Zarins A. Biochemical and metabolic abnormalities in articular cartilage from osteo-arthritic human hips. II. Correlation of morphology with biochemical and metabolic data. J Bone Joint Surg Am. 1971;53:523–37.
114. O'Driscoll SW, Marx RG, Beaton DE, Miura Y, Gallay SH, Fitzsimmons JS. Validation of a simple histological-histochemical cartilage scoring system. Tissue Eng. 2001;7:313–20.

115. O'Driscoll SW, Marx RG, Fitzsimmons JS, Beaton DE. Method for automated cartilage histomorphometry. Tissue Eng. 1999;5:13–23.
116. O'Driscoll SW, Saris DB, Ito Y, Fitzimmons JS. The chondrogenic potential of periosteum decreases with age. J Orthop Res. 2001;19:95–103.
117. Ostergaard K, Andersen CB, Petersen J, Bendtzen K, Salter DM. Validity of histopathological grading of articular cartilage from osteoarthritic knee joints. Ann Rheum Dis. 1999;58:208–13.
118. Ostergaard K, Petersen J, Andersen CB, Bendtzen K, Salter DM. Histologic/histochemical grading system for osteoarthritic articular cartilage: reproducibility and validity. Arthritis Rheum. 1997;40:1766–71.
119. Pearson RG, Kurien T, Shu KS, Scammell BE. Histopathology grading systems for characterisation of human knee osteoarthritis--reproducibility, variability, reliability, correlation, and validity. Osteoarthritis Cartilage. 2011;19:324–31.
120. Rutgers M, van Pelt MJ, Dhert WJ, Creemers LB, Saris DB. Evaluation of histological scoring systems for tissue-engineered, repaired and osteoarthritic cartilage. Osteoarthritis Cartilage. 2010;18:12–23.
121. Laverty S, Girard CA, Williams JM, Hunziker EB, Pritzker KP. The OARSI histopathology initiative - recommendations for histological assessments of osteoarthritis in the rabbit. Osteoarthritis Cartilage. 2010;18(Suppl 3):S53–65.
122. Mainil-Varlet P, Aigner T, Brittberg M, Bullough P, Hollander A, Hunziker E, Kandel R, Nehrer S, Pritzker K, Roberts S, Stauffer E, International Cartilage Repair S. Histological assessment of cartilage repair: a report by the Histology Endpoint Committee of the International Cartilage Repair Society (ICRS). J Bone Joint Surg Am. 2003;85-A(Suppl 2):45–57.
123. Mainil-Varlet P, Van Damme B, Nesic D, Knutsen G, Kandel R, Roberts S. A new histology scoring system for the assessment of the quality of human cartilage repair: ICRS II. Am J Sports Med. 2010;38:880–90.
124. Pritzker KP, Aigner T. Terminology of osteoarthritis cartilage and bone histopathology - a proposal for a consensus. Osteoarthritis Cartilage. 2010;18(Suppl 3):S7–9.
125. Bonasia DE, Marmotti A, Massa AD, Ferro A, Blonna D, Castoldi F, Rossi R. Intra- and inter-observer reliability of ten major histological scoring systems used for the evaluation of in vivo cartilage repair. Knee Surg Sports Traumatol Arthrosc. 2015;23:2484–93.
126. Pauli C, Whiteside R, Heras FL, Nesic D, Koziol J, Grogan SP, Matyas J, Pritzker KP, D'Lima DD, Lotz MK. Comparison of cartilage histopathology assessment systems on human knee joints at all stages of osteoarthritis development. Osteoarthritis Cartilage. 2012;20:476–85.
127. Longo UG, Forriol F, Maffulli N, Denaro V. Evaluation of histological scoring systems for tissue-engineered, repaired and osteoarthritic cartilage. Osteoarthritis Cartilage. 2010;18:12–23.
128. Roemer FW, Hunter DJ, Crema MD, Kwoh CK, Ochoa-Albiztegui E, Guermazi A. An illustrative overview of semi-quantitative MRI scoring of knee osteoarthritis: lessons learned from longitudinal observational studies. Osteoarthritis Cartilage. 2016;24:274–89.
129. Alizai H, Virayavanich W, Joseph GB, Nardo L, Liu F, Liebl H, Nevitt MC, Lynch JA, McCulloch CE, Link TM. Cartilage lesion score: comparison of a quantitative assessment score with established semiquantitative MR scoring systems. Radiology. 2014;271:479–87.
130. Hunter DJ, Lo GH, Gale D, Grainger AJ, Guermazi A, Conaghan PG. The reliability of a new scoring system for knee osteoarthritis MRI and the validity of bone marrow lesion assessment: BLOKS (Boston Leeds Osteoarthritis Knee Score). Ann Rheum Dis. 2008;67:206–11.
131. Grogan SP, Barbero A, Winkelmann V, Rieser F, Fitzsimmons JS, O'Driscoll S, Martin I, Mainil-Varlet P. Visual histological grading system for the evaluation of in vitro-generated neocartilage. Tissue Eng. 2006;12:2141–9.
132. Zilkens C, Miese FR, Crumbiegel C, Kim YJ, Herten M, Antoch G, Krauspe R, Bittersohl B. Magnetic resonance imaging and histology of ovine hip joint cartilage in two age populations: a sheep model with assumed healthy cartilage. Skelet Radiol. 2013;42:699–705.
133. Baum T, Joseph GB, Karampinos DC, Jungmann PM, Link TM, Bauer JS. Cartilage and meniscal T2 relaxation time as non-invasive biomarker for knee osteoarthritis and cartilage repair procedures. Osteoarthritis Cartilage. 2013;21:1474–84.
134. Mannicke N, Schone M, Oelze M, Raum K. Articular cartilage degeneration classification by means of high-frequency ultrasound. Osteoarthritis Cartilage. 2014;22:1577–82.
135. Kleemann RU, Krocker D, Cedraro A, Tuischer J, Duda GN. Altered cartilage mechanics and histology in knee osteoarthritis: relation to clinical assessment (ICRS Grade). Osteoarthritis Cartilage. 2005;13:958–63.
136. Gahunia HK, Babyn P, Lemaire C, Kessler MJ, Pritzker KP. Osteoarthritis staging: comparison between magnetic resonance imaging, gross pathology and histopathology in the rhesus macaque. Osteoarthritis Cartilage. 1995;3:169–80.
137. Custers RJ, Creemers LB, Verbout AJ, van Rijen MH, Dhert WJ, Saris DB. Reliability, reproducibility and variability of the traditional Histologic/Histochemical Grading System vs the new OARSI Osteoarthritis Cartilage Histopathology

Assessment System. Osteoarthritis Cartilage. 2007;15:1241–8.
138. Chu CR, Williams A, Tolliver D, Kwoh CK, Bruno S 3rd, Irrgang JJ. Clinical optical coherence tomography of early articular cartilage degeneration in patients with degenerative meniscal tears. Arthritis Rheum. 2010;62:1412–20.
139. Mankin HJ, Lippiello L. Biochemical and metabolic abnormalities in articular cartilage from osteo-arthritic human hips. J Bone Joint Surg Am. 1970;52:424–34.
140. Saarakkala S, Julkunen P, Kiviranta P, Makitalo J, Jurvelin JS, Korhonen RK. Depth-wise progression of osteoarthritis in human articular cartilage: investigation of composition, structure and biomechanics. Osteoarthritis Cartilage. 2010;18:73–81.
141. Aigner T, Cook JL, Gerwin N, Glasson SS, Laverty S, Little CB, McIlwraith W, Kraus VB. Histopathology atlas of animal model systems - overview of guiding principles. Osteoarthritis Cartilage. 2010;18(Suppl 3):S2–6.
142. Pritzker KP. Animal models for osteoarthritis: processes, problems and prospects. Ann Rheum Dis. 1994;53:406–20.
143. Cook JL, Hung CT, Kuroki K, Stoker AM, Cook CR, Pfeiffer FM, Sherman SL, Stannard JP. Animal models of cartilage repair. Bone Joint Res. 2014;3:89–94.
144. Tang C, Jin C, Li X, Li J, Du X, et al. Evaluation of an autologous bone mesenchymal stem cell-derived extracellular matrix scaffold in a Rabbit and Minipig model of cartilage repair. Med Sci Monit. 2019;25:7342–50.
145. Azizi S, Farsinejad A, Kheirandish R, Fatemi H. Intra-articular effects of combined xenogenous serum rich in growth factors (SRGF) and vitamin C on histopathology grading and staging of osteoarthritis in rat model. Transfus Clin Biol. 2019;26(1):3–9.
146. Domínguez Pérez JM, Fernández-Sarmiento JA, Aguilar García D, Granados Machuca MDM, Morgaz Rodríguez J, et al. Cartilage regeneration using a novel autologous growth factors-based matrix for full-thickness defects in sheep. Knee Surg Sports Traumatol Arthrosc. 2019;27(3):950–61.
147. Chen FS, Frenkel SR, Di Cesare PE. Repair of articular cartilage defects: part I. Basic Science of cartilage healing. Am J Orthop (Belle Mead NJ). 1999;28:31–3.
148. Frenkel SR, Di Cesare PE. Degradation and repair of articular cartilage. Front Biosci. 1999;4:D671–85.
149. Behzadi C, Welsch GH, Laqmani A, Henes FO, Kaul MG, Schoen G, Adam G, Regier M. Comparison of T2* relaxation times of articular cartilage of the knee in elite professional football players and age- and BMI-matched amateur athletes. Eur J Radiol. 2017;86:105–11.
150. Peers SC, Maerz T, Baker EA, Shetty A, Xia Y, Puwal S, Marcantonio D, Keyes D, Guettler J. T1ρ magnetic resonance imaging for detection of early cartilage changes in knees of asymptomatic collegiate female impact and nonimpact athletes. Clin J Sport Med. 2014;24(3):218–25.
151. Bywaters EG, Dorling J. Amyloid deposits in articular cartilage. Ann Rheum Dis. 1970;29:294–306.
152. Athanasou NA, Sallie B. Localized deposition of amyloid in articular cartilage. Histopathology. 1992;20:41–6.
153. Di Franco M, Coari G, Bonucci E. A morphological study of bone and articular cartilage in ochronosis. Virchows Arch. 2000;436:74–81.
154. Pritzker KP. Articular pathology of gout, calcium pyrophosphate dihydrate, and basic calcium phosphate crystal deposition arthropathies. In: Terkeltaub R, editor. Gout & other crystal arthropathies. Philadelphia: Elsevier, Saunders; 2012. p. 1–19.
155. Bolduc JA, Collins JA, Loeser RF. Reactive oxygen species, aging and articular cartilage homeostasis. Free Radic Biol Med. 2018; https://doi.org/10.1016/j.freeradbiomed.2018.08.038. Epub ahead of print.
156. van der Korst JK, Willekens FL, Lansink AG, Henrichs AM. Age-associated glycopeptide pigment in human costal cartilage. Am J Pathol. 1977;89:605–20.
157. Tsukahara Y, Nasu T. Ceroid-like pigment in age changes of human cartilage. Acta Pathol Jpn. 1974;24:357–69.
158. Das S, Goswami RP, Ghosh A, Ghosh P, Lahiri D, Basu K. Temporal evolution of urate crystal deposition over articular cartilage after successful urate-lowering therapy in patients with gout: an ultras onographic perspective. Mod Rheumatol. 2017;27(3):518–23.
159. Thiele RG, Schlesinger N. Ultrasonography shows disappearance of monosodium urate crystal deposition on hyaline cartilage after sustained normouricemia is achieved. Rheumatol Int. 2010;30(4):495–503.
160. Davies LC, Blain EJ, Gilbert SJ, Caterson B, Duance VC. The potential of IGF-1 and TGFbeta1 for promoting "adult" articular cartilage repair: an in vitro study. Tissue Eng Part A. 2008;14:1251–61.
161. Eisenstein R, Kuettner KE, Neapolitan C, Soble LW, Sorgente N. The resistance of certain tissues to invasion. III. Cartilage extracts inhibit the growth of fibroblasts and endothelial cells in culture. Am J Pathol. 1975;81:337–48.
162. Crawford MD, Kim HT. New-onset synovial chondromatosis after total knee arthroplasty. J Arthroplasty. 2013;28(375):e371–4.
163. Bozkurt M, Ugurlu M, Dogan M, Tosun N. Synovial chondromatosis of four compartments of the knee: medial and lateral tibiofemoral spaces, patellofemo-

ral joint and proximal tibiofibular joint. Knee Surg Sports Traumatol Arthrosc. 2007;15:753–5.
164. Grynpas MD, Eyre DR, Kirschner DA. Collagen type II differs from type I in native molecular packing. Biochim Biophys Acta. 1980;626:346–55.
165. Czitrom AA. Allograft reconstruction after tumor surgery in the appendicular skeleton. In: Czitrom AA, Gross AE, editors. Allografts in orthopaedic practice. Baltimore: Williams & Wilkins; 1992. p. 83–119.
166. McGoveran BM, Pritzker KP, Shasha N, Price J, Gross AE. Long-term chondrocyte viability in a fresh osteochondral allograft. J Knee Surg. 2002;15:97–100.
167. Pritzker KP, Gross AE, Langer F, Luk SC, Houpt JB. Articular cartilage transplantation. Hum Pathol. 1977;8:635–51.
168. Sherman SL, Garrity J, Bauer K, Cook J, Stannard J, Bugbee W. Fresh osteochondral allograft transplantation for the knee: current concepts. J Am Acad Orthop Surg. 2014;22:121–33.
169. Robert H. Chondral repair of the knee joint using mosaicplasty. Orthop Traumatol Surg Res. 2011;97:418–29.
170. Ulstein S, Aroen A, Rotterud JH, Loken S, Engebretsen L, Heir S. Microfracture technique versus osteochondral autologous transplantation mosaicplasty in patients with articular chondral lesions of the knee: a prospective randomized trial with long-term follow-up. Knee Surg Sports Traumatol Arthrosc. 2014;22:1207–15.
171. Goyal D, Keyhani S, Goyal A, Lee EH, Hui JH, Vaziri AS. Evidence-based status of osteochondral cylinder transfer techniques: a systematic review of level I and II studies. Arthroscopy. 2014;30:497–505.
172. Quarch VM, Enderle E, Lotz J, Frosch KH. Fate of large donor site defects in osteochondral transfer procedures in the knee joint with and without TruFit plugs. Arch Orthop Trauma Surg. 2014;134:657–66.
173. Anderson JA, Little D, Toth AP, Moorman CT 3rd, Tucker BS, Ciccotti MG, Guilak F. Stem cell therapies for knee cartilage repair: the current status of preclinical and clinical studies. Am J Sports Med. 2014;42:2253–61.
174. Jeon JE, Vaquette C, Klein TJ, Hutmacher DW. Perspectives in multiphasic osteochondral tissue engineering. Anat Rec (Hoboken). 2014;297:26–35.
175. Lee JK, Responte DJ, Cissell DD, JC H, Nolta JA, Athanasiou KA. Clinical translation of stem cells: insight for cartilage therapies. Crit Rev Biotechnol. 2014;34:89–100.
176. Lopa S, Madry H. Bioinspired scaffolds for osteochondral regeneration. Tissue Eng Part A. 2014;20:2052–76.
177. Orth P, Rey-Rico A, Venkatesan JK, Madry H, Cucchiarini M. Current perspectives in stem cell research for knee cartilage repair. Stem Cells Cloning. 2014;7:1–17.
178. Demoor M, Ollitrault D, Gomez-Leduc T, Bouyoucef M, Hervieu M, Fabre H, Lafont J, Denoix JM, Audigie F, Mallein-Gerin F, Legendre F, Galera P. Cartilage tissue engineering: molecular control of chondrocyte differentiation for proper cartilage matrix reconstruction. Biochim Biophys Acta. 2014;1840:2414–40.
179. Lo KW, Jiang T, Gagnon KA, Nelson C, Laurencin CT. Small-molecule based musculoskeletal regenerative engineering. Trends Biotechnol. 2014;32:74–81.
180. Kos P, Varga F, Handl M, Kautzner J, Chudacek V, Drzik M, Povysil C, Trc T, Amler E, Hanus M. Correlation of dynamic impact testing, histopathology and visual macroscopic assessment in human osteoarthritic cartilage. Int Orthop. 2011;35:1733–9.
181. Temple-Wong MM, Bae WC, Chen MQ, Bugbee WD, Amiel D, Coutts RD, Lotz M, Sah RL. Biomechanical, structural, and biochemical indices of degenerative and osteoarthritic deterioration of adult human articular cartilage of the femoral condyle. Osteoarthritis Cartilage. 2009;17:1469–76.
182. Grogan SP, Aklin B, Frenz M, Brunner T, Schaffner T, Mainil-Varlet P. In vitro model for the study of necrosis and apoptosis in native cartilage. J Pathol. 2002;198:5–13.
183. Deponti D, Di Giancamillo A, Scotti C, Peretti GM, Martin I. Animal models for meniscus repair and regeneration. J Tissue Eng Regen Med. 2015;9:512–27.
184. Longo UG, Rizzello G, Berton A, Fumo C, Battaglia G, Khan WS, Denaro V. A review of preclinical and clinical studies using synthetic materials for meniscus replacement. Curr Stem Cell Res Ther. 2013;8:438–43.
185. Scotti C, Hirschmann MT, Antinolfi P, Martin I, Peretti GM. Meniscus repair and regeneration: review on current methods and research potential. Eur Cell Mater. 2013;26:150–70.
186. Ghazi Zadeh L, Chevrier A, Farr J, Rodeo SA, Buschmann MD. Augmentation techniques for meniscus repair. J Knee Surg. 2018;31(1):99–116.
187. Ferrari MB, Murphy CP, Gomes JLE. Meniscus repair in children and adolescents: a systematic review of treatment approaches, meniscal healing, and outcomes. J Knee Surg. 2018; https://doi.org/10.1055/s-0038-1653943. Epub ahead of print.
188. Kaminski R, Kulinski K, Kozar-Kaminska K, Wielgus M, Langner M, Wasko MK, Kowalczewski J, Pomianowski S. A prospective, randomized, double-blind, parallel-group, placebo-controlled study evaluating meniscal healing, clinical outcomes, and safety in patients undergoing meniscal repair of unstable, complete vertical meniscal tears (Bucket

Handle) augmented with platelet-rich plasma. Biomed Res Int. 2018;2018:9315815. eCollection 2018.
189. Bilgen B, Jayasuriya CT, Owens BD. Current concepts in meniscus tissue engineering and repair. Adv Healthc Mater. 2018;7(11):e1701407. Epub 2018.
190. Blake MH, Johnson DL. Knee meniscus injuries: common problems and solutions. Clin Sports Med. 2018;37(2):293–306.
191. Braun HJ, Gold GE. Diagnosis of osteoarthritis: imaging. Bone. 2012;51:278–88.
192. Monson NL, Haughton VM, Modl JM, Sether LA, Ho KC. Normal and degenerating articular cartilage: in vitro correlation of MR imaging and histologic findings. J Magn Reson Imaging. 1992;2:41–5.
193. McKenzie CA, Williams A, Prasad PV, Burstein D. Three-dimensional delayed gadolinium-enhanced MRI of cartilage (dGEMRIC) at 1.5T and 3.0T. J Magn Reson Imaging. 2006;24:928–33.
194. Zbyn S, Mlynarik V, Juras V, Szomolanyi P, Trattnig S, Sodium MR. Imaging of articular cartilage pathologies. Curr Radiol Rep. 2014;2:41.
195. Kinnunen J, Kokkonen HT, Kovanen V, Hauta-Kasari M, Vahimaa P, Lammi MJ, Toyras J, Jurvelin JS. Nondestructive fluorescence-based quantification of threose-induced collagen cross-linking in bovine articular cartilage. J Biomed Opt. 2012;17:97003.
196. Nieminen HJ, Ylitalo T, Karhula S, Suuronen JP, Kauppinen S, Serimaa R, Haeggstrom E, Pritzker KP, Valkealahti M, Lehenkari P, Finnila M, Saarakkala S. Determining collagen distribution in articular cartilage using contrast-enhanced micro-computed tomography. Osteoarthritis Cartilage. 2015;23:1613–21.
197. Finnila MA, Thevenot J, Aho OM, Tiitu V, Rautiainen J, Kauppinen S, Nieminen MT, Pritzker K, Valkealahti M, Lehenkari P, Saarakkala S. Association between subchondral bone structure and osteoarthritis histopathological grade. J Orthop Res. 2017;35:785–92.
198. Muratovic D, Cicuttini F, Wluka A, Findlay D, Wang Y, Otto S, Taylor D, Humphries J, Lee Y, Labrinidis A, Williams R, Kuliwaba J. Bone marrow lesions detected by specific combination of MRI sequences are associated with severity of osteochondral degeneration. Arthritis Res Ther. 2016;18:54.
199. Waldstein W, Perino G, Gilbert SL, Maher SA, Windhager R, Boettner F. OARSI osteoarthritis cartilage histopathology assessment system: a biomechanical evaluation in the human knee. J Orthop Res. 2016;34:135–40.

Part VII

Research in Articular Cartilage Repair and Cartilage Bioengineering

Human-Derived Cells in Chondral or Osteochondral Repair

16

Brent Mollon, Rita Kandel, and John S. Theodoropoulos

16.1 Introduction

Chondral or osteochondral (OC) lesions of the knee are common in those seeking treatment by orthopedic surgeons and are identified in over 60% of knees in a large cohort undergoing arthroscopy [1, 2]. These lesions can be disabling, often limiting function of a young, active, and productive group of the population. However, the surgical treatment of articular cartilage defects remains a challenging area with poor long-term results [3].

Articular cartilage is an avascular tissue composed of chondrocytes arranged within an extracellular matrix (ECM) of proteoglycans and collagen [4]. The function of cartilage is to produce a low-friction surface that, along with the meniscus in the knee, also bears load [5]. The homeostasis of articular cartilage is complex, and our understanding of the interplay between joint mechanics, hormones, growth factors, and aging is evolving. An understanding of these mechanisms helps us understand the pathologic degradation of articular cartilage. Under normal conditions, the balance between matrix synthesis and breakdown is maintained by chondrocytes. In simplified terms, a chondral lesion represents a derangement in homeostasis, with destructive forces outpacing the ability of chondrocytes to synthesize replacement matrix. Once the process of degeneration is underway, the ability of hyaline cartilage to repair itself is limited.

Clinically, cartilage defects can be classified according to the International Cartilage Repair Society (ICRS) classification [6]. This arthroscopic grading system categorizes cartilage pathology into one of five grades based on depth. Grade 0 represents normal cartilage; Grade 1

Funding Supported by Canadian Institutes of Health Research (CIHR) grant support.

B. Mollon, MD, FRCSC, MSc (✉)
Department of Orthopaedics,
Orillia Soldiers' Memorial Hospital,
Orillia, ON, Canada

Simcoe-Muskoka Orthopaedics, Orillia, ON, Canada

R. Kandel, MD
Department of Laboratory Medicine and Pathology,
Department of Surgery, and Institute of Biomaterials and Biomedical Engineering, University of Toronto,
Toronto, ON, Canada

Department of Pathology and Laboratory Medicine,
Mount Sinai Hospital, Toronto, ON, Canada

Lunenfeld-Tanenbaum Research Institute,
Mount Sinai Hospital, Toronto, ON, Canada

J. S. Theodoropoulos, MD, FRCSC, MSc
Division of Orthopaedic Surgery,
University of Toronto, Toronto, ON, Canada

University of Toronto Orthopaedic Sports Medicine Program, Women's College Hospital, Toronto, ON, Canada

Division of Orthopaedic Surgery, Women's College Hospital and Mount Sinai Hospital, Toronto, ON, Canada

H. K. Gahunia et al. (eds.), *Articular Cartilage of the Knee*,
https://doi.org/10.1007/978-1-4939-7587-7_16

lesions represent softening of the cartilage or superficial cracks; Grade 2 lesions extend down to less than 50% of cartilage depth; Grade 3 lesions extend beyond 50% of cartilage depth as far as (but not through) subchondral bone; Grade 4 lesions represent OC lesions. Lesions can be further described based on size and location, with larger lesions and those involving weight-bearing surfaces thought to be more symptomatic [7]. For further details refer to Appendix A.

As of yet, none of the current treatment modalities adequately reproduce the low-friction properties of cartilage that enable it to resist wear over time. As a result, there are nonetheless, a myriad of clinical options as to the treatment of cartilage defects within the knee. Palliative procedures such as arthroscopic chondroplasty attempt to shave off loose chondral edges that are thought to catch within a joint and cause pain [4]. While useful for short-term pain relief, these procedures do not repair the chondral lesion which over time can expand and progress to osteoarthritis (OA). Stimulatory procedures such as microfracture attempt to induce fibrocartilaginous tissue formation within the defect by breaching the subchondral bone and releasing stimulatory factors into the joint from the blood and/or bone marrow [8]. However, fibrocartilage (composed predominantly of type I collagen) is biomechanically inferior to hyaline cartilage (composed of predominantly type II collagen), and the ability of this procedure to halt or slow the development of OA is unclear [3, 9]. Transplant-type procedures, including both auto- and allo- OC transplants, attempt to fill the defect with cartilage taken from non-weight-bearing surfaces within the patient's knee or from a donor. However, donor-site mortality in autograft procedures and the potential for disease transmission in allograft transplant procedures are disadvantages of these procedures [4, 10]. Additionally, the long-term durability of the grafts is unclear, and the technical challenges inherent in these procedures (such as adequately matching the depth and curvature of cartilage between the graft and adjacent host cartilage) may lead to variable clinical results [4]. Limiting clinical use of the above options is the relative lack of high-quality, comparative clinical studies demonstrating long-term outcomes. While the importance of relieving pain and regaining function in the short-term is an important consideration for patients, attention is shifting to identifying procedures that will prevent the longer-term sequela of cartilage injury, the development of OA.

An ideal cartilage repair technique would result in the replacement of the damaged cartilage with chondrocytes and ECM similar to hyaline cartilage that is well integrated into the surrounding cartilage and has homeostatic capabilities similar to native tissue. Much hope lies in the area of tissue engineering to achieve this goal. The goal of creating hyaline cartilage within a knee should theoretically improve joint mechanics and slow or even halt the progression toward OA. The aim of this chapter is to provide an understanding of the underlying theory and current practice of using human-derived cells and tissue engineering for the treatment of chondral and OC lesions. The current clinical data supporting these approaches and an understanding of the limitations of this science will be presented.

16.2 Tissue Engineering

16.2.1 Principles

Current research efforts are directed at augmenting allograft or autograft chondrocyte transplants in order to improve the quality of transplanted tissue and its integration. However, there is great interest in advancing the field of tissue engineering, so it can be used to repair joint defects. The goals of tissue engineering are directed toward reconstituting the structure and function of human tissues [11]. However, the underlying principles of tissue engineering are foreign to many clinicians, and the rapid evolution of the field can complicate an understanding of these new advances.

Tissue engineering has made it possible to create biologically active, two- or three-dimensional cartilage-like tissue to fill a chondral lesion, complete with chondrocytes and a supporting ECM. This process requires three basic

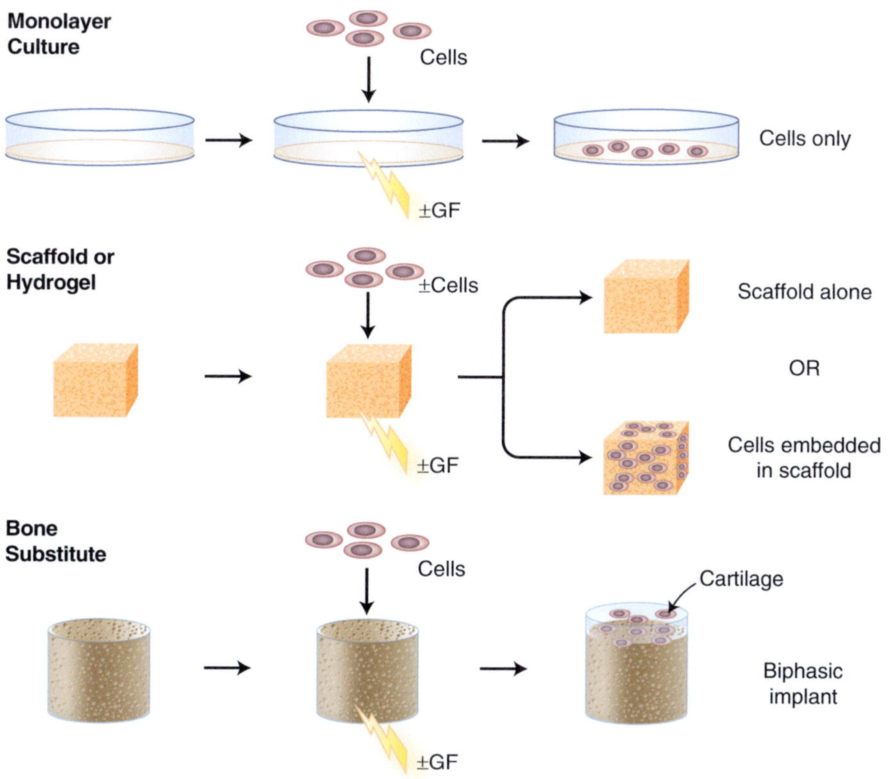

Fig. 16.1 Overview of cartilage engineering. (This diagram demonstrates the approaches for cartilage tissue engineering. The three main components (chondrocyte cell source, biomaterial, and/or growth factors) are utilized to produce one of three end products: chondrocytes, cell-seeded scaffold, or biphasic implant (cartilage overtop a bone substitute))

components: first, viable cells; second, appropriate structural matrix or scaffold that facilitates formation of cartilage matrix; and third, the chemical and/or mechanical factors that encourage appropriate growth of the cells in vivo or in vitro on the scaffold (Fig. 16.1) [11]. The ultimate goal of the above components is the eventual integration of the engineered tissue into the host [11]. This chapter will focus on only one of the three components of tissue engineering, the cells. An in-depth exploration of scaffolds and growth factors can be found in Chap. 17 and will be only described here as it relates to chondrocyte culture and ultimately cartilage matrix production.

An example of one tissue engineering approach under commercial development is that of NeoCart® (Histogenics, Waltham, MA) [12, 13]. The autologous chondrocytes used in this approach are obtained arthroscopically from the patient's knee by an orthopedic surgeon. Once obtained the chondrocytes are cultured on a bovine collagen gel/sponge construct, which serves as the scaffold. Additionally, hydrostatic pressure is introduced in vitro during the culturing process via a bioreactor, which applies mechanical stimulation to induce matrix synthesis. The result is a three-dimensional structure containing chondrocytes with an ECM that resembles hyaline-like cartilage in vivo. While this description is simplified, it nonetheless illustrates the components of tissue engineering and its role in creating clinical solutions to treat cartilage defects. The final product can be sized and fit into a cartilage defect through a mini-arthrotomy (or in some cases arthroscopy) and secured with a collagen/polyethylene glycol-based glue [13].

16.2.2 Definitions

In an attempt to standardize and clarify future discussions on tissue engineering, the following definitions should be understood. "Growth" is considered an increase in volume due to an accumulation of cells and matrix similar to that present in the original object [14]. "Remodeling" represents a change in the properties of a tissue due to a change in the structure or composition of that tissue. "Maturation" represents the process of remodeling to achieve the functional properties attributed to adult tissues. "Differentiation" refers to the adoption of a different phenotype by a cell, often by specialization of a previously pluri- or multipotent cell. "Stem cells" are those cells with a capacity for self-renewal and, under appropriate circumstances, the ability to differentiate into more specialized cellular lineages [14].

16.3 Human Cells in Chondral Repair

While there are several methods under ongoing investigation, the underlying goal of all cellular approaches to cartilage tissue engineering is to ultimately have or generate chondrocytes capable of creating hyaline cartilage that can integrate into the surrounding cartilage and underlying bone [15]. The sources of chondrocytes or precursor cells capable of differentiating into a chondrocyte lineage are varied. They include primarily obtained chondrocytes (e.g., direct OC transplantation), passaged chondrocytes or stem cells that can be induced to differentiate to chondrocytes including induced pluripotent cells, mesenchymal stromal cells, and embryonic stem cells. These cells, from most specialized to least specialized, will be explored in order.

16.3.1 Chondrocytes and Articular Cartilage: Properties

The only cellular component of human cartilage is the chondrocyte [16]. This cell initially arises from undifferentiated mesenchymal cells. During growth, chondrocytes proliferate and synthesize large amounts of cartilage matrix. The dry weight of this matrix is composed of 60% collagen (type II predominant), 25% proteoglycans (PG: molecules with a protein core and negatively charged glycosaminoglycan (GAG) chains), and 15% other molecules and glycoproteins (which are thought to be involved in matrix organization) [16, 18]. The dry weight of the various matrix components varies with cartilage health and aging. The remainder of the weight of cartilage is water which makes up 80% of the "wet weight" [16]. This liquid carries gases, metabolites, ions, and proteins allowing for diffusion of nutrients and small amounts of oxygen. For an in-depth understanding of articular cartilage structure, function, growth, and development, please refer to Chaps. 1 and 2 of this book.

The cartilage undergoes maturation until adulthood. The cellularity of articular cartilage decreases by 50% in an adult when compared to fetal tissues [19–21]. Additionally, the dry weight of cartilage increases as the collagen composition of the matrix increases to adult values [20, 21]. The cartilage develops a zonal organization of superficial, middle, deep, and calcified layers by adulthood [22, 23]. In the superficial zone (SZ), chondrocytes appear flattened and are arranged parallel to the joint surface [17]. Additionally, the ECM is composed of higher amounts of collagen and water and lower amounts of proteoglycans compared to other zones, giving the SZ a greater tensile stiffness and ability to resist shear forces [5]. The chondrocytes in the SZ are also believed to be involved in boundary lubrication, secreting molecules like proteoglycan 4 (a glycoprotein also known as lubricin) to decrease friction within the joint [24, 25]. The middle zone (MZ) represents 40–60% of articular cartilage and is composed of larger, randomly oriented collagen fibrils [26]. The PG concentration is higher than in the SZ, providing it with the ability to withstand compressive forces [27]. MZ chondrocytes exhibit a round shape and are more metabolically active than in the SZ [26]. The MZ is rich in collagen type II and aggrecan, but other proteins such as cartilage intermediate protein and small leucine-rich PGs are present [28–32].

The deep zone (DZ) of articular cartilage is composed of spherical chondrocytes. It has the largest collagen fibrils leading to the lowest water content of any of the zones of articular cartilage, despite the highest PG content and lowest collagen content [17]. The collagen fibrils are oriented perpendicular to the joint surface. DZ chondrocytes share phenotypic similarities with growth plate hypertrophic chondrocytes, such as expression of collagen type X, alkaline phosphatase, and other proteins that have been implicated in the regulation of cartilage calcification [33, 34]. The zone of calcified cartilage (ZCC), the mineralized region of the DZ of cartilage, interdigitates with the underlying bone and anchors hyaline cartilage to the bone [35]. The DZ–ZCC interface is maintained in part by collagen fibrils organized perpendicular to the joint surface that bridges these two cartilage zones [27, 28]. At the interface between the hyaline and calcified cartilage is the tidemark, and studies of tetracycline incorporation have demonstrated that the tidemark advances slowly in the hyaline cartilage [36]. As ZCC thickness remains relatively constant through life in healthy cartilage, a control mechanism, not yet elucidated, must be present to ensure that cartilage calcification occurs at the same rate as its replacement by bone [14, 35, 37, 38]. Mineralization-related molecules such as osteopontin expression have been implicated in limiting the size of mineral deposits [14]. Recreating this interface is likely critical to tissue-engineered functionality as the calcified cartilage serves to distribute forces and prevents shearing of the hyaline cartilage from the bone [36].

Cartilage maturation represents a dynamic process and has profound implications for biological cartilage repair. The zonal orientation, the increase in dry weight, and the sevenfold increase in collagen crosslinks in adult cartilage are thought to result in a 180% increase in the compressive and 450% increase in the tensile modulus of cartilage [20, 21]. Additionally, the ZCC is thought to be critical for the long-term survival of cartilage as it represents the anchor between the bone and cartilage [14]. The complex organization of cartilage, the weight-bearing environment of a joint, the changes in the other joint tissues, and the presence of inflammatory cytokines present a daunting challenge for successful cartilage repair.

16.3.2 Marrow Stimulation Techniques

Perhaps the simplest use of human cells in cartilage regeneration falls under the heading "marrow stimulation techniques." This group includes abrasion arthroplasty, OC drilling, and microfracture [4]. All of these procedures seek to breach the subchondral plate to allow for release of chondroprogenitor cells and formation of a blood clot in the defect [8]. These cells then form fibrocartilage consisting primarily of type I collagen [4]. For the detailed description of the abovementioned technique, refer to Chap. 11.

Of the above techniques, microfracture is the more commonly performed procedure, and it can be utilized in localized lesions less than 2 cm^2 lesions [39]. This is an arthroscopic procedure where loose pieces of cartilage are debrided and the subchondral bone is then breached using an awl or drill to a depth of 2–4 mm. Holes are made 2–3 mm apart from each other, with the size and distribution of these holes thought to influence repair [4, 40]. Bone marrow stroma and blood can be seen leaking from the holes, representing the release of progenitor cells into the defect.

The complications attributed to these procedures are minimal. However, the fibrocartilage created is inferior to hyaline cartilage. Recent efforts have focused on developing ways of modifying this response to favor more hyaline-like tissue formation [41]. At present, marrow stimulation techniques represent a procedure intended to relieve pain and, at most, postpone the progression toward OA [3].

16.3.3 Autogenic and Allogenic Osteochondral Transplant

Given the complexity of mature adult articular cartilage, it is understandable that early attempts to repair an OC lesion with tissue that structurally and histologically matches native cartilage were in the form of tissue taken from non-weight-bearing zones within a patient's own knee (autogenic transplant) or removed from a cadaver (allogenic transplant). Osteochondral autograft transplantation (OAT) involves the transfer of an OC plug from a non-weight-bearing portion of the joint (e.g., lateral or medial trochlea, intercondylar notch) into the defect [42]. This approach is indicated for the treatment of focal OC lesions of the femoral condyle measuring between 1 and 2 cm^2 in size. In larger lesions, multiple OC plugs may be transplanted into the OC defect (a procedure termed "mosaicplasty"). A lesion greater than 2 cm^2 is a relative contraindication to this procedure. Osteochondral allograft transplantation represents a treatment alternative to autograft when lesions are larger than 2 cm^2 [44]. Ideally, cold-stored or fresh allografts should be utilized within 4 weeks of harvest to maximize chondrocyte viability and cartilage biomechanical properties [43]. Fresh-frozen grafts are an alternative, but the freezing has been shown to decrease chondrocyte viability and damage ECM, and thus are not preferred [4].

The above procedures can be performed via arthroscopy or arthrotomy. The host OC lesion is identified, smoothened, and rounded to accept a press-fit graft. The subchondral bone is drilled to encourage progenitor cell release at the base of the graft. A graft is then selected and harvested with the intention that the graft will match the lesion in terms of size, depth, and overall cartilage morphology. The graft is then press-fit into the lesion [45]. Autogenic donor sites may be left untreated or filled with a matrix to encourage OC repair with the intent of decreasing graft-site morbidity [e.g., TruFit Bone Graft Substitute Plugs (Smith and Nephew, Andover, MA], but this is still controversial.

Osteochondral transplant procedures are not without potential complications. Concern remains over donor site morbidity, which ultimately limits the size of OC lesion that can be treated with this technique [4, 46]. Use of allograft tissue raises the concern of disease transmission, increased risk of infection, requires access to a bone bank and can be difficult to schedule electively due to variable access to allografts [45]. Additionally, in both procedures, the ability to appropriately size the graft and match to host cartilage shape can be technically challenging [46]. If the graft is left proud or is subsided relative to the surrounding native cartilage, then a stress riser will be created, leading to point loading and increased wear at that site [47, 48]. One way to circumvent many of these problems is the use of biphasic implants in which cartilage formed on and integrated with a bone substitute could be generated in culture, shaped to mimic the defect, and then implanted [39, 48, 49].

16.3.4 Autologous Chondrocyte Implantation

In an attempt to repair cartilage using cells thought to be capable of producing hyaline cartilage without the morbidity associated with autograft and issues with allograft, autologous chondrocyte implantation (ACI) evolved as an alternative [50, 51, 146]. The first clinical results of this treatment were reported by Brittberg et al. [50]. Cartilage is obtained via arthroscopic biopsy, the chondrocytes isolated and cultured in monolayer. The chondrocyte suspension is then placed in the defect, and a watertight periosteal patch is placed over the defect and sutured to adjacent cartilage to hold the cells in place [50]. This process requires two operations 6–8 weeks apart and is indicated for focal lesions from 2 to 10 cm^2 in size [4].

Although clinical results are generally favorable for this procedure, several drawbacks of the classical ACI procedure have been identified. Clinically, the risks of this procedure include arthrofibrosis, delamination of the graft, and periosteal hypertrophy [12, 53]. From a histological point of view, some studies have questioned the ability of ACI to reliably produce hyaline-like cartilage [53, 54]. For example, animal models have suggested that the periosteal patch along with release of progenitor cells when the subchondral bone is breached may be the factors that encourage healing instead of the implanted chondrocytes [56, 57]. Furthermore, it is thought that culturing chondrocytes in monolayers, so-called passaged chondrocytes, encourages dedifferentiation to cells with a fibroblast-like morphology and decreased capacity to produce a hyaline-like matrix [55, 56, 58, 59, 60]. Much research is now directed at improving the above approach. One such modification, termed "characterized chondrocyte implantation" (CCI), utilizes chondrocyte marker profiles to select for cells that are more likely to produce hyaline cartilage. A 5-year outcome study has identified a subgroup of patients who have improved repair after CCI compared to microfracture [57]. Others focus on utilizing synthetic patches to minimize the number of operations required and/or the utilization of growth factors during cell expansion in order to improve the ability of chondrocytes to produce hyaline cartilage while minimizing complications [52, 68].

As noted above that passaged chondrocyte cells change their phenotype but interestingly, these cells have the potential to undergo redifferentiation under appropriate conditions [61, 62]. One such technique involves co-culturing with primary (or non-passaged) chondrocytes [63]. Investigators have shown that passaged human chondrocytes when cultured with xenogeneic primary chondrocytes encourage redifferentiation of the human cells and reacquisition of the ability to form hyaline cartilage [63]. These cells could then be used to redifferentiate other passaged chondrocytes, thus forming a stable phenotype which could be utilized in ACI procedures [63]. The mechanism underlying this redifferentiation is unclear but may be related to paracrine signaling, direct cell-cell communication, or regulation by the ECM [64–66].

Tissue engineering principles have also attempted to recreate the zonal architecture of mature cartilage in a number of different ways either by multilayering chondrocytes from the different zones of cartilage, selective isolation of chondrocytes from zones of cartilage, or the use of scaffolds that favor zonal differentiation [67, 68]. Generating hyaline cartilage with the architectural complexity of native articular cartilage is an area of intensive investigation and has yet to be solved.

The continuing evolution of ACI procedures through tissue engineering to attempt to overcome these limitations has resulted in several subsequent "generations" of cartilage repair procedures [69]. These represent application of more complex tissue engineering principles but have less clinical evidence as to their efficacy, and, for some approaches, only animal studies exist. As there appears to be little consensus regarding what advances are required to designate an improvement within a given generation, we propose the following list shown in Table 16.1 as modified from other investigators [69, 70]. The first-generation procedure uses periosteal patches to implant chondrocytes cultured in monolayer as described above [70]. Second-generation cartilage repair techniques utilize absorbable scaffolds and chondrocytes; the scaffolds provide support and a more biologic three-dimensional infrastructure for chondrocyte growth. Third-generation treatments utilize xeno/allogenic chondrocytes, enhancements in scaffold technology (chondro-conductive and inductive matrix), mechanical-like conditioning to the chondrocytes or the production of biphasic grafts [70]. Fourth-generation approaches represent a further evolution to include the use of stem cells to generate chondrocytes and/or the utilization of gene therapy to encourage chondrogenesis [71].

As alluded to in third- and fourth-generation procedures, researchers are looking toward other sources or cell types capable of producing chondrocytes in hopes of identifying one that will produce large amounts of hyaline cartilage, while also reducing patient morbidity or the need for multiple operations. In broad terms, the two main cell types capable of differentiating into chondrocytes are mesenchymal stromal cells (MSCs) and embryonic stem cells (ESCs).

Table 16.1 Evolution of Autologous Chondrocyte Implantation: Cartilage Repair Approaches

Generation	Description	Defining Features
1	Autogenous chondrocytes are obtained via arthroscopy, expanded in culture, and reimplanted under a patch (e.g., periosteum, collagen, or synthetic material) during a second operation	Use of chondrocytes; Patch required
2	Autogenous chondrocytes (± selection) are obtained via arthroscopy, chondrocytes are placed on a scaffold, and the chondrocyte/scaffold complex is inserted into the defect at a later operation	Use of scaffolds; No patch required
3	Introduces either chondro-conductive or chondro-inductive scaffolds, xeno/allogeneic cells, biphasic graft constructs, or mechanically conditioned chondrocytes during the culturing process	Utilizes two or three components of tissue engineering (introduces growth factors/mechanical conditioning) *or* introduces other cell types (non-stem cell) *or* attempts to reproduce zonal architecture of mature cartilage
4	Utilizes mesenchymal stromal cells, stem cells, or gene therapy to generate chondrocytes	Stem cells/gene therapy for chondrogenesis

Reprinted with the authors' permission [69]

Definition of cartilage repair generations: Note that with each subsequent generation, the advances are intended to either: produce hyaline cartilage more consistently, improve graft integration, decrease donor morbidity, and/or decrease the number of procedures

16.4 Mesenchymal Stromal Cells

Mesenchymal stromal cells are multipotent cells that have the potential to differentiate into osteocyte, adipocyte, and chondrocyte lineages under the proper conditions [71]. MSCs are also defined by their ability to express certain surface molecules (i.e., CD73, CD105, CD90) and grow as adherent fibroblast-like cells in monolayer culture in vitro [72, 73]. The term mesenchymal "stromal cell" has replaced mesenchymal "stem cell" as these cells are ultimately restricted in the cells into which they can differentiate [74]. Nonetheless, MSCs represent precursor cells to chondrocytes, and thus, it is hoped that these cells may be utilized to encourage chondral repair.

A detailed protocol to collect, isolate, and grow mesenchymal stromal cells is beyond the scope of this article [See Reference [75] for details of the protocol]. A brief overview of this process is as follows: The cells are obtained via aspiration from bone marrow or enzymatic degradation of tissue (e.g., adipose tissue). The cells are then expanded in culture. Flow cytometry can be used to sort for cells that express MSC surface markers, and "stemness" can be demonstrated by inducing differentiation into adipocytes, osteoblasts, and chondrocytes under the appropriate culture conditions [73].

16.4.1 Bone Marrow-Derived Mesenchymal Stromal Cells

The bone marrow represents the main source of MSCs (so-called bmMSCs), although they can be obtained from other sources including the umbilical cord, adipose tissue, synovial membrane, and articular cartilage [75]. It is known that human MSCs cultured from different sites express different types and densities of cell surface proteins/markers [75]. Some surface antigens appear to be specific to a certain MSC source. For example, tissue nonspecific alkaline phosphatase (TNAP) is exclusively found on bmMSCs, whereas CD34+ is identified only on adipose tissue-derived MSCs, and stage-specific embryonic antigen 4 (SSEA-4) is expressed by placenta-derived MSCs [76–78]. Complicating matters, surface antigen profiles differ between in vivo and in vitro cells. CD271, for example, is found on high levels of native bmMSCs but not after in vitro culture [78]. This area of research is still evolving, and surface mapping may one day allow researchers to select for cells with enhanced chrondrogenic potential. For example, Battula et al. used monoclonal antibodies to identify antigens associated with rapidly growing bmMSCs: CD271 and CD56 [79]. Cells that expressed both antigens proliferated more than 30 times faster than an unsorted pool of bmMSCs. Additionally, cells that expressed CD271, CD56, as well as TNAP preferably generated chondrocytes while displaying decreased adipogenic potential but unchanged myogenic, osteogenic, and neurogenic potential relative to an undifferentiated bmMSCs pool. Thus, while preferentially sorting MSCs based on cell surface antigens represents an exciting method to select for proliferating cells with chondrogenic potential, additional work is required before it can be applied clinically.

The strategies for the utilization of MSCs in the human knee or for cartilage regeneration theoretically include two categories, with some overlap between them. The first is using MSCs applied to chondral defects via direct (i.e., intraarticular) or indirect (i.e., intravenous) injection. The second is the utilization of MSCs in tissue engineering which involves inducing differentiation of the cells to chondrocytes either prior to placing in the scaffold or while the cells are in the scaffold to create chondrocyte impregnated grafts. While clinical research trials are underway and available data on the above is expanding, the majority of published data focuses on the former group and utilizes bmMSCs [75, 80–82, 147]. For example, Wakitani et al. utilized culture expanded autologous bmMSCs embedded on a collagen sheet for the treatment of patellofemoral joint chondral defects involving the femur, patella, or both [79]. The bmMSCs were transplanted into the defect and secured with a periosteal graft or synovium (similar to first-generation ACI techniques), with symptomatic improvement noted for as long as 27 months [80]. Long-term follow-up studies have confirmed this to be a safe procedure without development of tumor or infections in a group of 40 patients over 11 years [81]. In an observational cohort study by Nejadnik et al., ACI was compared with a group that received a similar treatment using autologous bmMSCs instead of chondrocytes, the authors concluded there was no difference in clinical outcome between groups at 24 months after operation [81]. These results suggest at the very least equivalence in outcome between implantation of chondrocytes or bmMSCs in ACI-type procedures in terms of short-term symptomatic relief. Additionally, the above studies obtained bmMSCs via an iliac crest aspirate [82–86], thus potentially allowing for single-stage ACI-type procedure to be performed on the affected knee.

The clinical trials have yet to show a favorable benefit of bmMSCs over chondrocytes in traditional ACI-type procedures in terms of histological appearance. While biopsies obtained during second look arthroscopies suggest the presence of hyaline-like cartilage in both the bmMSCs and ACI group in one trial [81], this is based on a small subset of the original study population requiring arthroscopy for symptomatic knees. Thus, any histologic superiority of bmMSCs over earlier generation ACI techniques is still unclear.

16.4.2 Adipose-Derived Stromal Cells

As a potential alternative to bmMSCs, it has been shown that adipose-derived stromal cells (ASC) display chondrogenic potential [83, 84, 148–150]. The isolation procedure consists of harvesting adipose tissue from the patient, and stem cells are isolated via enzymatic digestion of the tissue followed by cell culture expansion. The resulting population of ASCs is very similar to bmMSCs [85]. However, there are important differences between them to consider. Firstly, bmMSCs display more human leukocyte antigens (HLA-ABC) than ASCs, and thus ASCs might be more appropriate for use in allogenic transplant procedures. Secondly, differentiation toward a chondrocyte lineage may be affected by differing sensitivities to growth factors. For example, aggrecan upregulation is found to occur with transforming growth factor (TGF)-β3 administration to bmMSCs, whereas bone morphogenic protein-6 (BMP-6) upregulates aggrecan in ASCs [88]. Thus, tissue engineering processes may need to be modified in order to maximize chondrogenic potential. Thirdly, current evidence suggests that human-derived bmMSCs have a greater capacity for chondrogenesis, whereas human-derived ASCs have a greater capacity for adipogenesis [87, 88]. This reduced potential for chondrogenesis may be independent of our current culture methods and be intrinsic to the ASC, with these cells showing a reduced gene expression for BMPs while also lacking TGF-β1 receptor expression [89]. The seemingly superior chondrogenic potential of bmMSCs has led some researchers to suggest that this cell source is more appropriate for cartilage engineering than ASCs [90]. Others point out that the abundant availability of adipose tissue makes low morbidity, large-quantity tissue harvests possible, which may compensate for its lower chondrogenic potential [90]. Clinical studies will be required to determine the optimal source of MSCs.

16.4.3 Muscle-Derived Multipotent Cells

The muscle has been identified as a plentiful source of MSCs, and its utility in regenerating articular cartilage has been explored in animal models [91]. There are three sources of muscle-derived stem cells (MDSCs). Pericytes, cells associated with capillaries, are involved in vascular maintenance but are also known for their ability to generate mesenchymal tissues in vivo [92, 93]. As these cells are present in all tissues and have similar in vivo differentiation capabilities and surface markers to MSCs [94], some investigators believe pericytes represent a source of multipotential cells which can be mobilized from the vasculature to aid in tissue repair [92]. Satellite cells are found alongside muscle fibers and divide in response to injury. While most satellite cells are committed to myogenesis, myoendothelial cells have been shown to be able to differentiate into all mesenchymal lineages in vivo [93]. The third potential source of MDSCs is from a traumatized muscle and can be debrided during surgeries for orthopedic trauma [95]. Injured muscle contains a high amount of multipotent cells [95], which are thought to be released in response to injury in order to participate in the regeneration of skeletal muscle [92]. Although these cells are not thought to represent true stem cells (in that they may have not been in a dormant state prior to injury), there are little differences between multipotent cells harvested at injury, other forms of MDSCs, and even bmMSCs [92, 96].

The utility of MDSCs in chondral repair has been explored in a few animal models to date. For example, Adachi et al. utilized allogenic MDSCs in a rabbit model with a full-thickness articular cartilage defect [96]. They found viable MDSCs, and the repair tissue consisted of type II collagen at 4 weeks, concluding that allogenic MDSCs are a viable option for the treatment of cartilage defects. However, this is a short-term study and a longer trial (> 6 months) will be necessary. Other researchers have attempted to enhance this process by gene therapy. For example, Kuroda et al. concluded that MDSCs genetically engineered to express BMP-4 also expressed type II collagen as early as 4 weeks after transplantation into a full-thickness cartilage defect in rats [97]. This is an exciting alternative cell source, but additional work must be done to confirm the suitability of MDSCs for cartilage repair.

16.4.4 Other Sources of Mesenchymal-Like Cells in Chondrogenesis

Umbilical cord matrix cells have been shown to have mesenchymal-like differentiation capacities, including the ability to differentiate into chondrocytes [98]. Umbilical cord matrix-derived stromal cells (ucMSC) are progenitor cells obtained from the "Wharton's jelly" of the umbilical cord [83], a matrix composed primarily of mucopolysaccharides designed to protect the umbilical blood vessels from mechanical force

[99]. Despite having chondrocyte differentiation potential, current research implies ucMSC-derived chondrocytes produce fibrous tissue instead of hyaline-like cartilage [100–102]. Although modification of growth factors and/or culture techniques may ultimately allow for hyaline-like cartilage formation, other sources have more potential as sites for isolating MSCs suitable for use in chondral repair.

The human synovium also has cells with substantial chondrogenic potential and represents a reservoir of articular cartilage-destined precursor cells [102–105]. Indeed, a comparison of adipose-derived cells, bmMSCs, muscle-derived cells, and synovial-derived cells had a superior potential for chondrogenesis [104] and produced larger cartilage aggregates over time when compared with bmMSCs. Synovium-derived mesenchymal stem cells (SMSCs) have yet to be used clinically, and the requirement for a two-staged procedure has made SMSCs less appealing to some clinicians.

16.4.5 Embryonic Stem Cells

Another cell source is the embryonic stem cells [ESCs; or human ESCs (hESCs)]. Representing the least differentiated cell line available, ESCs are able to proliferate in an undifferentiated state for a prolonged period [106]. Importantly for cartilage regeneration, ESCs are capable of differentiating into any mature cell in the body, including chondrocytes [107, 108]. Indeed, the chondrogenic potential of ESCs was first noted histologically in teratomas, which are tumors with components of all three germ layers [110].

ESCs are obtained from the inner cell mass of blastocyst-stage embryos [106]. From there, the progression from undifferentiated ESCs to chondrocytes can take one of two paths. The first path utilizes the formation of an embryoid body (EB) to select for mesodermal cells capable of chondrogenesis. An EB forms as a result of the tendency of ESCs to self-aggregate in vitro and subsequently differentiate into the three germ layers as cells proliferate. Mesodermal cells can subsequently be isolated, cultured in the presence chondrogenic growth factors [platelet-derived growth factor (PDGF)-bb, TGF-β, BMP], and encouraged toward a chondrocyte lineage [109–111]. Although simple in theory, several challenges arise when utilizing this technique to produce a clinically safe chondrocyte cell line from ESCs. As is common when manipulating pluripotent cells, it is difficult to guarantee a pure population of cells of the lineage of interest. Although it is possible to generate chondrocytes, they are often contaminated with other cell types [111–113]. While it is reasonable to assert that ESCs differentiate into mature cell lineages, evidence exists to suggest that ESCs that have differentiated to chondrocytes can undergo differentiation into other lineages such as skeletal muscle, adipocytes, and epithelial cells [113]. Complicating matters, the factors involved in regulating cell phenotype are varied and involve factors in addition to growth factors. For example, the size of the EB has even been shown to impact cellular differentiation, with EBs larger than 100 microns in size having a tendency toward hematopoietic or endothelial differentiation, whereas those smaller than 100 microns are more likely to develop into chondrocytes [114]. Our understanding of the factors involved in influencing cellular heterogeneity during the differentiation process is evolving, and new technologies are being developed to address these issues [115–118].

The second method, a two-step procedure, for differentiating ESCs into chondrocytes involves first transforming ESCs into MSCs. By utilizing MSCs as an intermediary stage, the tumorigenic potential of ESCs is theoretically lost, thus making this an attractive clinical option. The transformation of ESCs into MSCs can be accomplished several ways [117–120]. The basic principles include culturing human ESCs in an environment that encourages MSC formation (e.g., proper growth factors and medium). MSC cells can be sorted using cell surface antigens and flow cytometry (i.e., CD105+/CD24-) or by plating the cells in MSC permissive conditions such as hydrogels [119]. This latter approach does not necessarily require the formation of an embryoid body, although some researchers allow

EB formation prior to MSC formation. Once MSCs are obtained, the path toward chondrogenesis occurs as previously described.

Induced pluripotent stem cells (iPSCs) is an alternate method of creating cells with ESC-like properties. As originally described, transducing mouse fibroblasts with the transcription factors Oct3/4, Sox2, Klf4, and c-Myc, cells can be transformed into ESC-like pluripotent stem cells [121]. IPSC express ES cell marker genes and demonstrate ESC-like growth capabilities, including potential for teratoma formation. Since the first studies by Takahashi and Yamanaka [121], many other cell types have been induced to acquire ESC-like phenotype [122]. Wei et al. described the trans-differentiation of human chondrocytes into iPSCs [123], and recently, Wood et al. generated iPSCs from human ACL [151].

In keeping with tissue engineering principles, the successful differentiation of ESCs into a viable chondrocyte population requires appropriate culture conditions and growth factors. For example, studies using human or murine cells have demonstrated improved chondrogenic differentiation in ESCs cultured in a high-density micromass system or on electrospun nanofibers [124, 125]. Growth factors such as TGF-β and BMP-2 have been shown to be inducers of chondrogenic differentiation of hESCs [111, 112, 126, 127]. Nonetheless, additional work is required to advance our understanding in this area. The utilization of growth factors to support chondrogenesis has led to variable results, reflecting the complex effects of growth factors on different cells in different stages of differentiation, in addition to confounding factors such as culture conditions [113, 127–129].

While the utilization of hESCs holds promise, much work is required to understand the factors involved in producing a clinically suitable, homogenous chondrocyte population [130–133]. Indeed, no trial in humans has as yet been published, although animal studies have been reported [131, 134, 135]. Clinically, obtaining a pure population of cells that are able to differentiate homogenously into a chondrocyte lineage in a safe manner has been challenging. Undifferentiated residual ESCs are known to be tumorigenic as they are capable of forming teratomas in vivo [135, 136]. Nonetheless, our understanding of conditions that influences teratoma formation continues to evolve. For example, joint immobility may encourage tumor formation while joint mobility encourages regeneration [135]. Additionally, other animal studies have suggested that injection of ESCs into a joint cavity results in teratoma formation, while localized injection into OC defects does not. In addition, the development of DNA alterations and genomic instability in iPSCs are issues that need to be addressed before these cells can be considered for use on cartilage repair [108]. Thus, while ESCs represent a potential human cell for chondrocyte repair, it is not currently a viable clinical option. Additionally, concerns over the ethical use of stem cell technology have led to the cautious development of ESCs for clinical treatment and will likely be a prominent issue even if reliable chondrogenesis can be achieved.

16.5 Clinical Impact

Despite exciting research developments leading to generating a viable chondrocyte population with clinical utility, it has yet to translate into measurable clinical gains. Currently, the main focus of tissue engineering has been on improving ACI techniques. The utilization of some newer sources of chondrocytes (e.g., MSCs, stem cells) has yet to translate into clinical studies. Nonetheless, the current landscape of clinical trials will be explored.

Many systematic reviews on ACI have been published, but only a few will be highlighted [137–141]. Vasiliadis et al. conducted a systematic review of randomized trials comparing ACI treatment to other treatment options (e.g., microfracture) [138]. Of the nine trials identified, they found no superiority of ACI over other treatments but concluded overall that available evidence was too heterogeneous and of too poor quality to make any definitive clinical recommendations. A similar review of nine studies was conducted by Vavken et al. [139]. Their data suggest that among high-quality trials, ACI results in better tissue quality and clinical outcomes. Nonetheless, they acknowledge the absolute differences between groups are quite small and may not be of clinical importance. They concluded additional research is required.

A review of level I and II evidence with similar inclusion criteria by Harris et al. elaborated on some differences between studies [140]. Of seven studies comparing microfracture to ACI, they found three trials showed better clinical results with ACI after 1 to 3 years follow-up, one study reporting better results after microfracture at 2 years, and three trials reporting no difference after 1 to 5 years. They noted the only predictive factor of better clinical outcomes with ACI when compared to other treatments was a defect size of > 4 cm^2. They also noted no apparent difference between first- and second-generation ACI techniques or between open and arthroscopic techniques. There was, however, a trend toward greater complication rates in open procedures performed with a periosteal patch (i.e., first-generation ACI).

Considering the high cost associated with engineering chondrocytes, there has only been one study focusing on the cost-effectiveness of these therapies. Clar et al. [137] conducted such a trial, but ultimately they were unable to generate concrete conclusions due to the insufficient evidence present. They acknowledge that, if ACI were able to produce more durable hyaline cartilage, then the long-term clinical benefits may outweigh the initial costs. However, long-term studies are required to support the assertion that the hyaline cartilage generated results in improved long-term biomechanical properties that delay or prevent the development of OA.

One must also consider the complications of a procedure before making a recommendation. Harris et al. reviewed all failures and complications from ACI therapies published in 82 studies [141]. They found an overall failure rate of 5.8% with a mean time to failure at 22 months. This failure rate was higher for periosteal-patched ACIs (7.7%), with rates decreasing in all arthroscopic procedures (3.3%) or those using second-generation ACI techniques (0.83%). Overall unplanned reoperation rates were 27% in periosteal-patched ACIs, which decreased to 5% in second-generation ACI and to 1.4% in all arthroscopic second-generation ACI techniques. This study would suggest that while it has been difficult to identify functional benefits to evolving ACI techniques, the overall complication rates and need for reoperation have decreased in all arthroscopic and second-generation techniques.

Available data on third-generation techniques are mostly limited to prospective safety trials [142, 143]. A randomized controlled trial to establish the safety of using the cartilage autograft implantation system (morselized cartilage) (CAIS; DePuy Mitek, Inc., Raynham, MA) was compared to microfracture in 29 patients [142]. This procedure utilized minced autologous hyaline cartilage placed on an absorbable polyglycolic acid-polycaprolactone scaffold and affixed using absorbable polydioxanone staples. The authors found significant improvements in the clinical rating scales utilizing the International Knee Documentation Committee [IKDC] and Knee Injury and Osteoarthritis Outcome Score [KOOS] at the 24-month follow-up. Complications were found to be similar between groups. From this they concluded the CAIS is safe and effective but acknowledged their study was limited by a small sample size and may have been influenced by differences between study populations (more patients with acute onset of symptoms, more men, and more full-time workers in the CAIS group). Crawford et al. presented a prospective trial to evaluate the safety of the third-generation NeoCart procedure (see section "Tissue Engineering – Principles" of this chapter) [13]. They enrolled eight patients and found overall improvement in pain, function, and range of motion at 2 years. Defect fill (as measured by MRI) was found to be 67–100% in six patients, 33–66% in one patient, and less than 33% in one patient. No serious complications were associated with the implant. The significance of these findings is limited by a small sample size and lack of a control group. None of the above two trials discussed the histology of the repair tissue (i.e., fibrocartilage vs. hyaline-like cartilage).

16.6 Future Directions

Despite effort and research evaluating the use of cellular therapies to regenerate chondral defects, no true clinical benefit of newer-generation ACI technologies over older techniques like microfracture has been established [139, 140, 144, 146]. The literature supporting a biomechanically superior tissue filling the defect in ACI has yet to be shown clinically in long-term trials [138, 140]. Results of third- and fourth-generation techniques are beginning to be published [142, 143]. Additionally, the use of other cell types for chondrogenesis has yet to be utilized in humans due to novelty (i.e., synovial-derived chondrocytes) and concerns for safety (i.e., embryonic stem cells). Clearly at this time, many of the potential cellular sources described above are still experimental and may be decades away from clinical practice, if at all. Indeed, many questions still need to be answered. Which cells most easily undergo chondrogenic differentiation and under what circumstances? Which cell when differentiated to a chondrocyte produces a matrix most similar to native hyaline cartilage, and will this tissue decrease the risk of developing arthritis in those with OC lesions? How will our evolving understanding of growth factors and scaffolds impact OC repair? [48]. As integration can be an issue, are biphasic implants the best way to treat cartilage defects? Also, do we need to recapitulate cartilage zonal organization with a deep calcified zone to facilitate integration and weight bearing? Will this approach be suitable to use in an arthritic joint with bony architecture changes and in the presence of inflammation and cytokines? What should the rehabilitation process look like? Nevertheless, there have been many advances in our understanding of the issues related to cartilage repair which can now be the focus of future investigations.

16.7 Conclusions

While our understanding of the requirements for successful cartilage tissue engineering is expanding, the clinical impact of this work is yet to be seen. As evidence of the usefulness of these techniques mounts, clinical use of cartilage tissue engineering will expand, evidence-based medicine must be used to determine efficacy, and these considerations must include other factors such as cost-effectiveness, ease of cell harvest and growth, and quality of the cartilage produced. Thus, many complex factors yet to be appreciated will ultimately help guide which advances will take it beyond the bench to the bedside. In spite of all this, cartilage tissue engineering represents a potentially powerful tool for the clinician to treat chondral defects.

References

1. Widuchowski W, Widuchowski J, Trzaska T. Articular cartilage defects: study of 25,124 knee arthroscopies. Knee. 2007;14(3):177–82.
2. Curl WW, Krome J, Gordon ES, Rushing J, Smith BP, Poehling GG. Cartilage injuries: a review of 31,516 knee arthroscopies. Arthroscopy. 1997;13(4):456–60.
3. Browne JE, Branch TP. Surgical alternatives for treatment of articular cartilage lesions. J Am Acad Orthop Surg. 2000;8(3):180–9.
4. Angel MJ, Sgaglione NA, Latterman C. Articular cartilage lesions/osteoarthritis. In: Kibler WB, editor. Orthopaedic knowledge update: Sports Medicine. 4th ed; 2011. p. 155–71.
5. Buckwalter JA, Mankin HJ. Articular cartilage. Part I: Tissue design and chondrocyte-matrix interactions. J Bone Joint Surg Am. 1997;79-A:600–11.
6. Brittberg M, Winalski CS. Evaluation of cartilage injuries and repair. J Bone Joint Surg Am. 2003;85:58–69.
7. Noyes FR, Stabler CLA. system for grading articular cartilage lesions at arthroscopy. Am J Sports Med. 1989;17(4):505–13.
8. Mithoefer K, Williams RJI, Warren RF, Potter HG, Spock CR, Jones EC, et al. The microfracture technique for the treatment of articular cartilage lesions in the knee: a prospective cohort study. J Bone Joint Surg Am. 2005;87:1911–20.
9. Gobbi A, Nunag P, Malinowski K. Treatment of full thickness chondral lesions of the knee with microfracture in a group of athletes. Knee Surg Sports Traumatol Arthrosc. 2005;13(3):213–21.
10. Hangody L, Kish G, Karpati Z, Szerb I, Udvarhelyi I. Arthroscopic autogenous osteochondral mosaicplasty for the treatment of femoral condylar articular defects. A preliminary report. Knee Surg Sports Traumatol Arthrosc. 1997;5(4):262–7.
11. Hunziker EB. Articular cartilage repair: basic science and clinical progress. A review of the cur-

rent status and prospects. Osteoarthritis Cartilage. 2002;10(6):432–63.
12. Safran MR, Kim H, Zaffagnini S. The use of scaffolds in the management of articular cartilage injury. J Am Acad Orthop Surg. 2008;16(6):306–11.
13. Crawford DC, Heveran CM, Cannon WD Jr, Foo LF, Potter HG. An autologous cartilage tissue implant NeoCart for treatment of grade III chondral injury to the distal femur: prospective clinical safety trial at 2 years. Am J Sports Med. 2009;37(7):1334–43.
14. Mikos AG, Herring SW, Ochareon P, Elisseeff J, HH L, Kandel R, et al. Engineering complex tissues. Tissue Eng. 2006;12(12):3307–39.
15. Buckwalter JA, Woo SL, Goldberg VM, Hadley EC, Booth F, Oegema TR, et al. Soft-tissue aging and musculoskeletal function. J Bone Joint Surg Am. 1993;75(10):1533–48.
16. Buckwalter JA, Mankin HJ, Grodzinsky AJ. Articular cartilage and osteoarthritis. Instr Course Lect. 2005;54:465–80.
17. Quinn TM, Hunziker EB, Häuselmann HJ. Variation of cell and matrix morphologies in articular cartilage among locations in the adult human knee. Osteoarthritis Cartilage. 2005;13(8):672–8.
18. Jadin KD, Wong BL, Bae WC, Li KW, Williamson AK, Schumacher BL, et al. Depth-varying density and organization of chondrocytes in immature and mature bovine articular cartilage assessed by 3d imaging and analysis. J Histochem Cytochem. 2005;53(9):1109–19.
19. Williamson AK, Chen AC, Masuda K, Thonar EJ, Sah RL. Tensile mechanical properties of bovine articular cartilage: variations with growth and relationships to collagen network components. J Orthop Res. 2003;21(5):872–80.
20. Williamson AK, Chen AC, Sah RL. Compressive properties and function-composition relationships of developing bovine articular cartilage. J Orthop Res. 2001;19(6):1113–21.
21. Jadin KD, Bae WC, Schumacher BL, Sah RL. Three-dimensional (3-D) imaging of chondrocytes in articular cartilage: growth-associated changes in cell organization. Biomaterials. 2007;28(2):230–9.
22. Hunziker EB, Kapfinger E, Geiss J. The structural architecture of adult mammalian articular cartilage evolves by a synchronized process of tissue resorption and neoformation during postnatal development. Osteoarthritis Cartilage. 2007;15(4):403–13.
23. Schmidt TA, Gastelum NS, Nguyen QT, Schumacher BL, Sah RL. Boundary lubrication of articular cartilage: role of synovial fluid constituents. Arthritis Rheum. 2007;56(3):882–91.
24. Schumacher BL, Block JA, Schmid TM, Aydelotte MB, Kuettner KE. A novel proteoglycan synthesized and secreted by chondrocytes of the superficial zone of articular cartilage. Arch Biochem Biophys. 1994;311(1):144–52.
25. Hasler EM, Herzog W, JZ W, Muller W, Wyss U. Articular cartilage biomechanics: theoretical models, material properties, and biosynthetic response. Crit Rev Biomed Eng. 1999;27(6):415–88.
26. Poole AR, Kojima T, Yasuda T, Mwale F, Kobayashi M, Laverty S. Composition and structure of articular cartilage: a template for tissue repair. Clin Orthop Relat Res. 2001;391(Suppl):S26–33.
27. Goldring MB, Marcu KB. Cartilage homeostasis in health and rheumatic diseases. Arthritis Res Ther. 2009;11(3):224.
28. Heinegard D, Larsson T, Sommarin Y, Franzen A, Paulsson M, Hedbom E. Two novel matrix proteins isolated from articular cartilage show wide distributions among connective tissues. J Biol Chem. 1986;261(29):13866–72.
29. Poole AR, Webber C, Pidoux I, Choi H, Rosenberg LC. Localization of a dermatan sulfate proteoglycan (DS-PGII) in cartilage and the presence of an immunologically related species in other tissues. J Histochem Cytochem. 1986;34(5):619–5.
30. Bianco P, Fisher LW, Young MF, Termine JD, Robey PG. Expression and localization of the two small proteoglycans biglycan and decorin in developing human skeletal and non-skeletal tissues. J Histochem Cytochem. 1990;38(11):1549–63.
31. Miosge N, Flachsbart K, Goetz W, Schultz W, Kresse H, Herken R. Light and electron microscopical immunohistochemical localization of the small proteoglycan core proteins decorin and biglycan in human knee joint cartilage. Histochem J. 1994;26(12):939–45.
32. Gannon JM, Walker G, Fischer M, Carpenter R, Thompson RC Jr, Oegema TR Jr. Localization of type X collagen in canine growth plate and adult canine articular cartilage. J Orthop Res. 1991;9(4):485–94.
33. Miao D, Scutt A. Histochemical localization of alkaline phosphatase activity in decalcified bone and cartilage. J Histochem Cytochem. 2002;50(3):333–40.
34. Oegema J, Carpenter RJ, Hofmeister F, Thompson J. The interaction of the zone of calcified cartilage and subchondral bone in osteoarthritis. Microsc Res Tech. 1997;37(4):324–32.
35. Revell PA, Pirie C, Amir G, Rashad S, Walker F. Metabolic activity in the calcified zone of cartilage: observations on tetracycline labelled articular cartilage in human osteoarthritic hips. Rheumatol Int. 1990;10(4):143–7.
36. Bullough PG, Jagannath A. The morphology of the calcification front in articular cartilage. Its significance in joint function. J Bone Joint Surg Br. 1983;65(1):72–8.
37. Sun Y, Kandel R. Deep zone articular chondrocytes in vitro express genes that show specific changes with mineralization. J Bone Miner Res. 1999;14(11):1916–25.
38. Allan KS, Pilliar RM, Wang J, Grynpas MD, Kandel RA. Formation of biphasic constructs containing cartilage with a calcified zone interface. Tissue Eng. 2007;13(1):167–77.

39. Williams RJ III, Harnly HW. Microfracture: indications, technique, and results. Instr Course Lect. 2007;56:419–28.
40. Chen H, Hoemann CD, Sun J, Chevrier A, McKee MD, Shive MS, et al. Depth of subchondral perforation influences the outcome of bone marrow stimulation cartilage repair. J Orthop Res. 2011;29(8):1178–84.
41. Hoemann CD, Hurtig M, Rossomacha E, Sun J, Chevrier A, Shive MS, et al. Chitosan-glycerol phosphate/blood implants improve hyaline cartilage repair in ovine microfracture defects. J Bone Joint Surg Am. 2005;87(12):2671–86.
42. Barber FA, Chow JC. Arthroscopic chondral osseous autograft transplantation (COR procedure) for femoral defects. Arthroscopy. 2006;22(1):10–6.
43. Williams SK, Amiel D, Ball ST, Allen RT, Wong VW, Chen AC, et al. Prolonged storage effects on the articular cartilage of fresh human osteochondral allografts. J Bone Joint Surg Am. 2003;85-A(11):2111–20.
44. Gross AE, Kim W, Las HF, Backstein D, Safir O, Pritzker KP. Fresh osteochondral allografts for posttraumatic knee defects: long-term followup. Clin Orthop Relat Res. 2008;466(8):1863–70.
45. Miniaci A, Martineau PA. Technical aspects of osteochondral autograft transplantation. Instr Course Lect. 2007;56:447–55.
46. Wu JZ, Herzog W, Hasler EM. Inadequate placement of osteochondral plugs may induce abnormal stress-strain distributions in articular cartilage - finite element simulations. Med Eng Phys. 2002;24(2):85–97.
47. Koh JL, Wirsing K, Lautenschlager E, Zhang LO. The effect of graft height mismatch on contact pressure following osteochondral grafting: a biomechanical study. Am J Sports Med. 2004;32(2):317–20.
48. Pilliar RM, Kandel RA, Grynpas MD, Zalzal P, Hurtig M. Osteochondral defect repair using a novel tissue engineering approach: sheep model study. Technol Health Care. 2007;15(1):47–56.
49. Theodoropoulos JS, De Croos JN, Park SS, Pilliar R, Kandel RA. Integration of tissue-engineered cartilage with host cartilage: an in vitro model. Clin Orthop Relat Res. 2011;469(10):2785–95.
50. Brittberg M, Lindahl A, Nilsson A, Ohlsson C, Isaksson O, Peterson L. Treatment of deep cartilage defects in the knee with autologous chondrocyte transplantation. N Engl J Med. 1994;331(14):889–95.
51. Dewan AK, Gibson MA, Elisseeff JH, Trice ME. Evolution of autologous chondrocyte repair and comparison to other cartilage repair techniques. Biomed Res Int. 2014;2014:272481.
52. Breinan HA, Martin SD, Hsu HP, Spector M. Healing of canine articular cartilage defects treated with microfracture, a type-II collagen matrix, or cultured autologous chondrocytes. J Orthop Res. 2000;18(5):781–9.
53. Grigolo B, Roseti L, De FL, Piacentini A, Cattini L, Manfredini M, et al. Molecular and immunohistological characterization of human cartilage two years following autologous cell transplantation. J Bone Joint Surg Am. 2005;87(1):46–57.
54. Richardson JB, Caterson B, Evans EH, Ashton BA, Roberts S. Repair of human articular cartilage after implantation of autologous chondrocytes. J Bone Joint Surg Br. 1999;81(6):1064–8.
55. Getgood A, Brooks R, Fortier L, Rushton N. Articular cartilage tissue engineering: today's research, tomorrow's practice? J Bone Joint Surg Br. 2009;91(5):565–76.
56. Dorotka R, Bindreiter U, Macfelda K, Windberger U, Nehrer S. Marrow stimulation and chondrocyte transplantation using a collagen matrix for cartilage repair. Osteoarthritis Cartilage. 2005;13(8):655–64.
57. Vanlauwe J, Saris DB, Victor J, Almqvist KF, Bellemans J, Luyten FP, et al. Five-year outcome of characterized chondrocyte implantation versus microfracture for symptomatic cartilage defects of the knee: early treatment matters. Am J Sports Med. 2011;39(12):2566–74.
58. Barbero A, Grogan S, Schafer D, Heberer M, Mainil-Varlet P, Martin I. Age related changes in human articular chondrocyte yield, proliferation and post-expansion chondrogenic capacity. Osteoarthritis Cartilage. 2004;12(6):476–84.
59. Barbero A, Ploegert S, Heberer M, Martin I. Plasticity of clonal populations of dedifferentiated adult human articular chondrocytes. Arthritis Rheum. 2003;48(5):1315–25.
60. Holtzer H, Abbott J, Lash J, Holtzer S. The loss of phenotypic traits by differentiated cells in vitro, i. Dedifferentiation of cartilage cells. Proc Natl Acad Sci U S A. 1960;46(12):1533–42.
61. Gan L, Kandel RA. vitro cartilage tissue formation by Co-culture of primary and passaged chondrocytes. Tissue Eng. 2007;13(4):831–42.
62. Ahmed N, Taylor DW, Wunder J, Nagy A, Gross AE, Kandel RA. Passaged human chondrocytes accumulate extracellular matrix when induced by bovine chondrocytes. J Tissue Eng Regen Med. 2010;4(3):233–41.
63. Ahmed N, Gan L, Nagy A, Zheng J, Wang C, Kandel RA. Cartilage tissue formation using redifferentiated passaged chondrocytes in vitro. Tissue Eng Part A. 2009;Part(3):665–73.
64. Hwang NS, Varghese S, Puleo C, Zhang Z, Elisseeff J. Morphogenetic signals from chondrocytes promote chondrogenic and osteogenic differentiation of mesenchymal stem cells. J Cell Physiol. 2007;212(2):281–4.
65. Guillotin B, Bourget C, Remy-Zolgadri M, Bareille R, Fernandez P, Conrad V, et al. Human primary endothelial cells stimulate human osteoprogenitor cell differentiation. Cell Physiol Biochem. 2004;14(4–6):325–32.
66. Dell'Accio F, De BC, Luyten FP. Microenvironment and phenotypic stability specify tissue formation by human articular cartilage-derived cells in vivo. Exp Cell Res. 2003;287(1):16–27.

67. Jiang J, Tang A, Ateshian GA, Guo XE, Hung CT, Bioactive LHH. stratified polymer ceramic-hydrogel scaffold for integrative osteochondral repair. Ann Biomed Eng. 2010;38(6):2183–96.
68. Hettrich CM, Crawford D, Rodeo SA. Cartilage repair: third-generation cell-based technologies--basic science, surgical techniques, clinical outcomes. Sports Med Arthrosc Rev. 2008;16(4):230–5.
69. Mollon B, Kandel R, Chahal J, Theodoropoulos J. The clinical status of cartilage tissue regeneration in humans. Osteoarthritis Cartilage. 2013;21(12):1824–33.
70. Kessler MW, Ackerman G, Dines JS, Grande D. Emerging technologies and fourth generation issues in cartilage repair. Sports Med Arthrosc Rev. 2008;16(4):246–54.
71. Pittenger MF, Mackay AM, Beck SC, Jaiswal RK, Douglas R, Mosca JD, et al. Multilineage potential of adult human mesenchymal stem cells. Science. 1999;284(5411):143–7.
72. Dominici M, Le BK, Mueller I, Slaper-Cortenbach I, Marini F, Krause D, et al. Minimal criteria for defining multipotent mesenchymal stromal cells. The International Society for Cellular Therapy position statement. Cytotherapy. 2006;8(4):315–7.
73. Keating A. Mesenchymal stromal cells. Curr Opin Hematol. 2006;13(6):419–25.
74. Aicher WK, Buhring HJ, Hart M, Rolauffs B, Badke A, Klein G. Regeneration of cartilage and bone by defined subsets of mesenchymal stromal cells - potential and pitfalls. Adv Drug Deliv Rev. 2011;63(4–5):342–51.
75. Maumus M, Peyrafitte JA, D'Angelo R, Fournier-Wirth C, Bouloumie A, Casteilla L, et al. Native human adipose stromal cells: localization, morphology and phenotype. Int J Obes. 2011;35(9):1141–53.
76. Battula VL, Bareiss PM, Treml S, Conrad S, Albert I, Hojak S, et al. Human placenta and bone marrow derived MSC cultured in serum-free, b-FGF-containing medium express cell surface frizzled-9 and SSEA-4 and give rise to multilineage differentiation. Differentiation. 2007;75(4):279–91.
77. Buhring HJ, Battula VL, Treml S, Schewe B, Kanz L, Vogel W. Novel markers for the prospective isolation of human MSC. Ann N Y Acad Sci. 2007;1106:262–71.
78. Battula VL, Treml S, Bareiss PM, Gieseke F, Roelofs H, de Zwart P, et al. Isolation of functionally distinct mesenchymal stem cell subsets using antibodies against CD56, CD271, and mesenchymal stem cell antigen-1. Haematologica. 2009;94(2):173–84.
79. Wakitani S, Nawata M, Tensho K, Okabe T, Machida H, Ohgushi H. Repair of articular cartilage defects in the patello-femoral joint with autologous bone marrow mesenchymal cell transplantation: three case reports involving nine defects in five knees. J Tissue Eng Regen Med. 2007;1(1):74–9.
80. Wakitani S, Okabe T, Horibe S, Mitsuoka T, Saito M, Koyama T, et al. Safety of autologous bone marrow-derived mesenchymal stem cell transplantation for cartilage repair in 41 patients with 45 joints followed for up to 11 years and 5 months. J Tissue Eng Regen Med. 2011;5(2):146–50.
81. Nejadnik H, Hui JH, Feng Choong EP, Tai BC, Lee EH. Autologous bone marrow-derived mesenchymal stem cells versus autologous chondrocyte implantation: an observational cohort study. Am J Sports Med. 2010;38(6):1110–6.
82. Xu Y, Balooch G, Chiou M, Bekerman E, Ritchie RO, Longaker MT. Analysis of the material properties of early chondrogenic differentiated adipose-derived stromal cells (ASC) using an in vitro three-dimensional micromass culture system. Biochem Biophys Res Commun. 2007;359(2):311–6.
83. Wagner W, Wein F, Seckinger A, Frankhauser M, Wirkner U, Krause U, et al. Comparative characteristics of mesenchymal stem cells from human bone marrow, adipose tissue, and umbilical cord blood. Exp Hematol. 2005;33(11):1402–16.
84. De Francesco F, Ricci G, D' Andrea F, Nicoletti GF, Ferraro GA. Human Adipose Stem Cells: From Bench to Bed-Side. Tissue Eng B Rev. 2015;21(6):572–84.
85. Diekman BO, Rowland CR, Lennon DP, Caplan AI, Guilak F. Chondrogenesis of adult stem cells from adipose tissue and bone marrow: induction by growth factors and cartilage-derived matrix. Tissue Eng. 2010;Part(2):523–33.
86. Huang JI, Kazmi N, Durbhakula MM, Hering TM, Yoo JU, Johnstone B. Chondrogenic potential of progenitor cells derived from human bone marrow and adipose tissue: a patient-matched comparison. J Orthop Res. 2005;23(6):1383–9.
87. Liu TM, Martina M, Hutmacher DW, Hui JH, Lee EH, Lim B. Identification of common pathways mediating differentiation of bone marrow- and adipose tissue-derived human mesenchymal stem cells into three mesenchymal lineages. Stem Cells. 2007;25(3):750–60.
88. Henning T, Lorenz H, Thiel A, Goetzke K, Dickhut A, Geiger F, et al. Reduced chondrogenic potential of adipose tissue derived stromal cells correlates with an altered TGFbeta receptor and BMP profile and is overcome by BMP-6. J Cell Physiol. 2007;211:682–91.
89. Afizah H, Yang Z, Hui JH, Ouyang HW, Lee EHA. comparison between the chondrogenic potential of human bone marrow stem cells (BMSCs) and adipose-derived stem cells (ADSCs) taken from the same donors. Tissue Eng. 2007;13(4):659–66.
90. Hildner F, Albrecht C, Gabriel C, Redl H, van Griensven M. State of the art and future perspectives of articular cartilage regeneration: a focus on adipose-derived stem cells and platelet-derived products. J Tissue Eng Regen Med. 2011;5(4):e36–51.
91. Jackson WM, Nesti LJ, Tuan RS. Potential therapeutic applications of muscle-derived mesenchymal stem and progenitor cells. Expert Opin Biol Ther. 2010;10(4):505–17.
92. Farrington-Rock C, Crofts NJ, Doherty MJ, Ashton BA, Griffin-Jones C, Canfield AE. Chondrogenic

and adipogenic potential of microvascular pericytes. Circulation. 2004;110(15):2226–32.
93. Crisan M, Yap S, Casteilla L, Chen CW, Corselli M, Park TS, et al. A perivascular origin for mesenchymal stem cells in multiple human organs. Cell Stem Cell. 2008;3(3):301–13.
94. Nesti LJ, Jackson WM, Shanti RM, Koehler SM, Aragon AB, Bailey JR, et al. Differentiation potential of multipotent progenitor cells derived from war-traumatized muscle tissue. J Bone Joint Surg Am. 2008;90(11):2390–8.
95. Jackson WM, Aragon AB, Djouad F, Song Y, Koehler SM, Nesti LJ, et al. Mesenchymal progenitor cells derived from traumatized human muscle. J Tissue Eng Regen Med. 2009;3(2):129–38.
96. Adachi N, Sato K, Usas A, Fu FH, Ochi M, Han CW, et al. Muscle derived, cell based ex vivo gene therapy for treatment of full thickness articular cartilage defects. J Rheumatol. 2002;29(9):1920–30.
97. Kuroda R, Usas A, Kubo S, Corsi K, Peng H, Rose T, et al. Cartilage repair using bone morphogenetic protein 4 and muscle-derived stem cells. Arthritis Rheum. 2006;54(2):433–42.
98. Can A, Karahuseyinoglu S. Concise review: human umbilical cord stroma with regard to the source of fetus-derived stem cells. Stem Cells. 2007;25(11):2886–95.
99. Meyer FA, Laver-Rudich Z, Tanenbaum R. Evidence for a mechanical coupling of glycoprotein microfibrils with collagen fibrils in Wharton's jelly. Biochim Biophys Acta. 1983;755(3):376–87.
100. Wang L, Tran I, Seshareddy K, Weiss ML, Detamore MS. A comparison of human bone marrow-derived mesenchymal stem cells and human umbilical cord-derived mesenchymal stromal cells for cartilage tissue engineering. Tissue Eng Part A. 2009;15(8):2259–66.
101. Hildner F, Wolbank S, Redl H, van Griensven M, Peterbauer A. How chondrogenic are human umbilical cord matrix cells? A comparison to adipose-derived stem cells. J Tissue Eng Regen Med. 2010;4(3):242–5.
102. Koyama E, Shibukawa Y, Nagayama M, Sugito H, Young B, Yuasa T, et al. A distinct cohort of progenitor cells participates in synovial joint and articular cartilage formation during mouse limb skeletogenesis. Dev Biol. 2008;316(1):62–73.
103. Kim MJ, Son MJ, Son MY, Seol B, Kim J, Park J, et al. Generation of human induced pluripotent stem cells from osteoarthritis patient-derived synovial cells. Arthritis Rheum. 2011;63(10):3010–21.
104. Sakaguchi Y, Sekiya I, Yagishita K, Muneta T. Comparison of human stem cells derived from various mesenchymal tissues: superiority of synovium as a cell source. Arthritis Rheum. 2005;52(8):2521–9.
105. Shirasawa S, Sekiya I, Sakaguchi Y, Yagishita K, Ichinose S, Muneta T. In vitro chondrogenesis of human synovium-derived mesenchymal stem cells: optimal condition and comparison with bone marrow-derived cells. J Cell Biochem. 2006;97(1):84–97.
106. Thomson JA, Itskovitz-Eldor J, Shapiro SS, Waknitz MA, Swiergiel JJ, Marshall VS, et al. Embryonic stem cell lines derived from human blastocysts. Science. 1998;282(5391):1145–7.
107. Odorico JS, Kaufman DS, Thomson JA. Multilineage differentiation from human embryonic stem cell lines. Stem Cells. 2001;19(3):193–204.
108. Toh WS, Lee EH, Cao T. Potential of human embryonic stem cells in cartilage tissue engineering and regenerative medicine. Stem Cell Rev. 2011;7(3):544–59.
109. Francioli SE, Martin I, Sie CP, Hagg R, Tommasini R, Candrian C, et al. Growth factors for clinical-scale expansion of human articular chondrocytes: relevance for automated bioreactor systems. Tissue Eng. 2007;13(6):1227–34.
110. Toh WS, Guo XM, Choo AB, Lu K, Lee EH, Cao T. Differentiation and enrichment of expandable chondrogenic cells from human embryonic stem cells in vitro. J Cell Mol Med. 2009;13(9B):3570–90.
111. Koay EJ, Hoben GM, Athanasiou KA. Tissue engineering with chondrogenically differentiated human embryonic stem cells. Stem Cells. 2007;25(9):2183–90.
112. Toh WS, Yang Z, Liu H, Heng BC, Lee EH, Cao T. Effects of culture conditions and bone morphogenetic protein 2 on extent of chondrogenesis from human embryonic stem cells. Stem Cells. 2007;25(4):950–60.
113. Hegert C, Kramer J, Hargus G, Muller J, Guan K, Wobus AM, et al. Differentiation plasticity of chondrocytes derived from mouse embryonic stem cells. J Cell Sci. 2002;115(23):4617–28.
114. Messana JM, Hwang NS, Coburn J, Elisseeff JH, Zhang Z. Size of the embryoid body influences chondrogenesis of mouse embryonic stem cells. J Tissue Eng Regen Med. 2008;2(8):499–506.
115. Gerecht-Nir S, Cohen S, Itskovitz-Eldor J. Bioreactor cultivation enhances the efficiency of human embryoid body (hEB) formation and differentiation. Biotechnol Bioeng. 2004;86(5):493–502.
116. Bratt-Leal AM, Carpenedo RL, McDevitt TC. Engineering the embryoid body microenvironment to direct embryonic stem cell differentiation. Biotechnol Prog. 2009;25(1):43–51.
117. Lian Q, Lye E, Suan YK, Khia Way TE, Salto-Tellez M, Liu TM, et al. Derivation of clinically compliant MSCs from CD105+, CD24- differentiated human ESCs. Stem Cells. 2007;25(2):425–36.
118. Cameron CM, Hu WS, Kaufman DS. Improved development of human embryonic stem cell-derived embryoid bodies by stirred vessel cultivation. Biotechnol Bioeng. 2006;94(5):938–48.
119. Hwang NS, Varghese S, Zhang Z, Elisseeff J. Chondrogenic differentiation of human embryonic stem cell-derived cells in arginine-glycine-aspartate-modified hydrogels. Tissue Eng. 2006;12(9):2695–706.

120. Lee EJ, Lee HN, Kang HJ, Kim KH, Hur J, Cho HJ. Novel embryoid body-based method to derive mesenchymal stem cells from human embryonic stem cells. Tissue Eng Part A. 2010;16(2):705–15.
121. Takahashi K, Yamanaka S. Induction of pluripotent stem cells from mouse embryonic and adult fibroblast cultures by defined factors. Cell. 2006;126(4):663–76.
122. Robinton DA, Daley GQ. The promise of induced pluripotent stem cells in research and therapy. Nature. 2012;481(7381):295–305.
123. Wei Y, Zeng W, Wan R, Wang J, Zhou Q, Qiu S, et al. Chondrogenic differentiation of induced pluripotent stem cells from osteoarthritic chondrocytes in alginate matrix. Eur Cell Mater. 2012;23:1–12.
124. Tanaka H, Murphy CL, Murphy C, Kimura M, Kawai S, Polak JM. Chondrogenic differentiation of murine embryonic stem cells: effects of culture conditions and dexamethasone. J Cell Biochem. 2004;93(3):454–62.
125. Nam J, Johnson J, Lannutti JJ, Agarwal S. Modulation of embryonic mesenchymal progenitor cell differentiation via control over pure mechanical modulus in electrospun nanofibers. Acta Biomater. 2011;7(4):1516–24.
126. Nakagawa T, Lee SY, Reddi AH. Induction of chondrogenesis from human embryonic stem cells without embryoid body formation by bone morphogenetic protein 7 and transforming growth factor beta1. Arthritis Rheum. 2009;60(12):3686–92.
127. zur Nieden NI, Kempka G, Rancourt DE, Ahr HJ. Induction of chondro-, osteo- and adipogenesis in embryonic stem cells by bone morphogenetic protein-2: effect of cofactors on differentiating lineages. BMC Dev Biol. 2005;5:1–15.
128. Yang Z, Sui L, Toh WS, Lee EH, Cao T. Stage-dependent effect of TGF-beta1 on chondrogenic differentiation of human embryonic stem cells. Stem Cells Dev. 2009;18(6):929–40.
129. Fecek C, Yao D, Kacorri A, Vasquez A, Iqbal S, Sheikh H, et al. Chondrogenic derivatives of embryonic stem cells seeded into 3D polycaprolactone scaffolds generated cartilage tissue in vivo. Tissue Eng Part A. 2008;14(8):1403–13.
130. Bai HY, Chen GA, Mao GH, Song TR, Wang YX. Three step derivation of cartilage like tissue from human embryonic stem cells by 2D-3D sequential culture in vitro and further implantation in vivo on alginate/PLGA scaffolds. J Biomed Mater Res A. 2010;94(2):539–46.
131. Hwang NS, Varghese S, Lee HJ, Zhang Z, Ye Z, Bae J, et al. In vivo commitment and functional tissue regeneration using human embryonic stem cell-derived mesenchymal cells. Proc Natl Acad Sci U S A. 2008;105(52):20641–6.
132. Toh WS, Lee EH, Guo XM, Chan JK, Yeow CH, Choo AB, et al. Cartilage repair using hyaluronan hydrogel-encapsulated human embryonic stem cell-derived chondrogenic cells. Biomaterials. 2010;31(27):6968–80.
133. Heng BC, Cao T, Lee EH. Directing stem cell differentiation into the chondrogenic lineage in vitro. Stem Cells. 2004;22(7):1152–67.
134. Nakajima M, Wakitani S, Harada Y, Tanigami A, Tomita N. In vivo mechanical condition plays an important role for appearance of cartilage tissue in ES cell transplanted joint. J Orthop Res. 2008;26(1):10–7.
135. Wakitani S, Aoki H, Harada Y, Sonobe M, Morita Y, Mu Y, et al. Embryonic stem cells form articular cartilage, not teratomas, in osteochondral defects of rat joints. Cell Transplant. 2004;13(4):331–6.
136. Wakitani S, Takaoka K, Hattori T, Miyazawa N, Iwanaga T, Takeda S, et al. Embryonic stem cells injected into the mouse knee joint form teratomas and subsequently destroy the joint. Rheumatology. 2003;42(1):162–5.
137. Clar C, Cummins E, McIntyre L, Thomas S, Lamb J, Bain L, et al. Clinical and cost-effectiveness of autologous chondrocyte implantation for cartilage defects in knee joints: systematic review and economic evaluation. Health Technol Assess. 2005;9(47):iii–v.
138. Vasiliadis HS, Wasiak J, Salanti G. Autologous chondrocyte implantation for the treatment of cartilage lesions of the knee: a systematic review of randomized studies. Knee Surg Sports Traumatol Arthrosc. 2010;18(12):1645–55.
139. Vavken P, Samartzis D. Effectiveness of autologous chondrocyte implantation in cartilage repair of the knee: a systematic review of controlled trials. Osteoarthritis Cartilage. 2010;18(6):857–63.
140. Harris JD, Siston RA, Brophy RH, Lattermann C, Carey JL, Flanigan DC. Failures, re-operations, and complications after autologous chondrocyte implantation–a systematic review. Osteoarthritis Cartilage. 2011;19(7):779–91.
141. Harris JD, Siston RA, Pan X, Flanigan DC. Autologous chondrocyte implantation: a systematic review. J Bone Joint Surg Am. 2010;92(12):2220–33.
142. Cole BJ, Farr J, Winalski CS, Hosea T, Richmond J, Mandelbaum B, et al. Outcomes after a single-stage procedure for cell-based cartilage repair: a prospective clinical safety trial with 2-year follow-up. Am J Sports Med. 2011;39(6):1170–9.
143. Yamasaki S, Mera H, Itokazu M, Hashimoto Y, Wakitani S. Cartilage repair with autologous bone marrow mesenchymal stem cell transplantation: review of preclinical and clinical studies. Cartilage. 2014;5(4):196–202.
144. Williams GM, Klisch SM, Sah RL. Bioengineering cartilage growth, maturation, and form. Pediatr Res. 2008;63(5):527–34.
145. Knutsen G, Drogset JO, Engebretsen L, Grøntvedt T, Ludvigsen TC, Løken S, Solheim E, Strand T, Johansen O. A randomized multicenter trial comparing autologous chondrocyte implantation with microfracture: long-term follow-up at 14 to 15 years. J Bone Joint Surg Am. 2016;98(16):1332–9.
146. Schlumberger M, Schuster P, Bülow HJ, Mayer P, Eichinger M, et al. Arthroscopic autolo-

gous chondrocyte implantation in the knee with an in situ crosslinking matrix: minimum 4-year clinical results of 15 cases and 1 histological evaluation. Arch Orthop Trauma Surg. 2019;139(11):1607–15.

147. Chahal J, Gómez-Aristizábal A, Shestopaloff K, Bhatt S, Chaboureau A, et al. Bone marrow mesenchymal stromal cell treatment in patients with osteoarthritis results in overall improvement in pain and symptoms and reduces synovial inflammation. Stem Cells Transl Med. 2019;8(8):746–57.

148. Roato I, Belisario DC, Compagno M, Lena A, Bistolfi A, et al. Concentrated adipose tissue infusion for the treatment of knee osteoarthritis: clinical and histological observations. Int Orthop. 2019;43(1):15–23.

149. Lee WS, Kim HJ, Kim KI, Kim GB, Jin W. Intra-articular injection of autologous adipose tissue-derived mesenchymal stem cells for the treatment of knee osteoarthritis: a phase IIb, randomized, placebo-controlled clinical trial. Stem Cells Transl Med. 2019;8(6):504–11.

150. Onoi Y, Hiranaka T, Nishida R, Takase K, Fujita M, et al. Second-look arthroscopic findings of cartilage and meniscus repair after injection of adipose-derived regenerative cells in knee osteoarthrits: Report of two cases. Regen Ther. 2019;11:212–16.

151. Woods S, Bates N, Dunn SL, Serracino-Inglott F, Hardingham TE, et al. Generation of human-induced pluripotent stem cells from anterior cruciate ligament. J Orthop Res. 2020;38(1):92–104.

Relevance of Engineered Scaffolds for Cartilage Repair

17

Mikael Starecki, Michael A. Gott, John A. Schwartz, Nicholas A. Sgaglione, and Daniel A. Grande

17.1 Introduction

Articular cartilage is a specialized connective tissue that allows for smooth, frictionless movement of the joints. The complex biomechanical properties and substantial durability of articular cartilage is attributed to its macromolecular composition and architecture as well as the integrity of its extracellular matrix (ECM) [1, 2]. Refer to Chap. 1 for an in-depth description of knee articular cartilage morphology and biochemical composition.

Articular cartilage injury caused by trauma, pathological conditions, or degeneration is the major cause of disability worldwide. Due to its avascular nature and consequent lack of access to a pool of potential reparative cells and humoral factors, once injured, adult articular cartilage has limited capability for self-repair and/or regeneration to its native state [3, 4]. Further, due to low chondrocyte to ECM ratio, especially in aging cartilage, the ability of the chondrocytes to repair the tissue is small [5–7]. However, in contrast to adults, the articular cartilage of children and adolescents has better healing capacity after injury. This is partly due to the presence of stem cells in the growth plate, which are able to divide and differentiate into chondrocytes, and partly due to the

M. Starecki, MD
Resurgens Orthopaedics, West Cobb, Marietta, GA, USA

Department of Orthopaedic Surgery, East-West Surgery Center, Wellstar Cobb Hospital and Wellstar Douglas Hospital, Austell, GA, USA

M. A. Gott, MD
Westchester Health Orthopaedics and Sports Medicine, Westchester Sport and Spine, White Plains Hospital, White Plains, NY, USA

J. A. Schwartz, MD
Orthopaedic Research Center, Colorado State University, Fort Collins, CO, USA

Orthopaedic Research Laboratory, Feinstein Institute for Medical Research, North Shore-LIJ Health System, Manhasset, NY, USA

N. A. Sgaglione, MD
Department of Orthopaedic Surgery, Long Island Jewish Medical Center, Northwell Health, New Hyde Park, NY, USA

Department of Molecular Medicine and Orthopaedic Surgery, Donald and Barbara Zucker School of Medicine at Hofstra-Northwell, Hempstead, NY, USA

D. A. Grande, PhD (✉)
Orthopaedic Research Laboratory, Feinstein Institute for Medical Research, North Shore-LIJ Health System, Manhasset, NY, USA

Center for Bioelectronic Medicine, Feinstein Institute for Medical Research, North Shore-LIJ Health System, Manhasset, NY, USA

Department of Molecular Medicine and Orthopaedic Surgery, Donald and Barbara Zucker School of Medicine at Hofstra-Northwell, Hempstead, NY, USA

Department of Orthopaedic Surgery, Long Island Jewish Medical Center, Northwell Health, New Hyde Park, NY, USA
e-mail: DGrande@northwell.edu

H. K. Gahunia et al. (eds.), *Articular Cartilage of the Knee*,
https://doi.org/10.1007/978-1-4939-7587-7_17

presence of a certain degree of vascularization within the articular cartilage that allows direct access of the nutrients to the cartilage.

Based on whether the injury penetrates through the underlying subchondral bone, defects of articular cartilage fall into two main categories, chondral or osteochondral (OC) defects [4]. Partial- or full-thickness cartilage defects that are limited to the uncalcified cartilage lack an inherent ability to heal spontaneously [8]; whereas, full-thickness cartilage defects that penetrate through the vascularized subchondral bone, referred to as an OC defect have access to the bone marrow-derived chondroprogenitor stem cells, enabling some degree of spontaneous repair through the formation of fibrocartilage [9].

Due to its limited ability to regenerate itself, several cartilage repair techniques have been utilized to relieve symptoms and functional limitations [9]. Current treatments for cartilage injury include, but are not limited to, abrasion/debridement, chondroplasty/arthroplasty/mosaicplasty, marrow stimulation techniques (i.e., multiple drilling or microfracture), OC autografting/allografting, and cell-based therapies using cultured autologous/allogeneic chondrocytes, stem cells, or a combination of both.

Initially, the concept of a tissue-engineered (TE) scaffold was to provide cells with a delivery system to maintain them within a defect site. In recent years, several innovative cartilage repair strategies using bioengineered, biocompatible, and bioabsorbable scaffolds have evolved. The implantation of the scaffold within a chondral or OC defect provides support for the local migration of chondrogenic or osteogenic cells that ultimately synthesize new ECM. These scaffolds play a vital role as a primary mechanical function to bear joint forces. The goals of this chapter are to highlight the key features of successful cartilage scaffolds and three-dimensional (3D) constructs, and to review scaffolds that are currently being investigated and clinically used.

17.2 Evolution of Articular Cartilage Repair Treatment Options

The investigation of scaffolds by the orthopedic community is the result of an ongoing process searching for a reliable way to treat damaged articular cartilage. Initial attempts at treating focal chondral defects used techniques to stimulate the bone marrow cells to differentiate into native chondrocytes by abrasion arthroplasty. In 1959, Pridie described a method of resurfacing osteoarthritis (OA) joints and introduced the principle of multiple drilling of subchondral bone to encourage the formation of fibrocartilaginous repair tissue [10]. This was followed in the 1990s by Steadman's procedure of microfracture (MFX) of the subchondral bone [11–14]. Multiple drilling and MFX procedures allowed the influx of blood and marrow-derived chondroprogenitor cells into the chondral defect followed by the blood clot formation and stimulation of the classical wound repair cascade; these techniques yielded the formation of a mixed tissue type but primarily fibrocartilage. However, compared with normal articular cartilage that is abundant in proteoglycans (PGs) and collagen type II, fibrocartilage repair tissue has inferior biochemical and biomechanical properties as it is abundant in collagen type I, which is poorly organized and susceptible to injury. Similar to untreated cartilage defects, the breakdown of fibrocartilage repair tissue over time and repetitive loading will lead to OA [8, 15–17].

Over the past 20 years, autologous chondrocyte implantation (ACI) procedure has become widespread for clinically treating focal cartilage defects as it aims to generate hyaline-like or hyaline cartilage repair tissue [5]. The ACI model was first tested by Grande et al. in rabbits [18] Although this surgical technique was first performed in Sweden in 1987, Brittberg et al. pioneered the clinical use of this technique and provided the first description of the procedure on human femoral condyle chondral defects in 1994 [19]. Further improvements in tissue engineering (TE) have contributed to the subsequent ACI generations (second, third, and fourth) which involve the combination of autologous chondrocytes with orthobiologic, resorbable biomaterials/scaffolds that secure the cells in the defect area and enhance their proliferation and differentiation [20–22].

The first and second ACI generation does not utilize a scaffold; however, instead of an autologous periosteal cover used in the first generation, a bioabsorbable collagen membrane cover is used in the second ACI generation. In third-generation ACI, chondrocytes are seeded onto a collagen scaffold used to fill the defect. The scaffold is attached to the defect using a fibrin glue. The matrix-induced autologous chondrocyte implantation (MACI) is a trademark for the commercially available scaffold originally produced by Genzyme, which was marketed by Aastrom Biosciences Inc. but now acquired by Vericel Corporation (Cambridge, MA, USA). The MACI autologous cellularized scaffold is comprised of collagen type I/III membrane manufactured from porcine peritoneal tissue, which is indicated for the repair of single or multiple symptomatic, full-thickness cartilage defects of the adult knee, with or without bone involvement. Whereas in the fourth ACI generation, the chondrocytes are seeded on a 3D scaffold that aids in preserving their chondrogenic phenotype [20].

17.3 Cartilage Tissue Engineering

From a basic science and TE standpoint, what integral components are necessary for the successful restoration of articular cartilage? The three key elements of approach of cartilage TE that provides an innovative approach for the repair of articular cartilage defects are as follows [20, 23–28]:

17.3.1 Viable Cells with Chondrogenic Potential

There are two cell populations that are capable of proliferation and differentiation into mature chondrocytes. One source is hyaline chondrocytes (autogenic or allogenic) that are harvested, cultured, and then seeded on the scaffold. Another source includes multipotent or pluripotent stem cell populations with chondrogenic potential. These stem cells may originate from various mesenchymal tissues such as bone marrow, synovium, adipose tissue, skeletal muscle, perichondrium, and periosteum [23, 29].

17.3.2 Orthobiologic Scaffolds

Next, filling a cartilage defect necessitates a biocompatible, biodegradable and biomechanically stable scaffold that houses and allows the viable cells to be delivered as well as provide and sustain a permissive environment for cellular functioning. It must also facilitate proper orientation of repaired tissue for a sufficient time to allow integration with the adjacent native articular cartilage.

17.3.3 Signaling Molecules and Growth Factor(s)

Growth factors play a very important role in TE for repairing articular cartilage and OC defects with a more successful outcome. Corroborated in animal studies, cell-assisted and growth-factor scaffolds produced much better results, while growth-factor-free scaffolds showed a much lower rate of healing [30–34].

With the use of reliable delivery systems, the use of growth factors has been suggested to improve the repair of cartilage [35]. Several hormonal and paracrine factors regulate the proliferation and differentiation of chondrocytes and cells with chondrogenic potential. The Transforming growth factor-beta (TGF-β) superfamily, the parathyroid hormone (PTH) related peptide Indian hedgehog (IH) loop, and a number of transcription factors, such as Sox and Runx, are involved in the regulation of chondrocyte proliferation and differentiation [36]. The delivery of TGF-β, with the use of alginate, for the treatment of OC defects in the rabbit knee showed an improvement in the repair of cartilage defects

[37]. Chitosan hydrogels have also been successfully used to deliver growth factors to chondrocytes [38]. These bioactive molecules in the form of growth factors stimulate the chondrogenic response and ensure proper growth of the articular cartilage ECM [30].

17.4 Tissue-Engineered Scaffolds for Cartilage Repair

Tissue engineering uses principles of cell and developmental biology, engineering and material science, suitable biochemical and physicochemical factors, and medicine to generate constructs that can successfully recapitulate the function of native tissues in terms of histology, 3D morphology, biochemistry, and biomechanics. Over the past two decades, the evolution of TE has led to innovative techniques including preparation of various clinically effective and safe orthobiologic scaffolds in the hope of improving articular cartilage healing, repair and regeneration. Through the development and ex vivo manufacture of implantable cartilage scaffolds, the goal of cartilage TE is to promote long-lasting, functional repair of chondral lesions which would then translate into patient's relief from joint pain and restoration of function.

These scaffolds provide an important supporting network for cartilage cells to adhere and proliferate, to direct cell differentiation/metabolism, and to mediate the cell-to-cell signaling and interaction [39–42] (Figs. 17.1 and 17.2).

17.4.1 Requirements for Cartilage Scaffolds

The physical and biochemical properties of scaffolds are critical for the success of the cartilage repair process, which involves chondrogenesis and creation of the cartilage ECM. Properties that should be considered when engineering scaffolds for articular cartilage repair is listed as follows:

17.4.1.1 Biocompatibility

Biocompatibility is important in characterizing biomaterials and involves two major principles: biosafety and biofunctionality. Scaffolds must be biocompatible or non-immunogenic. An inflammatory response to the scaffold would lead to rejection of the implant. A good scaffold is non-cytotoxic and able to form tissue with the host. This should be true in both the scaffold's native form and its degradation by-products. As the scaffold is slowly degraded and replaced by the host cells along with new ECM, the effect of the released chemical cross-linking agents and the levels of acidic by-products on the surrounding native tissue should be carefully investigated [43].

17.4.1.2 Biodegradability

Scaffolds should ideally be biodegradable in a predictable and uniform manner. The scaffold is implanted with the idea that it will eventually be replaced by native tissue, neocartilage, and ECM. Often the scaffold will degrade over time at the same rate with tissue formation. If the scaffold has degradation rate faster than cartilage regeneration, the mechanical strength of the material can be compromised, particularly if applied in the load-bearing region of the joint. Further, it is important to bear in mind that biocompatible scaffolds are possible to degrade over time but not all by-products of biodegradable scaffolds are biocompatible as some of the degraded by-products might not be compatible to the chondrocytes and/or cartilage tissue.

17.4.1.3 Permeability and Porosity

The TE scaffold is designed and fabricated in order to provide a proper architecture for cells to grow, proliferate, and differentiate as well as enhance and guide new tissue formation. In order for chondrocytes or chondrogenic cells to migrate through the scaffold, it needs to be permeable. Permeability will also allow for important growth factors to reach desired targets. Using precisely designed poly-epsilon-capro-

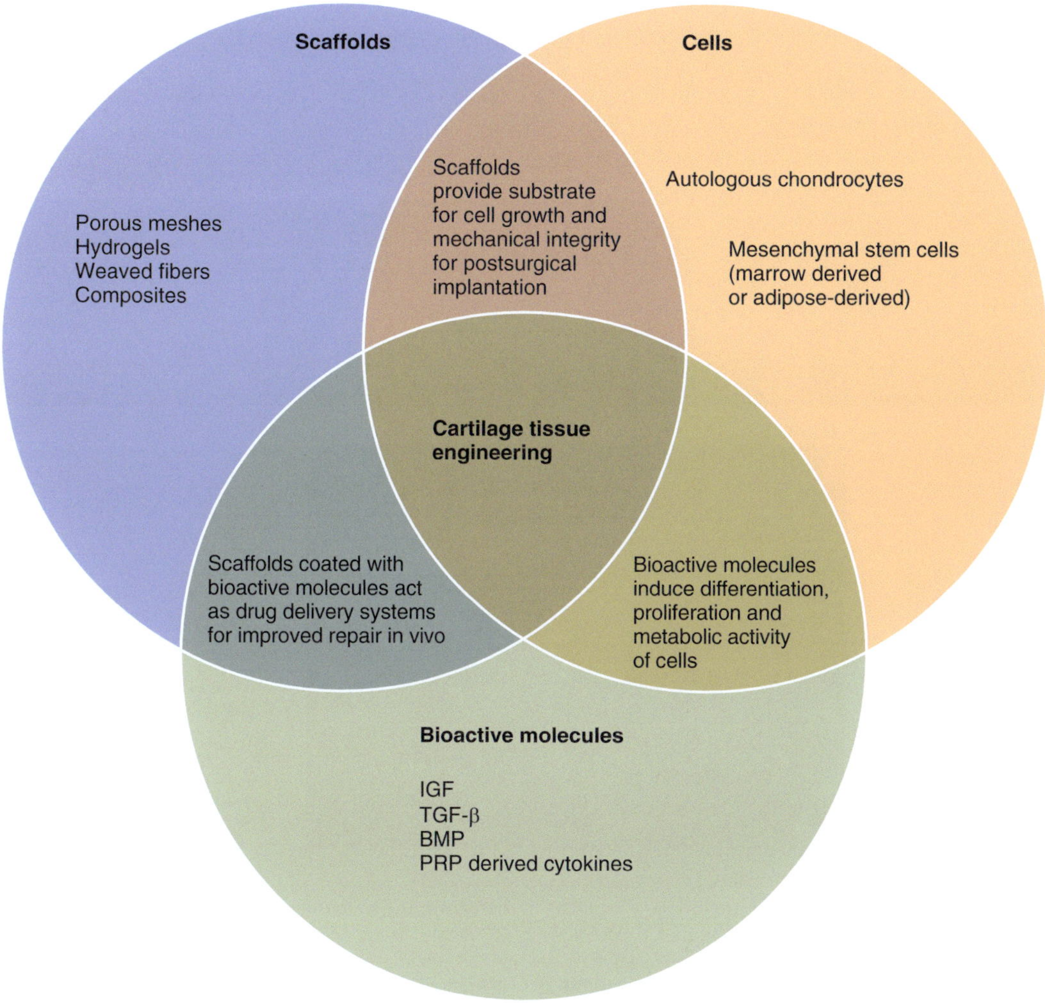

Fig. 17.1 The tripartite view of the field of tissue engineering as it applies to cartilage repair
IGF, *Insulin-like growth factor*; TGF-β, *Transforming growth factor-beta*; BMP, *Bone morphogenetic protein*; PRP, *Platelet-rich plasma*

lactone (PECL) scaffolds, in vitro investigation showed that permeability affects the chondrogenic performance of chondrocytes and bone marrow stromal cells in opposite ways [44]. PECL is a semicrystalline, biodegradable polyester which has a long time of degradation; however, the biodegradability, biocompatibility, and mechanical properties of the pure PECL have been shown to be suboptimal for bone TE applications [45].

Another essential factor in the design of the cartilage scaffold relates to its porosity and pore interconnectivity [46]. The scaffold should have sufficient porosity with adequate pore size to enable cell impregnation into and through the scaffold, cell-to-cell interaction, and the growth of repair tissue [47, 48]. Also, porosity allows cell growth as nutrient, oxygen and waste transport. Average pore size, pore size distribution, pore volume, pore interconnectivity, pore shape, and pore wall roughness are important parameters to consider while designing a scaffold [49]. It provides a porous biocompatible network into which the surrounding native tissue is induced and acts as a temporary template for the new tissue's growth and reorganization. Therefore, a fine balance between scaffold permeability, porosity, and stability is necessary.

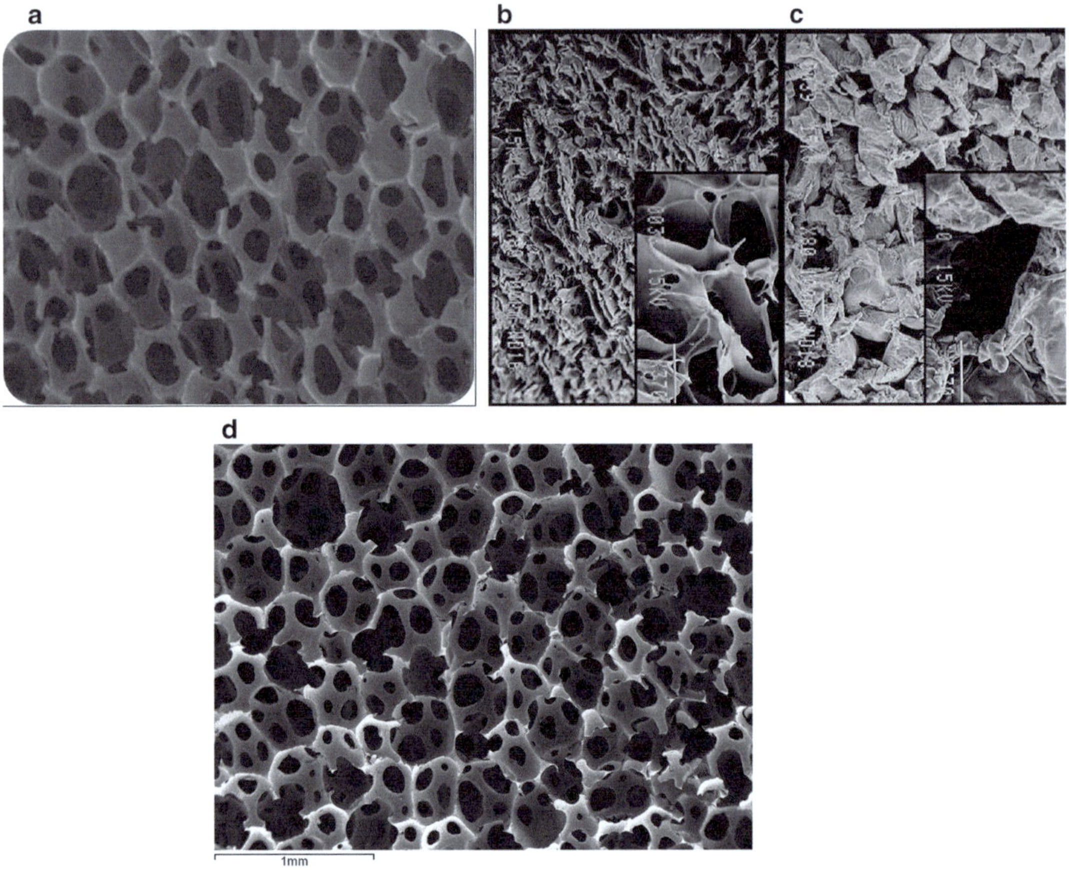

Fig. 17.2 Scanning Electron Microscopy of various tissue engineered (TE) scaffolds. (**a**) Biomerix (Biomerix Corporation, Fremont, CA, USA) biointegrative nondegradable matrix (magnification, 23×). (**b**) Cross-linked derivative of hyaluronic acid (HA) (magnification, 80×). (**c**) Poly-L-lactic acid (PLLA) / polyglycolic acid (PGA) 50/50 copolymer (magnification, 80×). (**d**) Biomerix degradable matrix (magnification, 35×)

17.4.1.4 Mechanical Stability

The biomechanical properties of the scaffold are critical to the success of the implant. The biostability of many scaffolds depends on the factors such as strength, elasticity, and absorption at the material interface and its chemical degradation [50]. It is essential to retain the mechanical strength of the scaffold structure after implantation for the regeneration of hyaline cartilage and bone in chondral and OC repair. Also, it is critical that the biomaterial scaffold temporarily withstands and conducts the loads and stresses that the new tissue will ultimately bear. The mechanical properties of bulk biomaterials are altered by their processing into scaffolds of various pore sizes and pore orientations, and further these properties will rapidly diminish as a function of implantation time [51]. A scaffold should be capable of maintaining the integrity of the impregnated cells (chondrocytes or stem cells) when subjected to external mechanical forces expected with everyday movement. Studies examining chondrocyte behavior showed cells cultured in vitro in a two-dimensional (2D) fashion or monolayer lose their chondrogenic phenotype. These cells were shown to regain their phenotype when cultured on a 3D scaffold [13–16].

17.4.1.5 Versatility

The versatility of a scaffold can be explained by the numerous possibilities of modification in its chemical structure through the substitution of its functional groups. A good scaffold should be versatile. It should be capable of aiding in the repair of full- and partial-thickness chondral lesions.

17.4.1.6 Durability and Retainability

A scaffold should be durable with adequate mechanical integrity to withstand both the implantation procedure and mechanical forces typically experienced during joint mobility. The scaffold's biomechanical load-bearing capability is especially critical during the period of post-transplantation till the regenerated tissue is able to withstand load-bearing. Further, the scaffold should be fabricated such that it is retained and confined at the site of implantation [52].

17.4.1.7 Reproducibility

In order for scaffolds to have a significant clinical impact, they need to be reproducible and readily available. This should be similar to the way any tool is available to the orthopedic surgeon. For example, while performing an anterior cruciate ligament (ACL) reconstruction in a 20-year-old athlete, the surgeon encounters a large isolated chondral defect on the medial femoral condyle. Current scaffolds necessitate the use of a two-stage procedure. The creation of a scaffold that could be cultured and prepared in the operating room (OR) in a method similar to platelet rich plasma (PRP) would be invaluable.

17.4.2 Types of Tissue-Engineered Scaffolds

Current matrices used for TE applications are fabricated from two main classes of biodegradable polymers based on their composition, namely natural material-based and synthetic-based scaffolds [53]. Each class of scaffolds is further divided into specific subsets or polymers and composite scaffold types.

17.4.2.1 Natural Material Scaffolds

Natural scaffolds are useful because they replicate a native environment that promotes cell adhesion and proliferation. Both protein- and carbohydrate-based scaffolds fall under the umbrella of natural material scaffolds.

A. Proteins-Based Scaffolds

Protein-based scaffolds include collagen membranes and fibrin.

Collagen

Collagen is the major protein that makes up the connective tissue [54]. Tropocollagen is the basic subunit of collagen. It is made up of three polypeptide chains wound together in a triple helix that forms collagen's tertiary structure. Ligands are important molecules attached to collagen. Ligands facilitate cell adhesion as well as cell migration, differentiation, and morphology [55, 56]. The availability of functional groups or ligands along collagen's backbone provides the potential for interaction with growth factors and other molecules. This capability adds another dimension to collagen's use as a tissue-engineered scaffold [57]. Using collagen fiber scaffolds to deliver *chondrocytes* in vivo in rabbits, it was reported that at 6 months a hyaline-like repair tissue was generated that was biochemically and mechanically similar to native articular cartilage [58].

The repair capability of shape-memory native collagen versus denatured collagen scaffolds with chondrocytes was investigated for full-thickness articular cartilage defects in the knee of New Zealand white rabbits [59]. The native collagen scaffolds showed a greater degree of chondrocyte proliferation, adhesion, and redifferentiation, as well as chondrocyte-matrix interaction compared to the denatured collagen scaffolds. Further, the native collagen scaffolds significantly maintained chondrocytes function, promoted cartilage and subchondral bone regeneration, compared with the denatured collagen scaffolds. This study suggests that collagen scaffolds with the triple-helical structure may have greater potential for articular cartilage repair.

Dorotka et al. used a collagen type I membrane scaffold to support cell migration and adhesion in a MFX defect in a goat model [60]. The study compared three groups: MFX alone, MFX combined with a collagen type I membrane scaffold, and MFX in combination with a chondrocyte-seeded scaffold. In this study, the chondrocyte-seeded scaffold was histologically superior. Furthermore, the addition of a collagen scaffold (without chondrocytes) showed improved healing to MFX alone [60, 61].

Fibrin

Fibrin is the major clot component that is formed at wound sites. Fibrin has been tested both as a stand-alone scaffold and a delivery substrate for chondrocytes, stem cells with chondrogenic potential, and/or growth factors [62–65]. Fibrin is a product of fibrinogen and thrombin. This reaction produces a natural 3D matrix that is biodegradable leaving behind non-toxic physiological substances. Studies by Fortier et al. and Nixon et al. successfully used 3D fibrin scaffolds in vitro and in vivo [63–66]. The study showed that chondrocytes and mesenchymal stem cells were supported by the 3D matrix and promoted healing in equine cartilage defects [63]. Another study by the same group combined insulin-like growth factor 1 (IGF-1) to the fibrin matrix in vitro. The addition of IGF-1 produced more tissue and increased ECM and collagen II production [66].

B. Carbohydrate-Based Scaffolds

The carbohydrate components specific to articular cartilage includes the aggrecans (a hydrophilic PG) and hyaluronic acid (HA), both of which are the major component of cartilage ECM. As such, carbohydrate-based scaffolds have been extensively explored in cartilage repair studies. Examples of carbohydrate-based scaffolds include alginate, agarose, HA, and chitosan [57].

Agarose and Alginate

Agarose and alginate are anionic carbohydrate/polysaccharide polymers derived from seaweed that form hydrogels. Since the past few years, injectable hydrogels with cells and bioactive molecules have been used as bioscaffolds for OC lesion treatment, repair, and regeneration [67–69]. Although agarose has been extensively used for in vitro studies, it does not resorb well and may elicit immunogenic response in vivo. When seaweed is placed in the presence of calcium cations, ionic bonding creates cross-linked alginate chains. The 3D alginate beads are created when cells are added to a calcium chloride solution. A 3D platform is important for chondrocyte structure and function. In vitro chondrocytes that are grown in a monolayer dedifferentiate and lose their phenotypic expression. These dedifferentiated chondrocytes when expanded and then seeded in 3D alginate cultures redifferentiated to the cartilage phenotype [70]. Mierisch et al. investigated the effect of alginate on rabbit chondrocytes in vitro and in vivo [35, 37]. Alginate promoted the expression of cartilage-specific genes and enabled the delivery of chondrocytes into OC defects [35]. Also, the use of alginate allowed the controlled delivery of TGF-β selectively to the defect site, hence avoiding systemic side effects [37]. Diduch et al. used alginated beads impregnated with mesenchymal stem cells to repair OC defects in a rabbit model [71]. However, alginate has had limited use clinically because of concerns with its biocompatibility [26].

Hyaluronic Acid

Hyaluronic acid (also known as hyaluronan) is a major component of cartilage ECM. It is a highly conserved glycosaminoglycan (GAG) that is also found throughout the body. In vitro, in vivo, and clinical studies have proven this molecule to be ideal for TE strategies in cartilage repair by stimulating chondrogenesis in mesenchymal stem cells [72–74]. *Hyaff-11* (Fidia Advanced Biopolymers Laboratories, Abano Terme, Italy) is the trademarked name for an esterified hyaluronan scaffold. Its ubiquitous nature in the human body makes it highly biocompatible. It has been shown to fully resorb in a controllable and predictable manner within 3 months. Its main by-product is HA. An extensive biocompatibility study by Campoccia et al. showed that its by-products are fully resorbed and do not elicit an inflammatory response [75]. Further, it can be used to culture chondrocytes in 3D culture conditions that mimic an in vivo situation. Chondrocyte culture exhibited their normal phenotype secreting proteins and molecules characteristic of hyaline cartilage [76–79]. In vivo animal models using autologous chondrocytes seeded on HA-based scaffolds have successfully regenerated hyaline cartilage. The engineered cartilage-like tissue was integrated with the surrounding native articular surface [80]. However, contrary to other studies, Knudson et al. reported that HA induced chondrocytic chondrolysis and perturbed the cartilage matrix homeostasis [81].

Chitosan

Chitosan, found naturally in the arthropod exoskeleton, is a polysaccharide that forms a hydrogel when cross-linked with chondroitin sulfate (CS) [82, 83]. It is a partially deacetylated derivative of chitin. Specifically, it is a bi-copolymer of glucosamine and N-acetylglucosamine. A chitosan-based scaffold has the potential of delivering growth factors as well as mature chondrocytes and chondrogenic mesenchymal stem cells [38, 64]. Chitosan is cationic and has a high charge density in solution. This allows it to "carry" biologically active anionic polysaccharides such as GAGs, deoxyribonucleic acid (DNA), and alginates. Chitosan's charge density is pH dependent, and a change in pH (i.e., from in vitro to in vivo) would allow for release of these compounds [85, 86]. Chitosan scaffold is biocompatible, biodegradable, bioactive, non-expensive, and non-immunogenic, with antibacterial capability [87]. Chitosan degradation products are non-toxic and are involved in the synthesis of articular cartilage [88]. They include CS, dermatan sulfate (DS), HA, keratan sulfate (KS), and glycosylated collagen type II [82]. In vitro studies have suggested that chitosan could promote the expression of cartilage matrix components and reduce inflammatory and catabolic mediator's production by chondrocytes [89]. Studies performed using sheep and rabbit chondral defect models showed improvements over the use of MFX alone [90, 91]. In OA-induced rabbit model, chitosan prevented cartilage degradation and synovial membrane inflammation. Several studies have also shown that chitosan could induce chondrogenic differentiation of mesenchymal stem cells [89].

17.4.2.2 Synthetic Polymer-Based Scaffolds

Polymeric scaffolds have been extensively used for articular cartilage TE. The mechanical and biologic properties of synthetic polymers can be tailored to varying engineering strategies and chondral defect dimensions [42, 43, 92]. The most widely used synthetic polymers include polylactic acid (PLA), PGA, polylactic co-glycolic acid (PLGA), and PECL. These compounds are appealing because they are relatively inexpensive and have already been accepted by the American Food and Drug Administration (FDA) for use in sutures [57]. Compared to natural scaffolds, synthetics can be configured to sustain weight-bearing forces making them more biomechanically stable. Further, these scaffolds have improved degradation properties allowing for a controlled release of growth factors as well as the ability to control the degradation rate of the scaffold itself [93, 94]. In addition, these compounds are easily produced, have "off-the-shelf" capabilities, and can be used to fill chondrocyte-donor sites.

In vitro studies have shown that bone marrow mesenchymal stem cell has the potential to differentiate into chondrocytes when cultured within PLA or PLA/alginate scaffolds in the presence of TGF-β [95]. In vivo studies in immature rabbit knees have shown that PGA-PLA copolymer absorbable pads with calcium alginate allowed the delivery of chondrocytes to the OC defects with indication of enhanced cartilage regeneration [93]. Photopolymerizing hydrogel systems using PLGA microspheres have provided a method to encapsulate cells and implant materials in a minimally invasive as well as provided a mode for controlled release of growth factors [96]. However, the major downside to synthetic scaffolds is their poor biocompatibility. They lack natural sites for cell adhesion, as well as porosity, inhibiting replacement of the scaffold by native cartilage cells. The by-products are acidic which can cause inflammation as well as chondrocyte death [97, 98]. Giant cell formation has also been observed with the use of synthetic scaffolds [99].

17.4.2.3 Hybrid and Biomimetic Zonal Scaffolds

Recently, advances in the cartilage construct design and fabrication techniques have enabled the strategic design of scaffolds with complex, biomimetic structures and properties [100–106]. Scaffolds can acquire better biocompatibility and mechanical adaptability by developing composite-, biomimetic-, and nano-materials [92, 107–113]. Examples of nanomaterials include electrospun nanofibers and emulsion nanoparticles which provide nanoscale features for biomaterials, more closely replicating the 3D ECM, providing better cell adhesion, integration, interaction, and signaling [109]. Several studies have described and developed scaffolds with hybrid and/or biomimetic zonal designs [46, 47, 114]. Advanced TE scaffold design for OC lesions includes biphasic, triphasic, and gradient configurations aimed to promote cartilage and bone layer formation with an interdigitating transitional zone at the bone-cartilage interface [115]. Cartilage TE constructs typically lack the complex spatial gradients of cell types and tissue organization for bone-soft tissue interface regeneration and the stratified zonal architecture present in adult articular cartilages. This has led to increased interest in bioprinting technologies and biofabrication strategies that makes it possible to generate zonal distributions of cells, matrix, and bioactive cues in 3D [116, 117]. Several fabrication processes have been developed to create microenvironments to facilitate and control cell adhesion and organization on a 3D scaffold. Using a novel 3D printing method, fabrication of highly porous 3D cytocompatible scaffold architectures based on cell-responsive polymeric inks, i.e., sodium alginate and gelatin (SA-Gel, 1:3 ratio) have shown excellent adhesion rate and growth behavior of chondrocytes in vitro [118]. Another study showed that 3D extrusion-based printing at high temperature and pressure results in an aligned effect on the polymer molecules, which in turn induced varying cell differentiation capacities as well as different cell morphology and orientation on scaffolds [119, 120]. Recent advances in nanotechnology and the four-dimensional (4D) printing have succeeded in creating a new range of materials to develop into the desired biological responses to the cellular level [121]. The 4D printing technology has extended the ability of active composite materials to change form and function after they are 3D printed, offering additional capabilities and performance-driven applications [122]. These 4D materials are developed by printing shape memory polymer fibers in an elastomeric matrix achieving a programmed action through the stimulation of the shape memory fibers. The time-dependent shape and/or functional changes realized with 4D fabrication techniques have shown great application potential for the development of scaffolds with high biocompatibility for articular cartilage and OC defect repair [121].

17.4.2.4 Commercialized Scaffolds

For a scaffold to perform optimally, several design considerations must be addressed, with an eye toward the eventual form, function, and tissue site. The chemical and mechanical properties of the scaffold must be tuned to optimize the interaction with cells and surrounding tissues. For complex TE, mass transport limitations, vascularization, and host tissue integration are important considerations. As the tissue architecture to be replaced becomes more complex and hierarchical, scaffold design must also match this complexity to recapitulate a functioning tissue.

The creation of ACI using bioengineered scaffolds emerged due to multiple drawbacks and limitations of the first-generation ACI such as cell leakage, uneven chondrocyte distribution from injection and graft failure, and finally periosteal flap hypertrophy [123]. The third-generation ACI was the first time a true scaffold was used and chondrocytes were impregnated on a tissue-engineered scaffold used to fill the defect. There are several examples of the third-generation scaffolds which are attached to the small defect using a fibrin glue or sutured to the chondral surface in the case of large defects. These include *Hyalograft C* (a benzylic ester of HA-based scaffold) [124], *MACI* scaffold (composed of a collagen type I/III membrane from porcine peritoneal tissue), and *BioSeed C* (a synthetic-based polymer fleece comprised of PGA/PLA and polydioxanone fleece with a fibrin fleece to evenly distribute cells) [20]. Further evolution of the TE technology led to the manufacture of a 3D scaffold which was used in the fourth generation. Mechanical stimulation of chondrocytes in 3D culture allows for maintenance of chondrogenic phenotype and creates a stable mature hyaline matrix [70, 125]. Examples of the fourth-generation ACI that are commercially available include *NeoCart*, *a* 3D scaffold that is a collagen type I matrix of bovine origin. Autologous chondrocytes are harvested and then seeded on this 3D scaffold in a hydrostatic bioreactor for 7 days [126]. *Cartipatch* is an alginate-cultured 3D scaffold that uses a combination of two polymers (agarose and alginate) with seeded autologous chondrocytes [127, 128]. *Alginate beads* are unique to the above two examples because this TE technology uses allogenic chondrocytes harvested from a cadaveric knee within 24 h of death. These chondrocytes are cultured and mixed with alginate to form beads [129]. Almqvist et al.'s study explores the possibility of freezing and storing these alginate beads to be used in the future in an "off-the-shelf" fashion [129]. Refer to Chap. 18 for an overview of the commercially available bioengineered cartilage grafts and clinical outcome.

17.5 Considerations and Future Directions

Modern TE concepts integrate cells, scaffolds, signalling molecules and growth factors. Various biomaterials are being explored for an optimally fabricated cartilage repair scaffold. Native biological materials and synthetic polymeric materials have their pros and cons. Nevertheless the unfavorable factors of these scaffolds can be overcome through either physical or biochemical modifications. Further, developing composite-, biomimetic-, and nanomaterials can enhance the biocompatibility and mechanical adaptability of the cartilage-engineered scaffolds.

The treatment of articular cartilage lesions is complicated, but novel TE approaches can improve the outcome. A TE approach is less invasive and reduces surgical time, periosteal hypertrophy, and morbidity. An optimal scaffold should not only satisfy the biological, biochemical, and biomechanical perspective to support and enhance the growth of hyaline-like repair tissue but should also be surgeon-friendly. The scaffold handling properties and implantation procedure should also be simple and conducive. Scaffold materials that are "off-the-shelf" and allow a one-step arthroscopic procedure are extremely attractive.

Although a plethora of devices and materials are being examined for their potential to deliver cells and growth factors to cartilage and OC lesions, and to act as scaffolds for ingrowth of new cartilage-like tissue, a reliable and reproducible way of treating cartilage defects still remains elusive to the orthopedic community. Technologies that allow cell homing to scaffolds with molecules such as TGF-β or stromal cell-derived factor-1 [SDF-1] represent the next leap forward to using scaffolds as an adjunct to microfracture chondroplasty. From the standpoint of TE, the future will be in the use of precisely engineered scaffolds utilizing 3D and 4D bioprinting to fabricate scaffolds with a structure that has the collagen "gothic" architecture of Benninghoff's arcades and other subtle design considerations that will allow improved performance. All of these issues will be dependent upon the further elucidation of the exact mechanisms of why cartilage repair is impaired and how scaffolds may be used to overcome this problem.

References

1. Simon TM, Jackson DW. Articular cartilage: injury pathways and treatment options. Sports Med Arthrosc. 2006;14(3):146–54.
2. Mankin HJ. The response of articular cartilage to mechanical injury. J Bone Joint Surg Am. 1982;64(3):460–6.
3. Marlovits S, et al. Cartilage repair: generations of autologous chondrocyte transplantation. Eur J Radiol. 2006;57(1):24–31.
4. Ahmed TA, Hincke MT. Strategies for articular cartilage lesion repair and functional restoration. Tissue Eng Part B Rev. 2010;16(3):305–29.
5. Frenkel SR, et al. Effects of nitric oxide on chondrocyte migration, adhesion, and cytoskeletal assembly. Arthritis Rheum. 1996;39(11):1905–12.

6. Frenkel SR, Di Cesare PE. Scaffolds for articular cartilage repair. Ann Biomed Eng. 2004;32(1):26–34.
7. Mankin H, Mow V, Buckwalter J, Iannotti J, Ratcliffe A. Orthopaedic basic science. In: Simon SR, editor. Form and function of articular cartilage. Rosemont, IL: American Academy of Orthopaedic Surgeon; 1994. p. 443–70.
8. Buckwalter JA, Mankin HJ. Articular cartilage: degeneration and osteoarthritis, repair, regeneration, and transplantation. Instr Course Lect. 1998;47:487–504.
9. Temenoff JS, Mikos AG. Review: tissue engineering for regeneration of articular cartilage. Biomaterials. 2000;21(5):431–40.
10. Pridie KH. A method of resurfacing osteoarthritic knee joints. J Bone Joint Surg (Br). 1959;41(3):618–9.
11. Steadman J, Rodkey W, Singleton S, Briggs K. Microfracture technique for full-thickness chondral defects: technique and clinical results. Oper Tech Orthop. 1997;7:300–4.
12. Steadman JR, Rodkey WG, Rodrigo JJ. Microfracture: surgical technique and rehabilitation to treat chondral defects. Clin Orthop Relat Res. 2001;391 Suppl:S362–9. Review. PMID: 11603719.
13. Frisbie DD, et al. Arthroscopic subchondral bone plate microfracture technique augments healing of large chondral defects in the radial carpal bone and medial femoral condyle of horses. Vet Surg. 1999;28(4):242–55.
14. Steadman JR, et al. The microfracture technique in the treatment of full-thickness chondral lesions of the knee in National Football League players. J Knee Surg. 2003;16(2):83–6.
15. Buckwalter JA, Mankin HJ. Articular cartilage: tissue design and chondrocyte-matrix interactions. Instr Course Lect. 1998;47:477–86.
16. Buckwalter JA, Mankin HJ. Articular cartilage repair and transplantation. Arthritis Rheum. 1998;41(8):1331–42.
17. Hunziker EB. Articular cartilage repair: basic science and clinical progress. A review of the current status and prospects. Osteoarthritis Cartilage. 2002;10(6):432–63.
18. Grande D, Pitman M, Peterson L, et al. The repair of experimentally produced defects in rabbit articular cartilage by autologous chondrocyte transplantation. J Orthop Res. 1989;7:208–19.
19. Brittberg M, et al. Treatment of deep cartilage defects in the knee with autologous chondrocyte transplantation. N Engl J Med. 1994;331(14):889–95.
20. Haleem AMC, Chu CR. Advances in tissue engineering techniques for articular cartilage repair. Oper Tech Orthop. 2010;20(2):76–89.
21. Williams Iii RJ, Brophy RH. Cartilage repair procedures: clinical approach and decision making. Instr Course Lect. 2008;57:553–61.
22. Brittberg M. Cell carriers as the next generation of cell therapy for cartilage repair: a review of the matrix-induced autologous chondrocyte implantation procedure. Am J Sports Med. 2010;38(6):1259–71.
23. Kessler MW, Grande DA. Tissue engineering and cartilage. Organogenesis. 2008;4(1):28–32.
24. Zhang L, Hu J, Athanasiou KA. The role of tissue engineering in articular cartilage repair and regeneration. Crit Rev Biomed Eng. 2009; 37(1–2):1–57.
25. Kock L, van Donkelaar CC, Ito K. Tissue engineering of functional articular cartilage: the current status. Cell Tissue Res. 2012;347(3):613–27.
26. Danisovic L, et al. The tissue engineering of articular cartilage: cells, scaffolds and stimulating factors. Exp Biol Med (Maywood). 2012;237(1):10–7.
27. Grande DA, Breitbart AS, Mason J, Paulino C, Laser J, Schwartz RE. Cartilage tissue engineering: current limitations and solutions. Clin Orthop Relat Res. 1999;367 Suppl:S176–85. PMID: 10546646.
28. Daher RJ, et al. New methods to diagnose and treat cartilage degeneration. Nat Rev Rheumatol. 2009;5(11):599–607.
29. Chiang H, Jiang CC. Repair of articular cartilage defects: review and perspectives. J Formos Med Assoc. 2009;108(2):87–101.
30. Gugjoo MB, Amarpal SGT, Aithal HP, Kinjavdekar P. Cartilage tissue engineering: role of mesenchymal stem cells along with growth factors & scaffolds. Indian J Med Res. 2016;144(3):339–47.
31. Fortier LA, Barker JU, Strauss EJ, et al. The role of growth factors in cartilage repair. Clin Orthop Relat Res. 2011;469(10):2706–15.
32. Gugjoo MB, Amarpal, Abdelbaset-Ismail A, et al. Mesenchymal stem cells with IGF-1 and TGF- β1 in laminin gel for osteochondral defects in rabbits. Biomed Pharmacother. 2017;93:1165–74.
33. Huang K, Li Q, Li Y, et al. Cartilage tissue regeneration: the roles of cells, stimulating factors and scaffolds. Curr Stem Cell Res Ther. 2018;13(7):547–67.
34. Yu DA, Han J, Kim BS. Stimulation of chondrogenic differentiation of mesenchymal stem cells. Int J Stem Cells. 2012;5(1):16–22.
35. Mierisch CM, et al. Transforming growth factor-beta in calcium alginate beads for the treatment of articular cartilage defects in the rabbit. Arthroscopy. 2002;18(8):892–900.
36. Brochhausen C, Lehmann M, Halstenberg S, et al. Signalling molecules and growth factors for tissue engineering of cartilage-what can we learn from the growth plate? J Tissue Eng Regen Med. 2009;3(6):416–29.
37. Mierisch CM, et al. Chondrocyte transplantation into articular cartilage defects with use of calcium alginate: the fate of the cells. J Bone Joint Surg Am. 2003;85-A(9):1757–67.

38. Chenite A, et al. Novel injectable neutral solutions of chitosan form biodegradable gels in situ. Biomaterials. 2000;21(21):2155–61.
39. Ge Z, et al. Functional biomaterials for cartilage regeneration. J Biomed Mater Res A. 2012;100(9):2526–36.
40. Stoop R. Smart biomaterials for tissue engineering of cartilage. Injury. 2008;39(Suppl 1):S77–87.
41. Safran MR, Kim H, Zaffagnini S. The use of scaffolds in the management of articular cartilage injury. J Am Acad Orthop Surg. 2008;16(6):306–11.
42. Cao, Z., Dou, C.; Dong S., Scaffolding biomaterials for cartilage regeneration. J Nanomater, 2014. 2014: p. 1–8.
43. Lu L, et al. Biodegradable polymer scaffolds for cartilage tissue engineering. Clin Orthop Relat Res. 2001;(391 Suppl):S251–70.
44. Kemppainen JM, Hollister SJ. Differential effects of designed scaffold permeability on chondrogenesis by chondrocytes and bone marrow stromal cells. Biomaterials. 2010;31(2):279–87.
45. Abedalwafa M, Wang F, Wang L, Li C. Biodegradable poly-epsilon-caprolactone (PCL) for tissue engineering applications : a review. Rev Adv Mater Sci. 2013;34:123–40.
46. Pan Z, et al. Effect of porosities of bilayered porous scaffolds on spontaneous osteochondral repair in cartilage tissue engineering. Regen Biomater. 2015;2(1):9–19.
47. Izadifar Z, Chen X, Kulyk W. Strategic design and fabrication of engineered scaffolds for articular cartilage repair. J Funct Biomater. 2012;3(4):799–838.
48. Rowland CR, Colucci LA, Guilak F. Fabrication of anatomically-shaped cartilage constructs using decellularized cartilage-derived matrix scaffolds. Biomaterials. 2016;91:57–72.
49. Coombes AG, Rizzi SC, Williamson M, et al. Precipitation casting of polycaprolactone for applications in tissue engineering and drug delivery. Biomaterials. 2004;25(2):315–25.
50. Nair LS, Laurencin CT. Biodegradable polymers as biomaterials. Prog Polym Sci. 2007; 32(8-9):762–98.
51. Anseth KS, Bowman CN, Brannon-Peppas L. Mechanical properties of hydrogels and their experimental determination. Biomaterials. 1996;17(17):1647–57.
52. Risbud MV, Sittinger M. Tissue engineering: advances in in vitro cartilage generation. Trends Biotechnol. 2002;20(8):351–6.
53. Kalkan R, Nwekwo CW, Adali T. The use of scaffolds in cartilage regeneration. Crit Rev Eukaryot Gene Expr. 2018;28(4):343–8.
54. Stenzel KH, Miyata T, Rubin AL. Collagen as a biomaterial. Annu Rev Biophys Bioeng. 1974;3(0):231–53.
55. Kleinman HK, Klebe RJ, Martin GR. Role of collagenous matrices in the adhesion and growth of cells. J Cell Biol. 1981;88(3):473–85.
56. Kleinman HK, et al. Binding of cell attachment protein to collagen: effect of chemical modifications. Ann N Y Acad Sci. 1978;312:436–8.
57. Getgood A, et al. Articular cartilage tissue engineering: today's research, tomorrow's practice? J Bone Joint Surg Br. 2009;91(5):565–76.
58. Frenkel SR, et al. Chondrocyte transplantation using a collagen bilayer matrix for cartilage repair. J Bone Joint Surg Br. 1997;79(5):831–6.
59. Jiang LB, Su DH, Liu P, et al. Shape-memory collagen scaffold for enhanced cartilage regeneration: native collagen versus denatured collagen. Osteoarthritis Cartilage. 2018;26(10):1389–99.
60. Dorotka R, et al. Marrow stimulation and chondrocyte transplantation using a collagen matrix for cartilage repair. Osteoarthritis Cartilage. 2005;13(8):655–64.
61. Dorotka R, et al. Repair of articular cartilage defects treated by microfracture and a three-dimensional collagen matrix. Biomaterials. 2005;26(17):3617–29.
62. Hendrickson DA, et al. Chondrocyte-fibrin matrix transplants for resurfacing extensive articular cartilage defects. J Orthop Res. 1994;12(4):485–97.
63. Fortier LA, et al. Coordinate upregulation of cartilage matrix synthesis in fibrin cultures supplemented with exogenous insulin-like growth factor-I. J Orthop Res. 1999;17(4):467–74.
64. Fortier LA, Nixon AJ, Lust G. Phenotypic expression of equine articular chondrocytes grown in three-dimensional cultures supplemented with supraphysiologic concentrations of insulin-like growth factor-1. Am J Vet Res. 2002;63(2):301–5.
65. Nixon AJ, Saxer RA, Brower-Toland BD. Exogenous insulin-like growth factor-I stimulates an autoinductive IGF-I autocrine/paracrine response in chondrocytes. J Orthop Res. 2001;19(1):26–32.
66. Nixon AJ, et al. Enhanced repair of extensive articular defects by insulin-like growth factor-I-laden fibrin composites. J Orthop Res. 1999;17(4):475–87.
67. Puertas-Bartolomé M, Benito-Garzón L, Olmeda-Lozano M. In situ cross-linkable polymer systems and composites for osteochondral regeneration. Adv Exp Med Biol. 2018;1058:327–55.
68. Ribeiro VP, Pina S, Oliveira JM, Reis RL. Silk fibroin-based hydrogels and scaffolds for osteochondral repair and regeneration. Adv Exp Med Biol. 2018;1058:305–25.
69. Conrad B, Han LH, Yang F. Gelatin-based microribbon hydrogels accelerate cartilage formation by mesenchymal stem cells in 3D. Tissue Eng Part A. 2018; https://doi.org/10.1089/ten.TEA.2018.0011. [Epub ahead of print].
70. Bonaventure J, et al. Reexpression of cartilage-specific genes by dedifferentiated human articular chondrocytes cultured in alginate beads. Exp Cell Res. 1994;212(1):97–104.
71. Diduch DR, et al. Marrow stromal cells embedded in alginate for repair of osteochondral defects. Arthroscopy. 2000;16(6):571–7.

72. Chen WY, Abatangelo G. Functions of hyaluronan in wound repair. Wound Repair Regen. 1999;7(2):79–89.
73. Marcacci M, et al. Articular cartilage engineering with Hyalograft C: 3-year clinical results. Clin Orthop Relat Res. 2005;435:96–105.
74. Kujawa MJ, Caplan AI. Hyaluronic acid bonded to cell-culture surfaces stimulates chondrogenesis in stage 24 limb mesenchyme cell cultures. Dev Biol. 1986;114(2):504–18.
75. Campoccia D, et al. Semisynthetic resorbable materials from hyaluronan esterification. Biomaterials. 1998;19(23):2101–27.
76. Aigner J, et al. Cartilage tissue engineering with novel nonwoven structured biomaterial based on hyaluronic acid benzyl ester. J Biomed Mater Res. 1998;42(2):172–81.
77. Brun P, et al. Chondrocyte aggregation and reorganization into three-dimensional scaffolds. J Biomed Mater Res. 1999;46(3):337–46.
78. Grigolo B, et al. Tissue engineering for cartilage repair: in vitro properties of a hyaluronan-derivative. Chir Organi Mov. 2003;88(4):351–5.
79. Grigolo B, et al. Evidence for redifferentiation of human chondrocytes grown on a hyaluronan-based biomaterial (HYAff 11): molecular, immunohistochemical and ultrastructural analysis. Biomaterials. 2002;23(4):1187–95.
80. Grigolo B, et al. Transplantation of chondrocytes seeded on a hyaluronan derivative (hyaff-11) into cartilage defects in rabbits. Biomaterials. 2001;22(17):2417–24.
81. Knudson W, et al. Hyaluronan oligosaccharides perturb cartilage matrix homeostasis and induce chondrocytic chondrolysis. Arthritis Rheum. 2000;43(5):1165–74.
82. Suh JK, Matthew HW. Application of chitosan-based polysaccharide biomaterials in cartilage tissue engineering: a review. Biomaterials. 2000;21(24):2589–98.
83. Lahiji A, et al. Chitosan supports the expression of extracellular matrix proteins in human osteoblasts and chondrocytes. J Biomed Mater Res. 2000;51(4):586–95.
84. Yuan D, Chen Z, Lin T, Luo X, Dong H, Feng G. Cartilage tissue engineering using combination of chitosan hydrogel and mesenchymal stem cells. J Chem. 2015;2015. 6 pages.
85. Gaserod O, Smidsrod O, Skjak-Braek G. Microcapsules of alginate-chitosan--I. A quantitative study of the interaction between alginate and chitosan. Biomaterials. 1998;19(20):1815–25.
86. Denuziere A, et al. Chitosan-chondroitin sulfate and chitosan-hyaluronate polyelectrolyte complexes: biological properties. Biomaterials. 1998;19(14):1275–85.
87. Oryan A, Sahvieh S. Effectiveness of chitosan scaffold in skin, bone and cartilage healing. Int J Biol Macromol. 2017;104(Pt A):1003–11.
88. Shamekhi MA, Rabiee A, Mirzadeh H, et al. Fabrication and characterization of hydrothermal cross-linked chitosan porous scaffolds for cartilage tissue engineering applications. Mater Sci Eng C Mater Biol Appl. 2017;80:532–42.
89. Comblain F, Rocasalbas G, Gauthier S, Henrotin Y. Chitosan: a promising polymer for cartilage repair and viscosupplementation. Biomed Mater Eng. 2017;28(s1):S209–15.
90. Hoemann CD, et al. Chitosan-glycerol phosphate/blood implants improve hyaline cartilage repair in ovine microfracture defects. J Bone Joint Surg Am. 2005;87(12):2671–86.
91. Hoemann CD, et al. Chitosan-glycerol phosphate/blood implants elicit hyaline cartilage repair integrated with porous subchondral bone in microdrilled rabbit defects. Osteoarthritis Cartilage. 2007;15(1):78–89.
92. Villarreal-Gomez LJ, et al. Electrospinning as a powerful technique for biomedical applications: a critically selected survey. J Biomater Sci Polym Ed. 2016;27(2):157–76.
93. Cohen SB, et al. The use of absorbable co-polymer pads with alginate and cells for articular cartilage repair in rabbits. Biomaterials. 2003;24(15):2653–60.
94. Capito RM, Spector M. Scaffold-based articular cartilage repair. IEEE Eng Med Biol Mag. 2003;22(5):42–50.
95. Caterson EJ, et al. Polymer/alginate amalgam for cartilage-tissue engineering. Ann N Y Acad Sci. 2002;961:134–8.
96. Elisseeff J, et al. Controlled-release of IGF-I and TGF-beta1 in a photopolymerizing hydrogel for cartilage tissue engineering. J Orthop Res. 2001;19(6):1098–104.
97. Gray ML, et al. Mechanical and physiochemical determinants of the chondrocyte biosynthetic response. J Orthop Res. 1988;6(6):777–92.
98. Grande DA, et al. Evaluation of matrix scaffolds for tissue engineering of articular cartilage grafts. J Biomed Mater Res. 1997;34(2):211–20.
99. Spain TL, Agrawal CM, Athanasiou KA. New technique to extend the useful life of a biodegradable cartilage implant. Tissue Eng. 1998;4(4):343–52.
100. Lim EH, Sardinha JP, Myers S. Nanotechnology biomimetic cartilage regenerative scaffolds. Arch Plast Surg. 2014;41(3):231–40.
101. Webber MJ, et al. A perspective on the clinical translation of scaffolds for tissue engineering biomimetic collagenous scaffold to tune inflammation by targeting macrophages. Ann Biomed Eng. 2015;43(3):641–56.
102. Smeriglio P, et al. 3D hydrogel scaffolds for articular chondrocyte culture and cartilage generation. J Vis Exp. 2015;(104). https://doi.org/10.3791/53085.
103. Ren K, et al. In-situ forming glycopolypeptide hydrogels as biomimetic scaffolds for cartilage tissue engineering. J Control Release. 2015;213:e64–5.

104. Gegg C, Yang F. Spatially patterned microribbon-based hydrogels induce zonally-organized cartilage regeneration by stem cells in 3D. Acta Biomater. 2019. pii: S1742-7061(19)30704-4. https://doi.org/10.1016/j.actbio.2019.10.025. [Epub ahead of print].
105. De Moor L, Beyls E, Declercq H. Scaffold free microtissue formation for enhanced cartilage repair. Ann Biomed Eng. 2019. https://doi.org/10.1007/s10439-019-02348-4. [Epub ahead of print].
106. Kon E, Filardo G, Brittberg M, Busacca M, Condello V, et al. A multilayer biomaterial for osteochondral regeneration shows superiority vs microfractures for the treatment of osteochondral lesions in a multicentre randomized trial at 2 years. Knee Surg Sports Traumatol Arthrosc. 2018;26(9):2704–15.
107. O'Brien CM, et al. Three-dimensional printing of nanomaterial scaffolds for complex tissue regeneration. Tissue Eng Part B Rev. 2015;21(1):103–14.
108. Jeznach O, Kołbuk D, Sajkiewicz P. Injectable hydrogels and nanocomposite hydrogels for cartilage regeneration. J Biomed Mater Res A. 2018; https://doi.org/10.1002/jbm.a.36449. [Epub ahead of print].
109. Manoukian OS, Dieck C, Milne T, et al. Nanomaterials/Nanoco mposites for osteochondral tissue. Adv Exp Med Biol. 2018;1058:79–95.
110. Schipani R, Nolan DR, Lally C, Kelly DJ. Integrating finite element modelling and 3D printing to engineer biomimetic polymeric scaffolds for tissue engineering. Connect Tissue Res. 2019:1–16. https://doi.org/10.1080/03008207.2019.1656720. [Epub ahead of print].
111. Wang J, Wang Y, Sun X, Liu D, Huang C, et al. Biomimetic cartilage scaffold with orientated porous structure of two factors for cartilage repair of knee osteoarthritis. Artif Cells Nanomed Biotechnol. 2019;47(1):1710–21.
112. Camarero-Espinosa S, Cooper-White JJ. Combinatorial presentation of cartilage-inspired peptides on nanopatterned surfaces enables directed differentiation of human mesenchymal stem cells towards distinct articular chondrogenic phenotypes. Biomaterials. 2019;210:105–15.
113. Owida HA, Yang R, Cen L, Kuiper NJ, Yang Y. Induction of zonal-specific cellular morphology and matrix synthesis for biomimetic cartilage regeneration using hybrid scaffolds. J R Soc Interface. 2018;15(143). pii: 20180310. https://doi.org/10.1098/rsif.2018.0310.
114. Pereira DR, Reis RL, Oliveira JM. Layered scaffolds for osteochondral tissue engineering. Adv Exp Med Biol. 2018;1058:193–218.
115. Spencer V, Illescas E, Maltes L, et al. Osteochondral tissue engineering: translational research and turning research into products. Adv Exp Med Biol. 2018;1058:373–90.
116. Goldstein TA, Epstein CJ, Schwartz J, et al. Feasibility of bioprinting with a modified desktop 3D printer. Tissue Eng Part C Methods. 2016; 22(12):1071–6.
117. Daly AC, Freeman FE, Gonzalez-Fernandez T, et al. 3D bioprinting for cartilage and osteochondral tissue engineering. Adv Healthc Mater. 2017;6(22). https://doi.org/10.1002/adhm.201700298. Epub 2017.
118. Kankala RK, Lu FJ, Liu CG, et al. Effect of Icariin on engineered 3D-printed porous scaffolds for cartilage repair. Materials (Basel). 2018;11(8):E1390. https://doi.org/10.3390/ma11081390.
119. Guo T, Ringel JP, Lim CG, et al. Three dimensional extrusion printing induces polymer molecule alignment and cell organization within engineered cartilage. J Biomed Mater Res A. 2018;106(8):2190–9.
120. Guo T, Lembong J, Zhang LG, Fisher JP. Three-dimensional printing articular cartilage: recapitulating the complexity of native tissue<sup/>. Tissue Eng Part B Rev. 2017;23(3):225–36.
121. Iulian A, Dan L, Camelia T, et al. Synthetic materials for osteochondral tissue engineering. Adv Exp Med Biol. 2018;1058:31–52.
122. Tibbits S. 4D printing: multi - material shape change. Archit Des. 2014;84:116–21.
123. Brittberg M. Autologous chondrocyte implantation--technique and long-term follow-up. Injury. 2008;39(Suppl 1):S40–9.
124. Gobbi A, et al. Patellofemoral full-thickness chondral defects treated with Hyalograft-C: a clinical, arthroscopic, and histologic review. Am J Sports Med. 2006;34(11):1763–73.
125. Waldman SD, et al. Long-term intermittent shear deformation improves the quality of cartilaginous tissue formed in vitro. J Orthop Res. 2003;21(4):590–6.
126. Crawford DC, et al. An autologous cartilage tissue implant NeoCart for treatment of grade III chondral injury to the distal femur: prospective clinical safety trial at 2 years. Am J Sports Med. 2009;37(7):1334–43.
127. Almqvist KF, et al. Treatment of cartilage defects in the knee using alginate beads containing human mature allogenic chondrocytes. Am J Sports Med. 2009;37(10):1920–9.
128. Dhollander AA, et al. Midterm results of the treatment of cartilage defects in the knee using alginate beads containing human mature allogenic chondrocytes. Am J Sports Med. 2012;40(1):75–82.
129. Almqvist KF, et al. Biological freezing of human articular chondrocytes. Osteoarthritis Cartilage. 2001;9(4):341–50.

Commercially Available Bioengineered Cartilage Grafts

18

Benedict A. Rogers, Jaskarndip Chahal, and Allan E. Gross

18.1 Introduction

The goals of managing patients with symptomatic chondral defects of the knee include optimizing clinical and functional outcomes, generating durable hyaline or hyaline-like cartilage with low procedure-associated morbidity, utilizing cost-effective technology, and ultimately delaying and/or preventing the development of secondary degenerative sequelae [1]. At the present time, there are no surgical repair techniques that have satisfied all of these requisite conditions, thereby resulting in a tremendous investment of time and financial resources on the development and evaluation of novel bioengineered constructs to optimize the cartilage repair process. Currently, there are a large number of products for cartilage repair within the biological pipeline from discovery to phase 3 clinical trials [1]. Through a combination of synthetic materials, scaffolds, and cell-based strategies, there are an increasing number of therapeutic options that will be available in the future.

Scaffolds are designed to be chondroconductive or chondroinductive and can be implanted as solid three-dimensional constructs (with or without cells) into osteochondral defects or in liquid form to augment marrow stimulation techniques [1]. Scaffolds act as a "biological net" as they have been developed to permit the migration and in-growth of cells followed by subsequent resorption and replacement with native repair tissue [1]. Ongoing challenges with scaffolding include maintenance within the defect, controlling the rate of degradation, and promoting repair tissue maturation [1, 2].

In contrast to scaffolds, *synthetic constructs* resurface a focal chondral defect and do not resorb over time. Ideally, these products would be cost-effective with minimal concern for disease transmission and/or immunogenic responses [1, 2]. Pertinent considerations for such implants

B. A. Rogers, MA, MSc, MRCGP, DipLMC, DipSEM, FRCS (Orth), PhD
Brighton and Sussex Medical School, Brighton, UK

Trauma and Orthopaedics Department, Brighton and Sussex University Hospitals NHS Trust, Brighton, UK

J. Chahal, MD, FRCSC, MSc, MBA
Division of Orthopaedic Surgery, University of Toronto, Toronto, ON, Canada

University of Toronto Orthopaedic Sports Medicine and University Health Network Arthritis Program, Toronto, ON, Canada

Division of Orthopaedic Surgery, Toronto Western Hospital and Women's College Hospital, Toronto, ON, Canada

A. E. Gross, MD, FRCSC, O ONT (✉)
Division of Orthopaedic Surgery, University of Toronto, Toronto, ON, Canada

Gluskin Granovsky Division of Orthopaedics, Joseph and Wolf Lebovic Health Complex, Mount Sinai Hospital, Toronto, ON, Canada
e-mail: Allan.Gross@sinaihealthsystem.ca

H. K. Gahunia et al. (eds.), *Articular Cartilage of the Knee*,
https://doi.org/10.1007/978-1-4939-7587-7_18

include their material properties, osteoconductivity, chondroconductivity, stability at the implant-bone interface, ability to withstand weight-bearing forces, and their coefficient of friction.

Existing or novel cell-based therapies may also be used in isolation or in combination with various scaffold products. Furthermore, there has been a recent emphasis on the use of autograft and allograft minced cartilage with or without scaffolds, as well as scaffold-based strategies to optimize outcomes following microfracture. The objective of this chapter is to provide an overview of the different types of commercially available bioengineered cartilage grafts including cell-based therapies, microfracture augmentation techniques, and the use of particulated articular cartilage, as well as examples of scaffold and synthetic materials that can be used in isolation. For an in-depth knowledge of cell-based and engineered cartilage constructs refer to Chaps. 16 and 17.

18.2 Microfracture Augmentation

The microfracture procedure is a form of bone marrow stimulation to enhance cartilage repair by taking advantage of the body's own healing potential [3]. A sharp awl (i.e., pick) is used arthroscopically through one of the arthroscopic skin portals, and a mallet is used to impact the awl at right angles into the subchondral bone at regular intervals (approximately ten holes per cm^2) with a depth of 2–3 mm. The penetration of the subchondral bone allows for the communication of the osteochondral defect with mesenchymal stem cells and growth factors from the bone marrow and eventually leads to the formation of fibrocartilaginous tissue that covers the cartilage lesion [4].

In an evidence-based systematic analysis on the efficacy of microfracture, several factors affecting functional outcomes were identified [5]. Positive prognostic factors included younger age (< 30–45 years), duration of symptoms < 12 months, lower body mass index, higher preoperative activity levels (Tegner > 4), lesions less than 2–4 cm^2, and the use of microfracture as a first-line procedure. Post microfracture, the repair cartilage volume plays a critical role in the durability of functional improvement in the knee. Mithoefer et al. [5] concluded that while microfracture provides effective short-term functional improvement of knee function, there is insufficient data on its long-term results. Additional shortcomings of the technique include limited hyaline repair tissue which is predominantly fibrocartilaginous or fibrous, variable repair cartilage volume, and possible functional deterioration over time [5].

Due to the *aforementioned* shortcomings associated with microfracture, there has been a focus on techniques that augment the microfracture procedure (i.e. microfracture 'plus') [6, 7]. At the present time, several commercially available scaffolds or techniques are being investigated as adjuncts including Chondrotissue®, Autologous Matrix-Induced Chondrogenesis – AMIC®, Gelrin C®, BST-CarGel®, and BioCartilage® [1] (Table 18.1).

18.2.1 Chondrotissue®

Chondrotissue® (BioTissue AG, Freiburg, Germany) is a freeze-dried nonwoven resorbable polyglycolic acid fleece that is infused with hyaluronic acid (Fig. 18.1) [8]. Prior to implantation, the scaffold is immersed in autologous serum and then sutured over a microfractured defect. The use of this implant is based on the rationale that hyaluronan supports the chondrogenic differentiation of human mesenchymal progenitors and that these progenitors are recruited by autologous serum [11]. Implantation in an ovine model demonstrated the formation of higher-quality cartilaginous repair tissue compared to microfracture alone [11]. Patrascu et al. reported the 2-year outcome of a single traumatic medial femoral condyle lesion treated with Chondrotissue® [12]. This case report demonstrated good pain relief, hyaline-like cartilage tissue formation, and good-to-excellent filling of the defect on Magnetic resonance imaging (MRI). Further investigation is required before this technology will be available for routine clinical use.

Table 18.1 To date commercially available scaffolds for microfracture augmentation

Procedure	Product	Component	Company/ location	Reference
Microfracture Augmentation	Chondrotissue®	Resorbable polyglycolic acid infused with hyaluronic acid	BioTissue AG, Freiburg, Germany	[8]
	Autologous matrix-induced Chondrogenesis® (AMIC®)	Chondro-Gide, a type I/III collagen bi-membrane	Chondro-Gide, Geistlich biomaterials, Switzerland	[8, 9]
	Gelrin C®	Bioabsorbable photopolymerized hydrogel of polyethylene glycol diacrylate bound to fibrinogen	Regentis, Haifa, Israel	[8]
	BST-CarGel®	Chitosan-glycerol phosphate-based scaffold	Smith and Nephew Inc., Massachusetts, USA	[1, 8]
	BioCartilage®	Desiccated micronized allogeneic cartilage extracellular matrix tissue allograft	Arthrex, Naples, Florida, USA	[10]

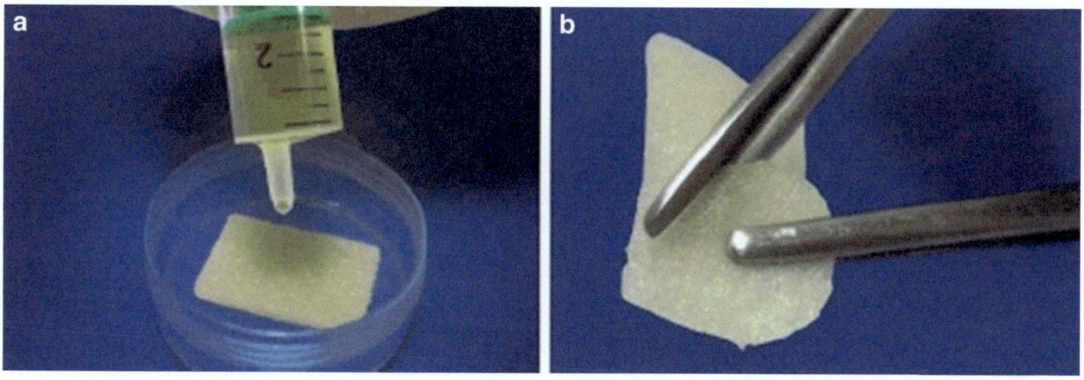

Fig. 18.1 (**a**, **b**) Preparation of Chondrotissue® prior to implantation for the management of a focal condylar defect in the knee (Image obtained with permission from http://www.sports-surgery.com/article.asp?article=122)

18.2.2 Autologous Matrix-Induced Chondrogenesis®

Autologous Matrix-Induced Chondrogenesis® (AMIC® Chondro-Gide, Geistlich Biomaterials, Switzerland) is a commonly used microfracture augmentation technique in Europe that utilizes Chondro-Gide, a type I/III collagen membrane, to stabilize the clot in a marrow-stimulated defect (Fig. 18.2a) [8, 9]. This membrane is secured with either fibrin glue or suture, and the procedure is performed with open surgery (Fig. 18.2b). Successful mid-term results have been reported in Europe thus far with patients demonstrating improved pain and function [10, 13–17]. While the original technique was performed with microfracture of the underlying defect, recent evidence has suggested that the subchondral stroma is better reached by drilling [8, 18]. As such, a 1.1 mm K-wire is used to create multiple drill holes with constant cooling applied so the subchondral bone is reached [14]. Volz et al. have demonstrated in a randomized trial with a 5-year follow-up that the AMIC procedure results in improved functional and radiologic outcomes. While results were not significantly different at 2-year follow-up, the microfracture patients had a deterioration over the ensuing 3 years implying that the AMIC group results in more stable outcomes over the long term [19].

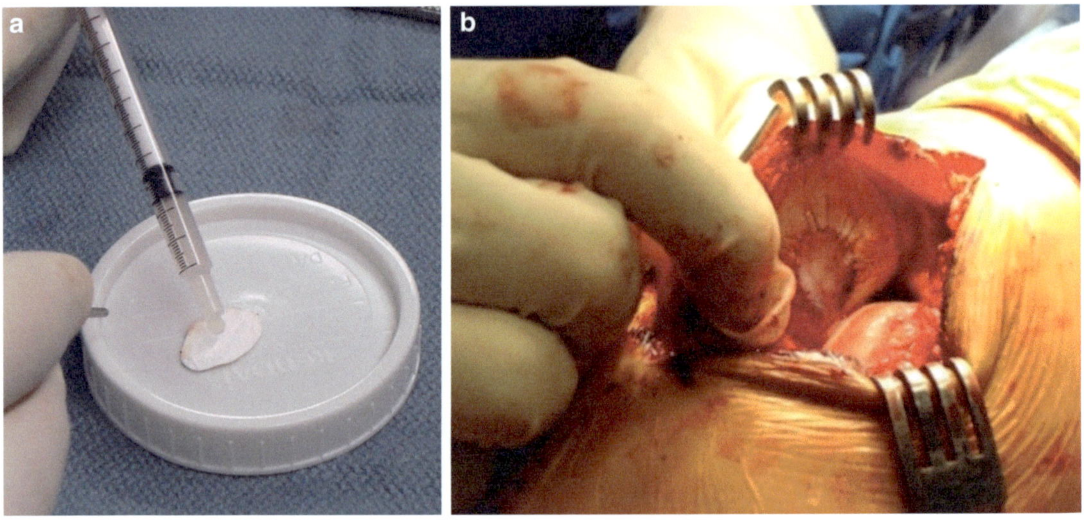

Fig. 18.2 (**a**) Preparation of Chondro-Gide collagen I/III bilayer to stabilize the clot in a marrow-stimulated defect. (**b**) Autologous Matrix-Induced Chondrogenesis® (AMIC) technique performed for a focal chondral defect of the patella

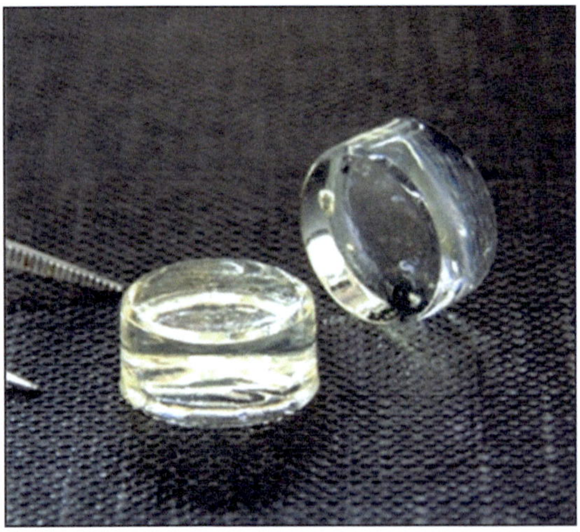

Fig. 18.3 Photo of Gelrin C scaffold (Image courtesy of Brian Cole MD MBA)

18.2.3 Gelrin C®

Gelrin C® (Regentis, Haifa, Israel) is a bioabsorbable photopolymerized hydrogel of polyethylene glycol diacrylate bound to fibrinogen that degrades within 6–12 months as new cartilage takes its place (Fig. 18.3) [8]. Gelrin C is injected into a previously microfractured defect as a liquid that polymerizes in situ, conforming to the lesion size, shape, and depth. Short exposed to ultraviolet light converts the liquid into a soft, elastomeric, semi-solid hydrogel implant, which integrates with the surrounding tissue and bone. In vitro, Gelrin C exhibits innate chondrogenic and osteoconductive potential and is nonimmunogenic. In an ovine model, it demonstrated type II collagen and proteoglycan synthesis in treated versus untreated defects [1]. This product is being investigated in an ongoing clinical trial in Israel [8].

18.2.4 BST-CarGel®

BST-CarGel® (Smith and Nephew, Andover, MA, USA) is a chitosan-glycerol phosphate-based scaffold whose active component is a polyglucosamine thrombogenic polysaccharide. With this technique, peripheral whole blood is mixed to BST-CarGel just before implantation into a microfractured defect which results in adhesion and polymerization of the construct [1, 8, 20]. This procedure causes the stem cells to move to the injured area and regenerate cartilaginous cells. The rationale for using chitosan as a scaffold is related to its thrombogenic, self-adhering, and resorbable properties; its use is also supported by basic science data in rabbits where chitosan-glycerol phosphate implants have demonstrated better integration of repaired tissue with the adjacent native tissue and more hyaline-like repair tissue than of subchondral bone drilling alone [1, 8, 20]. A randomized trial demonstrated improved MRI and histological morphology of chondral defects in patients treated with BST-CarGel® compared with microfracture alone. Despite this, there were no differences in clinical outcome scores [21]. Recently, a retrospective study was conducted in a cohort of 91 patients (total of 93 lesions) with articular cartilage defects in the knee who had undergone microfracture surgery with CarGel [22]. Investigation of the short-term clinical and radiographic outcomes of these patients showed few postoperative complications and significant reductions in pain and swelling after treatment.

18.2.5 BioCartilage®

BioCartilage (Arthrex, Naples, Florida, USA) is a desiccated, micronized allogeneic cartilage extracellular matrix allograft that is native to articular cartilage, including type II collagen, proteoglycans, and additional growth factors. BioCartilage has been developed for International Cartilage Repair Society (ICRS, now referred to as "International Cartilage Regeneration and Joint Preservation Society") grade III or IV articular cartilage lesions in conjunction with microfracture (Fig. 18.4). After successful BioCartilage augmented microfracture surgery, the T2 mapping properties of the repair tissue showed similarity to that of the adjacent native articular cartilage [23]. The micronized matrix granules provides a chondroconductive, biocompatible, resorbable material that has a particle size range of 100 to 300 μm, which improves handling and delivery into the defect and facilitates a greater surface area for attachment of mesenchymal stem cells (MSCs) in vivo [24, 25]. This freeze-dried tissue allograft is processed and packaged by the University of Miami Tissue Bank. Prior to utilization, BioCartilage® is combined with platelet-rich plasma (PRP) or bone marrow aspirate concentrate (BMAC). The resultant solution is added to a microfractured chondral lesion and "fixed" with fibrin glue. The addition of PRP or BMAC to the desiccated BioCartilage cells is beneficial due to the presence of anabolic factors [26]. When PRP has been combined with a collagen membrane or matrix, the formation of hyaline-like tissue was enhanced when performed in conjunction with microfracture [10].

A preclinical study in baboons demonstrated a complete regeneration of cartilage over International Cartilage Repair Society (ICRS) grade III lesions at 9 weeks and beyond in nine of ten baboons, while control subjects maintained open chondral lesions [27]. Chondrogenesis was observed when the BioCartilage® was placed directly adjacent to healthy cartilage; however, it did not exhibit osteogenesis. Furthermore, no adverse events or indications of infections or rejections of the human BioCartilage® were observed in the preclinical evaluation [27]. At the present time, there is no human data regarding the safety profile, incorporation, and early results following the use of BioCartilage in conjunction with the microfracture procedure.

18.3 Cell-Based Therapy

Cell-based technique for articular cartilage restoration uses culture-expanded cells (Table 18.2).

18.3.1 Carticel® and Matrix-Associated Chondrocyte Implantation®

Carticel® and matrix-associated chondrocyte implantation (MACI, Vericel Corporation, Cambridge, Massachusetts, USA) both represent two-stage cartilage restoration procedures that are commonly used in North America and Europe, respectively. Stage I involves confirmation that the lesion is suitable for an autologous chondrocyte implantation (ACI) procedure. Using an arthroscopic gouge or ring curet, two to three full-thickness chondral biopsy (each measuring 5 mm x 10 mm, size of a tic-tac) is obtained from the margins of the intercondylar notch.

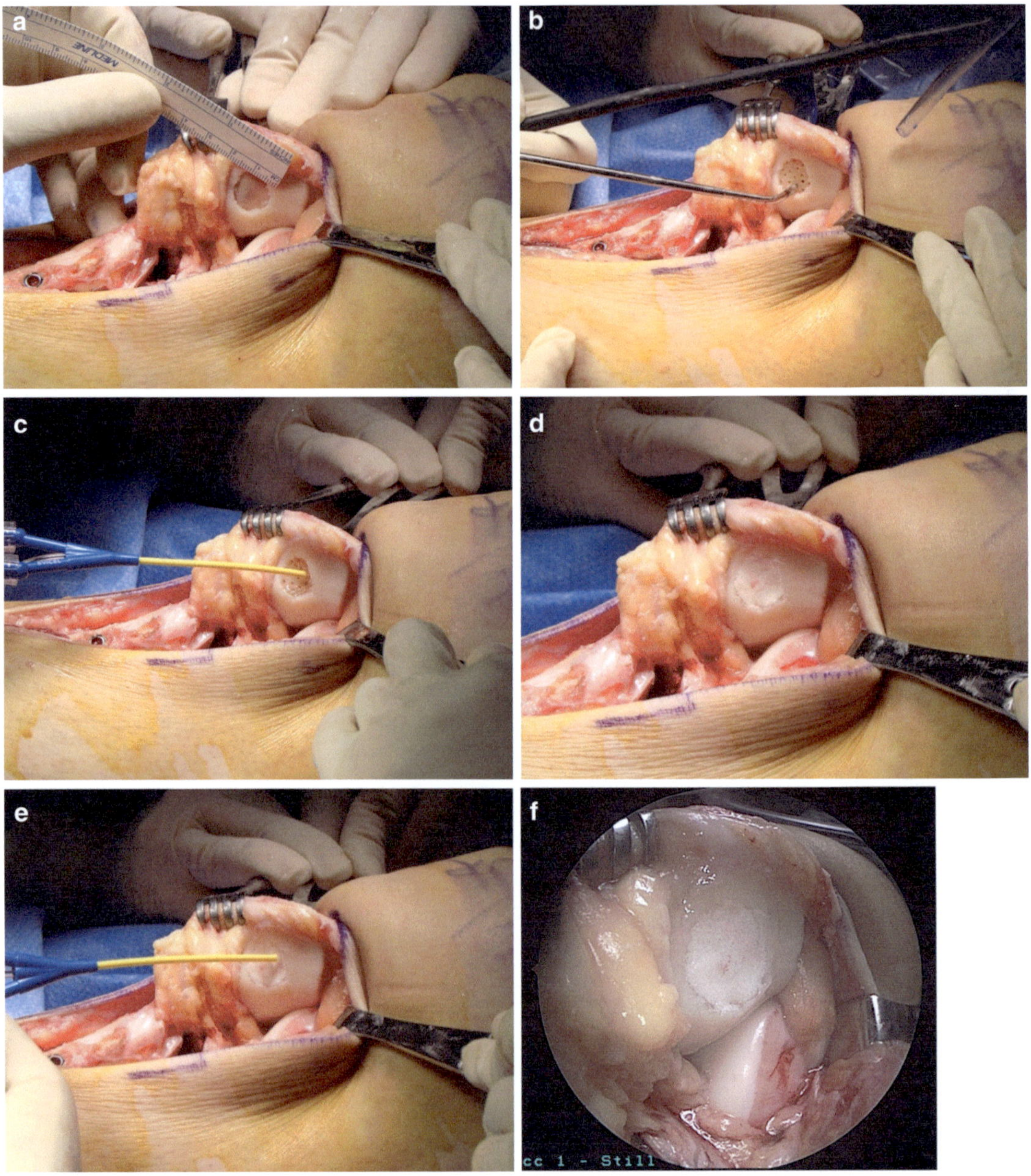

Fig. 18.4 Procedure involving the application of the BioCartilage® allograft to an isolated focal defect involving the patella. (**a**) Preparation and sizing of cartilage defect. (**b**) Microfracture of cartilage defect. (**c**) Application of fibrin glue at the base of the defect. (**d**) Application of BioCartilage® allograft. (**e**) Subsequent application of fibrin glue over repair site. (**f**) Final Biocartilage® construct (Images courtesy of Brian J Cole MD MBA)

Table 18.2 Cell-based two-stage articular cartilage restoration procedure for symptomatic chondral cartilage defect(s) of the knee

Procedure	Product	Component	Company/location	Reference
	Autologous chondrocyte implantation (Carticel®)	Placement of periosteal flap	Vericel Corporation, Cambridge, Massachusetts, USA	[28, 29]
Cell-based Therapy	Matrix-associated chondrocyte implantation® (Maci®)	Use porcine type I/III collagen bi-membrane	Vericel Corporation, Cambridge, Massachusetts, USA	[30, 31]
	ChondroCelect®	Placement of periosteal flap	TiGenix NV, Leuven, Belgium	[32–34]

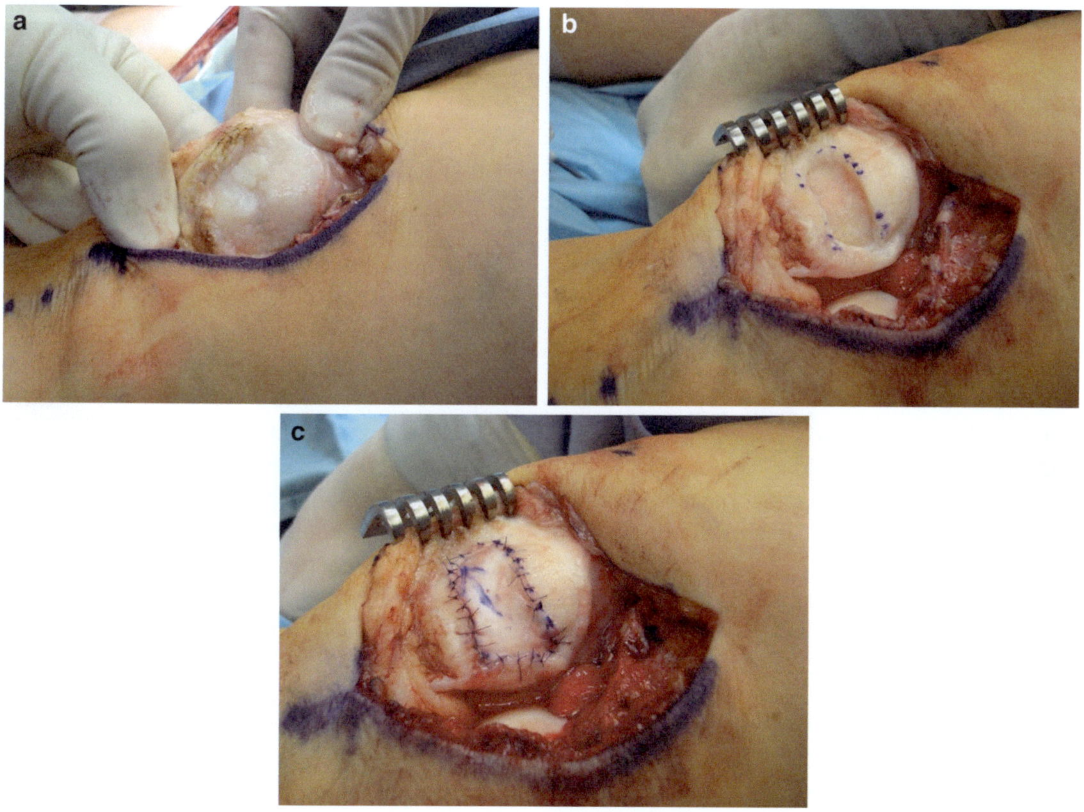

Fig. 18.5 Carticel procedure for the management of an isolated focal defect involving the patella. (**a**) Assessment of cartilage defect. (**b**) Defect sizing and creation of vertical walls at margins. (**c**) Collagen I–III bi-membrane sutured onto defect with 6–0 dyed Vicryl suture. Cultured chondrocytes are injected in a suspension through an opening in the construct which is subsequently closed (arrow) (Images courtesy of Brian J Cole, MD, MBA)

After a period of in vitro chondrocyte proliferation, cells are transplanted during a second-stage surgical procedure.

Carticel® (initially owned by Genzyme but now owned by Vericel Corporation) is an FDA-approved ACI treatment for damaged articular cartilage (Fig. 18.5). Unlike microfracture or similar bone marrow stimulation techniques, ACI has the potential to regenerate hyaline-like cartilage by culturing chondrocytes from a non-weight-bearing region of the articular surface [28, 29]. The procedure was developed over a decade ago for the treatment of symptomatic chondral defects of the knee and has further been adapted for use in the shoulder and ankle [35–37]. The original ACI technique, described by Brittberg et al., required the suturing of a periosteal membrane to the rim of the debrided chondral defect with cultured chondrocytes subsequently injected to fill the defect underneath the membrane [35]. The restoration of the congruity of the articular cartilage is often difficult using this technique, and grafts are slow to mature [29].

The matrix-induced autologous chondrocyte implantation technique has been developed with a porcine type I/III collagen bi-membrane (in place of the periosteal membrane), which is seeded with chondrocytes (Fig. 18.6) [30, 31]. One surface has a higher density of collagen fibers, affording a low-friction surface that appears smooth. The other membrane has a rough appearance with larger gaps between collagen fibers into which chondrocytes are seeded. The MACI membrane can be secured directly to the base of a prepared chondral defect with fibrin glue. MACI represents a procedure that does not require periosteal harvesting or suturing of the graft. The procedure is therefore attractive since it may be performed faster and through a less extensive exposure than conventional ACI. The MACI technique does not involve the injection of a suspension of chondrocytes below a membrane.

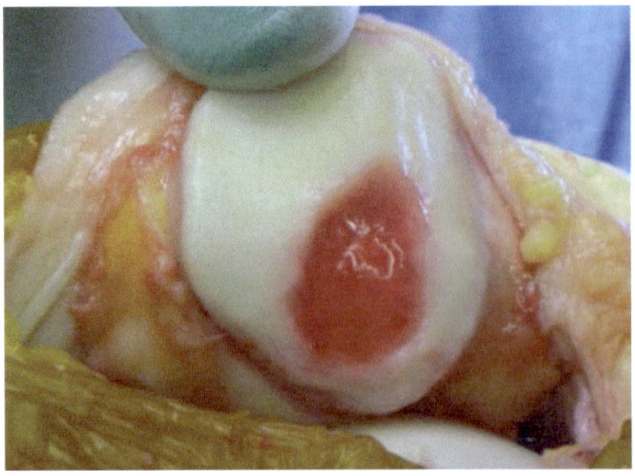

Fig. 18.6 Matrix-induced autologous chondrocyte implantation (MACI) procedure for the management of an isolated focal defect involving the patella

Therefore, unlike ACI with a periosteal membrane and ACI with a collagen membrane, there is no risk of leakage of chondrocytes and uneven distribution [38].

Autologous chondrocyte implantation produces hyaline-like repair tissue in full-thickness cartilage defects, and functional improvement with up to 10 years of follow-up has been demonstrated [29, 35, 39–43]. Preliminary clinical reports of the MACI technique have been encouraging [36, 44]. Bartlett et al. reported the results of a prospective randomized study comparing ACI (44 patients) versus MACI (47 patients) for osteochondral defects of the knee [45]. The comparative histological and clinical outcome scores for both techniques were similar at 1 year, with the frequency of reoperation in each group being 9%. The Summit Trial (level 1) in 2014 demonstrated that for defects larger than 3 cm^2, MACI resulted in improved clinical outcomes compared with microfracture at 2 years follow-up, despite similar structural repair [46].

Harris et al. [43] conducted a systematic review comprised of level I and II clinical studies to compare the efficacy of ACI with alternative treatments. Based on this review, complications were reported to be higher with open, periosteal-covered, first-generation techniques. Furthermore, younger patients with a shorter duration of preoperative symptoms and fewer surgical procedures had the best outcomes following both microfracture and ACI. Defect size more than 4 cm^2 was the only factor predictive of better outcomes when ACI was compared to osteochondral autograft transfer system (OATS) or microfracture.

Jungmann et al. conducted a level III retrospective cohort study that looked at both individual and environmental risk factors which were predictive of re-intervention after an index ACI procedure [47]. Of 813 patients who underwent an ACI procedure, 88 (21.3%) required re-intervention (debridement or revision cartilage surgery) at a mean time of 1.8 years. The four prognostic factors associated with a significantly higher risk for repeat surgery were female gender, previous surgeries of the affected joint, previous bone marrow stimulation, and previous periosteal patch-covered ACI. The lower re-intervention rates for the intermediate (overweight) body mass index (BMI) group (16.8%) suggest that a BMI higher than 30 (obesity, 25.0%) as well as increased physical activity of patients with low BMI (23.7%) is associated with an inferior outcome. Furthermore, the authors demonstrated that unlike that for microfracture, defect size was not a predictor of re-intervention following ACI. The authors highlighted that these facts are easily obtainable in the preoperative period when considering an ACI procedure. Finally, a recent case-control study by Pestka et al. [48] demonstrated that age- and defect-matched patients treated with ACI after a failed initial microfracture procedure were significantly more likely to have higher failure rates and lower Knee Injury and Osteoarthritis Outcome Score (KOOS) pain and KOOS activities of daily living (ADL) scores compared with patients whose first-line treatment was with ACI.

Limited data available on the use of ACI in early osteoarthritis suggest this intervention can reduce the patient's symptoms and increase function [49, 50]; however, these results are preliminary. Minas et al. reported a prospective case series of 155 knees (153 patients) that were treated with ACI [51]. The patients had on average over two large chondral defects per knee, and each defect had a mean size of 4.9 cm^2. Patient pain and function were assessed using Western Ontario and McMaster Universities Osteoarthritis Index (WOMAC), modified Cincinnati, 36-item Short-Form Health Survey (SF-36), Knee Society score, and satisfaction questionnaire. With up to 11 years of follow-up, 92% of patients were functioning well.

18.3.2 ChondroCelect®

ChondroCelect® (TiGenix NV, Leuven, Belgium) is a variation of the ACI procedure. Cellular markers are used to select out autologous chondrocytes that have been harvested from the patient. The selected chondrocytes are proposed to afford more potential for producing a higher-quality, more hyaline-like cartilage after transplantation [52, 53]. Cell lines are expanded, while their cartilage phenotype is maintained to enhance the ability to generate stable cartilage [32].

A single randomized study of 118 patients comparing ChondroCelect (performed with a periosteal patch) with microfracture has been reported [33, 34, 54]. Inclusion criteria included patient age between 18 and 50 years with a single symptomatic femoral condyle cartilage lesion between 1 and 5 cm^2. Exclusion criteria included patellofemoral cartilage lesions, osteochondritis dissecans (OCD), depth of lesion > 0.5 cm, prior meniscal transplant, prior mosaicplasty, and prior microfracture within the last 12 months. With a 3-year mean follow-up, significant differences favoring characterized chondrocyte implantation (CCI) were shown in overall KOOS ($P = 0.048$) and the subdomains of pain ($P = 0.044$) and quality of life (QoL) ($P = 0.036$). More CCI- than microfracture-treated patients were treatment responders (83% vs 62%, respectively). Histological examination of the repair biopsy at 12 months showed superior hyaline-like repair in the ChondroCelect® arm compared to the microfracture arm (computer-assisted histomorphometry, $P = 0.003$; overall histology score, $P = 0.010$). At 5-year follow-up, the average change from baseline in KOOS was not different between both groups. Subgroup analysis revealed that CCI resulted in better outcome in participants with time since the symptom onset of less than 3 years, which was statistically significant and clinically relevant [54]. ChondroCelect® is the first cell therapy product to be authorized in the European Union, and a beneficial cost utility of ACI with ChondroCelect®, measured using quality-adjusted life year (QALY), has been shown in comparison to microfracture [55].

The use of classic first-generation ACI has been associated with several limitations related to the complexity and the morbidity of the surgical procedure, as well as the frequent occurrence of periosteal hypertrophy [30, 56, 57]. More joint complications occurred after ACI implantation than after subchondral bone microfracture: more frequently symptomatic cartilage hypertrophy (27% versus 13%, possibly related to the implantation technique), joint swelling (22% versus

6.6%), joint effusion (24% versus 9.8%), and joint crepitation (18% versus 6.6%). Further, ACI was sometimes associated with flu-like syndrome (in 7.8% of patients), which did not occur with the microfracture technique.

18.4 Particulated Articular Cartilage Grafts

Lu et al. demonstrated that minced cartilage without cell culture served as an effective intraoperative cell source for cartilage repair [58]. The authors demonstrated that (a) there is an inverse relationship between cartilage fragment size and amount of cartilage outgrowth, (b) the highest level of cellular activity was localized at the minced cartilage edge, and (c) the amount of tissue required approximated one-tenth of the area of the entire defect to be treated [58]. It was hypothesized that chondrocytes in the cartilage pieces were able to "escape" from the extracellular matrix, migrate, multiply, and form the observed hyaline-like cartilage tissue matrix that integrated with the surrounding host tissue [58, 59].

Currently available products which utilize particulated articular cartilage in a single-stage setting include the Cartilage Autograft Implantation System (CAIS®: DePuy Mitek, Raynham, MA) and Zimmer® DeNovo® NT Natural Tissue Graft (DeNovo NT: Zimmer Biomet, Warsaw, Indiana) (Table 18.3). In regard to CAIS®, autogenous cartilage tissue from the margins of the intercondylar notch is processed intraoperatively and loaded onto a scaffold, and the resultant construct is fixed into place with bioabsorbable staples (Fig. 18.7) [59, 60]. With DeNovo NT, allogeneic juvenile cartilage tissue is processed in advance, is available "on the shelf," and is fixed in place using fibrin glue (Fig. 18.8) [61, 62]. With DeNovo NT, the use of allograft tissue allows for the treatment of very large defects, and the juvenile source of the chondrocytes has the potential for more robust cellular activity than older cartilage tissue [64–68]. The upshot for both CAIS® and DeNovo® NT products are small cartilage fragments which serve as a source of viable chondrocytes that can migrate into the surrounding matrix and collagen [1]. Within the context of tissue engineering, both technologies utilize two requisite features – (a) a bioactive component (i.e., cells or chondrocytes) which drives the biological process and (b) a biomaterial that serves as a carrier or scaffold which in turn provides architectural support and facilitates integration of repaired tissue with contiguous tissue [60]. In essence, the particulate nature of both grafts allows for an optimization of graft surface area for cartilage expansion, and the use of cells and scaffolds creates the potential for a chondroinductive and chondroconductive milieu, respectively [69].

18.4.1 Cartilage Autograft Implantation System – CAIS®

The CAIS® (DePuy Mitek, Raynham, MA) involves an instrument which arthroscopically harvests cartilage from an autogenous donor site

Table 18.3 Particulated articular cartilage one-stage restoration procedure for symptomatic chondral cartilage defect(s) of the knee

Procedure	Product	Articular Cartilage Source and Fixation	Company/ location	Reference
Particulated Articular Cartilage	Cartilage autograft implantation system (CAIS®)	Autogenous cartilage tissue obtained from the margins of the intercondylar notch, loaded onto a 3D scaffold consisting of 35% polycaprolactone and 65% polyglycolic acid with a polydiaxanone (PDO) mesh and fixed with bioabsorbable staples	DePuy Mitek, Raynham, MA, USA	[59, 60]
	Zimmer® DeNovo® NT Natural Tissue Graft	Allogeneic embryonic cartilage tissue fixed with fibrin glue	Zimmer Biomet, Warsaw, Indiana, USA	[61–63]

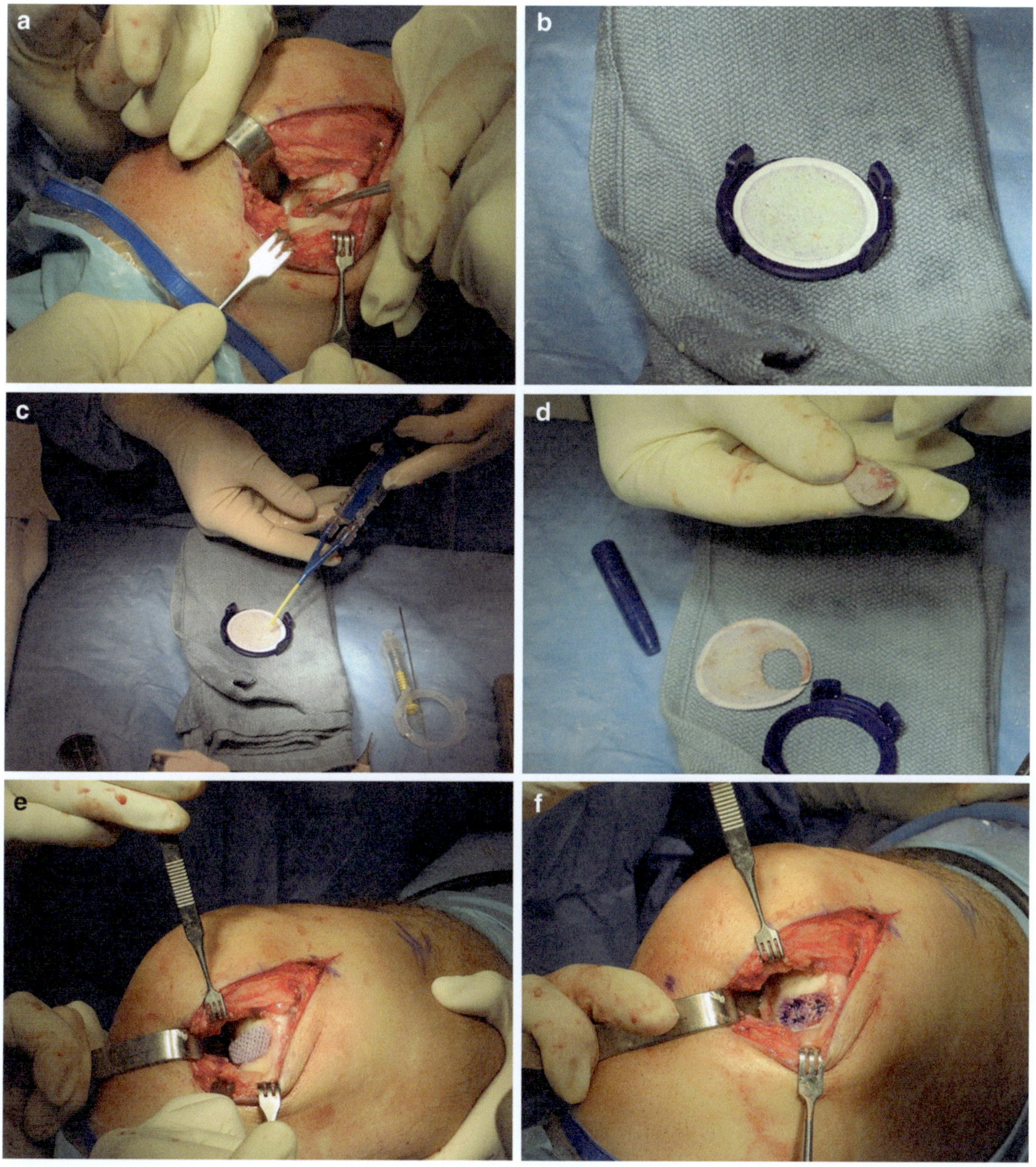

Fig. 18.7 Cartilage Autograft Implantation System (CAIS) procedure for the management of an isolated focal defect involving the medial femoral condyle of the knee. (**a**) Preparation and sizing of knee cartilage defect. (**b**) Harvested cartilage placed on the copolymer scaffold. (**c**) Application of fibrin glue. (**d**) The scaffold is sized and cut according to the prepared cartilage defect. (**e**) CAIS scaffold implant placed and fixed in situ. (**f**) In situ fixation with polydiaxanone (PDO) staples (Images courtesy of Brian J Cole MD MBA)

and distributes the cartilage fragments homogeneously onto an absorbable three-dimensional (3D) scaffold which consists of 35% polycaprolactone and 65% polyglycolic acid and is further reinforced with a polydiaxanone (PDO) mesh (Advanced Technologies and Regenerative Medicine, Raynham, MA) [59, 60]. This scaffold is a foam-like material that serves to keep the tissue fragments in place and provides a 3D environment for cartilage matrix generation. The

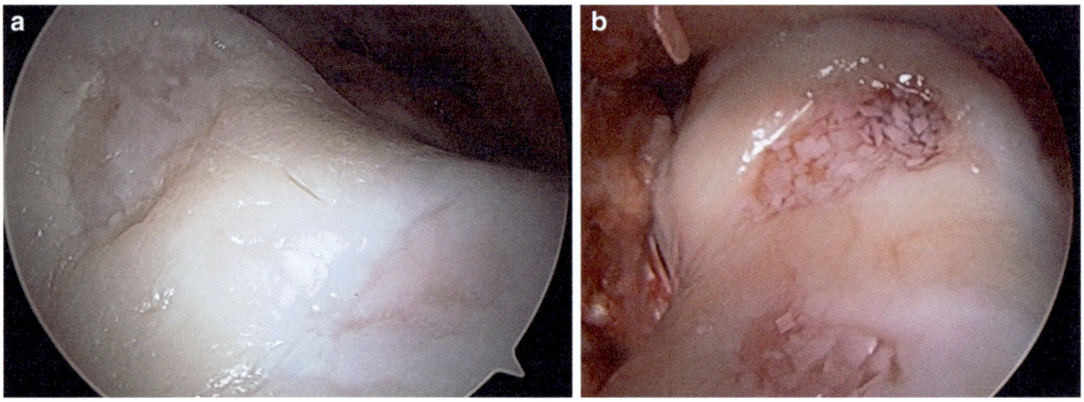

Fig. 18.8 Zimmer® DeNovo® NT Natural Tissue Graft (DeNovo NT) for the management of two focal defects involving the trochlea of the knee. (**a**) Arthroscopic visualization of two trochlear defects. (**b**) Application of DeNovo NT after defect debridement and sizing (Images courtesy of Brian J Cole MD MBA)

cartilage-scaffold construct is secured to the recipient site using PDO staples [1, 59].

Cole et al. conducted a proof of concept and safety randomized controlled trial in 29 patients where patient-reported outcomes and MRI findings were compared at a minimum of 2-year follow-up among patients treated with CAIS® and microfracture [60]. This study demonstrated that the SF-36, International Knee Documentation Committee (IKDC) score, and KOOS improved in both groups over a 24-month period. However, patients who were treated with CAIS had significantly higher overall IKDC score at 12 months postoperatively and had significantly higher scores on all five KOOS subscales at 24 months after surgery. MRI scans showed that patients treated with microfracture also had a higher incidence of intralesional osteophytes at 6 and 12 months postoperatively. A larger multicenter randomized trial comparing CAIS® and microfracture is currently in progress.

18.4.2 Zimmer® DeNovo® NT Natural Tissue Graft – DeNovo NT®

Zimmer® DeNovo® NT Natural Tissue Graft (DeNovo NT: Zimmer Biomet, Warsaw, Indiana) is considered a "minimally manipulated" human tissue allograft, regulated in the United States as a 361 HCT/P product similar to fresh osteochondral allograft, allograft meniscus transplants, and bone-tendon-bone allografts [59, 62]. It is available for clinical application without investigational device exemption [59]. The graft is prepared by removing live cartilage tissue from fresh cadaveric juvenile femoral condyles (up to age 13) and particulating them manually into cubes of approximately 1 cm^3 [62]. Thin aluminum foil is pressed into the defect to create a 3D mold. Once formed, the mold is removed, and its surface area is calculated – one package of DeNovo NT covers 2.5 cm^2. Following this, the medium in which the DeNovo NT is contained is aspirated, and the particulate cartilage fragments are transferred to the mold 1–2 mm apart. Fibrin glue is subsequently applied to the fragments of cartilage until the mold is filled to within 1 mm of its total depth. After a curing time of 3–10 min, fibrin glue is also applied to the base of the defect; the cartilage-fibrin glue construct is separated off the foil and is pressed into the defect [59, 61, 62].

The use of DeNovo NT in a clinical setting was first reported by Bonner et al. [61] where a patellar defect was successfully treated at 2-year follow-up as measured by the IKDC and postoperative MRI which demonstrated fill of the defect with repair tissue and near full resolution of preoperative subchondral bone edema. Subsequently, Farr and Yao [62] reported the results from the first 4 of 25 patients enrolled in a prospective single-arm cohort study investigating the use of DeNovo NT in patients with one or two chondral lesions on the femoral condyles or trochlea. Initial results demonstrated improvements in IKDC and KOOS scores at 2 years compared to baseline, as well as defect filling that persists to at least 2 years following surgery. There were also no complications and no evidence of graft rejection phenomena. Cole and Farr published the results of a 2-year prospective case series in 25 patients treated with DeNovo NT for chondral defects of the knee. Patients had improved KOOS scores over baseline and MRI T2-weighted scores were returning to a level approximating that of normal articular cartilage by 2 years [63].

18.5 Other Scaffold or Synthetic Materials

18.5.1 Biphasic Cartilage Scaffolds

There is increasing evidence that highlights the importance of subchondral bone in supporting a lasting repair of full-thickness chondral lesions, with a fully regenerated osseous architecture being associated with a favorable outcome [70, 71]. As a consequence, multilayered articular cartilage scaffolds, such as the Cartilage Repair Device® (CRD, Kensey Nash Corporation) and ChondroMimetic® (Orthomimetics, Cambridge, UK), have been developed. The production of biphasic or multiphasic composite scaffolds made of a cartilage layer and an underlying subchondral bone region is an evolving technology [72–74].

Variations in structural, chemical, and mechanical properties in the different layers of articular cartilage can be mimicked using a multilayered biphasic construct. Such a strategy is thought to improve the fixation of the engineered cartilage tissue into the joint lesion by the integration of the subchondral bone region into the host bone tissue. However, the quality of the subchondral bone below the cartilage defect may affect both the potential for regeneration and the longevity of the chondral repair [71].

An additional advantage of a multilayered construct is the disparate physiological requirements of chondrocytes (in the cartilage) and osteoblasts (in the subchondral bone) [75]. Chondrocytes must be protected from intimate contact with blood vessel formation [76, 77], whereas osteoblasts require vascularization [78–80].

The multiphasic composite produced by Kensey Nash Corporation consists of three parts, an upper collagen I fiber layer for articular cartilage repair, a hydrophobic interface, and a lower polylactic acid (PLA) part for bone repair, the whole structure mimicking the structure of an osteochondral plug. The construct combines a malleable matrix for cartilage repair and a solid mineralized matrix for the regeneration of the subchondral bone [81]. The two matrices were brought together in a proprietary method that bonds the two regions while maintaining the porosity at the interface. The cartilage-like layer has the potential to support the differentiation of mesenchymal stem cells [82, 83]. In vitro evidence supports the development of a good genetic, biochemical, and histological bioenvironment with this multiphasic construct; however, longer-term clinical results are awaited [84]. ChondroMimetic® implants in a caprine model demonstrated increased chondral and osseous fill of the defect when compared with empty defects at 12 weeks [1].

18.5.2 Hydrogels

Polyvinyl hydrogels have gained increase attention as synthetic materials that can be used for cartilage restoration [85]. An example of such product is Cartiva® (Carticept Medical Inc., Alpharetta, GA) which is a poly(vinyl alcohol) hydrogel developed for full-thickness chondral defects [86]. This material is optimized to closely resemble the wear, strength, and coefficient of friction properties of human articular cartilage [1]. Cartiva® is a synthetic material that, unlike a scaffold, is not designed to resorb or be replaced by native repair tissue over time. Furthermore, a proprietary technology is applied to the bone side of this hydrogel that induces bone ingrowth to facilitate long-term fixation into the defect [1]. A small case series of 15 patients treated arthroscopically with Cartiva resulted in 13 successful outcomes at 1 year as measured by the IKDC, with one case of loosening and one case of dislodgement. As per MRI, no implant expulsions were noted, and the analysis revealed that integration is not necessary for the device to be successful. Rather isolated implants surrounded by high-quality bone, a flush presentation and about 10% radial compression (diameter of implant site about 10% smaller than implant diameter) improve outcome in vivo. More data is required before synthetic hydrogels will be available for routine clinical use [85].

18.6 Conclusions

Given the plethora of treatment options available for focal chondral defects of the knee, a careful comparative evaluation of emerging products with established treatments will be required. Specifically, for a novel technology to be adopted, researchers must demonstrate biological and clinical efficacy, safety, feasibility (e.g., single-stage procedure), cost-effectiveness, and durability of any observed clinical improvements. Additionally, the Food and Drug Administration (FDA) has clearly indicated that individual level response or "responder" analyses are required for the evaluation and approval of medical devices and technologies in the context of cartilage repair [87]. Two different concepts have been developed to aid in the understanding of outcome scores at the individual level which include the "minimal clinically important difference" (MCID) and the "patient acceptable symptomatic state" (PASS) of pertinent patient-reported outcome measures. Finally, well-designed prospective comparative cohort studies, as well as multicenter randomized trials, will be needed to address the aforementioned requisites for the adoption of novel cartilage repair technologies.

References

1. McNickle AG, Provencher MT, Cole BJ. Overview of existing cartilage repair technology. Sports Med Arthrosc. 2008;16(4):196–201.
2. Cascio BM, Sharma B. The future of cartilage repair. YOTSM. 2008., Elsevier Inc;16:221–4.
3. Hurst JM, et al. Rehabilitation following microfracture for chondral injury in the knee. Clin Sports Med. 2010;29(2):257–65. viii.
4. Reinold MM, et al. Current concepts in the rehabilitation following articular cartilage repair procedures in the knee. J Orthop Sports Phys Ther. 2006;36(10):774–94.
5. Mithoefer K, et al. Clinical efficacy of the microfracture technique for articular cartilage repair in the knee: an evidence-based systematic analysis. Am J Sports Med. 2009;37(10):2053–63.
6. Pipino G, Risitano S, Alviano F, Wu EJ, Bonsi L, Vaccarisi DC, Indelli PF. Microfractures and hydrogel scaffolds in the treatment of osteochondral knee defects: A clinical and histological evaluation. J Clin Orthop Trauma. 2019;10(1):67–75.
7. Gwosdz J, Rosinski A, Chakrabarti M, Woodall BM, Elena N, McGahan PJ, Chen JL. Osteochondral Allograft Transplantation of the Medial Femoral Condyle With Orthobiologic Augmentation and Graft-Recipient Microfracture Preparation. Arthrosc Tech. 2019;8(3):e321–e329.
8. Gomoll AH. Microfracture and augments. J Knee Surg. 2012;25(1):9–15.
9. Cascio BM, Sharma B. The future of cartilage repair. Oper Tech Sports Med. 2008;16:221–4.
10. Dhollander AA, et al. Autologous matrix-induced chondrogenesis combined with platelet-rich plasma gel: technical description and a five pilot patients report. Knee Surg Sports Traumatol Arthrosc. 2011;19(4):536–42.
11. Erggelet C, et al. Formation of cartilage repair tissue in articular cartilage defects pretreated with microfracture and covered with cell-free polymer-based implants. J Orthop Res. 2009;27:1353–60.
12. Patrascu J, Freymann U, Kaps C. Repair of a posttraumatic cartilage defect with a cell-free polymer-based cartilage implant. J Bone Joint Surg Br. 2010;92:1160–3.
13. Benthien JP, Behrens P. Autologous matrix-induced chondrogenesis (AMIC). A one-step procedure for retropatellar articular resurfacing. Acta Orthop Belg. 2010;76(2):260–3.
14. Benthien JP, Behrens P. The treatment of chondral and osteochondral defects of the knee with autologous matrix-induced chondrogenesis (AMIC): method description and recent developments. Knee Surg Sports Traumatol Arthrosc. 2011;19(8):1316–9.
15. Gille J, et al. Outcome of autologous matrix induced chondrogenesis (AMIC) in cartilage knee surgery: data of the AMIC registry. Arch Orthop Trauma Surg. 2013;133(1):87–93.
16. Schiavone Panni A, Del Regno C, Mazzitelli G, D'Apolito R, Corona K, Vasso M. Good clinical results with autologous matrix-induced chondrogenesis (Amic) technique in large knee chondral defects. Knee Surg Sports Traumatol Arthrosc. 2018;26(4):1130–6.

17. Bertho P, Pauvert A, Pouderoux T, Robert H; Orthopaedics and Traumatology Society of Western France (SOO). Treatment of large deep osteochondritis lesions of the knee by autologous matrix-induced chondrogenesis (AMIC): Preliminary results in 13 patients. Orthop Traumatol Surg Res. 2018;104(5):695–700.
18. Chen H, et al. Drilling and microfracture lead to different bone structure and necrosis during bone-marrow stimulation for cartilage repair. J Orthop Res. 2009;27(11):1432–8.
19. Volz M, Schaumburger J, Frick H, Grifka J, Anders S. A randomized controlled trial demonstrating sustained benefit of Autologous Matrix-Induced Chondrogenesis over microfracture at five years. Int Orthop. 2017;41(4):797–804.
20. Holt K, Sorhaindo M, Coady C, Wong IH. Arthroscopic treatment of medial femoral knee osteochondral defect using subchondroplasty and chitosan-based scaffold. Arthrosc Tech. 2019;8(4):e413–e418.
21. Stanish WD, et al. A new gel implant for cartilage repair, in ISAKOS, 8th Biennial Congress. Brazil: Rio de Janeiro; 2011.
22. Steinwachs M, Cavalcanti N, Mauuva Venkatesh Reddy S, Werner C, Tschopp D, Choudur HN. Arthroscopic and open treatment of cartilage lesions with BST-CARGEL scaffold and microfracture: A cohort study of consecutive patients. Knee. 2019;26(1):174–84.
23. Carter AH, Guttierez N, Subhawong TK, Temple HT, Lesniak BP, Baraga MG, Jose J. MR imaging of BioCartilage augmented microfracture surgery utilizing 2D MOCART and KOOS scores. J Clin Orthop Trauma. 2018;9(2):146–52.
24. Fortier LA, Chapman HS, Pownder SL. BioCartilage improves cartilage repair compared with microfracture alone in an equine model of full-thickness cartilage loss. Am J Sports Med. 2016;44:2366–74.
25. Hirahara AM, Mueller KW Jr. BioCartilage: a new bio material to treat chondral lesions. Sports Med Arthrosc Rev. 2015;23:143–8.
26. Fortier L, Hackett CH, Cole BJ. The effects of platelet-rich plasma on cartilage: basic science and clinical application. Oper Tech Sports Med. 2011;19:154–9.
27. Malinin T, Temple HT, Carpenter EM. Induction of regeneration of articular cartilage defects by freeze dried particulate cartilage allografts. International Cartilage Repair Society. 2009. Miami.
28. Briggs TW, et al. Histological evaluation of chondral defects after autologous chondrocyte implantation of the knee. J Bone Joint Surg Br. 2003;85(7):1077–83.
29. Peterson L, et al. Autologous chondrocyte transplantation. Biomechanics and long-term durability. Am J Sports Med. 2002;30(1):2–12.
30. Bentley G, et al. A prospective, randomised comparison of autologous chondrocyte implantation versus mosaicplasty for osteochondral defects in the knee. J Bone Joint Surg Br. 2003;85(2):223–30.
31. Haddo O, et al. The use of chondrogide membrane in autologous chondrocyte implantation. Knee. 2004;11(1):51–5.
32. Benya PD, Shaffer JD. Dedifferentiated chondrocytes reexpress the differentiated collagen phenotype when cultured in agarose gels. Cell. 1982;30(1):215–24.
33. Saris DB, et al. Characterized chondrocyte implantation results in better structural repair when treating symptomatic cartilage defects of the knee in a randomized controlled trial versus microfracture. Am J Sports Med. 2008;36(2):235–46.
34. Saris DB, et al. Treatment of symptomatic cartilage defects of the knee: characterized chondrocyte implantation results in better clinical outcome at 36 months in a randomized trial compared to microfracture. Am J Sports Med. 2009;37:10S–9S.
35. Brittberg M, et al. Treatment of deep cartilage defects in the knee with autologous chondrocyte transplantation. N Engl J Med. 1994;331(14):889–95.
36. Cherubino P, et al. Autologous chondrocyte implantation using a bilayer collagen membrane: a preliminary report. J Orthop Surg (Hong Kong). 2003;11(1):10–5.
37. Romeo AA, et al. Autologous chondrocyte repair of an articular defect in the humeral head. Arthroscopy. 2002;18(8):925–9.
38. Sohn DH, et al. Effect of gravity on localization of chondrocytes implanted in cartilage defects. Clin Orthop Relat Res. 2002;394:254–62.
39. Brittberg M, et al. Articular cartilage engineering with autologous chondrocyte transplantation. A review of recent developments. J Bone Joint Surg Am. 2003;85-A(Suppl 3):109–15.
40. Minas T, Peterson L. Advanced techniques in autologous chondrocyte transplantation. Clin Sports Med. 1999;18(1):13–44. v-vi.
41. Peterson L, et al. Treatment of osteochondritis dissecans of the knee with autologous chondrocyte transplantation: results at two to ten years. J Bone Joint Surg Am. 2003;85-A(Suppl 2):17–24.
42. Peterson L, et al. Two- to 9-year outcome after autologous chondrocyte transplantation of the knee. Clin Orthop Relat Res. 2000;374:212–34.
43. Harris JD, et al. Autologous Chondrocyte Implantation: A Systematic Review. J Bone Joint Surg. 2010;92:2220–33.
44. Bartlett W, et al. Autologous chondrocyte implantation at the knee using a bilayer collagen membrane with bone graft. A preliminary report. J Bone Joint Surg Br. 2005;87:330–2.
45. Bartlett W, et al. Autologous chondrocyte implantation versus matrix-induced autologous chondrocyte implantation for osteochondral defects of the knee: a prospective, randomised study. J Bone Joint Surg Br. 2005;87:640–5.
46. Saris D, et al. Matrix-applied characterized autologous cultured chondrocytes versus microfracture: two-year follow-up of a prospective randomized trial. Am J Sports Med. June 2014;42:1384–94.

47. Jungmann PM, et al. Autologous chondrocyte implantation for treatment of cartilage defects of the knee: what predicts the need for reintervention? Am J Sports Med. 2012;40(1):58–67.
48. Pestka JM, et al. Clinical outcome of autologous chondrocyte implantation for failed microfracture treatment of full-thickness cartilage defects of the knee joint. Am J Sports Med. 2012;40(2):325–31.
49. Minas T. Autologous chondrocyte implantation in the arthritic knee. Orthopedics. 2003;26(9):945–7.
50. Saleh KJ, et al. Symposium. Operative treatment of patellofemoral arthritis. J Bone Joint Surg Am. 2005;87(3):659–71.
51. Minas T, et al. Autologous chondrocyte implantation for joint preservation in patients with early osteoarthritis. Clin Orthop Relat Res. 2010;468(1):147–57.
52. Dell'Accio F, De Bari C, Luyten FP. Molecular markers predictive of the capacity of expanded human articular chondrocytes to form stable cartilage in vivo. Arthritis Rheum. 2001;44(7):1608–19.
53. Dell'Accio F, De Bari C, Luyten FP. Microenvironment and phenotypic stability specify tissue formation by human articular cartilage-derived cells in vivo. Exp Cell Res. 2003;287(1):16–27.
54. Vanlauwe J, et al. Five-year outcome of characterized chondrocyte implantation versus microfracture for symptomatic cartilage defects of the knee: early treatment matters. Am J Sports Med. 2011;39(12):2566–74.
55. Gerlier L, et al. The cost utility of autologous chondrocytes implantation using ChondroCelect(R) in symptomatic knee cartilage lesions in Belgium. Pharmacoeconomics. 2010;28(12):1129–46.
56. Henderson I, et al. Autologous chondrocyte implantation for treatment of focal chondral defects of the knee--a clinical, arthroscopic, MRI and histologic evaluation at 2 years. Knee. 2005;12(3):209–16.
57. Henderson IJ, et al. Prospective clinical study of autologous chondrocyte implantation and correlation with MRI at three and 12 months. J Bone Joint Surg Br. 2003;85(7):1060–6.
58. Lu Y, et al. Minced cartilage without cell culture serves as an effective intraoperative cell source for cartilage repair. J Orthop Res. 2006;24(6):1261–70.
59. Farr J, et al. Particulated articular cartilage: CAIS and DeNovo NT. J Knee Surg. 2012;25(1):23–9.
60. Cole BJ, et al. Outcomes after a single-stage procedure for cell-based cartilage repair: a prospective clinical safety trial with 2-year follow-up. Am J Sports Med. 2011;39(6):1170–9.
61. Bonner KF, Daner W, Yao JQ. 2-year postoperative evaluation of a patient with a symptomatic full-thickness patellar cartilage defect repaired with particulated juvenile cartilage tissue. J Knee Surg. 2010;23(2):109–14.
62. Farr J, et al. Clinical Cartilage Restoration: Evolution and Overview. Clin Orthop Relat Res. 2011;469(10):2696–705.
63. Farr J, Tabet SK, Margerrison E, Cole BJ. Clinical, radiographic, and histological outcomes after cartilage repair with particulated juvenile articular cartilage: a 2-year prospective study. Am J Sports Med. 2014;42(6):1417–25.
64. Adkisson HD, et al. The potential of human allogeneic juvenile chondrocytes for restoration of articular cartilage. Am J Sports Med. 2010;38(7):1324–33.
65. Namba RS, et al. Spontaneous repair of superficial defects in articular cartilage in a fetal lamb model. J Bone Joint Surg Am. 1998;80(1):4–10.
66. Hinckel BB, Gomoll AH. Patellofemoral cartilage rest oration: indications, techniques, and outcomes of autologous chondrocytes implantation, matrix-Induced chondrocyte implantation, and particulated Juvenile Allograft Cartilage. J Knee Surg. 2018;31(3):212–26.
67. Yanke AB, Tilton AK, Wetters NG, Merkow DB, Cole BJ, NT DN. Particulated Juvenile Cartilage Implant. Sports Med Arthrosc Rev. 2015;23(3):125–9.
68. Buckwalter JA, Bowman GN, Albright JP, Wolf BR, Bollier M. Clinical outcomes of patellar chondral lesions treated with juvenile particulated cartilage allografts. Iowa Orthop J. 2014;34:44–9.
69. McCormick F, et al. Minced articular cartilage--basic science, surgical technique, and clinical application. Sports Med Arthrosc. 2008;16(4):217–20.
70. Sellers RS, et al. Repair of articular cartilage defects one year after treatment with recombinant human bone morphogenetic protein-2 (rhBMP-2). J Bone Joint Surg Am. 2000;82(2):151–60.
71. Chu CR, et al. Osteochondral repair using perichondrial cells. A 1-year study in rabbits. Clin Orthop Relat Res. 1997;340:220–9.
72. Mano JF, Reis RL. Osteochondral defects: present situation and tissue engineering approaches. J Tissue Eng Regen Med. 2007;1(4):261–73.
73. Martin I, et al. Osteochondral tissue engineering. J Biomech. 2007;40(4):750–65.
74. Radhakrishnan J, Manigandan A, Chinnaswam YP, Subramanian A, Sethuraman S. Gradient nano-engineered in situ forming composite hydrogel for osteochondral regeneration. Biomaterials. 2018;162:82–98.
75. Schumann D, Ekaputra AK, Lam CX, Hutmacher DW. Biomaterials/scaffolds. Design of bioactive, multiphasic PCL/collagen type I and type II-PCL-TCP/collagen composite scaffolds for functional tissue engineering of osteochondral repair tissue by using electrospinning and FDM techniques. Methods Mol Med. 2007;140:101–24.
76. Archer CW, Francis-West P. The chondrocyte. Int J Biochem Cell Biol. 2003;35(4):401–4.
77. Barbero A, et al. Plasticity of clonal populations of dedifferentiated adult human articular chondrocytes. Arthritis Rheum. 2003;48(5):1315–25.

78. Orban JM, Marra KG, Hollinger JO. Composition options for tissue-engineered bone. Tissue Eng. 2002;8(4):529–39.
79. Soker S, Machado M, Atala A. Systems for therapeutic angiogenesis in tissue engineering. World J Urol. 2000;18(1):10–8.
80. Brighton CT, Hunt RM. Early histological and ultrastructural changes in medullary fracture callus. J Bone Joint Surg Am. 1991;73(6):832–47.
81. Frenkel SR, et al. Regeneration of articular cartilage--evaluation of osteochondral defect repair in the rabbit using multiphasic implants. Osteoarthritis Cartilage. 2005;13(9):798–807.
82. DeLise AM, Fischer L, Tuan RS. Cellular interactions and signaling in cartilage development. Osteoarthritis Cartilage. 2000;8(5):309–34.
83. Reichert JC, et al. Fabrication of polycaprolactone collagen hydrogel constructs seeded with mesenchymal stem cells for bone regeneration. Biomed Mater. 2009;4(6):065001.
84. Heymer A, et al. Multiphasic collagen fibre-PLA composites seeded with human mesenchymal stem cells for osteochondral defect repair: an in vitro study. J Tissue Eng Regen Med. 2009;3(5):389–97.
85. Baker MI, et al. A review of polyvinyl alcohol and its uses in cartilage and orthopedic applications. J Biomed Mater Res B Appl Biomater. 2012;100(5):1451–7.
86. Sciarretta FV. 5 to 8 years follow-up of knee chondral defects treated by PVA-H hydrogel implants. Eur Rev Med Pharmacol Sci. 2013;17(22):3031–8.
87. U.S. Department of Health and Human Services Food and Drug Administration, C.o.D.E.a.R.C., Center for Biologics Evaluation and Research (CBER), Center for Devices and Radiological Health (CDRH). Guidance for industry patient-reported outcome measures: use in medical product development to support labeling claims. 2009 December 2009 August 12, 2011]; Available from: http://www.fda.gov/downloads/Drugs/GuidanceComplianceRegulatoryInformation/Guidances/UCM193282.pdf.

Part VIII

Future Prospects for Knee Articular Cartilage Therapy

Knee Articular Cartilage: Future Directions for Research and Practice

19

Harpal K. Gahunia, Allan E. Gross, and Kenneth P. H. Pritzker

19.1 Knee Articular Cartilage, Future Research Directions

Articular cartilage serves as a lubricated, wear-resistant, friction-reducing self-maintaining material that is slightly compressible to evenly distribute forces onto the bone. Articular cartilage macromolecular composition and architecture and its biomechanical properties are well adapted to withstand mechanical loads increasingly for a ten-decade lifetime. The three-dimensional (3D) orientation of the structural molecules and various levels of compartmentalization, namely, the horizontal zones from the articular surface to the underlying subchondral bone as well as interstitially from the surface of the chondrocytes, enable articular cartilage function by facilitating smooth knee movements by reducing friction and by absorbing the impact of loading. Coupled with the biomechanical function of articular cartilage in its entirety, articular cartilage lubrication mechanisms provide almost frictionless surfaces between moving joints and do this throughout life adapting to both age and arthritic disease.

A special feature of articular cartilage is the environment of the chondrocytes and pericellular matrix within chondrons and the extra-chondral territorial and interterritorial matrix domains that these cells regulate. These chondrocytes are the key cellular mediators for cartilage homeostasis that normally maintains a functional matrix by modulating extracellular matrix (ECM) synthesis and degradation. Past structural studies have focused on various component molecules; the future is likely to bring forth better understanding of the integration of these molecules as a material as well as the role of the chondrocytes in forming integrated matrix structures, clearing damaged molecules, and repairing and/or regenerating injured and diseased cartilage.

At the bioengineering front, for the past several decades, in vitro, ex vivo, and in vivo investigations have enhanced our understanding of the significance of biomechanical stimuli (such as hydrostatic pressure, stress, or compression) on knee articular cartilage biomechanics.

H. K. Gahunia, MSc, PhD (✉)
Orthopaedic Science Consulting Services, Oakville, ON, Canada
e-mail: harpal.gahunia@utoronto.ca

A. E. Gross, MD, FRCSC, O ONT
Division of Orthopaedic Surgery, University of Toronto, Toronto, ON, Canada

Gluskin Granovsky Division of Orthopaedics, Joseph and Wolf Lebovic Health Complex, Mount Sinai Hospital, Toronto, ON, Canada

K. P. H. Pritzker, MD, FRCPC
Department of Laboratory Medicine and Pathobiology, Department of Surgery, and Institute of Biomaterials and Biomedical Engineering, University of Toronto, Toronto, ON, Canada

Department of Pathology and Laboratory Medicine, Mount Sinai Hospital, Toronto, ON, Canada

H. K. Gahunia et al. (eds.), *Articular Cartilage of the Knee*,
https://doi.org/10.1007/978-1-4939-7587-7_19

Biomechanics plays a central role in articular cartilage embryogenesis, growth, development and maturation, homeostasis, aging, adaptation to disease, and repair and regeneration. During embryogenesis and childhood, mechanical stimuli positively influence chondrogenesis, articular cartilage matrix production through appositional and interstitial growth, and cartilage maturation by promotion of endochondral ossification. Intrinsic to the influence of mechanical loading is the maintenance of articular cartilage structure and chondrocyte phenotype. Both excessive as well as insufficient loading can have a negative impact on the articular cartilage integrity promoting onset and progression of cartilage degeneration.

Typically, following physiologic knee loading, a cascade of events is initiated by the hydrostatic pressure within the articular cartilage ECM interstitial fluid, which then induces shear pressure and tension due to the fluid flow subsequently causing the ECM compression and deformation. These biomechanical changes are then transmitted from ECM through the pericellular capsule and matrix to the chondrocytes which in turn are subjected to hydrostatic pressure, shear pressure with some tension, and compression. Functioning as a biological sensor, chondrocytes detect and transduce ECM mechanical signals. The resultant mechanical stimulation on the chondrocyte further initiates a cascade of events which signals elevated gene expression and the corresponding ECM protein production.

Future studies pertaining to the biomechanics of articular cartilage are likely to be directed to the thorough investigation of the nature of extreme nonphysiologic loading on the knee and its articular cartilage component. This will enable us to further understand the impact of biomechanics on the signaling cascade of the chondrocytes which critically influences its matrix microenvironment and ECM production. Reactive oxygen species (ROS), particularly singlet oxygen are of particular interest as signal molecules [1]. These studies pertaining to the impact of excessive or sudden, abrupt biomechanical loads on knee articular cartilage (chondrocytes and it's microenvironment, and ECM) will be particularly useful to understand better how well articular cartilage can withstand and function with these excessive loads. This will lead to strategies or exercises which can prevent knee injury that may be encountered during sports activities (competitive sports, dancing, and gymnastics as well as noncompetitive sports and recreational activities), occupation-related injuries, or early stages of cartilage diseases. Further, from the cartilage engineering and cartilage repair perspective, investigations on the optimal biomechanical stimuli and its associated signaling cascade under high-impact loads will lead to successful therapeutic strategies for cartilage regeneration and repair.

The knee is one of the joints most commonly injured during sport-related activities in children and adults. The most common sport-related articular cartilage injuries are due to overuse and high impact. An overuse cartilage injury is a consequence of repeated activity resulting in cartilage fatigue and wear and tear (such as professional runners). High-impact sports that can lead to articular cartilage damage are those resulting from a direct, forceful impact on the knee joint (such as a tackle in football, rugby, and wrestling). In children, articular cartilage is a highly organized structure which repeatedly undergoes growth and remodelling while maintaining the shape of the joint. Injury to any part of this complex system can disrupt the functional properties of cartilage, which may lead to further joint degeneration. Although articular cartilage has intrinsic capacity for repair and regeneration, the organized structure of immature cartilage is particularly difficult to restore or duplicate once it is damaged or lost. Future research on knee articular cartilage in children will address the problems of how to maintain articular function and limb growth and reduce rehabilitation time after cartilage injury. As well through genomic therapy, hereditary cartilage disorders will receive attention to prevent deformity and functional loss that accompanies these diseases.

An integral component to the success of cartilage maintenance and repair is the tight-coupling of articular cartilage lubrication with articular cartilage structure. Future investigation in cartilage lubrication mechanisms may shed light on better means to assess cartilage lubrication deficiency whether related to endogenous lubrication production or deleterious changes in cartilage matrix. In turn this will stimulate therapeutic strategies to restore lubrication quality after injury, as well as with age and disease. This research will be directed toward reducing progression of joint degeneration. Further, the application of lubricating molecules including novel molecules may facilitate in vitro cell-seeded and bioengineered matrices for implants.

Aging of articular cartilage is a normal phenomenon (part and parcel of the normal life cycle), but articular cartilage ages at different rates in different people. A continually growing body of basic science and clinical evidence demonstrates the efficacy of an active lifestyle on retarding the cartilage aging process. Aging cartilage has three features which contribute to degenerative loss of function: matrix dehydration, accumulation of abnormal molecules in the extracellular substance, and focal chondrocyte death. Matrix dehydration largely results from reduction of sulfate anions on proteoglycan molecules. Research is likely to follow two lines: substitution of natural or synthetic charged molecules into cartilage matrix and stimulation of chondrocytes to manufacture highly sulfated proteoglycans. Aging cartilage accumulates many different kinds of molecules, including endogenous molecules such as enzyme inhibitors exported from the chondrocyte cell membrane, matrix degradation products such as advanced glycation end products (AGEs'), amyloid, lipid oxidation products, e.g., lipofuschin, which cannot be cleared easily, and sparingly soluble calcium pyrophosphate dihydrate (CPPD) crystals. These molecules interfere with nutrient and waste diffusion, can make chondrocyte signaling less sensitive, and may degrade biomechanical function. Also, due to their high stiffness compared to healthy articular cartilage, crystal deposits potentially alter chondrocyte mechanotransduction as well as cartilage biomechanics, when present in high concentration [2]. Current research is aimed at pharmacologic strategies which can dissolve or clear these accumulated substances. Focal chondrocyte death may result from necrosis following repeated impact trauma or apoptosis associated with inflammation, osteoarthritis (OA), or other reactive stimuli or chondrocyte senescence related to decreased signaling or inadequate nutrition from diffusion. On the near horizon are strategies to upregulate chondrocyte reactivity including stimulating controlled mitotic division in adjacent chondrocytes.

Articular cartilage regeneration presents an important clinical challenge due to difficulty to replicate the physiologic and functional properties of the native cartilage [3–6]. To date, a large array of cell types (See Chap. 17) are available for cartilage cell therapy, and recently, the use of cranial neural crest-derived chondrocytes and oral stem cells for repair of cartilage lesions seems promising as a cell source for cartilage regeneration [7]. Repair of osteochondral lesions in the knee remains a challenge to the orthopedic surgeons, in particular treating young, active individuals [8, 9]. Knee joint surgery for injury and arthritis is focused on preserving articular cartilage where possible, restoring knee function and decreasing postsurgical rehabilitation time. These goals may require surgical intervention at an earlier phases of disease processes but equally will demand precision of assessment and choice of intervention. Arthroscopic mechanical chondroplasty of the knee performed in isolation of concurrent procedures has shown clinical efficacy in the treatment of focal articular cartilage defects [10]. Some novel materials will likely have a theranostics function, monitoring function and supplying agents to help cartilage maintain itself [11]. Theranostics, exosomes, nanosomes, and nanoparticles have the potential to noninvasively detect, track, and treat joint tissue lesions including cartilage, but choosing how much tissue to debride, where to place these particles, and the skill associated with the delivery method, all will remain the province of the surgeon [11, 12]. Reduced rehabilitation time will be achieved by more precise surgery, adjunctive pharmacologic and biologic agents to accelerate healing, and more precise physical modalities to assist rehabilitation.

Osteochondral allografts have proven to be an excellent option for the larger defects involving the cartilage and bone [5, 13–16]. Harvesting the tissue and storage until testing is complete has proven to be an obstacle for the orthopedic surgeon who under the present circumstances has to perform the procedure in a narrow window of time after testing has been completed but before cartilage death begins [17]. The chondrocytes start to die after 2 weeks, but grafts can still be used up to approximately 5 weeks after harvest [18]. Research into development of solutions that maintain chondrocyte viability beyond that time period is being carried out and clinical trials are under way [19, 20]. Although adequate information on surgical technique, lesion location, and morphology of cartilage repair is reported in current clinical studies on articular cartilage restoration of the knee, there is variation and incomplete reporting on lesion size, depth, and grading, which should be addressed in future clinical studies to facilitate comparison among surgical techniques [21].

Currently, cartilage engineering strategies use biocompatible, biodegradable, and structurally as well as mechanically stable scaffolds that can allow successful loading, infiltration, and attachment of appropriate cells as well as bioactive molecules that enhance cell attachment and growth. These sophisticated techniques are expensive and require prolonged rehabilitation time. In the long term, the research goal will be to assess the matrix and cells adjacent to the defect by noninvasive means and then to stimulate repair and regeneration from chondrocytes in the adjacent tissues noninvasively or by minimally invasive means. Enhanced collaboration with industrial partners interested in cartilage repair will provide the financial sources to enable more sophisticated and detailed investigation of cartilage repair strategies including the use of growth factors, gene therapy, and tissue engineering. Future studies in integrative cartilage repair, specifically on engineered graft or scaffold constitution and design strategies to facilitate integration of regenerated cartilage to the native cartilage and the underlying subchondral bone will ensure long-term success of the engineered graft or scaffold for cartilage repair. Integral to these engineered graft or scaffold design strategies is the ability to withstand physiological mechanical forces that the knee is subjected to daily.

Much attention can be expected for research in articular cartilage diagnostics. To date, excellent progress has been made in the hardware and software front, including automated techniques for the visualization, mapping, and compositional and functional imaging of normal, injured, or diseased articular cartilage [22–30]. Beyond linear improvement in modalities such as magnetic resonance imaging and ultrasound, advances can be expected in novel modalities to investigate cartilage structure such as optical coherence tomography and nuclear magnetic resonance (NMR) functional imaging under in vivo mechanical loading conditions [31]. Further, clinical imaging will integrate knowledge from experimental imaging that currently has resolution and contrast 2+ orders of magnitude better. With regard to histologic understanding of cartilage structure, advances can be expected in 3D imaging and better visualization of structures such as the chondron and their dynamic relationships to surrounding extracellular matrix [32, 33]. As well, subchondral bone changes may be an effective surrogate for the state of articular cartilage [34–36]. This will result in more precise and therapeutically more useful assessment of knee cartilage and adjacent structures. Imaging can be expected to advance from visualization of anatomical and histologic structures to characterization of biomaterial characteristics and their association with biomechanical stimuli. Artificial intelligence techniques will be deployed to objectively assess images enabling much more objective data to be assessed by the imager. This will be particularly important for assessment of disease progression in serial studies.

19.2 Knee Articular Cartilage and Osteoarthritis

The knee is highly mobile which has the consequence that other joint structures principally ligaments and capsules are highly influential on the health and function of cartilage. Ambulatory changes associated with aging, obesity, or joint tissue injury that occurs prior to the development of OA symptoms can eventually lead to clinical OA [37, 38]. Osteoarthritis affects all tissues of the knee, yet unless there is advanced pathology in a component other than articular cartilage, cruciate ligament, or meniscal tear, other tissues within the knee are seldom considered when assessing OA. This problem is likely to be addressed in future by dynamic imaging studies employing ultrasound and/or magnetic resonance imaging (MRI). Osteoarthritis biomarkers have a long history but to date are insensitive to assess progression of cartilage deterioration. Cartilage biomarkers are of two types, biochemical markers and imaging markers. Biochemical markers can reflect upregulated or downregulated chondrocyte activity or alternatively abnormal matrix end products released from cartilage reflecting disease progression. While individual markers may have limited value, a promising approach is the assessment of markers of different types [39]. Imaging biomarkers currently are relatively insensitive and still depend more or less on assessment of joint space narrowing. An alternative emerging approach uses increasing subchondral bone thickness and density as proxy biomarkers for OA progression [36]. Conservative therapy of OA is dependent in part on recognizing the knee cartilage injury before irrevocable structural changes have occurred. Central to this strategy is the detection of OA at an earlier stage, which is as much a public health family medicine issue as it is an issue of better diagnostic techniques. A strategy to consider is to deploy existing conservative therapy, e.g., stationary bicycle riding, earlier in the OA process. Low-impact exercise and weight loss provide benefit and constitute the foundation for the treatment of OA [40, 41]. Further consideration might be to condition adjacent muscles by physical techniques such as periodization of exercise supplemented by nutriceutical or pharmacologic strategies to enhance muscle strength [42, 43].

Regarding OA therapy that restores cartilage, the problems have been centered around diagnostic difficulty for early cartilage injury and the perceived lack of regenerative capacity of articular cartilage. With current imaging techniques, domains of cartilage injury as well as cartilage defects can be recognized. Regarding cartilage regeneration, many factors are known to stimulate chondrocyte growth and regeneration, and it is well known that articular chondrocytes can grow and produce matrix ex vivo [44]. One approach to restorative therapy is to deliver agents or even stem cells into cartilage to foster regeneration. These “delivery” approaches require novel techniques, perhaps employing novel ultrasonics [45, 46].

The above paragraphs provide only a glimpse of advances that the coming years may bring. Given the momentum of current investigators and building on past achievements, we can be very optimistic that the societal and individual burden of knee disease will be substantially reduced in the foreseeable future.

References

1. Heywood HK, Lee DA. Bioenergetic reprogramming of articular chondrocytes by exposure to exogenous and endogenous reactive oxygen species and its role in the anabolic response to low oxygen. J Tissue Eng Regen Med. 2016;11(8):2286–94.
2. Carlson AK, McCutchen CN, June RK. Mechanobiological implications of articular cartilage crystals. Curr Opin Rheumatol. 2017;29:157–62.
3. Carballo CB, Nakagawa Y, Sekiya I, Rodeo SA. Basic Science of Articular Cartilage. Clin Sports Med. 2017;36:413–25.
4. Brody LT. Knee osteoarthritis: Clinical connections to articular cartilage structure and function. Phys Ther Sport. 2015;16:301–16.
5. Brittberg M, Gomoll AH, Canseco JA, Far J, Lind M, Hui J. Cartilage repair in the degenerative ageing knee. Acta Orthop. 2016;87:26–38.
6. Mithoefer K. Complex articular cartilage restoration. Sports Med Arthrosc Rev. 2013;21:31–7.
7. Taïhi I, Nassif A, Isaac J, Fournier BP, Ferré F. Head to knee: cranial neural crest-derived cells as promising candidates for human cartilage repair. Stem Cells Int. 2019;2019:9310318. https://doi.org/10.1155/2019/9310318.
8. Murray IR, Benke MT, Mandelbaum BR. Management of knee articular cartilage injuries in athletes: chondroprotection, chondrofacilitation, and resurfacing. Knee Surg Sports Traumatol Arthrosc. 2016;24:1617–26.

9. York PJ, Wydra FB, Belton ME, Vidal AF. Joint Preservation Techniques in Orthopaedic Surgery. Sports Health. 2017;9(6):1941738117712203.
10. Anderson DE, Rose MB, Wille AJ, Wiedrick J, Crawford DC. Arthroscopic mechanical chondroplasty of the knee is beneficial for treatment of focal cartilage lesions in the absence of concurrent pathology. Orthop J Sports Med. 2017;5:2325967117707213.
11. Eichaker LR, Cho H, Duvall CL, Werfel TA, Hasty KA. Future nanomedicine for the diagnosis and treatment of osteoarthritis. Nanomedicine (Lond). 2014;9:2203–15.
12. Tao SC, Yuan T, Zhang YL, Yin WJ, Guo SC, Zhang CQ. Exosomes derived from miR-140-5p-overexpressing human synovial mesenchymal stem cells enhance cartilage tissue regeneration and prevent osteoarthritis of the knee in a rat model. Theranostics. 2017;7:180–95.
13. Raz G, Safir OA, Backstein DJ, Lee PT, Gross AE. Distal femoral fresh Osteochondral allografts: follow-up at a mean of twenty-two years. J Bone Joint Surg Am. 2014;96:1101–7.
14. Taylor DW, CB K, Taylor JE, Gross AE. Use of fresh osteochondral allograft in repair of distal femur after trauma. Mcgill J Med. 2011;13:22.
15. Gross AE, Kim W, Las Heras F, Backstein D, Safir O, Pritzker KP. Fresh Osteochondral allografts for posttraumatic knee defects: long-term followup. Clin Orthop Relat Res. 2008;466:1863–70.
16. Gross AE, Shasha N, Aubin P. Long-term followup of the use of fresh osteochondral allografts for post-traumatic knee defects. Clin Orthop Relat Res. 2005;435:79–87.
17. Nover AB, Stefani RM, Lee SL, Ateshian GA, Stoker AM, Cook JL, Hung CT. Long-term storage and preservation of tissue engineered articular cartilage. J Orthop Res. 2016;34:141–8.
18. Olivos-Meza A, Velasquillo Martinez C, Olivos Diaz B, Landa-Solis C, Brittberg M, Pichardo Bahena R, Ortega Sanchez C, Martinez V, Alvarez Lara E, Ibarra-Ponce de Leon JC. co-culture of dedifferentiated and primary human chondrocytes obtained from cadaveric donor enhance the histological quality of repair tissue: an in-vivo animal study. Cell Tissue Bank. 2017;18:369–81.
19. Cook JL, Stannard JP, Stoker AM, Bozynski CC, Kuroki K, Cook CR, Pfeiffer FM. Importance of donor chondrocyte viability for osteochondral allografts. Am J Sports Med. 2016;44:1260–8.
20. Cook JL, Stoker AM, Stannard JP, Kuroki K, Cook CR, Pfeiffer FM, Bozynski C, Hung CT. A novel system improves preservation of osteochondral allografts. Clin Orthop Relat Res. 2014;472:3404–14.
21. Jones KJ, Sheppard WL, Arshi A, Hinckel BB, Sherman SL. Articular Cartilage Lesion Characteristic Reporting Is Highly Variable in Clinical Outcomes Studies of the Knee. Cartilage. 2019;10(3):299-304.
22. Cashman PM, Kitney RI, Gariba MA, Carter ME. Automated techniques for visualization and mapping of articular cartilage in MR images of the osteoarthritic knee: a base technique for the assessment of microdamage and submicro damage. IEEE Trans Nanobioscience. 2002;1:42–51.
23. Behzadi C, Welsch GH, Laqmani A, Henes FO, Kaul MG, Schoen G, Adam G, Regier M. Comparison of T2* relaxation times of articular cartilage of the knee in elite professional football players and age- and BMI-matched amateur athletes. Eur J Radiol. 2017;86:105–11.
24. Bouhrara M, Reiter DA, Sexton KW, Bergeron CM, Zukley LM, Spencer RG. Clinical high-resolution mapping of the proteoglycan-bound water fraction in articular cartilage of the human knee joint. Magn Reson Imaging. 2017;43:1–5.
25. Fripp J, Crozier S, Warfield SK, Ourselin S. Automatic segmentation of articular cartilage in magnetic resonance images of the knee. Med Image Comput Comput Assist Interv. 2007;10:186–194.
26. Hayashi D, Li X, Murakami AM, Roemer FW, Trattnig S, Guermazi A. Understanding magnetic resonance imaging of knee cartilage repair: a focus on clinical relevance. Cartilage. 2017:1947603517710309. https://doi.org/10.1177/1947603517710309. [Epub ahead of print].
27. Fritz J, Fritz B, Zhang J, Thawait GK, Joshi DH, Pan L, Wang D. Simultaneous multislice accelerated turbo spin echo magnetic resonance imaging: comparison and combination with in-plane parallel imaging acceleration for high-resolution magnetic resonance imaging of the knee. Invest Radiol. 2017;52(9):529–37.
28. Guermazi A, Roemer FW, Alizai H, Winalski CS, Welsch G, Brittberg M, Trattnig S. State of the art: mr imaging after knee cartilage repair surgery. Radiology. 2015;277:23–43.
29. Jungmann PM, Welsch GH, Brittberg M, Trattnig S, Braun S, Imhoff AB, Salzmann GM. Magnetic resonance imaging score and classification system (amadeus) for assessment of preoperative cartilage defect severity. Cartilage. 2017;8:272–82.
30. Van Rossom S, Smith CR, Zevenbergen L, Thelen DG, Vanwanseele B, Van Assche D, Jonkers I. Knee cartilage thickness, t1rho and t2 relaxation time are related to articular cartilage loading in healthy adults. PLoS One. 2017;12:e0170002.
31. Rossler E, Mattea C, Saarakkala S, Lehenkari P, Finnila M, Rieppo L, Karhula S, Nieminen MT, Stapf S. Correlations of low-field NMR and variable-field NMR parameters with osteoarthritis in human articular cartilage under load. NMR Biomed 2017; 30(8). https://doi.org/10. 1002/nbm.3738. Epub 2017 May 24.
32. Karhula SS, Finnila MA, Lammi MJ, Ylarinne JH, Kauppinen S, Rieppo L, Pritzker KP, Nieminen HJ, Saarakkala S. Effects of articular cartilage constituents on phosphotungstic acid enhanced micro-computed tomography. PLoS One. 2017;12:e0171075.
33. Nieminen HJ, Gahunia HK, Pritzker KPH, Ylitalo T, Rieppo L, Karhula SS, Lehenkari P, Haeggstrom E, Saarakkala S. 3D histopathological grading of

osteochondral tissue using contrast-enhanced micro-computed tomography. Osteoarthritis Cartilage. 2017;25(10):1680–9.
34. Aho OM, Finnila M, Thevenot J, Saarakkala S, Lehenkari P. Subchondral bone histology and grading in osteoarthritis. PLoS One. 2017;12:e0173726.
35. Hirvasniemi J, Thevenot J, Guermazi A, Podlipska J, Roemer FW, Nieminen MT, Saarakkala S. Differences in tibial subchondral bone structure evaluated using plain radiographs between knees with and without cartilage damage or bone marrow lesions – the Oulu Knee Osteoarthritis study. Eur Radiol. 2017.
36. Finnila MAJ, Thevenot J, Aho OM, Tiitu V, Rautiainen J, Kauppinen S, Nieminen MT, Pritzker K, Valkealahti M, Lehenkari P, Saarakkala S. Association between subchondral bone structure and osteoarthritis histopathological grade. J Orthop Res. 2017;35:785–92.
37. Andriacchi TP, Favre J. The nature of in vivo mechanical signals that influence cartilage health and progression to knee osteoarthritis. Curr Rheumatol Rep. 2014;16:463.
38. Lepage SIM, Robson N, Gilmore H, Davis O, Hooper A, et al. Beyond cartilage repair: the role of the osteochondral unit in joint health and disease. Tissue Eng Part B Rev. 2019;25(2):114–25.
39. Ahmed A, Shamsi A, Bano B. Characterizing harmful advanced glycation end-products (AGEs) and ribosylated aggregates of yellow mustard seed phytocystatin: Effects of different monosaccharides, Spectrochimica acta Part A, Molecular and biomolecular. Spectroscopy. 2017;171:183–92.
40. Gahunia HK, Pritzker KP. Effect of exercise on articular cartilage. Orthop Clin North Am. 2012;43:187–99. v
41. Poddar SK, Widstrom L. Nonoperative Options for Management of Articular Cartilage Disease. Clin Sports Med. 2017;36:447–56.
42. Strohacker K, Fazzino D, Breslin WL, Xu X. The use of periodization in exercise prescriptions for inactive adults: a systematic review. Prev Med Rep. 2015;2:385–96.
43. Handschin C. Caloric restriction and exercise "mimetics": ready for prime time? Pharmacol Res. 2016;103:158–66.
44. Ondresik M, Azevedo Maia FR, da Silva Morais A, Gertrudes AC, Dias Bacelar AH, Correia C, Goncalves C, Radhouani H, Amandi Sousa R, Oliveira JM, Reis RL. Management of knee osteoarthritis. Current status and future trends. Biotechnol Bioeng. 2017;114:717–39.
45. Nieminen HJ, Ylitalo T, Suuronen JP, Rahunen K, Salmi A, Saarakkala S, Serimaa R, Haeggstrom E. Delivering agents locally into articular cartilage by intense mhz ultrasound. Ultrasound Med Biol. 2015;41:2259–65.
46. Nieminen HJ, Barreto G, Finnila MA, Garcia-Perez A, Salmi A, Ranjan S, Eklund KK, Pritzker KPH, Saarakkala S, Haeggstrom E. Laser-ultrasonic delivery of agents into articular cartilage. Sci Rep. 2017;7:3991.

Appendix A

Arthroscopic Classification Systems for Chondral Injuries and Repair

Several published reports have been proposed to assess articular cartilage lesions and the clinical outcome of cartilage repair. For the macroscopic evaluation of articular cartilage, arthroscopic scoring systems were developed to probe the status of articular cartilage. The easily implemented arthroscopic cartilage lesion classification system, developed by Outerbridge in 1961, separates the severity of the lesions into four grades, 1 through IV [1]. Outerbridge's classification system, originally designed to visualize and describe chondromalacia of the patella, is reproducible and reliable, and continues to be the most widely used [2–5]. To incorporate chondral lesions observed in the entire knee, Potter et al. modified Outerbridge's classification to an extended 5-point classification system [6]. Based on four separate and distinct variables, Noyes et al. proposed a chondral lesion classification system that provides a description of the articular surface, the extent (depth) of involvement, the diameter of the lesion, and the location of the lesion [7]. The International Cartilage Repair Society (ICRS), founded in 1997, has been instrumental in developing standardization system for the evaluation of articular cartilage injury and repair [8, 9]. In 2018, ICRS was renamed as "International Cartilage Regeneration and Joint Preservation Society." ICRS Cartilage Injury Evaluation Package consists of two parts [9]:

A: Patient Part:

1. ICRS injury questionnaire
2. The IKDC subjective knee evaluation form—2000

B: Surgeon Part:

1. ICRS – Knee surgery history registration
2. IKDC – Knee examination form – 2000
3. ICRS – Articular cartilage injury mapping system
4. ICRS – Articular cartilage injury classification
5. ICRS – Osteochondritis dissecans classification
6. ICRS – Cartilage repair assessment system

The arthroscopic ICRS classification system is reproducible and has shown good inter- and intra-observer reliability, as well as excellent validity as proven by high correlation of the histological assessment of the cartilage lesion depth with the arthroscopic assessment [10]. Oswestry Arthroscopic Scores (OAS) were developed in an attempt to simplify and focus the scoring system on clinical needs [11]. Both ICRS and OAS were found to be comparable; however, as the lesion size increases, their reliability decreases [12, 13]. The commonly used arthroscopic scoring systems to evaluate articular cartilage lesions or repair are listed below.

1. Outerbridge classification [1]
2. Modified Outerbridge classification [6]
3. Noyes classification [7]
4. International Cartilage Repair Society – Injury [8, 9]

H. K. Gahunia et al. (eds.), *Articular Cartilage of the Knee*,
https://doi.org/10.1007/978-1-4939-7587-7

5. International Cartilage Repair Society – Repair [8, 9]
6. Oswestry Arthroscopy Score [11]

Outerbridge Classification

Grade	Description of the Lesion
I	Softening and swelling of the cartilage
II	Fragmentation and fissuring in an area half an inch or less in diameter
III	Same as grade 2, but an area more than half an inch in diameter is involved
IV	Erosion of cartilage down to bone

Modified Outerbridge Classification

Grade	Description of the Lesion
0	Normal, intact cartilage
I	Superficial chondral softening, swelling, or blistering with intact cartilage surface
II	Superficial chondral fragmentation, ulceration, fibrillation, or fissuring involving an area ½ an inch or less in diameter and less than 50% of the cartilage depth
III	Deep chondral ulceration, fibrillation, or fissuring involving an area more than 50% or more of the cartilage depth but without exposure of the subchondral bone
IV	Full-thickness chondral wear with exposure of subchondral bone

Noyes Classification

Grade	Description of the chondral lesion
0	Normal, intact cartilage
1A	Cartilage surface intact with some remaining resilience
1B	Cartilage surface intact with some deformation
2A	Cartilage surface damaged (cracks, fibrillation, fissures, or fragmentation) with less than half of the cartilage thickness involved
2B	Depth of involvement greater than half of cartilage thickness but without exposed bone
3A	Bone exposed with surface intact
3B	Bone exposed with surface cavitation

ICRS - Articular Cartilage Injury Classification

Grade	Description of the Cartilage Lesion
0	Normal
1A	Superficial fibrillation or softening
1B	Superficial fissures and lacerations
2	Defect less than 50% of depth
3A	Defect more than 50% but not down to the calcified layer
3B	Defect more than 50% down to the calcified layer
3C	Defect down to but not through the subchondral bone plate
3D	Defect more than 50% with blisters
4A	Defect includes superficial subchondral bone plate
4B	Defect down to deep subchondral bone

ICRS - Articular Cartilage Repair Assessment

ICRS – Cartilage repair	Points
I. Degree of defect repair	
I Protocol A [(1)]	
* In level with surrounding cartilage	4
* 75% repair of defect depth	3
* 50% repair of defect depth	2
* 25% repair of defect depth	1
* 0% repair of defect depth	0
I Protocol B [(2)]	
* 100% survival of initially grafted surface	4
* 75% survival of initially grafted surface	3
* 50% survival of initially grafted surface	2
* 25% survival of initially grafted surface	1
* 0% (plugs are lost or broken)	0
II. Integration to border zone	
* Complete integration with surrounding cartilage	4
* Demarcating border <1 mm	3
* 3/4 of graft integrated, 1/4 with a notable border >1 mm width	2
* 1/2 of graft integrated with surrounding cartilage, 1/2 with a notable border >1 mm	1
* From no contact to 1/4 of graft integrated with surrounding cartilage	0
III. Macroscopic appearance	
* Intact smooth surface	4
* Fibrillated surface	3
* Small, scattered fissures, or cracks	2
* Several, small or few but large fissures	1
* Total degeneration of grafted area	0
Overall repair assessment	
Grade I: Normal	12 P
Grade II: Nearly normal	11–8 P
Grade III: Abnormal	7–4 P
Grade IV: Severely abnormal	3–1 P
(1) Protocol A:	*(2) Protocol B:*
* Autologous chondrocyte implantation (ACI);	* Mossaicplasty;
* Periosteal or perichondrial transplantation;	* Osteochondral autograft transfer (OAT);
* Subchondral drilling;	* Osteochondral allografts;
* Microfracturing;	* Others:
* Carbon fiber implants;	
* Others:	

Oswestry Arthroscopy Score

OAS	Points
Graft level with Surrounding Cartilage	
Level	2
Raised	1
Below	0
Integration with Surrounding Cartilage	
Complete	2
Minor disruption (< 25% of area)	1
Major disruption (> 25% of area)	0
Appearance of Surface	
Smooth	2
Fine fronds	1
Severe fronds/fibrillation	0
Color of Graft	
Pearly, hyaline-like	2
White	1
Yellow bone	0
Stiffness on Probing	
Normal compared to adjacent cartilage	2
Softer	1
Very soft/hard	0
Total	0–10

References

1. Outerbridge RE. The etiology of chondromalacia patellae. J Bone Joint Surg Br. 1961;43-B:752–7.
2. Outerbridge RE. The etiology of chondromalacia patellae. 1961. Clin Orthop Relat Res. 2001;389:5–8.
3. Cameron ML, Briggs KK, Steadman JR. Reproducibility and reliability of the outerbridge classification for grading chondral lesions of the knee arthroscopically. Am J Sports Med. 2003;31(1):83–6.
4. Slattery C, Kweon CY. Classifications in brief: outerbridge classification of chondral lesions. Clin Orthop Relat Res. 2018;476(10):2101–4.
5. Lasmar NP, Lasmar RC, Vieira RB, de Oliveira JR, Scarpa AC. Assessment of the reproducibility of the outerbridge and FSA classification for chondral lesions of the knee. Rev Bras Ortop. 2015;46(3):266–9.
6. Potter HG, Linklater JM, Allen AA, Hannafin JA, Haas SB. Magnetic resonance imaging of articular cartilage in the knee. An evaluation with use of fast-spin-echo imaging. J Bone Joint Surg Am. 1998;80(9):1276–84.
7. Noyes FR, Stabler CL. A system for grading articular cartilage lesions at arthroscopy. Am J Sports Med. 1989;17(4):505–13.
8. Brittberg M, Peterson L. Introduction of an articular cartilage classification – ICRS. Newsletter. 1998;1:5–8.

9. The ICRS Clinical Cartilage Injury Evaluation system-2000 was developed during ICRS 2000 Standards Workshop at Schloss Münchenwiler, Switzerland, January 27–30, 2000 and further discussed during the 3rd ICRS Meeting in Göteborg, Sweden, April 28, 2000. The participants in the Clinical Münchenwiler Evaluation Group were as follows: Chairman - Mats Brittberg, Sweden; Paolo Aglietti, Italy; Ralph Gambardella, USA; Laszlo Hangody, Hungary; Hans Jörg Hauselmann, Switzerland; Roland P Jakob, Switzerland; David Levine, USA; Stefan Lohmander, Sweden; Bert R Mandelbaum, USA; Lars Peterson, Sweden; Hans-Ulrich Staubli, Switzerland. https://cartilage.org/content/uploads/2014/10/ICRS_evaluation.pdf.
10. Dwyer T, Martin CR, Kendra R, Sermer C, Chahal J, et al. Reliability and validity of the arthroscopic international cartilage repair society classification system: correlation with histological assessment of depth. Arthroscopy. 2017;33(6):1219–24.
11. Smith GD, Taylor J, Almqvist KF, Erggelet C, Knutsen G, et al. Arthroscopic assessment of cartilage repair: a validation study of 2 scoring systems. Arthroscopy. 2005;21(12):1462–7.
12. Paatela T, Vasara A, Nurmi H, Kautiainen H, Kiviranta I. Assessment of cartilage repair quality with the international cartilage repair society score and the oswestry arthroscopy score. J Orthop Res. 2020;38(3):555–562.
13. van den Borne MP, Raijmakers NJ, Vanlauwe J, Victor J, de Jong SN, et al. International Cartilage Repair Society (ICRS) and Oswestry macroscopic cartilage evaluation scores validated for use in Autologous Chondrocyte Implantation (ACI) and microfracture. Osteoarthritis Cartilage. 2007;15(12):1397–402.

Appendix B

Clinical Outcome Scoring Systems

Knee joint–specific patient outcome self-reporting tools are used to follow patients after traumatic knee injuries, cartilage repair surgical procedure, disease progression (such as osteoarthritis – OA), or pharmacological clinical trials to gain insight into the patient's changing symptoms and function over time. These scoring systems are designed and validated for the various treatment modalities recommended for musculoskeletal disorders. The presence of several evaluation tools attests to the difficulty in the precise evaluation of these disorders whose impact may extend to the various aspects of knee health, functional impairment, and quality-of-life outcomes. These scoring tools were developed for patients to assess their view about their knee health either post-injury, to evaluate the efficacy of pharmacological intervention, preoperative, and post-surgery follow-up assessment (cartilage repair or knee arthroplasty) or during the course of disease such as osteoarthritis. These outcome tools are used to assess one or more of the following criteria: pain, symptoms, activity of daily living, sports, quality of life, and physical health value. These assessment tools have been used to assess patients with injuries to one or more knee structures (ligament, meniscus, articular cartilage, tendon, etc.).

The commonly used measures of knee function are listed below, some of which are included in this appendix:

1. Knee Injury and Osteoarthritis Outcome Score (KOOS)
2. Knee Injury and Osteoarthritis Outcome Score Physical Function Short Form (KOOS-PS)
3. Knee Outcome Survey Activities of Daily Living Scale (KOS-ADLS)
4. Lysholm Knee Scoring Scale
5. Oxford Knee Score (OKS)
6. International Knee Document Committee (IDKC) Score Subjective Knee Form
7. Activity Rating Scale (ARS)
8. Tegner Knee Scoring Scale (TAS)
9. Marx Activity Rating Scale (MARS)
10. 36-Item Short-Form Health Survey (SF-36)
11. Western Ontario and McMaster Universities Osteoarthritis Index (WOMAC)

H. K. Gahunia et al. (eds.), *Articular Cartilage of the Knee*,
https://doi.org/10.1007/978-1-4939-7587-7

Knee Injury and Osteoarthritis Outcome Score (KOOS)

The Knee Injury and Osteoarthritis Outcome Score (KOOS) is a patient outcome reporting tool that is widely used in both short-term and long-term patient outcomes at different intervals in subjects with knee injury and OA [1]. The intended populations for the use of KOOS include young and middle-aged people with posttraumatic OA, as well as those with injuries that may lead to posttraumatic OA (e.g., anterior cruciate ligament [ACL], meniscal, or chondral injury).

The survey questions are designed to assess the patient's opinion about their knee and to know how well they are able to perform their usual activities, including sports. Assessment pertains to changes from week to week induced by conservative treatment (pharmacological or physical therapy) or surgical intervention or due to primary knee injury as well as primary or post-traumatic OA treatment. It is widely used for research purposes in experimental studies and large-scale databases [2–4].

The KOOS holds five separately scored subscales:

1. Symptoms/Stiffness (S, 5/2 questions)
2. Pain (P, 9 questions)
3. Function in Daily Living (A, 17 questions)
4. Function in Sport and Recreation (SP, 5 questions)
5. Knee-Related Quality of Life (Q, 4 questions)

Symptoms (S)

These questions should be answered thinking of your **knee symptoms** during the **last week**.

S1. Do you have swelling in your knee?

☐ Never ☐ Rarely ☐ Sometimes ☐ Often ☐ Always

S2. Do you feel grinding, hear clicking or any other type of noise when your knee moves?

☐ Never ☐ Rarely ☐ Sometimes ☐ Often ☐ Always

S3. Does your knee catch or hang up when moving?

☐ Never ☐ Rarely ☐ Sometimes ☐ Often ☐ Always

S4. Can you straighten your knee fully?

☐ Always ☐ Often ☐ Sometimes ☐ Rarely ☐ Never

S5. Can you bend your knee fully?

☐ Always ☐ Often ☐ Sometimes ☐ Rarely ☐ Never

Stiffness (S)

The following questions concern the amount of **joint stiffness** you have experienced during the **last week** in your knee. Stiffness is a sensation of restriction or slowness in the ease with which you move your knee.

S6. How severe is your knee stiffness after first wakening in the morning?

☐ None ☐ Mild ☐ Moderate ☐ Severe ☐ Extreme

S7. How severe is your knee stiffness after sitting, lying or resting **later in the day**?

☐ None ☐ Mild ☐ Moderate ☐ Severe ☐ Extreme

Pain (P)

P1. How often do you experience knee pain?

☐ Never ☐ Monthly ☐ Weekly ☐ Daily ☐ Always

What amount of **knee pain** have you experienced the **last week** during the following activities?

P2. Twisting/pivoting on your knee

☐ None ☐ Mild ☐ Moderate ☐ Severe ☐ Extreme

P3. Straightening knee fully

☐ None ☐ Mild ☐ Moderate ☐ Severe ☐ Extreme

P4. Bending knee fully

☐ None ☐ Mild ☐ Moderate ☐ Severe ☐ Extreme

P5. Walking on flat surface

☐ None ☐ Mild ☐ Moderate ☐ Severe ☐ Extreme

P6. Going up or down stairs

☐ None ☐ Mild ☐ Moderate ☐ Severe ☐ Extreme

P7. At night while in bed

☐ None ☐ Mild ☐ Moderate ☐ Severe ☐ Extreme

P8. Sitting or lying

☐ None ☐ Mild ☐ Moderate ☐ Severe ☐ Extreme

P9. Standing upright

☐ None ☐ Mild ☐ Moderate ☐ Severe ☐ Extreme

Function, Daily Living (A)

The following questions concern your physical function. By this we mean your ability to move around and to look after yourself. For each of the following activities please indicate the **degree of difficulty** you have experienced in the **last week** due to your knee.

A1. Descending stairs

☐ None ☐ Mild ☐ Moderate ☐ Severe ☐ Extreme

A2. Ascending stairs

☐ None ☐ Mild ☐ Moderate ☐ Severe ☐ Extreme

For each of the following activities please indicate the **degree of difficulty** you have experienced in the **last week** due to your knee.

A3. Rising from sitting

☐ None ☐ Mild ☐ Moderate ☐ Severe ☐ Extreme

A4. Standing

☐ None ☐ Mild ☐ Moderate ☐ Severe ☐ Extreme

A5. Bending to floor/pick up an object

☐ None ☐ Mild ☐ Moderate ☐ Severe ☐ Extreme

A6. Walking on flat surface

☐ None ☐ Mild ☐ Moderate ☐ Severe ☐ Extreme

A7. Getting in/out of car

☐ None ☐ Mild ☐ Moderate ☐ Severe ☐ Extreme

A8. Going shopping

☐ None ☐ Mild ☐ Moderate ☐ Severe ☐ Extreme

A9. Putting on socks/stockings

☐ None ☐ Mild ☐ Moderate ☐ Severe ☐ Extreme

A10. Rising from bed

☐ None ☐ Mild ☐ Moderate ☐ Severe ☐ Extreme

A11. Taking off socks/stockings

☐ None ☐ Mild ☐ Moderate ☐ Severe ☐ Extreme

A12. Lying in bed (turning over, maintaining knee position)

☐ None ☐ Mild ☐ Moderate ☐ Severe ☐ Extreme

A13. Getting in/out of bath

☐ None ☐ Mild ☐ Moderate ☐ Severe ☐ Extreme

A14. Sitting

☐ None ☐ Mild ☐ Moderate ☐ Severe ☐ Extreme

A15. Getting on/off toilet

☐ None ☐ Mild ☐ Moderate ☐ Severe ☐ Extreme

For each of the following activities please indicate the **degree of difficulty** you have experienced in the **last week** due to your knee.

A16. Heavy domestic duties (moving heavy boxes, scrubbing floors, etc)

☐ None ☐ Mild ☐ Moderate ☐ Severe ☐ Extreme

A17. Light domestic duties (cooking, dusting, etc)

☐ None ☐ Mild ☐ Moderate ☐ Severe ☐ Extreme

Function, Sports and Recreational Activities (SP)

The following questions concern your physical function when being active on a higher level. The questions should be answered thinking of **what degree of difficulty** you have experienced during the **last week** due to your knee.

SP1. Squatting

□ None □ Mild □ Moderate □ Severe □ Extreme

SP2. Running

□ None □ Mild □ Moderate □ Severe □ Extreme

SP3. Jumping

□ None □ Mild □ Moderate □ Severe □ Extreme

SP4. Twisting/pivoting on your injured knee

□ None □ Mild □ Moderate □ Severe □ Extreme

SP5. Kneeling

□ None □ Mild □ Moderate □ Severe □ Extreme

Quality of Life (Q)

Q1. How often are you aware of your knee problem?

□ Never □ Monthly □ Weekly □ Daily □ Constantly

Q2. Have you modified your life style to avoid potentially damaging activities to your knee?

□ Not at all □ Mildly □ Moderately □ Severely □ Totally

Q3. How much are you troubled with lack of confidence in your knee?

□ Not at all □ Mildly □ Moderately □ Severely □ Extremely

Q4. In general, how much difficulty do you have with your knee?

□ None □ Mild □ Moderate □ Severe □ Extreme

Knee Outcome Survey: Activities of Daily Living Scale (KOS-ADLS)

The KOS-ADLS is a self-administered questionnaire that was designed as a knee-specific scale to assess the symptoms and functional limitations that patients with knee impairment experience while performing their usual daily activities [5, 6]. These are the activities that best describe them over the past 1 or 2 days [7–9]. The intended populations for the use of KOS-ADLS are patients undergoing physical therapy for various knee pathologies, such as ligament/meniscal injury, OA, and patellofemoral pain.

The KOS-ADLS is one of the subjective scales used to evaluate the overall health of a patient with various dysfunctions of the knee. The symptoms component includes eight questions pertaining to knee pain, stiffness, swelling, giving way, weakness, and limping. The responses are graded on a scale from 0 to 5, with 5 being no symptom and 0 being the highest limitation caused by the symptom.

The functional limitations component includes eight questions pertaining to walking, ascending and descending stairs, standing, kneeling, squatting, sitting, and rising from a chair. These are the activities that best describe them over the past 1 or 2 days prior to their self-evaluation. The responses are graded on a 0 to 5 scale, where 5 indicates no limitation and 0 indicates a high level of functional limitation.

The symptom and function scores are added to obtain the total score. The lower percentage indicates lower levels of function, higher limitation, and disability.

Symptoms

To what degree does each of the following symptoms affect your level of daily activity? (Circle one number on each line).

Symptoms	Never have	Have (but, does not affect activity)	Affects activity slightly	Affects activity moderately	Affects activity severely	Prevents all daily activity
Pain	5	4	3	2	1	0
Grinding or grating	5	4	3	2	1	0
Stiffness	5	4	3	2	1	0
Swelling	5	4	3	2	1	0
Slipping or partial giving way of knee	5	4	3	2	1	0
Buckling or full giving way of knee	5	4	3	2	1	0
Weakness	5	4	3	2	1	0
Limping	5	4	3	2	1	0

Functional Limitations with Activities of Daily Living

How does your knee affect your *ability to do the following activities?*
(Circle one number on each line).

Activities	Not difficult at all	Minimally difficult	Somewhat difficult	Fairly difficult	Very difficult	Unable to do
Walk	5	4	3	2	1	0
Go up stairs	5	4	3	2	1	0
Go down stairs	5	4	3	2	1	0
Stand	5	4	3	2	1	0
Kneel on the front of your knee	5	4	3	2	1	0
Squat	5	4	3	2	1	0
Sit with your knee bent	5	4	3	2	1	0
Rise from a chair	5	4	3	2	1	0

Lysholm Knee Score

The Lysholm Knee Score, first designed as an outcome assessment tool post knee ligament surgery in 1982 and modified in 1985, measures activities of daily living (ADLs) [10, 11]. Currently, Lysholm assessment tool has shown adequate reliability and responsiveness for assessing mobility in knee ligament injury, meniscal tears and articular cartilage lesions as well as traumatic knee dislocation, patellofemoral pain, patellar instability, and degenerative diseases [12–14].

The 8 specific activities that are evaluated are as follows:

1. Limp: if there is any limping and if so, how severe it is and whether it is constant or not
2. Using cane or crutches: as a support or the use of any other walking assistance
3. Locking sensation in the knee: if such sensation is experienced and how often
4. Giving way sensation from the knee: whether there is any instability in the knee, how often, and when that occurs
5. Pain: existence of pain and degree of discomfort caused by it
6. Swelling: existence and persistence after different degrees of activity
7. Climbing stairs: existence of any issues with climbing stairs
8. Squatting: whether the action is possible and to what extent

The symptoms of pain, swelling, and instability are scored according to the activity in which they occur. To produce an overall score on a point scale of 0–100, eight factors are rated. The factors of limp, support, and locking are worth a potential of 23 points; pain and instability, 25 points each; swelling and stair climbing, 10 points each; and squatting, 5 points. Scores closer to 0 indicate severe symptoms and little to no recovery after surgery; whereas, scores closer to 100 are indicative of very little to no knee symptoms and the patient will likely make a full recovery.

The overall final assignment of Lysholm Knee Score is as follows:

1. Excellent = 95 to 100 points
2. Good = 84 to 94 points
3. Fair = 65 to 83 points
4. Poor = less than 65 points

Lysholm Knee Score		
Factor	**Scale**	**Points**
Limp	None	5
	Slight or periodic	3
	Severe and constant	0
Support	None	5
	Stick or crutch	2
	Weight-bearing impossible	0
Locking	No locking/catching sensations	15
	Catching sensation but no locking	10
	Locking: occasionally	6
	Locking: frequently	2
	Locked joint on examination	0
Instability	Never giving way	25
	Rarely during athletics or other severe exertion	20
	Frequently during athletics or other severe exertion (or incapable of participation)	15
	Occasionally in daily activities	10
	Often in daily activities	5
	Every step	0
Pain	None	25
	Inconstant and slight during severe exertion	20
	Marked during severe exertion	15
	Marked on or after walking more 2 km	10
	Marked on or after walking less than 2 km	5
	Constant	0
Swelling	None	10
	On severe exertion	6
	On ordinary exertion	2
	Constant	0
Stair climbing	No problem	10
	Slightly impaired	6
	One step at a time	2
	Impossible	0
Squatting	No problem	5
	Slightly impaired	4
	Not beyond 90°	2
	Impossible	0

Oxford Knee Score (OKS)

The Oxford Knee Score (OKS) was specifically designed, developed, and validated to assess pain and function after total knee replacement (TKR) surgery (arthroplasty) [15]. In large-scale studies, the OKS has been ranked the best disease−/site-specific patient-reported outcome for assessing the result of knee arthroplasty. Currently, OKS has also been used to measure outcomes in pharmacological treatments, after osteotomies, following rehabilitation or with fractures [16].

The OKS is a short, reproducible 12-item patient-reported outcome that reflects the patient's assessment of their knee-related health status and benefits of treatment [17]. In the original version of OKS, each question (pertaining to knee pain or function) is followed by 5 responses with score ranging from 0 (impaired knee function, worst outcome) to 4 (good knee function, best outcome). The maximum score is 60, which reflects excellent function. The grading for OKS is as follows [15].

1. *Score 0 to 19:* May indicate severe knee arthritis. Patient is highly likely to require some form of surgical intervention.
2. *Score 20 to 29:* May indicate moderate to severe knee arthritis. Patient may require formal treatment.
3. *Score 30 to 39:* May indicate mild to moderate knee arthritis. Patient may benefit from non-surgical treatment, such as exercise, weight loss, and/or anti-inflammatory medication.
4. *Score 40 to 48:* May indicate satisfactory joint function. Patient may not require any formal treatment.
5. *Score 49 to 60:* Indicate excellent knee function.

Please answer the following 12 multiple-choice questions. *During the past 4 weeks......*

1. How would you **describe the pain** you usually have from your knee?

☐ None ☐ Very Mild ☐ Mild ☐ Moderate ☐ Severe

2. Have you had any **trouble washing and drying** yourself (all over) because of your knee?

☐ No trouble at all ☐ Very little trouble ☐ Moderate trouble ☐ Extreme difficulty ☐ Impossible to do

3. Have you had any **trouble getting in and out** of the car or using public transport because of your knee? (With or without a stick)

☐ No trouble at all ☐ Very little trouble ☐ Moderate trouble ☐ Extreme difficulty ☐ Impossible to do

4. For **how long** have you been able to **walk before pain** from your knee becomes severe? (With or without a stick)

☐ No pain >60 min ☐ 16 to 60 minutes ☐ 5 to 15 minutes ☐ Around the house only ☐ Not at all – pain severe on walking

5. After a meal (sat at a table), **how painful** has it been for you **to stand up** from a chair because of your knee?

☐ Not at all painful ☐ Slightly painful ☐ Moderately painful ☐ Very painful ☐ Unbearable

6. Have you been **limping** when walking, because of your knee?

☐ Rarely/never ☐ Sometimes or just at first ☐ Often, not just at first ☐ Most of the time ☐ All of the time

7. Could you **kneel** down and get up again afterwards?

☐ Yes, easily ☐ With little difficulty ☐ With moderate difficulty ☐ With extreme difficulty ☐ No, impossible

8. Have you been **troubled by pain** from your knee at night in bed?

□ No nights □ Only 1 or 2 nights □ Some nights □ Most nights □ Every night

9. How much has **pain** from your knee interfered with your **usual work**? (Including housework)

□ Not at all □ A little bit □ Moderately □ Greatly □ Totally

10. Have you felt that your **knee** might suddenly **"give away"** or let you down?

□ Rarely/never □ Sometimes or just at first □ Often, not just at first □ Most of the time □ All the time

11. Could you do **household shopping** on your own?

□ Yes, easily □ With little difficulty □ With moderate difficulty □ With extreme difficulty □ No, impossible

12. Could you **walk down** a flight of stairs?

□ Yes, easily □ With little difficulty □ With moderate difficulty □ With extreme difficulty □ No, impossible

International Knee Documentation Committee (IKDC) Subjective Knee Evaluation Form

The entire IKDC package includes several forms, which may be used individually as shown below:

1. Demographic Form
2. Current Health Assessment Form
3. Subjective Knee Evaluation Form
4. Knee History Form
5. Surgical Documentation Form
6. Knee Examination Form

The IKDC Subjective Knee Evaluation Form is a patient-reported knee-specific outcome measure that provide patients with an overall function score for the evaluation of knee treatments. The purpose of IKDC is to detect improvement or deterioration in symptoms, function, and sports activities due to knee impairment.

The intended populations for the use of IKDC are patients with a variety of knee conditions, including ligament injuries, meniscal injuries, articular cartilage lesions, and patellofemoral pain [6].

The questionnaire includes three categories pertaining to patient knee symptoms (7 items), sports activity (2 items), and function (2 items) [3, 4, 17–19]. The scores for the individual items (Questions 1 to 9 and 10B) are added, while response to item 10A "Function Prior to Knee Injury" is not included in the overall score. The maximum possible score is 87. The IKDC scores range from 0 points (lowest level of function or highest level of symptoms) to 100 points (highest level of function and lowest level of symptoms). To determine the IKDC score, the patient response number for each item is added and the total is divided by the maximum score of 87, which is then multiplied by 100 as shown below:

$$\text{IKDC Score} = \frac{\text{Sum of Items}}{\text{Maximum Possible Score}} \times 100$$

Symptoms:

These questions should be answered thinking of your **knee symptoms during the last week.** Grade symptoms at the highest activity level at which you think you could function without significant symptoms, even if you are not actually performing activities at this level.

1. What is the **highest level of activity** that you can perform **without significant knee pain**?

   4 □ Very strenuous activities like jumping or pivoting as in basketball or soccer

   3 □ Strenuous activities like heavy physical work, skiing or tennis

   2 □ Moderate activities like moderate physical work, running or jogging

   1 □ Light activities like walking, housework or yard work

   0 □ Unable to perform any of the above activities due to knee pain

2. During the **past 4 weeks**, or since your injury, **how often** have you had **pain**?

   Constant 0 □ 1 □ 2 □ 3 □ 4 □ 5 □ 6 □ 7 □ 8 □ 9 □ 10 □ Never

3. If you have **pain**, **how severe** is it?

   Worst pain 0 □ 1 □ 2 □ 3 □ 4 □ 5 □ 6 □ 7 □ 8 □ 9 □ 10 □ No pain

4. During the **past 4 weeks**, or since your injury, **how stiff or swollen** was your knee?

   4 □ Not at all

   3 □ Mildly

   2 □ Moderately

   1 □ Very

   0 □ Extremely

5. What is the **highest level of activity** you can perform **without significant swelling** in your knee?

   4 □ Very strenuous activities like jumping or pivoting as in basketball or soccer

   3 □ Strenuous activities like heavy physical work, skiing or tennis

   2 □ Moderate activities like moderate physical work, running or jogging

   1 □ Light activities like walking, housework or yard work

   0 □ Unable to perform any of the above activities due to knee swelling

6. During the **past 4 weeks**, or since your injury, **did your knee lock or catch**?

   0 □ Yes

   1 □ No

7. What is the **highest level of activity** you can perform **without** significant **giving way in your knee**?

   4 □ Very strenuous activities like jumping or pivoting as in basketball or soccer

   3 □ Strenuous activities like heavy physical work, skiing or tennis

   2 □ Moderate activities like moderate physical work, running or jogging

   1 □ Light activities like walking, housework or yard work

   0 □ Unable to perform any of the above activities due to giving way of the knee

Sports Activities:

8. What is the **highest level of activity** you can participate in on a **regular basis**?

4 □ Very strenuous activities like jumping or pivoting as in basketball or soccer
3 □ Strenuous activities like heavy physical work, skiing or tennis
2 □ Moderate activities like moderate physical work, running or jogging
1 □ Light activities like walking, housework or yard work
0 □ Unable to perform any of the above activities due to knee

9. How does your **knee affect your ability** to:

	Activity	No Difficulty	Minimal Difficulty	Moderate Difficulty	Extreme Difficulty	Unable to do
a.	Go up stairs	4 □	3 □	2 □	1 □	0 □
b.	Go down stairs	4 □	3 □	2 □	1 □	0 □
c.	Kneel on the front of your knee	4 □	3 □	2 □	1 □	0 □
d.	Squat	4 □	3 □	2 □	1 □	0 □
e.	Sit with your knee bent	4 □	3 □	2 □	1 □	0 □
f.	Rise from a chair	4 □	3 □	2 □	1 □	0 □
g.	Run straight ahead	4 □	3 □	2 □	1 □	0 □
h.	Jump and land on your involved leg	4 □	3 □	2 □	1 □	0 □
i.	Stop and start quickly	4 □	3 □	2 □	1 □	0 □

Function:

10. How would you **rate the function of your knee** on a scale of 0 to 10 with 10 being normal, excellent function and 0 being the inability to perform any of your usual daily activities which may include sports?

10A. Function Prior to Your Knee Injury

Couldn't Perform daily activities 0 □ 1 □ 2 □ 3 □ 4 □ 5 □ 6 □ 7 □ 8 □ 9 □ 10 □ No limitation in daily activities

10B. Current Function of Your Knee

Can't perform daily activities 0 □ 1 □ 2 □ 3 □ 4 □ 5 □ 6 □ 7 □ 8 □ 9 □ 10 □ No limitation in daily activities

Tegner Activity Scale (TAS)

Developed in 1985, the Tegner Activity Scale (TAS) was originally intended for patients with anterior cruciate ligament injuries and used in conjunction with the Lysholm Knee Scoring Scale [11]. TAS is currently used in knee tissue injury (ligament injury, meniscal tears, cartilage lesions), osteochondritis dissecans, traumatic knee dislocation, patellar instability, patellofemoral pain, knee osteoarthritis, and interventions in these conditions [17, 20].

TAS is a graduated list of activities of daily living, recreation, and competitive sports. Patients self-assess their level of activity before injury or surgery and at the current state, that is, moment of assessment. TAS ranges from a score of 0 to 10. A score of 0 represents a person on sick leave or disability pension due to knee issues, a score greater than 6 can be achieved only by individuals who participate in recreational or competitive sports, and a score of 10 is achieved by those who participate in national and international elite competitive sports.

Please checkmark the category that most closely represents your **highest activity** level during the **last year (choose one)**	
☐ **Level 10**	**Competitive sports**: national or international soccer, football, rugby (elite)
☐ **Level 9**	**Competitive sports**: lower divisions of soccer, football, rugby, ice hockey, wrestling, gymnastics, basketball
☐ **Level 8**	**Competitive sports**: racquetball, squash or badminton, track and field, jumping (athletics), downhill skiing
☐ **Level 7**	**Competitive sports**: tennis, running (athletics), motorcars, speedway, handball, basketball, cross-country running **Recreational sports**: soccer, football, rugby, ice hockey, squash, jumping (athletics), basketball, racquetball, cross-country running
☐ **Level 6**	**Recreational sports**: tennis, badminton, handball, racquetball, basketball, downhill skiing, jogging at least 5 times weekly
☐ **Level 5**	**Work**: heavy labor such as construction, forestry **Competitive sports**: cycling, cross-country skiing **Recreational sports**: jogging on uneven ground at least twice weekly
☐ **Level 4**	**Work**: moderately heavy labor such as truck driving, heavy domestic work **Recreational sports**: cycling, cross-country skiing, jogging on uneven ground at least twice weekly
☐ **Level 3**	**Work**: light labor such as nursing **Competitive and recreational sports**: swimming, walking/hiking in forest possible
☐ **Level 2**	**Work**: light labor Walking on uneven ground possible but impossible to back pack or hike in forest
☐ **Level 1**	**Work**: sedentary work spending much time seated or somewhat inactive (secretarial, etc.) Walking on even ground possible
☐ **Level 0**	Sick leave or disability pension because of knee problems

Marx Activity Rating Scale (MARS)

The Marx Activity Rating Scale was designed in 2001 to evaluate the activity level of patients in less than 1 minute and to supplement other general health- and site-specific patient-reported outcome measures [21]. MARS consists of four questions that assess four functional activities or actions (frequency of running, cutting involving changing directions while running, deceleration, and pivoting) based on the subjects "healthiest and most active state in the past year" [22, 23].

Each activity is scored on a 5-point scale of frequency ranging from 0 (less than 1 time in a month) to 4 (4 or more times in a week). The total score is obtained by summing the individual scores (range, 0–16). A higher score indicates more frequent participation, hence more functional demand on the knee and potentially a higher risk of injury.

Please indicate **how often** you **performed each activity** in your healthiest and most active state, in the past year.

Activity	Less Than One Time in a Month	One Time in a Month	One Time in a Week	2 or 3 Times in a Week	4 or More Times in a Week
Running: Running while playing a sports or jogging					
Cutting: Changing directions while running					
Decelerating: Coming to a quick stop while running					
Pivoting: Turning your body with your foot planted while playing a sport. For example, skiing, skating, kicking, throwing, hitting a ball (golf, tennis, squash), etc.					

Short-Form Health Survey - 36 Item (SF-36)

Originally published in 1992, the 36-item Short-Form Health Survey (SF-36) obtained from Medical Outcome Health Survey Study tool is a measure of health-related quality of life [24]. The SF-36 has been implemented to define disease conditions, to determine the effect of treatment, to differentiate the effect of different treatments, and to compare orthopedic conditions with other medical conditions [25].

The SF-36 is a subset of questions from longer instruments that were used as a benchmark in examining the validity of Medical Outcome Studies for knee assessment [26, 27]. The SF-36 covers eight health domains as shown:

1. Physical functioning (10 items)
2. Bodily pain (2 items)
3. Role limitations due to physical health problems (4 items)
4. Role limitations due to personal or emotional problems (4 items)
5. Emotional well-being (5 items)
6. Social functioning (2 items)
7. Energy/fatigue (4 items)
8. General health perceptions (5 items)

Choose one option for each questionnaire item.

Q1. **In general**, would you say your **health** is:

□ Excellent (1) □ Very good (2) □ Good (3) □ Fair (4) □ Poor (5)

Q2. **Compared to one year ago**, how would you rate your health in general **now**?

□ Much better (1) □ Somewhat better (2) □ About the same (3) □ Somewhat worst (4) □ Much worst (5)

The following items are about activities you might do during a typical day. Does **your health now limit you** in these activities? If so, how much?

Activities		Yes, limited a lot	Yes, limited a little	No, not limited at all
Q3.	**Vigorous activities**, such as running, lifting heavy objects, participating in strenuous sports	□ 1	□ 2	□ 3
Q4.	**Moderate activities**, such as moving a table, pushing a vacuum cleaner, bowling, or playing golf.	□ 1	□ 2	□ 3
Q5.	Lifting or carrying groceries	□ 1	□ 2	□ 3
Q6.	Climbing **several** flights of stairs	□ 1	□ 2	□ 3
Q7.	Climbing **one** flight of stairs.	□ 1	□ 2	□ 3
Q8.	Bending, kneeling, or stooping	□ 1	□ 2	□ 3
Q9.	Walking **more than a mile**	□ 1	□ 2	□ 3
Q10.	Walking **several blocks**	□ 1	□ 2	□ 3
Q11.	Walking **one block**	□ 1	□ 2	□ 3
Q12.	Bathing or dressing yourself	□ 1	□ 2	□ 3

During the past **4 weeks**, have you had any of the following problems with your work or other regular daily activities **as a result of your physical health?**

Q13. Cut down the **amount of time** you spent on work or other activities.

□ Yes (1) □ No (2)

Q14. **Accomplished less** than you would like

□ Yes (1) □ No (2)

Q15. **Were limited in the kind** of work or other activities.

□ Yes (1) □ No (2)

Q16. Had **difficulty** performing the work or other activities (for example, it took extra effort).

□ Yes (1) □ No (2)

During the **past 4 weeks**, have you had any of the following problems with your work or other regular daily activities **as a result of any emotional problems** (such as feeling depressed or anxious)?

Q17. Cut down the **amount of time** you spent on work or other activities.

□ Yes (1) □ No (2)

Q18. **Accomplished less** than you would like.

□ Yes (1) □ No (2)

Q19. Didn't do work or other activities as **carefully** as usual.

□ Yes (1) □ No (2)

Q20. During the **past 4 weeks**, to what extent has your physical health or emotional problems interfered with your normal social activities with family, friends, neighbors, or groups?

□ Not at all (1) □ Slightly (2) □ Moderately (3) □ Quite a bit (4) □ Extremely (5)

Q21. How much **bodily** pain have you had during the **past 4 weeks**?

☐ None (1) ☐ Very mild (2) ☐ Mild (3) ☐ Moderate (4) ☐ Severe (5) ☐ Very severe (6)

Q22. During the **past 4 weeks**, how much did **pain interfere** with your normal work (including both work outside the home and housework)?

☐ Not at all (1) ☐ A little bit (2) ☐ Moderately (3) ☐ Quite a bit (4) ☐ Extremely (5)

These questions are about how you feel and how things have been with you **during the past 4 weeks**. For each question, please give the one answer that comes closest to the way you have been feeling. How much of the time **during the past 4 weeks...**

	During the past 4 weeks	All of the time	Most of the time	A good bit of the time	Some of the time	A little of the time	None of the time
Q23.	Did you feel full of pep?	☐ 1	☐ 2	☐ 3	☐ 4	☐ 5	☐ 6
Q24.	Have you been a nervous person?	☐ 1	☐ 2	☐ 3	☐ 4	☐ 5	☐ 6
Q25.	Have you felt so down in the dumps that nothing could cheer your up?	☐ 1	☐ 2	☐ 3	☐ 4	☐ 5	☐ 6
Q26.	Have you felt calm and peaceful?	☐ 1	☐ 2	☐ 3	☐ 4	☐ 5	☐ 6
Q27.	Did you have a lot of energy?	☐ 1	☐ 2	☐ 3	☐ 4	☐ 5	☐ 6
Q28.	Have you felt downhearted and blue?	☐ 1	☐ 2	☐ 3	☐ 4	☐ 5	☐ 6
Q29.	Did you feel worn out?	☐ 1	☐ 2	☐ 3	☐ 4	☐ 5	☐ 6
Q30.	Have you been a happy person?	☐ 1	☐ 2	☐ 3	☐ 4	☐ 5	☐ 6
Q31.	Did you feel tired?	☐ 1	☐ 2	☐ 3	☐ 4	☐ 5	☐ 6

Q32. During the past **4 weeks**, how much of the time has **your physical health or emotional problems** interfered with your social activities (like visiting with friends, relatives, etc.)?

☐ All of the time (1) ☐ Most of the time (2) ☐ Some time (3) ☐ A little time (4) ☐ None of the time (5)

How TRUE or FALSE is **each** of the following statements for you

	Statement True or False	Definitely true	Mostly true	Don't know	Mostly false	Definitely false
Q33.	I seem to get sick a little easier than other people	☐ 1	☐ 2	☐ 3	☐ 4	☐ 5
Q34.	I am as healthy as anybody I know	☐ 1	☐ 2	☐ 3	☐ 4	☐ 5
Q35.	I expect my health to get worse	☐ 1	☐ 2	☐ 3	☐ 4	☐ 5
Q36.	My health is excellent	☐ 1	☐ 2	☐ 3	☐ 4	☐ 5

Western Ontario and McMaster Universities Osteoarthritis Index (WOMAC)

Developed in 1982, the Western Ontario and McMaster Universities Osteoarthritis Index (WOMAC), is a multidimensional, self-administered health status, patient-reported outcome measure tool for patients with OA of knee and/or hip [28]. The measure was developed to evaluate the outcome of OA clinical trials and total knee arthroscopy [28, 29].

WOMAC questionnaire consists of 24 items divided into 3 subscales:

1. Pain (5 items, score range 0–20) severity during various positions or movements such as

walking, using stairs, in bed, sitting or lying, and standing upright.
2. Joint stiffness severity (2 items, score range 0–8) after first waking and later in the day.
3. Difficulty performing daily physical functional activities (17 items, score range 0–68) such as using stairs, rising from sitting, standing, bending, walking, getting in/out of a car, shopping, putting on/taking off socks, rising from bed, lying in bed, getting in/out of bath, sitting, getting on/off toilet, heavy domestic duties, and light domestic duties.

The Likert version of the WOMAC is rated on an ordinal scale of 0–4, with lower scores indicating lower levels of symptoms or physical disability. Each subscale is summated to a maximum score of 20, 8, and 68, respectively.

Pain:

A. The following questions concern the **amount of pain** you are currently experiencing in your knees. For each situation, please enter the amount of pain you have experienced in the **past 48 hours**.

	None (0)	**Mild** (1)	**Moderate** (2)	**Severe** (3)	**Extreme** (4)
1. Walking on a flat surface	☐	☐	☐	☐	☐
2. Going up or down stairs	☐	☐	☐	☐	☐
3. At night while in bed	☐	☐	☐	☐	☐
4. Sitting or lying	☐	☐	☐	☐	☐
5. Standing upright	☐	☐	☐	☐	☐

B. Please describe the **level of pain** you have experienced in the **past 48 hours** for each one of your knees.

	None (0)	**Mild** (1)	**Moderate** (2)	**Severe** (3)	**Extreme** (4)
1. Right knee	☐	☐	☐	☐	☐
2. Left knee	☐	☐	☐	☐	☐

Stiffness:

1. How **severe** is your **stiffness after first awakening** in the morning?

None (0)	**Mild** (1)	**Moderate** (2)	**Severe** (3)	**Extreme** (4)
☐	☐	☐	☐	☐

2. How **severe** is your **stiffness** after sitting, lying, or resting **later in the day**?

None (0)	**Mild** (1)	**Moderate** (2)	**Severe** (3)	**Extreme** (4)
☐	☐	☐	☐	☐

Functional Limitation:

The following questions concern your **physical function**. By this we mean your ability to move around and to look after yourself. For each of the following activities, please indicate the **degree of difficulty** you have experienced in the **last 48 hours**, in your knees. What degree of difficulty do you have with:

	None (0)	Mild (1)	Moderate (2)	Severe (3)	Extreme (4)
1. Descending (going down) stairs	☐	☐	☐	☐	☐
2. Ascending (going up) stairs	☐	☐	☐	☐	☐
3. Rising from sitting	☐	☐	☐	☐	☐
4. Standing	☐	☐	☐	☐	☐
5. Bending to floor	☐	☐	☐	☐	☐
6. Walking on a flat surface	☐	☐	☐	☐	☐
7. Getting in/out of car	☐	☐	☐	☐	☐
8. Going shopping	☐	☐	☐	☐	☐
9. Putting on socks/stockings	☐	☐	☐	☐	☐
10. Rising from bed	☐	☐	☐	☐	☐
11. Taking off socks/stockings	☐	☐	☐	☐	☐
12. Lying in bed	☐	☐	☐	☐	☐
13. Getting in/out of bath	☐	☐	☐	☐	☐
14. Sitting	☐	☐	☐	☐	☐
15. Getting on/off toilet	☐	☐	☐	☐	☐
16. Heavy domestic duties (mowing the lawn, lifting heavy grocery bags)	☐	☐	☐	☐	☐
17. Light domestic duties (such as tidying a room, dusting, cooking)	☐	☐	☐	☐	☐

References

1. Knee injury and Osteoarthritis Outcome Score (KOOS), English version LK1.0. http://www.koos.nu/
2. Roos EM, Roos HP, Lohmander LS, Ekdahl C, Beynnon BD. Knee injury and osteoarthritis outcome score (KOOS) - development of a self-administered outcome measure. J Orthop Sports Phys Ther. 1998;28:88–96.
3. Roos EM, Roos HP, Ekdahl C, Lohmander LS. Knee injury and osteoarthritis outcome score (KOOS)-validation of a Swedish version. Scand J Med Sci Sports. 1998;8:439–48.
4. Roos EM, Lohmander LS. The Knee injury and Osteoarthritis Outcome Score (KOOS): from joint injury to osteoarthritis. Health Qual Life Outcomes. 2003;1:64.
5. Irrgang JJ, Snyder-Mackler L, Wainner RS, Fu FH, Harner CD. Development of a patient-reported measure of function of the knee. J Bone Joint Surg Am. 1998;80:1132–45.
6. Irrgang JJ, Anderson AF, Boland AL, Harner CD, Kurosaka M, et al. Development and validation of the international knee documentation committee subjective knee form. Am J Sports Med. 2001;29:600–13.
7. KOS-ADLS: https://sapphirept.com/wp-content/forms/Knee_Outcome_Survey_ADL_Scale_(KOSADLS).pdf.
8. KOS-ADLS: https://www.thompsonhealth.com/Portals/0/_RehabilitationServices/PT%20Mgmt%20of%20Knee/Knee_Outcome_Survey_ADLs_questionnaire.pdf.
9. Marx RG, Jones EC, Allen AA, Altchek DW, O'Brien SJ, et al. Reliability, validity, and responsiveness of four knee outcome scales for athletic patients. J Bone Joint Surg Am. 2001;83:1459–69.
10. Lysholm J, Gillquist J. Evaluation of knee ligament surgery results with special emphasis on use of a scoring scale. Am J Sports Med. 1982;10(3):150–4.
11. Tegner Y, Lysholm J. Rating systems in the evaluation of knee ligament injuries. Clin Orthop Relat Res. 1985;(198):43–9.
12. Barber-Westin SD, Noyes FR. Rating of athletic and daily functional activities. In: Noyes FR, Barber-Westin SD, editors. Noyes' knee disorders: surgery, rehabilitation, clinical outcomes. 2nd ed: Elsevier Inc; 2017.
13. Lysholm Knee Score: https://doi.org/10.1016/C2013-0-18673-4.
14. Lysholm Knee Score: https://www.mdapp.co/lysholm-score-for-knee-ligament-surgery-calculator-293/
15. Dawson J, Fitzpatrick R, Murray D, Carr A. Questionnaire on the perceptions of patients about total knee replacement. J Bone Joint Surg Br. 1998;80(1):63–9.
16. Murray D, Rogers K, Pandit H, Beard D, Carr A, Dawson J. The use of the Oxford Hip and Knee Scores. J Bone Joint Surg. 2007;89(8):1010–4.
17. Collins NJ, Misra D, Felson DT, Crossley KM, Roos EM. Measures of knee function: International Knee Documentation Committee (IKDC) Subjective Knee Evaluation Form, Knee Injury and Osteoarthritis Outcome Score (KOOS), Knee Injury and Osteoarthritis Outcome Score Physical Function Short Form (KOOS-PS), Knee Outcome Survey Activities of Daily Living Scale (KOS-ADL), Lysholm Knee Scoring Scale, Oxford Knee Score (OKS), Western Ontario and McMaster Universities Osteoarthritis Index (WOMAC), Activity Rating Scale (ARS), and Tegner Activity Score (TAS). Arthritis Care Res (Hoboken). 2011;63(Suppl 11):S208–28.
18. IKDC: http://www.orthopaedicscore.com/scorepages/international_knee_documentation_comitee.html.
19. IKDC: https://www.sportsmed.org/AOSSMIMIS/members/downloads/research/IKDCEnglishUS.pdf.
20. van Meer BL, Meuffels DE, Reijman M. A comparison of the standardized rating forms for evaluation of anterior cruciate ligament injured or reconstructed patients. In: The anterior cruciate ligament. 2nd ed; 2018. https://doi.org/10.1016/B978-0-323-38962-4.00120-X.
21. Marx RG, Stump TJ, Jones EC, Wickiewicz TL, Warren RF. Development and evaluation of an activity rating scale for disorders of the knee. Am J Sports Med. 2001;29(2):213–8.
22. MARS: https://www.aaos.org/uploadedFiles/PreProduction/Quality/Measures/pdf-MARX%20SCALE-%20english.pdf.
23. MARS: http://banffsportmed.com/wp-content/uploads/2018/01/Marx-Activity-Rating-Scale.pdf.
24. Ware JE Jr, Sherbourne CD. The MOS 36-item short-form health survey (SF-36). I. Conceptual framework and item selection. Med Care. 1992;30:473–83.
25. Patel AA, Donegan D, Albert T. The 36-item short form. J Am Acad Orthop Surg. 2007;15(2):126–34.
26. Hays RD, Sherbourne CD, Mazel RM. The RAND 36-Item Health Survey 1.0. Health Econ. 1993;2(3):217–27.
27. SF-36: https://www.rand.org/health-care/surveys_tools/mos/36-item-short-form/survey-instrument.html.
28. Bellamy N, Buchanan WW, Goldsmith CH, Campbell J, Stitt LW. Validation study of WOMAC: a health status instrument for measuring clinically important patient relevant outcomes to anti-rheumatic drug therapy in patients with osteoarthritis of the hip or knee. J Rheumatol. 1988;15:1833–40.
29. WOMAC: http://www.womac.org/womac/index.htm.

Appendix C

Magnetic Resonance Imaging Evaluation Systems for Chondral Injuries and Repair

Magnetic resonance imaging is a noninvasive, sensitive tool that provides excellent spatial and contrast resolution of both intra- and extra-articular cartilage structures of the knee. The evolution and advancement of MRI technology, both hardware and software, have enhanced the ability of MRI to identify biomarkers of articular cartilage morphology and biochemical composition changes associated with chondral/osteochondral knee injuries and diseased state. To assess the incidence and extent of knee cartilage injuries, and classify disease stage as well as to evaluate the status of articular cartilage pre- and post-surgical cartilage repair procedure, various qualitative and quantitative MR imaging sequences have been used, such as two-dimensional spin echo (2D SE) and fast spin echo (FSE) (conventional MRI), three-dimensional spoiled gradient echo (3D SPGR), and three-dimensional fast imaging employing steady-state acquisition (3D FIESTA) [1–10]. These techniques have been beneficial in providing diagnosis with a valid, reliable morphological distinction of intact, native articular cartilage from various cartilage lesions as well as the follow-up of nonsurgical treatment for asymptomatic or minimally symptomatic osteochondral lesions. Further, quantitative MR parameters, such as T2 relaxation values, has provided an important tool to assess early OA stage through its ability to clearly delineate native from injured or repaired articular cartilage surface within the superficial zone of articular cartilage. For the evaluation of cartilage repair, the ICRS recommended MRI sequences are:

Intermediate-weighted fast SE
- With fat saturation
- Without fat saturation (with moderate TE)

T2-weighted fast SE
- With fat saturation
- Without fat saturation (with moderate TE)

T1-weighted fast GRE
- With chemical fat saturation
- With water excitation

The MRI assessment parameters after microfracture and autologous autograft transplantation cartilage repair procedure are:

Microfracture procedures:
- Degree of defect filling
- Characteristic morphology of reparative tissue
- Status of cartilage delamination (Presence or absence)
- Extent of peripheral repair tissue integration with native cartilage
- Presence of fissure

Autologous autograft transplantations:
- Degree of defect filling
- Radial curvation restoration of knee surface
- Presence or absence of displacement
- Peripheral integration of repair tissue to native cartilage
- Peripheral integration of repair tissue to osseous components

H. K. Gahunia et al. (eds.), *Articular Cartilage of the Knee*,
https://doi.org/10.1007/978-1-4939-7587-7

- Mophologic characteristics of the repair site
- Integrity of host tissue

The three most commonly used MR classification systems for cartilage repair are:

1. International Cartilage Repair Society (ICRS) - Cartilage Repair Assessment System.
2. Two-dimensional Magnetic Resonance Observation of Cartilage Repair Tissue score (2D MOCART).
3. Three-dimensional Magnetic Resonance Observation of Cartilage Repair Tissue score (3D MOCART).

International Cartilage Repair Society: Articular Cartilage Repair Assessment

Grade	ICRS - Cartilage Repair
	Degree of Defect Repair
4	In level with surrounding cartilage
3	75% repair of defect depth
2	50% repair of defect depth
1	25% repair of defect depth
0	0% repair of defect depth
	Integration to Border Zone
4	Complete integration with surrounding cartilage
3	Demarcating border < 1mm
2	3/4 of graft integrated, 1/4 with a notable border > 1 mm width
1	1/2 of graft integrated with surrounding cartilage, 1/2 with a notable border > 1mm
0	From no contact to 1/4 of graft integrated with surrounding cartilage
	Macroscopic Appearance
4	Intact smooth surface
3	Fibrillated surface
2	Small, scattered fissures or cracks
1	Several, small or few but large fissures
0	Total degeneration of grafted area

ICRS Assessment of Cartilage Repair

Grade	ICRS - Overall Repair Assessment
12	Grade I: Normal Hyaline cartilage: excellent filling and integration
11–8	Grade II: Nearly normal Cartilaginous: good filling and integration
7–4	Grade III: Abnormal Fibrocartilaginous: inadequate filling and integration
3–1	Grade IV: Severely abnormal Fibrous: None to very poor repair

Two-Dimensional Magnetic Resonance Observation of Cartilage Repair Tissue (2D-MOCART) Score (Marlovits et al. [11])

1. **Degree of defect repair and filling**
   - Complete (on a level with adjacent cartilage)
   - Hypertrophy (over the level of the adjacent cartilage)
   - Incomplete (under the level of the adjacent cartilage; underfilling)
     - > 50% of the adjacent cartilage
     - < 50% of the adjacent cartilage
   - Subchondral bone exposed (complete delamination or dislocation and/or loose body)
2. **Integration of cartilage repair tissue to border zone**
   - Complete (complete integration with adjacent cartilage)
   - Incomplete (incomplete integration with adjacent cartilage)
   - Demarcating border visible (split-like)
   - Defect visible

- < 50% of the length of the repair tissue
- > 50% of the length of the repair tissue

3. **Surface of the repair tissue**
   - Surface intact (lamina splendens intact)
   - Surface damaged (fibrillations, fissures, and ulcerations)
     - < 50% of repair tissue depth
     - > 50% of repair tissue depth or total degeneration
4. **Structure of whole repair tissue**
   - Homogeneous
   - Inhomogeneous or cleft formation
5. **Signal intensity of repair tissue**

   Dual T2-FSE
   - Isointense
   - Moderately hyperintense
   - Markedly hyperintense

   3D–GE-FS
   - Isointense
   - Moderately hypointense
   - Markedly hypointense
6. **Constitution of subchondral lamina**
   - Intact
   - Not intact
7. **Status of subchondral bone**
   - Intact
   - Non-intact (edema, granulation tissue, cysts, sclerosis)
8. **Possible adhesions**
   - No
   - Yes
9. **Possible joint effusion**
   - No
   - Yes

Three-Dimensional Magnetic Resonance Observation of Cartilage Repair Tissue (3D–MOCART) Score

(Welsch et al. [12])

1. **Defect fill** *(defect repair and filling in relation to the adjacent native cartilage)*
   - 0%
   - 0–25%
   - 25–50%
   - 50–75%
   - 75–100%
   - 100%
   - 100–125%
   - 125–150%
   - 150–200%
   - > 200%

   Localization (whole area of cartilage repair)
   - > 50%
   - < 50%

   Anatomic location
   - Central
   - Peripheral
   - Weight bearing
   - Non-weight bearing
2. **Cartilage interface** *(repair tissue integration with adjacent native cartilage – 2 MR planes)*

   Sagittal plane (*femur, patella, trochlea, tibia*)
   - Complete
   - Demarcating border visible (split-like)
   - Defect visible
     - < 50%
     - > 50%

   Coronal plane *(femur, tibia);* **axial plane** *(patella, trochlea)*
   - Complete
   - Demarcating border visible (split-like)
   - Defect visible
     - < 50%
     - > 50%

   Localization
   - Whole area of cartilage repair
     - > 50%
     - < 50%
   - Weight bearing
   - Non-weight bearing
3. **Bone interface** *(Transplant tissue - possible periosteal flap - integration to subchondral bone)*
   - Complete
   - Partial delamination
   - Complete delamination
   - Delamination

   Localization
   - Weight bearing
   - Non-weight bearing

4. **Repair tissue surface** *(constitution of the surface of the repair tissue)*
    - Surface intact
    - Surface damaged
        - < 50% of depth
        - > 50% of depth
    - Adhesions

    Localization
    - Whole area of cartilage repair
        - > 50%
        - < 50%
    - Central
    - Peripheral
    - Weight bearing
    - Non-weight bearing
5. **Repair tissue structure** *(constitution of the whole repair tissue)*
    - Homogeneous
    - Inhomogeneous or cleft formation

    Localization
    - Whole area of cartilage repair
        - > 50%
        - < 50%
    - Central
    - Peripheral
    - Weight bearing
    - Non-weight bearing
6. **Signal intensity** *(MR signal intensity of repair tissue relative to adjacent native cartilage)*
    - Normal (¼ *identical to adjacent native cartilage)*
    - Nearly normal (¼ slight areas of signal alterations)
    - Abnormal (¼ *large areas of signal alteration)*

    Localization
    - Central
    - Peripheral
    - Weight bearing
    - Non-weight bearing
7. **Subchondral lamina** *(constitution of the subchondral lamina)*
    - Intact
    - Not intact

    Localization
    - Whole area of cartilage repair
        - > 50%
        - < 50%
    - Central
    - Peripheral
    - Weight bearing
    - Non-weight bearing
8. **Chondral osteophytes** *(osteophytes within the cartilage repair area)*
    - Absent
    - Osteophytes
        - < 50% of repair tissue
        - > 50% of repair tissue

    Localization

    Size: ——mm (plane: ——) _ —— mm (plane: ——)
    - Central
    - Peripheral
    - Weight bearing
    - Non-weight bearing
9. **Bone marrow edema** *(maximum size and localization in relation to the cartilage repair tissue and other alterations assessed in the 3D MOCART score)*
    - Absent
    - Small (< 1 cm)
    - Medium (< 2 cm)
    - Large (< 4 cm)
    - Diffuse localization

    Size: ——mm (plane: ——) _ —— mm (plane: ——)
    - Central
    - Peripheral
    - Weight bearing
    - Non-weight bearing
    - Relation to other alterations within this score of variable No. ——
10. **Subchondral bone** (constitution of the subchondral bone)
    - Intact
    - Granulation tissue
    - Cyst

    Localization
    - Whole area of cartilage repair

    - > 50%
    - < 50%
  - Central
  - Peripheral
  - Weight bearing
  - Non-weight bearing
11. **Effusion** *(approx. size of joint effusion visualized in all planes)*
  - Absent
  - Small
  - Medium
  - Large

References

1. Windschuh J, Zaiss M, Ehses P, Lee JS, Jerschow A, et al. Assessment of frequency drift on CEST MRI and dynamic correction: application to gagCEST at 7 T. Magn Reson Med. 2019;81(1):573–82.
2. Trattnig S, Raudner M, Schreiner M, Roemer F, Bohndorf K. Biochemical cartilage imaging-update 2019. Radiologe. 2019;59(8):742–9.
3. Nebelung S, Post M, Knobe M, Tingart M, Emans P, et al. Detection of Early-Stage Degeneration in Human Articular Cartilage by Multiparametric MR Imaging Mapping of Tissue Functionality. Sci Rep. 2019;9(1):5895.
4. Juras V, Mlynarik V, Szomolanyi P, Valkovič L, Trattnig S. Magnetic Resonance Imaging of the Musculoskeletal System at 7T: Morphological Imaging and Beyond. Top Magn Reson Imaging. 2019;28(3):125–35.
5. Martín Noguerol T, Raya JG, Wessell DE, Vilanova JC, Rossi I, et al. Functional MRI for evaluation of hyaline cartilage extracellular matrix, a physiopathological-based approach. Br J Radiol. 2019;92(1103):20190443. https://doi.org/10.1259/bjr.20190443.
6. Li Z, Wang H, Lu Y, Jiang M, Chen Z, et al. Diagnostic value of T1ρ and T2 mapping sequences of 3D fat-suppressed spoiled gradient (FS SPGR-3D) 3.0-T magnetic resonance imaging for osteoarthritis. Medicine (Baltimore). 2019;98(1):e13834.
7. Colotti R, Omoumi P, Bonanno G, Ledoux JB, van Heeswijk RB. Isotropic three-dimensional T2 mapping of knee cartilage: Development and validation. J Magn Reson Imaging. 2018;47(2):362–71.
8. Joseph GB, Nevitt MC, McCulloch CE, Neumann J, Lynch JA, et al. Associations between molecular biomarkers and MR-based cartilage composition and knee joint morphology: data from the Osteoarthritis Initiative. Osteoarthr Cartil. 2018;26(8):1070–7.
9. Wyss M, Manoliu A, Marcon M, Spinner G, Luechinger R, et al. Clinical Magnetic Resonance Imaging of the Knee at 7 T: Optimization of Fat Suppression. Investig Radiol. 2019;54(3):160–8.
10. Fritz J, Ahlawat S, Fritz B, Thawait GK, Stern SE, et al. 10-Min 3D Turbo Spin Echo MRI of the Knee in Children: Arthroscopy-Validated Accuracy for the Diagnosis of Internal Derangement. J Magn Reson Imaging. 2019;49(7):e139–51.
11. Marlovits S, Singer P, Zeller P, Mandl I, Haller J, Trattnig S. Magnetic resonance observation of cartilage repair tissue (MOCART) for the evaluation of autologous chondrocyte transplantation: determination of interobserver variability and correlation to clinical outcome after 2 years. Eur J Radiol. 2006;57(1):16–23.
12. Welsch GH, Zak L, Mamisch TC, Paul D, Lauer L, Mauerer A, Marlovits S, Trattnig S. Advanced morphological 3D magnetic resonance observation of cartilage repair tissue (MOCART) scoring using a new isotropic 3D proton-density, turbo spin echo sequence with variable flip angle distribution (PD-SPACE) compared to an isotropic 3D steady-state free precession sequence (True-FISP) and standard 2D sequences. J Magn Reson Imaging. 2011;33(1):180–8.

Appendix D

Histological Scoring Systems for Chondral / Osteochondral Repair and Disease

Histological evaluation of knee articular cartilage in injury, disease, and therapy is the gold standard for a valid, reliable, reproducible, and objective evaluation of repaired and regenerated tissue as well as assessment of osteoarthritic knee. To date, several histological scoring systems to assess cartilaginous repair tissue and evaluate the disease state have been created, described, validated, and modified, some of which have been established as the key scoring systems.

Articular cartilage is vulnerable to injuries and degenerative diseases over time. Cartilage repair refers to the healing of injured cartilage or its replacement through cell proliferation and synthesis of new extracellular matrix [1, 2]. Regeneration, on the other hand, refers to the formation of an entirely new surface that essentially duplicates the native articular cartilage [2, 3]. Osteochondral cartilage repair/regeneration has been the focus of current research efforts which includes transplantation of cells, use of various biological grafts, use of bioactive agents, and/or use of biologically compatible, implant matrices [4]. The histological assessment of soft repair tissue is one of the most important outcome measures for the evaluation of the success of cartilage repair treatment [5]. For a successful cartilage repair/regeneration assessment from a histological viewpoint, it is crucial to carefully evaluate the conventional scoring system by taking the experimental design into account [3, 6–10]. Reflecting elementary and complex cartilage repair scoring systems, Orth and Madry outlined the individual parameter characteristic of chondral or osteochondral repair tissue, as shown in Table 1 [11]. To date, several histological scoring systems have been used to describe the quality of cartilage repair/regeneration (in vivo and in vitro) in OA joints and with the use of bioengineered implants [1, 3–9]. A comprehensive approach to histologically evaluate OC repair includes assessment of the repair tissue in the following areas: (1) native cartilage adjacent to defect, (2) tissue characteristics at the defect margin (bonding of native cartilage with the repair tissue), (3) repair tissue in OC defect at the level of uncalcified articular cartilage (above tidemark), (4) repair tissue in OC defect at the level of subchondral bone (below tidemark), and (5) tissue characteristics adjacent to the fixation device, if present [10].

H. K. Gahunia et al. (eds.), *Articular Cartilage of the Knee*,
https://doi.org/10.1007/978-1-4939-7587-7

Table 1 Schematic diagram of the individual parameter characteristic of chondral or osteochondral repair tissue as reflected by various cartilage repair scoring systems [11]

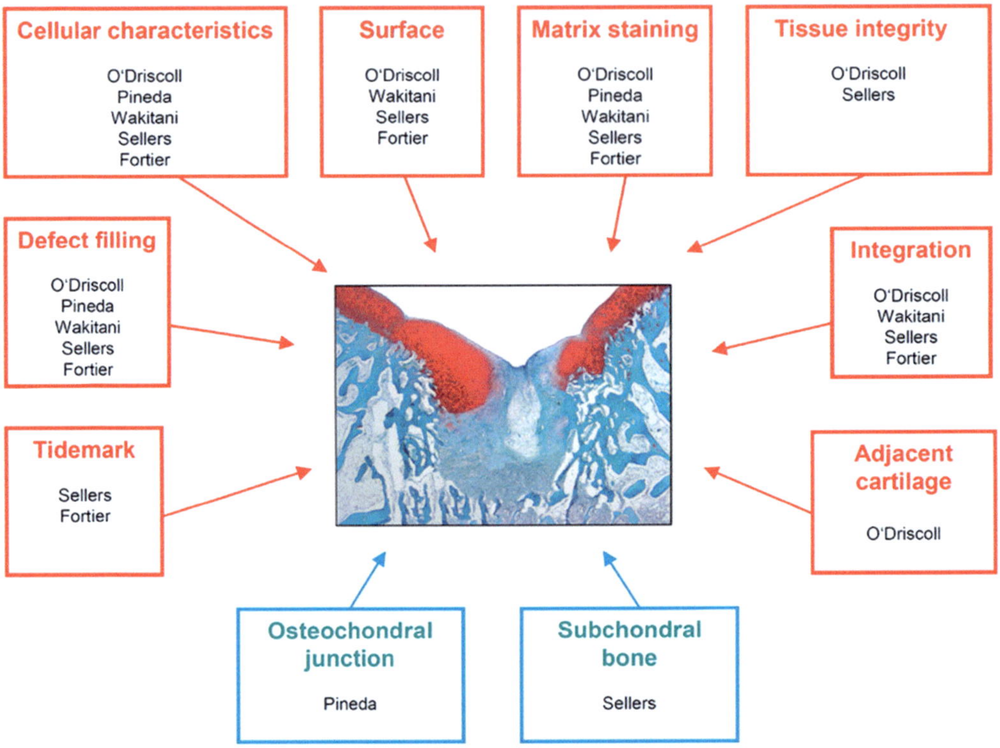

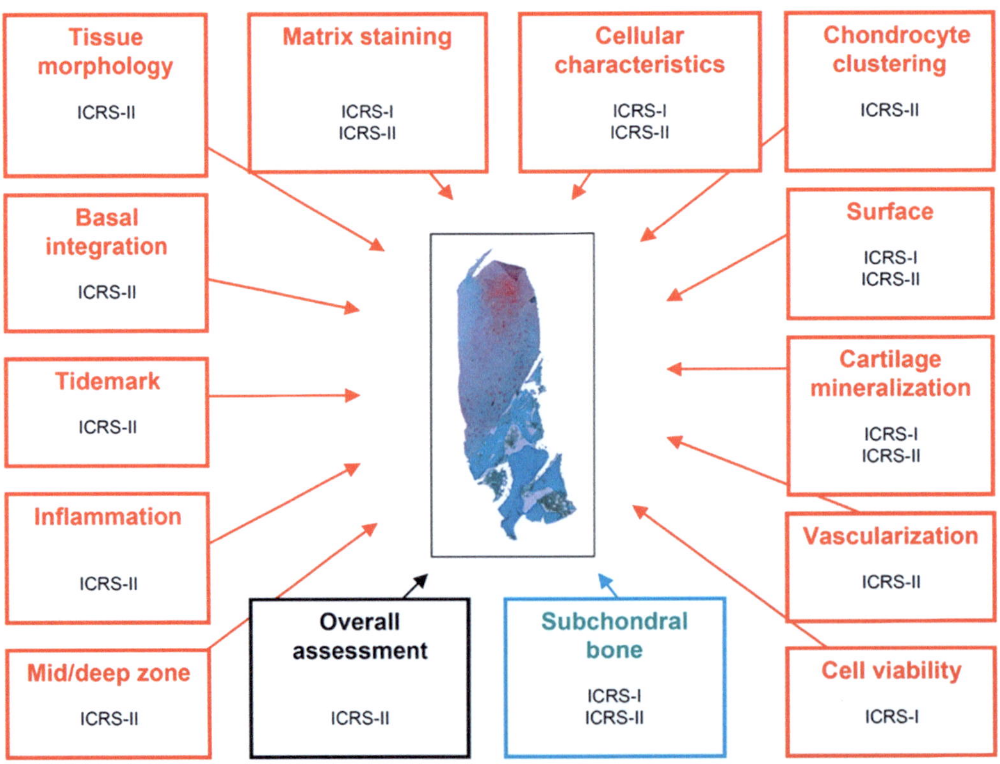

International Cartilage Repair Society - I: Histological Scoring System (Mainil-Varlet et al. [6])

Repair Tissue Morphology	Score
Surface	
Smooth/continuous	3
Discontinuities/irregularities	0
Matrix	
Hyaline	3
Mixture: Hyaline/fibrocartilage	2
Fibrocartilage	1
Fibrous tissue	0
Cell Distribution	
Columnar	3
Mixed/columnar clusters	2
Clusters	1
Individual cells/disorganized	0
Cell Population Viability	
Predominantly viable	3
Partially viable	1
< 10% viable	0
Subchondral Bone	
Normal	3
Bone necrosis/granulation tissue	1
Detached/fracture/callus at base	0
Cartilage Mineralization	
Normal	3
Abnormal/inappropriate location	0

International Cartilage Repair Society - II: Histological Scoring System (Mainil-Varlet et al. [7])

Features	Percent
Tissue Morphology (Viewed Under Polarized Light)	
Full-thickness collagen fibers	0%
Normal cartilage birefringence	100%
Matrix Staining (Metachromasia)	
No staining	0%
Full metachromasia	100%
Cell Morphology	
No round/oval cells	0%
Mostly round/oval cells	100%
Chondrocyte Clustering (Four or More Grouped Cells)	
Present	0%
Absent	100%
Surface Architecture	
Delamination or major irregularity	0%
Smooth surface	100%
Basal Integration	
No integration	0%
Complete integration	100%
Formation of a Tidemark	
No calcification front	0%
Tidemark	100%
Subchondral Bone Abnormalities/Marrow Fibrosis	
Abnormal	0%
Normal marrow	100%
Inflammation	
Present	0%
Absent	100%
Abnormal Calcification/Ossification	
Present	0%
Absent	100%
Vascularization (Within the Repaired Tissue)	
Present	0%
Absent	100%
Surface/Superficial Assessment	
Total loss or complete disruption	0%
Resembles intact articular cartilage	100%
Mid/deep Zone Assessment	
Fibrous tissue	0%
Normal hyaline cartilage	100%
Overall Assessment	
Bad (fibrous tissue)	0%
Good (hyaline cartilage)	100%

Assessment of Osteochondral Repair and Regeneration: Histological Scoring System (Gahunia [10])

Osteochondral Repair and Regeneration Scoring System

A. Native Cartilage Evaluation

Structural integrity
- Normal structure (3)
- Slight disorganization (2)
- Moderately disorganization (1)
- Severe disorganization (0)

Cellularity
- Normal (3)
- Diffuse hypercellular (2)
- Cloning/clustering (1)
- Hypocellular (0)

B. Defect Margin Integration to Native Cartilage

Tissue characteristics
- Very good cartilaginous integration (3)
- Good fibrocartilaginous integration (2)
- Fibrous integration (1)
- No integration (0)

Tissue cell type/organization
- Normal cartilaginous ECM (5)
- Slightly disorganized cartilaginous (4)
- Disorganized cartilaginous and fibrous ECM (3)
- Organized fibrous ECM (2)
- Disorganized fibrous ECM (1)
- Empty space between native and regenerated tissue (0)

C. Repair Tissue Evaluation (Above Tidemark)

Repair tissue characteristics
- Normal cartilaginous ECM (5)
- Slightly disorganized ECM (4)
- Disorganized chondrocytic (3)
- Organized fibrous ECM (2)
- Disorganized fibrous ECM (1)
- No regenerated tissue (0)

Safranin O matrix staining
- Normal (3)
- Slight reduction (2)
- Moderate reduction (1)
- Severe reduction or none (0)

Surface continuity:
- Smooth and continuous (3)
- Slightly discontinuous (2)
- Moderately discontinuous (1)
- Severely discontinuous (0)

Defect repair tissue filling
- 100% (4)
- > 75% and < 100% (3)
- > 50% and < 75% (2)
- > 25% and < 50% (1)
- < 25% (0)

Defect area vascularization (above tidemark)
- No vascularization (3)
- Mild vascularization (2)
- Moderate vascularization (1)
- Severe vascularization (0)

Infarcted granulation (Necrosis)
- Absent (2)
- Moderate (1)
- Severe (0)

D. Subchondral Bone Evaluation (Below Tidemark)

Predominant tissue
- Osseous (3)
- Cartilaginous (2)
- Fibrous tissue (1)
- No tissue (0)

Signs of bone repair/osteogenesis
- Mature bone (4)
- Mainly mature bone and minimally immature (3)
- 50:50 mature and immature bone (2)
- New bone only (1)
- No osteogenesis (0)

Neovascularization
- Normal (3)
- Mild (2)
- Moderate (1)
- Severe or none (0)

Infarcted granulation tissue
- Absent (3)
- Mild (2)
- Moderate (1)
- Severe (0)

E. Repair Tissue Surrounding Implant Tissue Characteristics
- Trabecular (4)
- Osteogenic (3)
- Osteogenic and fibrous (2)
- Fibrous (1)
- None (0)

Osteolysis
- None (3)
- Mild (2)
- Moderate (1)
- Severe (0)

Inflammatory indices
- None (3)
- Mild (2)
- Moderate (1)
- Severe (0)

Histopathological Scoring System for Osteoarthritic Articular Cartilage

Osteoarthritis (OA) often present as secondary OA due to primary inflammatory, infectious, and traumatic etiologies. The radiographic hallmarks of OA include asymmetric loss of articular cartilage resulting in joint space narrowing, followed by subchondral sclerosis, cysts, eburnation, and osteophyte formation. Early signs of OA are reflected as undulations on the articular cartilage surface. This is followed by cartilage surface irregularities and structural changes in the zone 1 extracellular matrix. Several OA histopathogical scoring systems have been proposed to date [3, 5, 12–16]. Gahunia et al. developed a scoring system to evaluate the structural integrity of articular cartilage surface and cartilage zones during various OA stages [12, 13].

Osteoarthritic Articular Cartilage: Histopathological Scoring System (Gahunia [12, 13])

Osteoarthritic Articular Cartilage Assessment

A. Articular Cartilage Surface Integrity

Smooth and continuous (0)
Slightly discontinuous (1)
Moderately discontinuous (2)
Severely discontinuous (3)

B. Articular Cartilage – Zone 1

Cellularity

Normal (0)
Diffuse hypercellular (1)
Cloning/clustering (2)
Hypocellular (3)

Fibrillation(s)

Absent (0)
Few (1)
Several (2)

Fissure(s)

Absent (0)
Present (1)

Fibrous tissue

Absent (0)
Present (1)

C. Articular Cartilage – Zone 2

Cellularity

Normal (0)
Diffuse hypercellular (1)
Cloning/clustering (2)
Hypocellular (3)

Extracellular matrix

Normal (0)
Slightly disorganized (1)
Moderately disorganized (2)
Severely disorganized (3)

Fissure(s)

Absent (0)
Present only Zone – 2 upper half (1)
Present up to Zone – 2 lower half (2)

Fibrous tissue

Absent (0)
Present – focal area (1)
Present – throughout (2)

D. Articular Cartilage – Zone 3

Cellularity

Normal (0)
Diffuse hypercellular (1)
Cloning/clustering (2)
Hypocellular (3)

Extracellular matrix

Normal (0)
Slightly disorganized (1)
Moderately disorganized (2)
Severely disorganized (3)

Fissure(s)

Absent (0)
Present only Zone – 3 upper half (1)
Present up to Zone – 3 lower half (2)

Fibrous tissue

Absent (0)
Present – focal area (1)
Present – throughout (2)

E. Articular Cartilage – Zone 4 (Below Tidemark)

Extracellular matrix

Normal (0)
Slightly disorganized (1)
Moderately disorganized (2)
Severely disorganized (3)

Vascular infiltration

No vascularization (0)
Mild vascularization (1)
Moderate vascularization (2)
Severe vascularization (3)

Fibrous tissue

Absent (0)
Present – focal area (1)
Present – throughout (2)

F. Tidemark

Present – Only one (0)
Multiplication (duplication or reduplication (1)

G. Subchondral Bone Evaluation

Subchondral sclerosis

None (0)
Mild (1)
Moderate (2)
Severe (3)

Granulation tissue

Absent (0)
Moderate (1)
Severe (2)

References

1. Bobic V, Noble J. Articular cartilage--to repair or not to repair. J Bone joint Surg Br. 2000;82:165–166.
2. Pritzker KPH. Posttraumatic cartilage hypertrophy: edema or repair? J Rheumatol. 1991;18:314–315.
3. Pritzker KPH, Gay S, Jimenez SA, Ostergaard K, Pelletier JP, Revell PA, Salter D, van den Berg WB. Osteoarthritis cartilage histopathology: grading and staging. Osteoarthritis Cartilage. 2006;14:13–29.
4. Updates in Cartilage Repair. Proceedings of the 4th Symposium of the International Cartilage Repair Society. Toronto, Canada, June 2002. J Bone Joint Surg Am. 2003;85-A Suppl 2:1–141., 85–A 1–141.
5. Rutgers M, van Pelt MJ, Dhert WJ, Creemers LB, Saris DB. Evaluation of histological scoring systems for tissue-engineered, repaired and osteoarthritic cartilage. Osteoarthritis Cartilage. 2010;18:12–23.
6. Mainil-Varlet P, Aigner T, Brittberg M, Bullough P, Hollander A, Hunziker E, Kandel R, Nehrer S, Pritzker K, Roberts S, Stauffer E. International Cartilage Repair Society: Histological assessment of cartilage repair: a report by the Histology Endpoint Committee of the International Cartilage Repair Society (ICRS). J Bone Joint Surg Am. 2003;85-A:45–57
7. Mainil-Varlet P, Van Damme B, Nesic D, Knutsen G, Kandel R, Roberts S. A new histology scoring system for the assessment of the quality of human cartilage repair: ICRS II. Am J Sports Med. 2010;38:880–890.
8. Hoemann C, Kandel R, Roberts S, Saris DB, Creemers L, Mainil-Varlet P, Méthot S, Hollander AP, Buschmann MD. International Cartilage Repair Society (ICRS) recommended guidelines for histological endpoints for cartilage repair studies in Animal models and clinical trials. Cartilage. 2011;2:153–172.
9. O'Driscoll SW, Keeley FW, Salter RB. Durability of regenerated articular cartilage produced by free autogenous periosteal grafts in major full-thickness defects in joint surfaces under the influence of continuous passive motion. A follow-up report at one year. J Bone Joint Surg Am. 1988;70(4):595–606.
10. Gahunia HK. Histological assessment of osteochondral repair and regeneration, International Cartilage Repair Society 2002, 4th Symposium.
11. Orth P, Madry H. Complex and elementary histological scoring systems for articular cartilage repair. Histol Histopathol. 2015;30(8):911–9.
12. Gahunia HK, Karhula S, Ylitalo T, Hæggström E, Pritzker KPH, Saarakkala S, Nieminen HJ. 3D–Histopathological grading of articular cartilage using contrast-enhanced high-resolution micro-CT. Osteoarthritis Cartilage. 2016;24:S277–8
13. Nieminen HJ, Gahunia HK, Pritzker KPH, Ylitalo T, Rieppo L, Karhula SS, Lehenkari P, Hæggström E, Saarakkala S. 3D histopathological grading of osteochondral tissue using contrast-enhanced microcomputed tomography. Osteoarthritis Cartilage. 2017;25(10):1680–1689.
14. Mankin HJ, Dorfman H, Lippiello L, Zarins A. Biochemical and metabolic abnormalities in articular cartilage from osteo-arthritic human hips. II. Correlation of morphology with biochemical and metabolic data. J Bone Joint Surg Am. 1971;53(3):523–37.
15. Pearson RG, Kurien T, Shu KS, Scammell BE. Histopathology grading systems for characterisation of human knee osteoarthritis--reproducibility, variability, reliability, correlation, and validity. Osteoarthritis Cartilage. 2011;19(3):324–31.
16. Pauli C, Whiteside R, Heras FL, Nesic D, Koziol J, et al. Comparison of cartilage histopathology assessment systems on human knee joints at all stages of osteoarthritis development. Osteoarthritis Cartilage. 2012;20(6):476–85.

Index

H. K. Gahunia et al. (eds.), *Articular Cartilage of the Knee*,
https://doi.org/10.1007/978-1-4939-7587-7

MIX
Papier aus verantwortungsvollen Quellen
Paper from responsible sources
FSC® C105338

If you have any concerns about our products,
you can contact us on
ProductSafety@springernature.com

In case Publisher is established outside the EU,
the EU authorized representative is:
Springer Nature Customer Service Center GmbH
Europaplatz 3, 69115 Heidelberg, Germany

Printed by Libri Plureos GmbH
in Hamburg, Germany